ANNUAL REVIEW OF PUBLIC HEALTH

ANNUAL REVIEW OF PUBLIC HEALTH

VOLUME 17, 1996

GILBERT S. OMENN, *Editor*

University of Washington

JONATHAN E. FIELDING, *Associate Editor*

University of California at Los Angeles

LESTER B. LAVE, *Associate Editor*

Carnegie Mellon University

http://annurev.org   science@annurev.org   415-493-4400

ANNUAL REVIEWS INC.   4139 EL CAMINO WAY   P.O. BOX 10139   PALO ALTO, CALIFORNIA 94303-0139

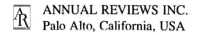 ANNUAL REVIEWS INC.
Palo Alto, California, USA

International Standard Serial Number: 0163–7525
International Standard Book Number: 0–8243–2717–9

Annual Review and publication titles are registered trademarks of Annual Reviews Inc.

∞ The paper used in this publication meets the minimum requirements of
American National Standard for Information Sciences—Permanence of Paper
for Printed Library Materials, ANSI Z39.48-1984.

Annual Reviews Inc. and the Editors of its publications assume no responsibility for the
statements expressed by the contributors to this *Review*.

Typesetting by Kachina Typesetting Inc., Tempe, Arizona; John Olson, President;
Jeannie Kaarle, Typesetting Coordinator; and by the Annual Reviews Inc. Editorial Staff

PRINTED AND BOUND IN THE UNITED STATES OF AMERICA

PREFACE

Public health and the mission of health promotion and disease prevention are gaining ground in the United States and around the world. The concept that populations and communities are units of organization and units of responsibility for health professionals is a core value of public health. The approaches of assessment, policy development, and assurance bring some order to planning and implementing programs at all levels of government and community. The rapid expansion of managed care may remove what for so long were characterized as "perverse economic incentives" for excess medical care, while challenging us to monitor the quality and sufficiency of managed care and help build ties to public health. Attention to smoking prevention, gun control, prevention of violence, global eradication of specific infectious diseases, and application of new genetic technologies in public health all reflect the vigor of public health sciences and public health practice.

In the United States, there is a renewed burst of interest in establishing schools of public health. The 1995 annual meeting of the American Public Health Association had a session on this topic that drew a packed room of individuals representing some 30 universities. Some already have programs in preventive medicine in their medical schools accredited by the Council for Education in Public Health. For them to expand into full-fledged schools of public health is a natural growth opportunity, in a pattern well established by schools like my own at the University of Washington. In other settings, universities with a strong program in health policy or in environmental health are examining their capacity to develop complementary strengths in epidemiology, biostatistics, health administration/health management, environmental health sciences, and social and behavioral sciences. With 27 fully accredited schools in only 20 states at present, too many states lack an academic partner for a triangular relationship with the Centers for Disease Control and Prevention and the state and local health departments. It is ironic that the Association of American Medical Colleges, besieged by financial and organizational challenges in the clinical world, would hear their president call for pulling schools of public health back into medical schools—during the same week as the discussion at the APHA pointing to a vibrant future for academic public health.

Far better, I say, that medicine and public health both be strong and be partners in addressing the compelling needs of ill and injured patients, led by the medical schools, and promotion of better health and prevention of disease and injury, led by the schools of public health. There is plenty of ground for cooperation and synergy. Prevention, after all, requires a reinforcing strategy that combines community-based prevention (a.k.a. public health) with properly targeted clinical preventive services and with social and economic policies that enhance healthy behaviors and discourage unhealthy behaviors of individuals and of companies and communities. This three-pronged prevention strategy is the framework for advocacy by the Partnership for Prevention—a national coalition of many health care, academic, federal and state government, managed care, pharmaceutical, and insurance sponsors.

In this setting of political and organizational ferment and with remarkable advances from biology, epidemiology, and the social sciences, the *Annual Review of Public Health* has an important niche. In a two-year ongoing cycle, we consider the developments and needs across the breadth of public health, choose topics that provide what we ourselves would be eager to read and hope others will make time to read, invite leading authors to prepare knowledgeable reviews, provide an editorial effort that we hope matches the expectations of our readers, and publish a volume that I think is timely and of lasting value. You can make your own judgment.

We organize our reviews under five headings: Epidemiology and Biostatistics; Environmental and Occupational Health; Behavioral Aspects of Health; Public Health Practice; and Health Services and Health Policy. We seek a balance of reviews in the five areas, yet we know and you surely recognize that some of these topics bridge two or more fields. That is, itself, a sign of the interconnectedness of our academic and practice roles across the breadth of public health. We work hard to make the articles readable and relevant to colleagues in public health practice, health care professional fields, and policy fields, as well as academic public health. Over the course of several volumes we try to provide reasonably comprehenseive coverage of the continuing and emerging challenges of our field.

In this Volume 17 we have two mini-symposia that may be of special interest. The Symposium on Public Health Aspects of Ophthalmic Disease (glaucoma, cataract, diabetic retinopathy) illustrates how epidemiology can guide approaches to all areas of clinical practice in medicine and surgery. The Symposium on Cancers of Special Importance to Women (lung, breast, ovarian, cervix) critically assesses risk factors and demonstrates the potential to marry biological, social, and environmental approaches to understand clinical conditions and to mobilize appropriate and cost-effective treatments and preventive interventions. We have a long way to go in assuring a public health perspective in clinical investigation and clinical care, including recognition through mechanistic studies of the heterogeneity of essentially all common diseases—heterogeneity that surely requires a strategy to identify subgroups requiring different kinds of preventive and therapeutic interventions. We thank the special editors for the mini-symposia, Dean Al Sommer of Johns Hopkins and Professor Jennifer Kelsey of Stanford.

Finally, as I complete my seventh and final volume as Editor, I want to thank asssociate editors Jonathan Fielding and Lester Lave, who have served so effectively in those roles with Lester Breslow and with me since the beginning of this Annual Reviews series. All of us also contributed as authors. Jonathan has already taken over the reins for Volume 18. Our current and previous members of the Editorial Advisory Board and our Annual Reviews staff, led now by Hilda Gould, have made this work a particularly rewarding endeavor. To Bill Kaufman, long a guiding force as publisher of the Annual Reviews, a special thanks. My own editorial assistant, Jean Knight, has been a lifesaver and a terrific partner in this role.

I promise you all that I will continue as a devoted reader of the *Annual Review of Public Health*.

GILBERT S. OMENN
EDITOR

Annual Review of Public Health
Volume 17 (1996)

CONTENTS

SOME RELATED ARTICLES FROM OTHER ANNUAL REVIEWS

From the *Annual Review of Genetics,* Volume 29 (1995):

DNA Repair in Humans, A Sancar

Genetics of Hereditary Colorectal Cancers, A de la Chapelle and P Peltomäki

Ecological Population Genetics: The Interface between Genes and the Environment, AA Hoffmann, CM Sgrò, and SH Lawler

The Human Genome: Organization and Evolutionary History, G Bernardi

Genetic Variation and Aging, JW Curtsinger, HH Fukui, AA Khazaeli, A Kirscher, SD Pletcher, DEL Promislow, and M Tatar

From the *Annual Review of Medicine,* Volume 47 (1996):

Ethical Issues of Fertility and Reproduction, PA Baird

Pulmonary Complications of HIV Infection, JF Murray

Alcohol, Coronary Disease, and Hypertension, AL Klatsky

Harnessing the Power of the Placebo Effect and Renaming It "Remembered Wellness," H Benson and R Friedman

Clinical Implications of the p53 Gene, D Sidransky and M Hollstein

The Geneticist's Approach to Complex Disease, S Ghosh and FS Collins

Apolipoprotein E Alleles as Risk Factors in Alzheimer's Disease, AD Roses

Evaluation of Diagnostic Tests, HC Sox Jr.

The Epidemiology of Psychiatric Disorders and the de facto Mental Health Care System, GS Norquist and DA Regier

Nicotine Addiction and Treatment, JE Rose

From the *Annual Review of Nutrition,* Volume 16 (1996):

Regulation of Carbohydrate and Fat Metabolism During and After Exercise, JO Holloszy and W Kohrt

Oxidized Low Density Lipoproteins in Atherogenesis: Role of Dietary Modification, PD Reaven and JL Witztum

Antioxidants in Human Health and Disease, B Halliwell

Folic Acid and the Prevention of Birth Defects, CE Butterworth Jr and A Bendich

Regulation of Metabolism by Retinoic Acid and Its Nuclear Receptors, M Pfahl and F Chytil

Control of Human Appetite: Implications for the Intake of Dietary Fat, JE Blundell, CL Lawton, JR Cotton, and JI Macdiarmid

Dietary Change and Traditional Food Systems of Indigenous Peoples, HV Kuhnlein and O Receveur

Cholesterol Policy and the Primary Prevention of Coronary Disease: Reflections on Clinical and Population Strategies, CD Naylor and JM Paterson

From the Annual Review of Psychology, Volume 47 (1996):

Expert and Exceptional Performance: Evidence of Maximal Adaptation to Task Constraints, KA Ericsson and AC Lehmann

Teams in Organizations: Recent Research on Performance and Effectiveness, RA Guzzo and MW Dickson

Methodological Issues in Psychopathology Research, KJ Sher and TJ Trull

Environmental Psychology 1989–1994, E Sundstrom, PA Bell, PL Busby, and C Asmus

Covariance Structure Analysis: Statistical Practice, Theory, and Directions, PM Bentler and P Dudgeon

From the Annual Review of Sociology, Volume 22 (1996):

An Introduction To Categorical Data Analysis, D Sloane and SP Morgan

Focus Groups, D Morgan

Comparative Medical Systems, D Mechanic and DA Rochefort

Law and Inequality: Race, Gender, and, Of Course, Class, C Seron and F Munger

Mass Media Effects on Violent Behavior, RB Felson

For the convenience of readers, a detachable order form/envelope is bound into the back of this volume

Annu. Rev. Public Health. 1996. 17:1–23

UNDERSTANDING RESEARCH SYNTHESIS (META-ANALYSIS)

Frederick Mosteller and Graham A. Colditz

Technology Assessment Group, Harvard School of Public Health, Boston, Massachusetts 02115

KEY WORDS: meta-analysis, review, research synthesis, overview, study design, heterogeneity

---

ABSTRACT

Synthesis of research findings has long been a part of reviewing and summarizing a field of study. Public health decisions are made on the available evidence. We summarize the approaches to research synthesis that draw on the best available evidence and the use of quantitative summaries through meta-analysis. We focus on observational studies. Heterogeneity offers the potential to observe a relation across study populations and circumstances. We emphasize the benefits of heterogeneity in overviews and the need to explore and describe the sources of heterogeneity. Random effects approaches to combining data are recommended, and the use of regression approaches is emphasized. Excluding studies with extreme results may bias a research synthesis and underestimate the true variance of the results, thus contributing to misleading inference. Thorough searching is the best guard against publication bias. We conclude with guidelines for combining epidemiological studies.

INTRODUCTION

The synthesis of research findings has long been a central part of a research review. It offers the potential to identify areas of agreement in a field of science and those areas with discrepancies, or that require further research. With the explosion in scientific publications, the field of research synthesis has formalized approaches to combining data from published studies. Over the past decade a number of comprehensive texts have been published that address statistical issues in combining data (49, 46, 68), the use of meta-analysis for exploration of new issues beyond those addressed in the primary studies (27), and more generally summarized the many issues in research

1

synthesis (28, 60, 72). The most complete technical discussion of meta-analysis is contained in the *Handbook of Research Synthesis* (28). In addition, the US Preventive Services Task Force (74) offers an extended collection of examples where a consistent set of criteria was applied to evaluate the strength of evidence supporting efficacy of preventive services. The Oxford study of obstetrics (12) also summarizes in volume 1 the methodologic issues encountered when developing a database that encompasses an entire field of medicine and public health. We do not attempt to summarize the breadth of material in these texts but focus on issues arising from the application of research synthesis in the public health setting and in observational epidemiological studies in particular.

Recently, through the Potsdam Consultation (83), guidelines have been published for the systematic review of randomized controlled trials (25). However, the Potsdam Consultation, despite an initial intention to address both clinical trials and observational studies, did not offer guidelines for synthesis of data from epidemiologic studies. While we await such formal guidelines, it is important to understand that many public health policy decisions are made on the available evidence whether strong or weak. A research synthesis potentially offers a systematic approach to presenting the data. In this review, we summarize several of the key issues faced when undertaking a research synthesis of observational data. We first review the development of meta-analysis and the key features that comprise a quantitative research synthesis. These include the protocol for study identification and explicit inclusion and exclusion criteria. We emphasize the strength of research synthesis to produce answers to new questions that cannot be addressed easily in individual studies. Further, we emphasize the benefits of heterogeneity among reports from the primary research studies. Among the goals of research synthesis is identifying sources of heterogeneity. Because evidence bearing on important public health issues is not always available from randomized controlled trials, we emphasize the "best evidence" approach to research synthesis. After briefly reviewing the history of meta-analysis, with particular emphasis on its application to observational data, we review key issues in the application of the methods of research synthesis. These include choosing an outcome measure, assessing the quality of the primary studies, and models for combining data. Recent developments in the application of regression models to meta-analysis are reviewed as is the potential impact of deleting studies with extreme results. Publication bias and approaches to minimize it are considered. We then discuss the desirability of single large studies, recent results comparing meta-analyses with outcomes of large studies, and developments in the application of meta-analytic methods to diagnostic tests. We conclude with recommendations for combining observational studies that, if implemented consistently, may improve the standards of research synthesis.

NAMING THE METHODS: RESEARCH SYNTHESIS vs META-ANALYSIS

The information explosion requires that we develop and apply a set of tools to facilitate the synthesis of data from a large number of studies when setting policy either at the bedside, at the level of funding patient care, or for research or priorities for the implementation of public health prevention strategies. Accordingly, the field of statistics has provided a rich set of approaches to combining data. Less well defined are the circumstances for the application of specific quantitative methods or what constitutes a robust meta-analysis.

With the evolution of this approach to synthesis of the existing research has emerged a name for the undertaking. Some refer to this as meta-analysis, others as overview, quantitative literature review, and research integration or research synthesis. Ironically, some may be turned off by the name chosen and the implications that go with the name.

Consequently, we prefer to consider the undertaking as a research synthesis, which can include narrative reviews where appropriate, and perhaps meta-analysis may be reserved for some specific set of methods for combining data. Although one of the tools for research synthesis is the set of quantitative methods to combine data, the more important feature is the protocol for study identification, along with explicit inclusion and exclusion criteria, regardless of the final decision on whether or how to statistically combine results from the primary studies.

AN EXAMPLE   The Institute of Medicine was charged by the US Congress to summarize the strength of evidence concerning the association between herbicide exposure during Vietnam service and diseases or conditions associated with such exposure. To assess whether a statistical association of disease with herbicide exposure exists, the committee (*a*) systematically reviewed and summarized available evidence relating herbicide exposure and each disease, and (*b*) summarized the evidence in tables according to study design and type of exposure (occupational, environmental, or Vietnam service) (52). Assessment did not focus on causality but on consistency of the association observed in the published studies. Four categories of evidence were then used to classify the associations. These were (*a*) sufficient evidence, (*b*) limited/suggestive evidence, (*c*) inadequate/insufficient evidence to determine whether an association exists, and (*d*) limited/suggestive evidence of no association. The criteria used for these classifications are summarized in Table 1. Although no formal combining of study results was undertaken to estimate the magnitude of an association, the systematic review of the literature offers those bodies that set public policy a clear view of the studies, their features, and their results. A similar approach was used by the Institute of Medicine to summa-

Table 1 Levels of evidence

1. *Sufficient evidence of an association*
Evidence is sufficient to conclude that there is a positive association. That is, a positive association has been observed between herbicides and the outcome in studies in which chance, bias,
and confounding could be ruled out with reasonable confidence. For example, if several
small studies that are free from bias and confounding show an association that is consistent
in magnitude and direction, there may be sufficient evidence for an association.

2. *Limited/suggestive evidence of an association*
Evidence is suggestive of an association between herbicides and the outcome but is limited because chance, bias, and confounding could not be ruled out with confidence. For example, at
least one high-quality study shows a positive association, but the results of other studies are
inconsistent.

3. *Inadequate/insufficient evidence to determine whether an association exists*
The available studies are of insufficient quality, consistency, or statistical power to permit a
conclusion regarding the presence or absence of an association. For example, studies fail to
control for confounding, have inadequate exposure assessment, or fail to address latency.

4. *Limited/suggestive evidence of no association*
There are several adequate studies covering the full range of levels of exposure that human
beings are known to encounter, that are mutually consistent in not showing a positive association between exposure to herbicides and the outcome at any level of exposure. A conclusion of "no association" is inevitably limited to the conditions, level of exposure, and
length of observation covered by the available studies. In addition, the possibility of a very
small elevation in risk at the levels of exposure studied can never be excluded.

rize evidence supporting causal associations between vaccines and adverse
events (51).

HOW RESEARCH SYNTHESIS MAY PRODUCE ANSWERS TO NEW QUESTIONS

Research synthesis is uniquely able to evaluate the influences of study level
attributes and to combine evidence over a broad domain. No single study can
hope to have the breadth of a research synthesis. Research synthesis can
investigate study level attributes such as study design (24, 65, 84), trends in
results over calendar time (20), the impact of covariate adjustment (19), study
quality, and the identification of research gaps or "silences" that require new
primary studies.

In a recent commentary, Berlin (7) presents a number of examples where
meta-analysis has addressed variability in study populations including clinical
characteristics and has identified important relations between treatment or

patient characteristics and the association under study. For example, he cites a meta-analysis that quantified the dose-response relation between cigarette smoking and risk of stroke (80), as well as a number of examples from occupational epidemiology where the meta-analysis of data across studies informs the dose-response relation.

BENEFITS OF HETEROGENEITY

Berlin (7) in commenting on Colditz et al (21) on heterogeneity, among other matters, gives applications that show that

1. heterogeneity in epidemiologic data is usual rather than exceptional;
2. the heterogeneity should be analyzed but interpreted with caution in the spirit of exploratory data analysis;
3. insights may come from effects of study design, exposure measurements, or changes in study populations; and
4. sources of heterogeneity are most easily interpreted when they have been established as important in advance of the analysis so that the findings become confirmatory rather than exploratory.

We should also note that when outcomes occur consistently across different populations, the heterogeneity of the populations and of the circumstances gives encouragement about the robustness of the effect.

Among the many goals of research synthesis are estimating an overall association, or magnitude of effect, and identifying sources of heterogeneity among results from the primary studies. When quantifying the magnitude of an association, we are usually addressing a question or hypothesis defined in advance of the analysis. On the other hand, when exploring data compiled for a meta-analysis to identify factors that may explain variation among studies, we move to an exploratory data analysis mode. Assessing and reporting heterogeneity is often ignored in meta-analysis of epidemiologic studies. All meta-analyses of epidemiologic data should estimate the magnitude of the among-study variance in addition to giving the methods used to assess it. We describe some of these methods in the section "methods for combining data."

BEST EVIDENCE

In developing recommendations for including or excluding certain tests in the annual medical check-up, the Canadian Task Force found it valuable to separate the strength of recommendation itself from the degree of the supporting evidence (11). This made it possible to exercise responsible professional judgment in the absence of strong empirical evidence while alerting the reader to the degree and quality of support. For example, the Task Force could give a strong recommendation while noting the weakness of its empirical support.

When evidence from randomized clinical trials, for much the same treatments on much the same populations, are carried out for much the same endpoints, opposition to or reservations about meta-analysis or research synthesis are much lighter than when we apply the methods to observational studies. One major problem in comparing treatments is achieving the a priori equivalence of groups to be compared (a problem that exists also in the analysis of a single observational study). The distinguished educational researcher Robert E Slavin (82) regards "best evidence synthesis" as a good device for combining information from studies. Under this plan, if randomized trials are not available, we do the best we can with observational studies, or in the weakest instances with anecdotal reports. By paying close attention to the details of the studies, Slavin (82) hopes to gain from weaker studies some of the benefits we get from covariates, stratification, or variation in study design in balanced experiments. Thus a worker using "best evidence synthesis" with weak data is encouraged to report more details about the studies examined than when the studies are strong.

In discussing this paper, Letzel (59) notes that purposes of epidemiologic investigations differ and that the quality of data required varies. For instance, in drug safety (a) identifying new drug risks, (b) new risk factors for known adverse drug effects, and (c) for quantifying known risks, investigators accept different levels of formality, and so best evidence synthesis may be satisfactory for some kinds of studies such as (a) and (b) above and not for others such as (c). And he reminds us too that "best evidence may still be no evidence" (p. 21).

HISTORY OF EPIDEMIOLOGIC APPLICATIONS OF META-ANALYSIS

Olkin gives a brief history of methods for combining data from individual studies (69). He traces methods from the combining of results from five studies of effectiveness of inoculation for enteric fever (39), to methods used in agricultural research (17, 18) and the social sciences. Despite early applications of meta-analysis by Beecher in anesthesia research (1), and in summarizing surgical research (42), it was not until the 1980s that the methods received wider application within the health sciences (63, 77). An early application in surgery by Gilbert et al illustrates both using classical analysis of variance and Bayesian methods for combining information in applications. They use random-effects models to study the magnitude of improvements in outcomes of surgery related to innovations (42).

Applications of combining epidemiologic data to strengthen inference go back at least to the 1964 quantitative review by MacMahon & Hutchison in which they combined data from 10 studies of intrauterine X-ray exposure and risk of childhood cancer (64). Five of the ten studies showed an elevated relative risk, though only two were statistically significant. Further, the studies with relative risk estimates <1 tended to be smaller. The test for heterogeneity among the ten studies was not significant. Using an inverse-variance weight they computed the average relative risk and confidence interval. The weighted average was 1.42, a statistically significant increase in risk of childhood cancer after exposure to X rays in utero.

More recently, meta-analysis has been applied to a wide range of topics in epidemiologic investigations (see, for example, a summary of studies from 1991 and 1992 in Reference 21). These topics include diet and cancer (48), exogenous hormones in relation to risk of breast (22) and ovarian cancer (45), cholesterol and heart disease (58), safety implications of bicycle paths (41), effectiveness of interventions aimed at increasing the use of seat belts (55), applications in the assessment of health technologies (86), and vaccine efficacy and side effects (51). Some applications have aimed only to describe an overall association. Others have used meta-analytic methods to describe variation among study results, either due to measures of "dose" across studies (47), quality of the epidemiologic measures used in the original studies of exercise and heart disease (6), or study design in relation to alcohol intake and risk of breast cancer (62).

These examples typify the broad range of applications for meta-analysis. However, considerable debate continues as to the merits of meta-analysis of observational studies. Importantly, Greenland emphasizes the merits of meta-analysis to contribute to knowledge through studying features across studies that may account for the variation in results, and so explain the heterogeneity among studies (44).

Although randomization in clinical trials assures the investigator that bias is minimized, in observational studies bias and unmeasured confounding always remain as concerns. No amount of careful combining of data from studies can overcome inherent deficiencies in the original data. Based on this concern, Shapiro argues that we should not proceed with meta-analysis of observational data (79). On the other hand, Petitti argues that the systematic review of the literature may make explicit some important features of a body of research that could be missed with a more traditional narrative review (71). This, of course, is a key feature of research synthesis. A formal synthesis with explicit criteria, be they for ranking quality or excluding studies, offers a technique to explore conditions under which various estimated effects occur.

CHOOSING AN OUTCOME MEASURE

When possible, an outcome measure should be chosen for a research synthesis that means the most to the problem at hand and to the intended audience. Of course, this may not always be a choice the analyst is free to make. The data reported in the original research papers will in large part determine the type of outcome measure that can be extracted from the studies and included in the research synthesis.

From a public health perspective, the overall outcome measure may be change in mortality, in survival, or in length of hospital stay. For example, in an evaluation of interventions to encourage use of seat belts, the percentage increase in use is the relevant measure. These measures are more directly relevant to the user of a research synthesis than some of the alternative measures referred to as effect size (a standardized measure of effects) that have been developed to deal with studies that report a wide range of outcome measures. When the analyst is faced with this situation, other measures of effect are possible. These include the probability of improvement for patients on the new therapy compared to some standard therapy (or program)—the Mann-Whitney statistic summarizes this measure across numerous types of data (23). The Mann-Whitney statistic ranges from 0 to 1.0; 0.5 means that the patients from the two groups have equal chance of improving their performance. More generally, the probability estimated by the Mann-Whitney statistic reflects a clinically meaningful outcome that should be readily interpreted. Alternative standardized measures of effect have been proposed by a range of analysts and may be applied if a more direct measure of outcome is not available across the studies included in a research synthesis (see Chapters 16 and 17 in Reference 28 for statistical details). Later we refer to methods for analyzing studies that provide results on more than one outcome.

QUALITY

Although many have suggested using the quality of studies to adjust their reported outcomes or to weight them in meta-analysis, these ideas have not been given a strong statistical basis and are not currently being used in that manner. Wortman (88) describes two methods of rating quality. One (89) is based on various threats to validity of the studies along the lines of Campbell & Stanley (10) and Cook & Campbell (26), and the other is based on a scoring of features of a clinical trial by Chalmers et al (13, 15).

The Oxford study of obstetrics observed that the task of assessing quality over many studies was enormous and chose to score studies on three key dimensions of potential bias (12). These were control of selection bias on entry (quality of random allocation); control of selection bias after entry (the extent to which the primary analysis includes every person entered into the study); and bias in assessing outcome (the extent to which the outcome assessment was blind to treatment).

Although we have a quality scoring system for randomized controlled trials (13,15), we do not have one (or several) for observational studies of various forms. Colditz et al (24) and Miller et al (65) did make suggestions for possible adjustments to outcomes based on the design of the studies, but this proposal has not caught on.

Greenland (44) argues against using the summed quality scores because he feels this mixes up different effects. Therefore he would analyze quality according to the individual components of quality rating. Attempts to use either the summed quality scores or the individual component scores leading to the total quality scores for randomized trials as defined by Chalmers and colleagues (13, 15) failed to find a difference in outcome or variability of outcome in Emerson et al (35), even though the data were adequate to show a substantial gain in average quality score over a 30-year period.

Some investigators have proposed using quality-weighted averages of outcomes. Detsky et al (32) suggest that the field is not ready to provide such weights or adjustments. The main methods in use for checking effects of quality are to analyze subgroups of studies categorized by quality, or by omitting the lowest quality studies to determine whether differences in quality are associated with differences in outcomes.

MODELS FOR COMBINING DATA

When combining data from several investigations, one must have a statistic to use for combining, such as the risk difference, the risk ratio, or the odds ratio (for the latter two, the logarithm of the statistic is much used). In addition, one needs a model for the combining. The models in most use are called fixed effects and random effects.

FIXED EFFECTS The attitude in using fixed-effects models is that each study estimates exactly the same value of effect—thus if we could have an infinite sample size from each study, then the same outcome would have been observed to many decimal places. When one considers the differing populations being treated and the differing treatments actually being offered, it is hard to believe that each study will have exactly the same outcome especially when the measurements are very accurate. If, however, this were the true situation, then we would get the smallest variance of the weighted average by using weights that are proportional to the reciprocals of the variances of the outcomes from the individual studies. (We have to estimate these variances.)

RANDOM EFFECTS   Because the fixed-effects approach often is not appropriate, a broader model is much used, a two-stage sampling model. We think of
Stage 1 as choosing a set of studies, or equivalently a set of means, from a
distribution with a mean and variance μ and σ_A^2. Then each study in the sample
is thought of as being carried out according to the sampling and method of
investigation actually used. The study, when analyzed, produces a random
error centered on the particular study's true mean. By an analysis such as the
DerSimonian & Laird approach (31), or an alternative source (57), we can
estimate the variance among the study means. And then the weights can be
chosen inversely as the variances. If the among-studies variance is σ_A^2 and the
variance associated with the uncertainty of study i as carried out in the field
is σ_A^2, then the variance of the observation Xi for the size of effect in study i
is $\sigma_A^2 + \sigma_i^2$.

Figure 1 illustrates with a numerical example the two-stage sampling operation associated with the random-effects model. The distribution of true mean
effects associated with the illustrated studies has been arbitrarily chosen to
have grand mean $\mu = 0$ and among-studies standard deviation $\sigma_A = 1$. In a
sample of four studies, the true means, which in practice are unknown, happen
to be $\mu_1 = -1.5$, $\mu_2 = 1$, $\mu_3 = -0.5$, and $\mu_4 = 2$. The sampling variability of the
observation X_i associated with study i when executed is taken to be (these are
estimated in practice) $\sigma_1 = 1/4$, $\sigma_2 = 3/4$, $\sigma_3 = 1/2$, $\sigma_4 = 3/8$ and the observed
values in this example are $X_1 = -1.8$, $X_2 = 1.9$, $X_3 = -0.3$, and $X_4 = 1.5$. Although
the figure has been drawn with fairly symmetrical and Gaussian-appearing
densities, these are not requirements for the approach.

The optimum weights for the X_i's in the random effects model are propor-
tional to $W_i = 1/(\sigma_A^2 + \sigma_i^2)$. In the example, the estimate of μ (whose true value
is 0) would be $\hat{\mu} = \Sigma W_i X_i / \Sigma W_i = .183$. The standard deviation of the estimate
is $1/\sqrt{\Sigma W_i} = .554$.

Had we been assuming fixed effects, the optimum estimate would have
used weights proportional to $w_i = 1/\sigma_i^2$ and the estimate would have been
$\Sigma w_i X_i / \Sigma w_i = -.552$, with standard deviation $1/\sqrt{\Sigma w_i} = .186$. Investigators naturally find this smaller standard deviation more attractive than the more real-
istic .554 given by the random effects model. In the example the normalized
weights for fixed effects and random effects differ considerably as illustrated
in Table 2.

The weights for fixed effects vary by a factor of nearly 10, whereas the ratio
of largest to smallest weight is only about 1.5 for the random effects method.
This equalizing feature often leads to objections because very large studies
may not be given much more weight than small ones. The reason is that a new
study brings new information about the distribution of true means that, in the

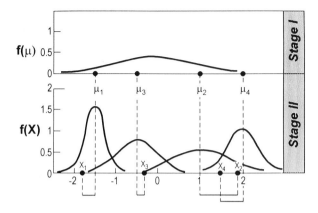

Figure 1 In Stage 1, from the population of studies with mean treatment effect μ and standard deviation σ_A, four studies are drawn for illustration (here the population has μ = 0, σ_A = 1). These drawings determine the associated unknown true means $\mu_1, \mu_2, \mu_3, \mu_4$. The studies are carried out with varying standard deviations $\sigma_1, \sigma_2, \sigma_3, \sigma_4$ (which may be partly due to different sample sizes) as shown in the Stage 2 diagram. The actual numerical outcomes of the studies are X_1, X_2, X_3, X_4. Notice that although $\mu_2 < \mu_4$, it turned out that $X_4 < X_2$ because of sampling variation.

fixed effects model, is totally discounted because of the initial assumption of equality.

The empirical variance of observations has itself great variability, and so sometimes we may find small variability among the outcomes, X_i, of the studies even though their true means, μ_i, differ. When this happens—less variability in the X_i than expected even if the true means were all alike—the DerSimonian & Laird approach treats the data as if fixed effects applied. This is not the same as believing in the assumption, but more like fitting a straight line even though the true function is probably curved. But when there is more variability than expected, the method estimates σ_A^2 and uses the estimate in the weighting.

The DerSimonian & Laird method adapts to the data. With k studies, use first the fixed-effect weights to get a provisional mean $\hat{\mu} = \sum_{i=1}^{k} w_i X_i / \sum w_i$.

Then compute a measure of heterogeneity, Q, which has a chi-square distribution with $k-1$ degrees of freedom when all the studies estimate the same quantity: $Q = \Sigma w_i (X_i - \hat{\mu})^2$. If the observed value of Q is less than $k-1$, use the weights of the model for fixed effects, i.e. $\hat{\mu}$. If Q is larger than $k-1$, use the weights W_1 appropriate for the random effects model. Then the needed estimate

Table 2 Normalized weights for the example in Figure 1

	Studies				
	1	2	3	4	Total
Fixed effects $w_i/\Sigma w_i$	.554	.062	.138	.246	1.0
Random effects $W_i/\Sigma W_i$	.289	.196	.246	.269	1.0

of σ_A^2 is given by $\dfrac{Q-(k-1)}{(\Sigma w_i - \Sigma w_i^2 / \Sigma w_i)}$. If the decision following the evaluation of Q is regarded as a test of significance, the significance level of approximately 0.5 is being used rather than the more customary 0.05. The DerSimonian & Laird method may not be optimal statistically, because of the association between a proportion and its variance. This would lead to incorrect answers in some situations. Other random-effects methods are available (36).

Some people think it unwise to combine estimates when the fixed-effects situation does not apply. Another attitude is that while it is good to try to remove variability due to study design or other characteristics due to the studies, we can use the final result to consider how variable the outcome of the application of the method may be in a new situation: roughly $\hat{\mu} \pm 2\hat{\sigma}_A$. So knowing something about the among-study variances gives warning about the uncertainty of the true effect in a new situation. [See Colditz et al (19) for illustration.]

Neither the fixed-effects nor the random-effects model represents the real situation, because we do not have a way to sample randomly from the true distributions. Instead we are sampling from the studies that occurred—or, if we have them all, from a process that produced these particular studies. And so the real situation is more like that of the paleontologist or geologist who report on the samples that emerge.

Nevertheless, the two-stage model allows for variability among studies and allows one to take account of study level variables; it seems more realistic than the fixed-effects model.

Vote-Counting

Among many ways of combining information from several studies, the sign test is a possible candidate. For example, if method A was superior to method B in 8 of 8 studies, then the two-sided significance level is $2/2^8 = 1/2^7 = 1/64$. This method treats all studies as of equal merit.

Unfortunately, many people regard counting the number of *significant* effects as a good way of summarizing data in a meta-analysis, but it is not. Large studies are likely to find significant results, and small ones not so likely. Counting *significant* effects uses data in a wasteful way and so is not recommended.

APPLICATION OF REGRESSION MODELS: SINGLE AND MULTIPLE OUTCOMES

Sometimes the meta-analyst has information on study-level covariates that may partly or wholly explain heterogeneity among study results. When relevant covariate information is available for the studies in a research synthesis, one should use appropriate statistical methods to study the effects of these covariates on the heterogeneous study results. For the analysis of data arising from a single study, regression methods serve this role. Special modifications of regression models are needed to adapt them for application to meta-analysis.

Berlin & Antman (8) discuss some general issues that arise in the application of regression methods to meta-analysis, and Berlin et al (9) consider methods for the (fixed-effects and random-effects) regression meta-analysis of epidemiologic dose-response data. Bayesian regression models have also been proposed for meta-analysis (33, 66).

Berkey et al (5) present a random-effects regression model that can supplement the random-effects model of DerSimonian & Laird (31) for the synthesis of 2 x 2 tables, allowing the inclusion of covariates that may explain heterogeneity. The method can also be used for the regression meta-analysis of continuous outcome variables. Just as the random-effects model of DerSimonian & Laird (31) reduces to a fixed-effects analysis when the data are homogeneous, the random-effects regression model (5) reduces to a fixed-effects regression model when the covariates in the model explain all the heterogeneity. Candidates for study-level covariates in these regression models include factors such as study design and study quality, but also include factors that are related to the treatment being evaluated (at what point in time, or for how long, does the trial protocol indicate the treatment is to be administered) or to the patients (their mean age, measures of how sick the patients are in each trial, the percentages of the cohort who are smokers or obese in an observational study). Thus, the application of regression methods to research synthesis can provide answers to new questions, as well as describing/adjusting/controlling for covariate differences among the studies.

When the research papers on a particular topic each provide results on more than one endpoint or outcome, a separate synthesis (or separate regression) of the results from each endpoint is often performed. Because these multiple endpoints are usually correlated, a simultaneous analysis that takes their correlation into account should add efficiency and accuracy. Raudenbush et al (73) showed how to analyze the effect sizes (a standardized or scale-free estimate of treatment difference) for each of the outcomes jointly in a single regression model that allows for adjustment of study-level covariates. This method applies to the meta-analysis of continuous multiple-outcomes that are measured on each subject, such as systolic and diastolic blood pressures. Gleser & Olkin (43) illustrate this method, along with univariate (separate outcomes) approaches and composite effect sizes, for the synthesis of correlated effect sizes using data from studies of the effects of coaching on SAT-Math and SAT-Verbal scores.

More recent methods (3, 4) for the regression-synthesis of multiple outcomes keep the measured outcomes in their original units, simplifying the interpretation of the results and providing other benefits. Gleser & Olkin (43) and Berkey et al (3) also consider the analysis of multiple (more than two) treatments as well as multiple endpoints. A difficulty with applying these methods for analyzing multiple endpoints is that the correlations among the outcomes are generally not provided by the published reports, and thus estimates must be obtained from external sources or from the subject-level data of one (or more) of the studies in the meta-analysis.

A different type of multiple endpoint arises when each trial or study reports survival proportions at a series of time points. Dear (29) extended the method of Raudenbush et al (73) to survival analysis, showing how to estimate the correlations among the serial survivorships and allowing the survival proportions reported at multiple times by the trials to be analyzed together. A potential problem with all of the above multiple-outcome methods is that they are based upon fixed-effects models. Using the regression models for continuous multiple outcomes (3, 4) indicates that these fixed-effects models may seriously underestimate the standard errors of regression coefficients when the unexplained (by regression) heterogeneity is substantial. Thus, until random-effects models are available for the simultaneous analysis of multiple endpoints, one may benefit more by doing separate random-effects analyses (5, 31) whenever the fixed-effects multiple-outcomes model is found to be inadequate for a particular application.

Finally, Berlin et al (9) discuss methods for meta-analyzing dose-response studies, a different type of multiple endpoint, in which each study provides a series of dose-specific relative risks, with one category serving as the common reference group. Those authors consider both fixed- and random-effects models for epidemiologic dose-response studies. Regarding the synthesis of correlated multiple outcomes, a major obstacle is the unavailability of the correlations that are needed in the estimation. Primary studies should, in the future, provide estimates of correlations among their (two or more) endpoints. This is a reasonable idea, even if the study is never to be included in a meta-analysis, so that readers can judge how independent are the reported findings on more than one outcome. Future methodological research needs to focus on random-effects regression models for multiple outcomes. Meta-regression methods provide a valuable device for accounting for the effects of study-level covariates in meta-analysis.

DELETING STUDIES WITH EXTREME RESULTS

Reviewing meta-analysis of epidemiologic data we note that assessing and reporting heterogeneity is often ignored. Further, excluding studies from meta-analysis because of observed heterogeneity is not uncommon (21). In a simulation we assessed the effect of removing the largest (or smallest) observations from a sample. If the studies had been drawn from normal distributions, then removing an extreme quarter of them would create bias of about 0.4 of a standard deviation. Further, by removing 25% of the data the variance is reduced by more than 40%. We conclude that removal of data can be dangerous for inference and should be avoided. It can easily lead to over-assurance about the precision of the results by suppression of among-study variation as well as bias. [Here we are not discussing two-sided trimming with suitable inferential tools to improve robustness (36a).]

PUBLICATION BIAS

Publication bias names the phenomenon in which studies with positive results are more likely to be published than are those with null or negative results. When this bias is present it can distort the interpretation of a research synthesis. Begg & Berlin summarize much of the work on this issue and report their own meta-analytic investigations of the magnitude of this bias in medicine (2). Several approaches to dealing with this potential problem have been suggested, including the file drawer calculation, and the creation of registers of clinical trials. These are discussed briefly in the following sections.

Rosenthal (75) introduced an attractive idea for quantifying the possible effect of publication bias. He formulated the problem as arising because investigators left studies without statistically significant results (or with negative results) in their file drawers instead of publishing them. He asked how many nonsignificant studies would be required to reduce an observed statistically significant meta-analysis to nonsignificance. If the number is unreasonably large, the observed result is regarded as good evidence for an effect. The method is not very stable, and Orwin (70) suggested an improvement. Iyengar & Greenhouse (50) have analyzed various approaches including a maximum likelihood approach that leads to heavy computing but offers more flexibility in the models and valuable information about the uncertainty of the parameters estimated for the model.

REGISTERS   Simes suggested that a register of all trials on oncology therapies would aid in identifying the population of studies and so avoid bias, or at least quantify the potential for bias in a research synthesis (81). In obstetrics, the Oxford group has created and analyzed a large data base of trials using the registry approach. Though this approach offers one response to the potential of publication bias, the implementation and maintenance of up-to-date registers of ongoing studies is likely to be expensive and, if not complete, may not resolve the underlying issue. The Cochrane Collaboration, however, may find registries a useful device in their attempt to locate all trials in medicine, and so it may turn out to be practical. Archie Cochrane was a physician who wanted to collect and analyze all the randomized trials in medicine; William G Cochran was a statistician who with G Udny Yule did early work on combining information from several investigations, especially in agriculture. Although several approaches to identification of publication bias have been proposed, experience with the peer review process suggests that if unpublished studies are identified for inclusion in a research synthesis, these unpublished studies should be handled separately. We no longer live in a time when articles are accepted in heavily reviewed journals without modification. Now it is commonplace for nearly every article to be rewritten before publication and for even the conclusions to be changed before publication, and so we cannot regard peer-reviewed articles as coming from the same population as the unpublished articles. For example, Lipsey & Wilson (61) compared effect size in published and unpublished articles on psychological, educational, and behavioral treatments and found published articles averaged 0.53 whereas unpublished gave 0.39 (in 92 articles where the author supplied the comparison).

A register can help in some settings, but the costs of establishing such a structure and the methods for maintaining a register are not clear. Unless well maintained, a register of all studies that are initiated will not add much to the field beyond a thorough search. Thorough searching is the best safeguard against publication bias.

SINGLE LARGE DEFINITIVE STUDY

The small number of mega-trials in clinical medicine offers an opportunity to compare a meta-analysis of published data from a series of smaller trials to the results of a huge study. Examples include streptokinase, intravenous nitroglycerin, and magnesium in the treatment of acute myocardial infarction (54), and BCG in prevention of tuberculosis (20). Though the concept of a huge simple trial has appeal, evidence suggests that the implementation of such a study may be far from simple (16). This is particularly so if the study includes elaborations such as a factorial design, as was the case in the magnesium study (ISIS-4) (54). Essentially, when several treatments and activities have to be decided on, a system can readily become overloaded, and often choices must be made by the deliverers of care about the priorities of different activities. For both intravenous nitroglycerin (90) and magnesium (85), meta-analysis of published small studies indicated that treatment improved survival. The mega trial ISIS-4 failed to confirm this treatment benefit for either therapy (54, 91). Some have argued that factors such as publication bias may explain some of the differences observed between mega-trials and meta-analyses published prior to the huge trial (34). Though one potential explanation, publication bias alone does not account for the discrepancy. For streptokinase, the two mega-trials each are consistent with the meta-analysis. For BCG, a huge trial using passive follow-up and acknowledged to miss at least 50% of all cases of tuberculosis, failed to show a protective effect observed in numerous other trials and case-control evaluations of BCG (20). For magnesium, the patients in ISIS-4 did not appear to be as sick as the patients in the earlier trials, and the treatment was administered later, relative to the onset of the patients chest pain, in ISIS-4 than in earlier trials. Another relevant factor is that, by the time ISIS-4 was conducted, the majority of patients were also receiving aspirin and thrombolytic therapy, perhaps reducing the marginal benefit of magnesium as it would be implemented in more current clinical practice. It is hard to allow for changes wrought by the dynamics of care.

Large trials are often not simple to implement and potentially sacrifice rigor of protocol implementation for apparent statistical benefits from huge numbers and thoughtful designs. A similar effort implemented across numerous smaller studies may offer greater potential to identify factors that contribute to the efficacy of a therapy.

For example, if afterthought suggests that some features of a trial need adjusting, we would regret having committed a huge sample to it. Some research would be welcome on appropriate sample sizes considering the likely possibilities of needing changes in design after a trial is completed.

COMPARING META-ANALYSES WITH OUTCOMES OF LARGE STUDIES

Do meta-analytic results agree with those of large trials? Villar et al (87) reviewed 30 meta-analyses (including 185 randomized controlled trials) from the pregnancy and childbirth module of the Cochrane database (37). They compared the meta-analysis result computed after removing the largest experiment with the result of the largest experiment (always over 1000 trials). In 24 of 30 comparisons the direction of treatment effect agreed. Other comparisons they made are more difficult to interpret; Flournoy & Olkin (40) regard this study as a useful first step in research on comparing a composite of small studies with a large one. A parallel overlapping study with an overlap of a third of the studies (14) found 24 of 27 pairs of estimates in the same direction and having overlapping confidence intervals, and 25 in the same direction.

DIAGNOSIS: CURRENT MOVEMENT IN THIS FIELD

Diagnostic tests have applications in public health prevention programs in addition to specific clinical settings. Therefore, we briefly review progress in this area, though we acknowledge that the application of meta-analytic methods is often constrained by the poor quality of the underlying evaluations of diagnostic tests. In this setting one is estimating a relationship [like a receiver operating characteristic curve (ROC)] rather than a location (like the difference in performance of two treatments), making for a much more difficult undertaking.

Irwig and colleagues have reviewed the steps in undertaking a meta-analysis of diagnostic tests, and they provide guidelines for conducting and reporting meta-analyses of test accuracy (53). Shapiro reviews the graphical and quantitative methods for summarizing diagnostic test accuracy, assessing the adequacy of the summary, and studying the effect of differences in study design, patient characteristics, or implementation of the diagnostic test on reported diagnostic accuracy (78). In an accompanying article, Rutter & Gatsonis review regression approaches to meta-analysis of diagnostic test data, summarizing methods and illustrating with examples of data presentation (76).

A recent thorough application of these methods, reported in the *American Journal of Epidemiology*, demonstrates the complexity of combining data on test performance and shows how a careful research synthesis can inform public health policy. Fahey et al combined data from 59 studies of the efficacy of PAP smears to estimate a summary receiver operating characteristic curve (38). They observed that specificity (percent of negative test results in women without cervical cancer) in the 90 to 95% range corresponded to sensitivity (percent of positive test results in those with cervical cancer) in the 20 to 35% range. Pap test accuracy was not associated with reported study characteristics or dimensions of quality that they were able to investigate.

Variation among the primary studies in the threshold used to classify results is a key feature of quantitative research synthesis of diagnostic test performance. One approach that takes this into account is that of Karduan & Karduan (56) and Moses et al (67) in which a summary ROC curve is estimated. Future primary studies should pay more attention to the methodologic standards for the conduct and reporting of diagnostic test evaluations.

GUIDELINES FOR COMBINING OBSERVATIONAL STUDIES

The need for guidelines for research synthesis is clearly argued by Cook et al who emphasize that guidelines are an integral part of the research process and will lead to improvement in the conduct and reporting of these studies (25). This argument parallels the experience with guidelines for the conduct and reporting of randomized controlled trials. Reporting appears to have improved since the publication of guidelines (30). For example, in a review of study quality and the outcomes of clinical trials, Emerson and colleagues noted that the quality of studies in medicine (as measured by the Chalmers score) has improved over time, though much room for improvement remains.

CONCLUSIONS

In principle, the guidelines for meta-analysis of observational data should at the minimum follow those for clinical trials (25). Features include the protocol development, searching strategy, study selection and listing of rejected studies, methodologic quality assessment, data extraction, analysis, evaluation of heterogeneity, subgroup analysis, presentation of results, interpretation, and dissemination.

Specific features of observational data that should be addressed include study design and the dual purposes of research synthesis, first to summarize an association and secondly to describe those factors that contribute to heterogeneity among the outcomes of the studies. We recommend that results should not be combined across study design but summarized separately for each design.

The assumption that the true effect size has a common true value for all study situations is very strong, impossible to verify, and surely wrong. The issue is not whether the observed results differ significantly from one another, but whether the population effects are exactly equal. Heterogeneity in epidemiologic data is usual rather than exceptional. We recommend that meta-analysts do not focus on tests of significance for homogeneity (say, at the 5% level), but rather quantify estimates of among-study variance. Heterogeneity should be interpreted with caution in the spirit of exploratory data analysis. (Because of the high variance of estimates of variance, this calculation may sometimes suggest a negative variance!) Sources of heterogeneity are most easily interpreted when they have been established in advance of the analysis so that findings become confirmatory rather than explanatory.

We recommend the use of the random-effects model for combining epidemiologic data because if homogeneity is observed, we will be guided to the homogeneous effects model, and if not, we will be guided to a model allowing for heterogeneity.

Deleting studies from a meta-analysis because of extreme published results is a risky approach to dealing with heterogeneity. It may substantially bias the mean estimate and underestimate the true variance. Often, studies that appear to be outliers can be explained by some difference in study design, patient characteristics, or treatment regimen. Setting aside studies without cause is generally dangerous for inference and is discouraged.

Because a major problem in observational studies is achieving a priori equivalence of the groups to be compared, a detailed summary of characteristics should be reported for each of the studies considered. These details may help assure the reader that design, the characteristics of the cohort, exposure dose, and covariates included (or excluded) from a study do not contribute greatly to the among-study variation in results. And if they do contribute, then the research synthesis can formally incorporate analysis on these factors.

Quality may be used as a covariate to explain variation among study results. As of this writing, no analytic procedure offers grounds for quality weighting.

ACKNOWLEDGMENTS

We thank Catherine S Berkey for contributing the material on applications of regression models and for providing helpful comments on earlier drafts, and Carol A Leighton for manuscript preparation.

Literature Cited

1. Beecher HK. 1955. The powerful placebo. *JAMA* 159:1602–6
2. Begg CB, Berlin JA. 1988. Publication bias: a problem in interpreting medical data. *J. R. Stat. Soc. A* 151:419–63
3. Berkey C, Anderson J, Hoaglin D. 1995. Multiple-outcome meta-analysis of clinical trials. *Stat. Med.* In press
4. Berkey C, Antczak-Bouckoms A, Hoaglin D, Mosteller F, Pihlstrom B. 1995. Multiple-outcomes meta-analysis of treatments for periodontal disease. *J. Dent. Res.* 74:1030–39
5. Berkey C, Hoaglin D, Mosteller F, Colditz G. 1995. A random-effects regression model for meta-analysis. *Stat. Med.* 14:395–411

6. Berlin JA, Colditz GA. 1990. A meta-analysis of physical activity in the prevention of coronary heart disease. *Am. J. Epidemiol.* 132:612–28
7. Berlin JA. 1995. The benefits of heterogeneity in meta-analysis of data from epidemiologic studies. Invited commentary. *Am. J. Epidemiol.* 142:383–87
8. Berlin JA, Antman E. 1994. Advantages and limitations of metaanalytic regressions of clinical trials data. *Online J. Curr. Clin. Trials*, Vol. 3
9. Berlin JA, Longnecker MP, Greenland S. 1993. Meta-analysis of epidemiologic dose-response data. *Epidemiology* 4:218–28
10. Campbell DT, Stanley JC. 1966. *Ex-*

perimental and Quasi-Experimental Designs for Research. Chicago: Rand McNally

11. Can. Task Force Period. Health Exam. 1979. The periodic health examination. *Can. Med. Assoc. J.* 121:1194–254

12. Chalmers I, Enkin M, Keirse MJNC. 1989. *Effective Care in Pregnancy and Childbirth.* Oxford: Oxford Univ. Press

13. Chalmers TC, Berrier J, Sacks HS, Levin H, Reitman D, Nagalingham R. 1987. Meta-analysis of clinical trials as a scientific discipline. II. Replicate variability and comparison of studies that agree and disagree. *Stat. Med.* 6:733–44

14. Chalmers TC, Lau J, Cappelleri JC, Schmid CH. 1994. Comparing results from the largest studies with meta-analyses of smaller studies. Abstr. 44A. Meet. Cochrane Collab. Hamilton, Ontario. *Control. Clin. Trials* 15(3S):63S

15. Chalmers TC, Smith H Jr., Blackburn B, Silverman B, Schroeder B, et al. 1981. A method for assessing the quality of a randomized control trial. *Control. Clin. Trials* 2:31–49

16. Charlton BG. 1994. Practice guidelines and practical judgement: the role of mega-trials, meta-analysis and consensus. *Br. J. Gen. Pract.* 44:290–91

17. Cochran WG. 1937. Problems arising in the analysis of a series of similar experiments. *J. R. Stat. Soc. Suppl.* 4: 102–18

18. Cochran WG. 1954. The combination of estimates from different experiments. *Biometrics* 10:101–29

19. Colditz GA, Berkey CS, Mosteller F, Brewer TF, Wilson ME, et al. 1995. The efficacy of Bacillus Calmette-Guerin in vaccination of newborn and infants in the prevention of tuberculosis: meta-analysis of the published literature. *Pediatrics* 96:29–35

20. Colditz GA, Brewer TF, Berkey CS, Wilson ME, Burdick E, et al. 1994. The efficacy of bacillus calmette-guerin vaccination in the prevention of tuberculosis: meta-analysis of the published literature. *JAMA* 271:698–702

21. Colditz GA, Burdick E, Mosteller F. 1995. Commentary on heterogeneity in meta-analysis of data from epidemiologic studies. *Am. J. Epidemiol.* 142: 371–82

22. Colditz GA, Egan KM, Stampfer MJ. 1993. Hormone replacement therapy and risk of breast cancer: Results from epidemiologic studies. *Am. J. Obstet. Gyn.* 168:1473–80

23. Colditz GA, Miller JN, Mosteller F. 1988. Measuring gain in the evaluation of medical technology: The probability of a better outcome. *Int. J. Technol. Assess. Health Care* 4:637–42

24. Colditz GA, Miller JN, Mosteller F. 1989. How study design affects outcomes in comparisons of therapy. 1. Medical. *Stat. Med.* 8:441–54

25. Cook DJ, Sackett DL, Spitzer WO. 1995. Methodologic guidelines for systematic reviews of randomized control trials in health care from the Potsdam consultation on meta-analysis. *J. Clin. Epidemiol.* 48:161–71

26. Cook TD, Campbell DT. 1979. *Quasi-Experimentation: Design and Analysis Issues for Field Settings.* Boston: Houghton Mifflin

27. Cook TD, Cooper H, Cordray DS, Hartmann H, Hedges LV, et al. 1992. *Meta-Analysis for Explanation: A Casebook.* New York: Russell Sage Found.

28. Cooper H, Hedges LV, eds. 1994. *The Handbook of Research Synthesis.* New York: Russell Sage Found.

29. Dear KBG. 1994. Iterative generalized least squares for meta-analysis of survival data at multiple times. *Biometrics* 50:989–1002

30. DerSimonian R, Charette LJ, McPeek B, Mosteller F. 1982. Reporting on methods in clinical trials. *N. Engl. J. Med.* 306:1332–37

31. DerSimonian R, Laird N. 1986. Meta-analysis in clinical trials. *Control. Clin. Trials* 7:177–88

32. Detsky AS, Naylor CD, O'Rourke K, McGreer A, L'Abbe KA. 1992. Incorporating variations in the quality of individual randomized trials into meta-analysis. *J. Clin. Epidemiol.* 45: 255–65

33. DuMouchel W. 1990. Bayesian meta-analysis. In *Statistical Methodology in Pharmaceutical Sciences,* ed. D Berry, pp. 509–29. New York: Marcel Dekker

34. Egger M, Smith GD. 1995. Misleading meta-analysis. Lessons from "an effective, safe, simple" intervention that wasn't. *Br. Med. J.* 310:752–54

35. Emerson JD, Burdick E, Hoaglin DC, Mosteller F, Chalmers TC. 1990. An empirical study of the possible relation of treatment differences to quality scores in controlled randomized clinical trials. *Control. Clin. Trials* 11:339–52

36. Emerson JH, Hoaglin DC, Mosteller F. 1993. A modified random-effects procedure for combining risk difference in sets of 2 x 2 tables from clinical trials. *J. Ital. Stat. Soc.* 2:269-290

36a. Emerson JH, Hoaglin DC, Mosteller F. 1996. Simple robust procedures for combining risk differences in sets of 2 $\times$ 2 tables. *Stat. Med.* In press

37. Enkin MW, Keirse MHNC, Renfrew MJ, Neilson JP, eds. 1993. *Pregnancy and Childbirth Module: Cochrane Database of Systematic Reviews* (Cochrane updates on disk). Oxford: Update Software: Disk issue 2.
38. Fahey MT, Irwig L, Macaskill P. 1995. Meta-analysis of pap test accuracy. *Am. J. Epidemiol.* 141:680–89
39. Fisher RA. 1932. *Statistical Methods for Research Workers*, p. 39. Edinburgh: Oliver & Body.
40. Flournoy N, Olkin I. 1995. Do small trials square with large ones? *Lancet* 345:741–42
41. Garder P, Leden L, Thedeen T. 1994. Safety implications of bicycle paths at signalized intersections. *Accid. Anal. Prev.* 26:429–39
42. Gilbert JP, McPeek B, Mosteller F. 1977. Progress in surgery and anesthesia: benefits and risks of innovative therapy. In *Costs Risk and Benefits of Surgery*, ed. JP Bunker, BA Barnes, F Mosteller, pp. 130–38; App. 9-II, pp. 156–58 (classical ANOVA); App. 9-III, pp. 158–61 (Bayesian inference); data analysis App. 9-IV, pp. 161–63). Oxford: Oxford Univ. Press
43. Gleser L, Olkin I. 1994. Stochastically dependent effect sizes. In *The Handbook of Research Synthesis,* ed. H Cooper, L Hedges, pp. 339–55. New York: Russell Sage Found.
44. Greenland S. 1994. Invited commentary: A critical look at some popular meta-analytic methods. *Am. J. Epidemiol.* 140:290–96
45. Hankinson SE, Colditz GA, Hunter DJ, Spencer TL, Rosner B, Stampfer MJ. 1992. A quantitative assessment of oral contraceptive use and risks of ovarian cancer. *Obstet. Gynecol.* 80:708–14
46. Hedges LV, Olkin I. 1985. *Statistical Methods for Meta-Analysis.* Orlando, Fl: Academic
47. Hertz-Piccotto I, Neutra RR. 1994. Resolving discrepancies among studies: the influence of dose on effect size. *Epidemiology* 5:156–63
48. Howe GR, Hirohata T, Hislop TG, Iscovich JM, Yuan JM, et al. 1990. Dietary factors and risk of breast cancer: combined analysis of 12 case-control studies. *J. Natl. Cancer Inst..* 82:561–69
49. Hunter JE, Schmidt FL. 1990. *Methods of Meta-Analysis: Correcting Error and Bias in Research Findings.* Newbury Park, CA: Sage
50. Iyengar S, Greenhouse JB. 1988. Selection models and the file drawer problem. *Stat. Sci.* 3:109–35
51. Inst. Med. 1991. Committee to review the adverse effects of Pertussis and Rubella vaccines. *Adverse Effects of Pertussis and Rubella Vaccines.* Washington, DC: Natl. Acad. Press
52. Inst. Med. 1994. Committee to review the health effects in Vietnam veterans of exposure to herbicides. *Veterans and Agent Orange: Health Effects of Herbicides used in Vietnam.* Washington, DC: Natl. Acad. Press
53. Irwig L, Gatsonis C, Lau J, Colditz G, Chalmers T, Mosteller F. 1994. Guidelines for meta-analyses evaluating diagnostic tests. *Ann. Intern. Med.* 120; 667–76
54. ISIS-4 Collaborative Group. 1995. ISIS-4: a randomised factorial trial assessing early oral captopril, oral mononitrate, and intravenous magnesium sulphate in 58050 patients with suspected cute myocardial infarction. *Lancet* 345:669–85
55. Johnston JJ, Hendricks SA, Fike JM. 1994. Effectiveness of behavioral safety belt interventions. *Accid. Anal. Prev.* 26:315–23
56. Kardaun JWPF, Kardaun OJWF. 1990. Comparative diagnostic performance of three radiological procedures for the detection of lumbar disk herniation. *Methods Info. Med.* 29:12–22
57. Laird NM, Mosteller F. 1990. Some statistical methods for combining experimental results. *Int. J. Technol. Assess. Health Care* 6:5–30
58. Law MR, Wald NJ, Thompson SG. 1994. By how much and how quickly does reduction in serum cholesterol concentration lower risk of ischemic heart disease? *Br. Med. J.* 308:367–73
59. Letzel H. 1995. "Best evidence synthesis: An intelligent alternative to meta-analysis": Discussion. A case of "Either-Or" or "As well". *J. Clin. Epidemiol.* 48:19–21
60. Light RJ, Pillemer DB. 1984. *Summing Up: The Science of Reviewing Research.* Cambridge, MA: Harvard Univ. Press
61. Lipsey MW, Wilson DB. 1993. The efficacy of psychological, educational, and behavioral treatment. Confirmation from meta-analysis. *Am. Psychol.* 48: 1181–209
62. Longnecker MP, Berlin JA, Orza MJ, Chalmers TC. 1988. A meta-analysis of alcohol consumption in relation to risk of breast cancer. *JAMA* 260:652–65
63. Louis TA, Fineberg HV, Mosteller F. 1985. Findings for public health from meta-analysis. *Annu. Rev. Public Health* 6:1–20
64. MacMahon B, Hutchison GB. 1964. Prenatal X-ray and children's cancer: A

review. *Acta Unio Internationalis Contra Cancrum* 20:1172–74

65. Miller JN, Colditz GA, Mosteller F. 1989. How study design affects outcomes in comparisons of therapy. II. Surgical. *Stat. Med.* 8:455–66
66. Morris CN, Normand SL. 1992. Hierarchical models for combining information and for meta-analysis. In *Bayesian Statistics*, 4:321–44. Oxford: Oxford Univ. Press
67. Moses LE, Shapiro D, Littenberg B. 1993. Combining independent studies of a diagnostic test into a summary (ROC) curve: data-analytic approaches and some additional considerations. *Stat. Med.* 12:1293–316
68. Natl. Res. Counc. 1992. *On combining information: statistical issues and opportunities for research.* Washington, DC: Natl. Acad. Sci. Press
69. Olkin I. 1995. Statistical and theoretical considerations in meta-analysis. *J. Clin. Epidemiol.* 48:133–46
70. Orwin R. 1983. A fail-safe N for effect size in meta-analysis. *J. Educ. Stat.* 8:157–59
71. Petitti DB. 1994. Of babies and bathwater. *Am. J. Epidemiol.* 140:779–82
72. Petitti DB. 1994. *Meta-Analysis, Decision Analysis and Cost-Effectiveness Analysis in Medicine: Methods for Quantitative Synthesis in Medicine.* Oxford: Oxford Univ. Press
73. Raudenbush S, Becker B, Kalaian H. 1988. Modeling multivariate effect sizes. *Psychol. Bull.* 103:111–20
74. Rep. US Prev. Serv. Task Force. 1989. *Guide to clinical preventive services.* Baltimore: Williams & Wilkins
75. Rosenthal R. 1979. The "file drawer problem" and tolerance for null results. *Psychol. Bull.* 86:638–41
76. Rutter CM, Gatsonis CA. 1995. Regression methods for meta-analysis of diagnostic test data. *Acad. Radiol.* 2:S48–S56
77. Sacks HS, Berrier J, Reitman D, Ancona-Berk VA, Chalmers TC. 1987. Meta-analysis of randomized controlled studies. *N. Engl. J. Med.* 316:450–55
78. Shapiro DE. 1995. Issues in combining independent estimates of the sensitivity and specificity of a diagnostic test. *Acad. Radiol.* 2:S37–S47
79. Shapiro S. 1994. Meta-analysis/Shmeta-analysis. *Am. J. Epidemiol.* 140:771–78
80. Shinton R, Beevers G. 1989. Meta-analysis of relation between cigarette smoking and stroke. *Br. Med. J.* 298:789–94
81. Simes RJ. 1986. Publication bias: the case for an international registry of clinical trials. *J. Clin. Oncol.* 4:1529–41
82. Slavin RE. 1995. Best evidence synthesis: An intelligent alternative to meta-analysis. *J. Clin. Epidemiol.* 48:9–18
83. Spitzer WO, ed. 1995. The Potsdam International Consultation on meta-analysis. *J. Clin. Epidemiol.* 48:1–171
84. Stampfer MJ, Colditz GA. 1991. Estrogen replacement therapy and coronary heart disease: a quantitative assessment of the epidemiologic evidence. *Prev. Med.* 20:47–63
85. Teo KK, Yusuf S, Collins R, Held PH, Peto R. 1991. Effects of intravenous magnesium in suspected acute myocardial infarction: overview of randomized trials. *Br. Med. J.* 303:1499–503
86. US Congr. Off. Technol. Assess. 1995. *Tools for evaluating health technologies: Five background papers.* BP-H-142. Washington, DC: US GPO
87. Villar V, Carroli G, Belizn JM. 1995. Predictive ability of meta-analyses of randomized controlled trials. *Lancet* 345:772–76
88. Wortman PM. 1994. Judging research quality. In *The Handbook of Research Synthesis*, ed. H Cooper, L Hedges, pp. 97–109. New York: Russell Sage Found.
89. Wortman PM. 1983. Evaluation research: A methodological perspective. *Annu. Rev. Psychol.* 34:223–60
90. Yusuf S, Collins R, MacMahon S, Peto R. 1988. Effect of intravenous nitrates on mortality in acute myocardial infarction: overview of the randomised trials. *Lancet* 1:1088–92
91. Yusuf S, Flather M. 1995. Magnesium in acute myocardial infarction. *Br. Med. J.* 310:751–52

Annu. Rev. Public Health. 1996. 17:25–46

DISABILITY AS A PUBLIC HEALTH OUTCOME IN THE AGING POPULATION[1]

Jack M. Guralnik[1], Linda P. Fried[2], and Marcel E. Salive[1]

[1]Epidemiology, Demography, and Biometry Program, National Institute on Aging, Bethesda, Maryland 20892; [2]Departments of Medicine and Epidemiology, The Johns Hopkins Medical Institutions, Baltimore, Maryland 21205

KEY WORDS: aging, disability, functional status, frailty, functional assessment

---

ABSTRACT

Improvements in life expectancy in the twentieth century have resulted from major declines in mortality at younger ages, but it is less well recognized that mortality declines at older ages have also played a substantial role in prolonging expectation of life. A person reaching age 65 in 1900 could expect to live an additional 11.9 years. Life expectancy at age 65 rose to 14.4 years by 1960 and then increased by about three years in the next three decades, reaching 17.5 years in 1992 (56, 70). As a greater proportion of the population survives to very old ages, the public health impact of the burden of disease and disability and related utilization of medical care and need for supportive and long-term care has become an important concern. In particular, the ability of the older person to function independently in the community is a critically important public health issue. A growing body of research in the last decade has addressed the measurement of disability, factors related to its onset, consequences of disability, and the potential for preventive interventions. This article summarizes the state of the art in these areas and discusses their public health relevance.

ASSESSING FUNCTIONING IN OLDER POPULATIONS

A wide range of instruments has been developed for assessing physical functioning and disability in older persons. The assessment of disability was first used to identify functional impairments in persons with serious chronic

---

diseases such as cancer (53) and stroke (55), particularly in institutional settings. In the past two decades these measures have been increasingly used to characterize older persons in various settings and for many purposes, including clinical assessment, clinical research, and community-based epidemiological studies. Disability is generally assessed through self-report or proxy report of difficulty or need for help in basic self-care tasks, more complex tasks necessary for living independently in the community, and tasks related to mobility and other more basic movements of the body. Additionally, physical performance measures, which objectively assess various aspects of physical functioning, have been used recently to supplement self-report of disability.

Basic self-care activities such as bathing, dressing, transferring from a bed to a chair, using the toilet, and eating are commonly referred to as activities of daily living (ADLs) (55) and are the most frequently used indicators of physical disability. These measures reflect a substantial degree of disability, and, in general, the more ADLs with which a person has difficulty, the more severe his or her disability. The prevalence of difficulty or need for help in performing ADLs is lower than other measures of disability, and ADLs work well to identify the most severely disabled individuals.

Disability has also been measured in relation to the ability to perform instrumental activities of daily living (IADLs), tasks considered necessary for independent living in the community. These tasks are generally considered to be more difficult and complex than those in the self-care domain and include activities such as shopping, preparing food, housekeeping, doing laundry, using transportation, taking medications, handling money, and using the telephone (64).

In addition to ADLs and IADLs, a wide variety of other measures of self-reported functional status have been developed (1, 9, 52). The assessment of mobility is an especially important part of functional evaluations. Mobility can be evaluated by self-report using a hierarchical approach, starting with simple mobility tasks such as transferring from a bed to a chair and progressing through walking short and longer distances, and climbing stairs. Surveys can also be used to assess more basic functions related to range of motion, strength and endurance (69), as well as the higher end of the functional spectrum, including vigorous exercise and walking medium and long distances (73).

A number of survey batteries that assess multiple domains of functional status have been developed, some specific to functioning and others designed to measure overall health status. For example, the Functional Status Questionnaire assesses physical function, psychological function, and social-role function (48). The Sickness Impact Profile, a general health status evaluation instrument, contains a large proportion of items that assess aspects of physical functioning and disability, including domains of mobility and confinement, movement of the body, personal hygiene, ambulation, usual daily work, and household management (4).

THE PREVALENCE OF DISABILITY IN THE OLDER POPULATION

Traditionally, public health officials evaluate the status of a population using total and cause-specific mortality rates and disease incidence and prevalence rates. Measures of disability add an important perspective on the health status of older populations. Although the presence of disease is certainly important, the functional consequences of disease in older people have major implications for quality of life, need for supportive services, and ultimately, need for long-term care, whether at home or in an institution. Disability status may reflect severity of disease, and measuring disability offers an important approach to summarizing the overall impact of multiple co-existing chronic conditions.

The largest national prevalence survey of disability was administered to more than 41 million persons as part of the 1990 United States Census long form (62). A two-part question asked first about difficulty in going outside alone (mobility disability) and second about taking care of personal needs such as bathing, dressing, or getting around in the home (ADL disability). Overall, an estimated 13.2 million Americans (70.5 per 1000 persons) age 16 years and older had a mobility or ADL disability, about half of whom were 65 years and older. Among those age 65 years and older, 16% had difficulty with mobility-related activities and 12% had difficulty with ADLs. A number of large national surveys in the 1980s specifically assessed disability in the older population (94). In analyses that evaluated ADL disability rates for a set of items common to all these surveys (bathing, dressing, eating, transferring, and toileting), it was found that the prevalence of *receiving help* with one or more of these ADLs ranged from 5.0 to 8.1% of noninstitutionalized adults age 65 years and older (94).

Both national and local surveys of representative older populations show consistent associations of disability with demographic characteristics. Prevalence of disability increases substantially with increasing age, is more common in women than men in age groups above age 75 years, is higher in those with lower education and income levels, and is somewhat higher in ethnic minorities (12, 13, 31). In longitudinal studies, men and women have similar incidence rates of disability, but women survive longer after becoming disabled, which accounts for the higher prevalence of disability in older women (85).

Surveys of disability in the older community-based population do not capture its full magnitude because a substantial proportion of the disabled population resides in nursing homes. Of nursing home residents age 65 years and older, over 90% are dependent in one or more ADLs and two thirds are reported to have memory impairment or disorientation (46). In 1987, an estimated 6.8% of persons ages 65 years and older used a nursing home at some time during the year, including 8.2% of women and 4.7% of men (21). Use of nursing homes increases dramatically with increasing age. Less than 1.5% of persons ages 65 to 69 used a nursing home in 1987. In the age group 85 to 89 years, one fourth of women and one fifth of men used a nursing home, and among those age 90 years and older, 46% of women and 31% of men used a nursing home in 1987. With the use of data from both the National Health Interview Survey and the National Nursing Home Survey, estimates of the impact of disability in the total older population have been made, including those dwelling in both the community and nursing homes (45, 80). Overall, 15% of men and 22% of women either live at home and need the help of another person with ADLs or IADLs or are resident in a nursing home (80). About 10% of men and women ages 65 to 74 years are dependent at home or live in a nursing home, but this figure rises to 46% of men and 62% of women in the 85 and older age group.

Measuring disability prevalence in a single population over time and making comparisons between populations would be important for understanding trends or differences in the public health impact of poor health in older persons. However, assessments have not always been standardized to the point where these comparisons can be readily made. Different surveys may assess the same disability items but may ask questions in a slightly different manner, translations of questionnaires may yield slightly different questions, and cultural differences in the way questions are interpreted and answered may also lead to different responses.

The U.S. National Long-Term Care Survey has been administered in an identical manner at three times in the 1980s (66). Analyses of these data have shown a modest decline in the prevalence of disability in ADLs and IADLs, although this decline was not uniform across all strata of disability. An effort has been made to develop instruments that can lead to useful comparisons of disability across countries, but this work is still in its early stages (20). In comparing local community disability rates even when the same instrument is administered, caution must be used in interpreting the data because out-migration of disabled individuals may occur from different communities at different rates. This was demonstrated in the communities of the Established Populations for the Epidemiologic Study of the Elderly (EPESE) (13). Prevalence of disability in the East Boston site was substantially higher than for the two rural counties in Iowa. However, this prevalence was related in part to greater use of home health care in East Boston (10), allowing individuals to remain in the community, whereas in Iowa persons were much more likely to leave the community and enter nursing homes (23). Thus, cross-sectional data revealed a greater proportion of disabled individuals in the East Boston community, but longitudinal follow-up revealed that older persons in East Boston may not have been in poorer health but were simply more likely to remain in the community when they became disabled.

SOCIAL AND HEALTH CONSEQUENCES OF DISABILITY

Disability in older persons affects both their quality of life and need for care, and has a major impact on their families and the entire health care system. Physical disability is associated with restrictions that affect all aspects of daily life. For example, in the Women's Health and Aging Study, a community-based study that recruited the one third most disabled women living in the community, it was found that in a typical week 34% of these disabled women did not go beyond their neighborhood, including 15% who didn't leave their homes, and that 12% stopped using rooms in their homes because of their disabilities (38).

The burden of care related to disability in the older population goes well beyond that received in nursing homes. Figure 1 combines data from the National Nursing Home Survey and the Supplement on Aging of the National Health Interview Survey to depict the type of care received according to disability level. A majority of persons with disability in IADLs receive only

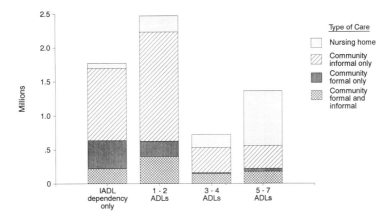

Figure 1   Number of persons who receive nursing home care and informal and formal care in the community according to level of disability. Community-dwelling persons represented in this figure reported actually receiving help for one or more activities of daily living (ADLs) or instrumental activities of daily living (IADLs). ADLs include bathing, dressing, eating, transferring, walking, using the toilet, and continence. IADLs include preparing meals, shopping, managing money, doing light housework, doing heavy housework, and getting outside. Source: Reference 45.

informal care (unpaid care provided by family, friends, and neighbors), with very few residing in nursing homes. The institutionalized proportion rises with the severity of disability, reaching 59% in persons with dependency in 5 to 7 ADLs, an indicator of severe disability. However, even at this high level of disability, more than one third of persons live at home and receive a combination of formal and informal care. Figure 1 clearly illustrates the importance of informal care in meeting the daily needs of older persons with lesser degrees of disability. Although those with disability in IADLs often meet their needs with formal care alone, few persons with one or two ADLs and almost no one with three or more ADLs reside in the community using only formal care.

Living arrangements of older persons in the community who develop disability play an important role in determining the source of their care and their eventual ability to remain in the community. The most likely source of informal care is, first, the spouse, if living and capable, followed by children and others. The magnitude of the reliance of older disabled people on informal care, illustrated in Figure 1, is of major public health concern for the future as the older population expands and the availability of informal care resources, especially from children, contracts.

Longitudinal epidemiologic studies have demonstrated that disability in older persons is a predictor of numerous important outcomes. In fact, in most prospective analyses in aging cohorts, disability is the strongest predictor of adverse outcomes after age. Because disability is an excellent marker for the overall burden and severity of disease in the older person, it is a strong predictor of future mortality. This has been found in both community-dwelling populations (6, 14, 58, 93) as well as in institutions, where those who are severely disabled are more likely to die than those with less disability (15). In the disabled community-dwelling population, there is also a strong mortality gradient according to the degree of disability. Two-year follow-up data from the National Long-Term Care Survey showed mortality rates rising from 15.2% in those with IADL disability only to 20.7% in those with disability in one or two ADLs, 24% in those with three or four ADLs, and 37.2% in those with five or six ADLs (65). In the EPESE communities, four-year all-cause mortality rates were four to six times higher in those age 70 years and older with ADL disability compared with persons who were nondisabled. Additionally, those with mobility disability, defined as the need for help in climbing stairs and/or walking 1/2 mile, were 2.5 times as likely to die as those with no disability (14). Even after adjusting for demographic characteristics, behavioral risk factors such as smoking and weight status, and several chronic diseases, disability continues to be an important predictor of mortality.

Disability status is a strong predictor of other health outcomes, including further declines in functioning (8, 65), increased number of acute illnesses, and increased risk of falls and injuries (9, 26). Performance on objective measures of functioning is highly predictive of falls both within an institution (88) and in the community (71, 87). Disability is also a predictor of health care utilization, including increased risk for recurrent hospitalization, greater use of outpatient care (26), and institutionalization (7, 23, 33, 79). Mor and colleagues (68) have also shown that functional status and change in function over time are associated with increased hospital use and cost of care. Other researchers have demonstrated a clear relationship between disability level and use of physician services (92) and paid home care (84).

Contrary to the belief that disability progresses in an inexorable downhill course, multiple longitudinal studies have demonstrated that it is not rare for individuals to report less disability in follow-up evaluations than they have reported at baseline. In the Alameda County Study, for example, 13% of men and 20% of women improved in functioning over a six-year period (85). In the National Long-Term Care Survey, 18% of older adults with one or two ADL disabilities did not report disability two years later (65). The probability of recovery decreased, however, with increasing disability at baseline. In those with three or more ADL disabilities, less than 6% reported no ADL disability two years later. The likelihood of improvement also decreases with longer duration of disability (8).

DISEASE AND DISABILITY

Compared to the extensive research devoted to understanding the pathophysiology and risk factors for specific diseases, relatively little work has examined the risk factors for functional decrements in aging. Most disability in older adults is caused by chronic conditions, injuries, and disuse. A theoretical framework for the pathway from disease to disability, which includes intermediate steps such as impairment and functional limitation, has been proposed by the World Health Organization (98) and the Institute of Medicine (47). In recent years, a number of epidemiologic and clinical investigations have explored the relationship of disease and disability in the older population and increased our understanding of the impact of specific diseases and the effect of co-occurrence of multiple chronic conditions on disability. However, the intricacies of the pathway from disease to disability, the mechanisms whereby specific diseases cause disability, and the manner in which multiple diseases interact to cause disability all need further study.

In evaluating a patient presenting with a new stroke or hip fracture, the physician may clearly understand the cause of the patient's disability. However, changing the perspective and trying to understand why an individual presenting with disability who has multiple chronic conditions has reached his or her level of functioning is often not so simple. Going a step further and attempting to understand the diseases responsible for disability from a population perspective is a particular challenge. In addition to the difficulty in understanding the interaction of multiple co-occurring conditions, unraveling the pathway from disease to disability is difficult because disability may represent decline in several different aspects of functioning, each of which may be affected by a different disease (27). The pathway from disease to disability can be influenced by many nondisease factors such as depression and social support. In addition, disability itself may lead to further disability or to new chronic medical conditions, which can then cause more disability.

Population-based studies of older populations have been used to demonstrate both the cross-sectional and longitudinal association of specific chronic diseases with disability. This has been done for a nationally representative sample using the Longitudinal Study of Aging (5, 44, 67) and for major cohort studies such as the Framingham Heart Study (35, 49, 72), the Study of Osteoporotic Fractures (17), the Cardiovascular Health Study (19, 27), and the Alameda County Study (39, 85). A number of chronic conditions of aging have consistently been found to be strongly related to disability. These include heart disease (especially myocardial infarction, angina, and congestive heart failure), osteoarthritis (especially arthritis of the knees), hip fracture, diabetes, intermittent claudication, stroke, chronic obstructive pulmonary disease, visual impairment, hearing impairment, depression, and cognitive impairment.

Several studies have attempted to improve our understanding of the relative impact of specific diseases on population disability. In an important early study (24), Ford and colleagues estimated that arthritis was responsible for 34% of physical disability in the older population. Stroke, visual impairment, heart disease, and dementia taken together accounted for half of disability, with the final 15% accounted for by peripheral vascular disease, lung disease, depression, diabetes, hearing impairment, and hypertension. Kosorok and colleagues (57) estimated the number of days of restricted activity attributed to specific diseases and conditions using data from the National Health Interview Survey. This population of community-dwelling older adults reported an average of 31 restricted activity days per person per year. Of these, 18% were associated with falls, 14% with heart disease, 12% with arthritis, and smaller percentages with atherosclerosis, diabetes, malignancies, and osteoporosis.

Using data from over 5000 participants in the Cardiovascular Health Study, Ettinger and colleagues (19) described disabilities reported by this population and the diseases that participants stated were the causes of specific disabilities in up to 17 tasks. Arthritis was the most commonly reported cause of disability, followed by heart disease, injury, old age, lung disease, and stroke. Arthritis was reported to be the cause of difficulty in a wide range of specific tasks, in contrast to other conditions that appear to have a more specific relationship with certain disabilities. For example, heart disease was reported to be associated with difficulty in activities requiring endurance, and stroke with upper extremity and self-care tasks. The validity of self-report of the disease responsible for disability is not known at this time, but the kind of information attainable from such a study may be useful from a public health as well as clinical point of view. If we can ascertain in a valid manner the specific underlying causes of disability in older people who may have multiple conditions, much interesting new research may be done in this field. Studies of the natural history of disability would be enhanced by being able to take into account the primary diseases underlying an individual's disabilities, and our understanding of potentially modifiable risk factors that affect the progression of disability could be considerably refined by knowing how these factors affect specific disease-disability combinations.

Another valuable innovation in this area is the estimation of population attributable risk of disability. This approach is analogous to estimating population attributable risk of disease as a reflection of the impact of specific risk factors. The estimation of the population attributable risk of specific diseases for disability is related to both the strength of the association between those diseases and disability, and the prevalence of the specific diseases. Guccione and colleagues (35) used the Framingham Heart Study cohort to examine the relationship of physician-diagnosed medical conditions and seven functional activities related to IADLs and mobility. The disease-disability relationship was examined after adjusting for age, sex, and comorbidity. Stroke was associated with disability in all seven tasks; hip fracture and depression were associated with disability in five tasks; and other conditions, including knee osteoarthritis, heart disease, congestive heart failure, and chronic obstructive pulmonary disease, were each associated with disability in four tasks. Population attributable risks were presented separately for each of the seven tasks. For example, attributable risk of specific diseases for difficulty in walking a mile was as follows: knee osteoarthritis, 15%; depression, 10%; stroke, 9%; heart disease, 9%; intermittent claudication, 7%; hip fracture, 5%; chronic obstructive pulmonary disease, 5%; diabetes, 4%; and congestive heart failure, 2%.

Although from a public health perspective it would be desirable to understand the impact of specific diseases on *overall* disability status, there is evidence that a great deal of information can be lost in aggregating a variety of heterogenous measures of disability into a single disability outcome measure. Using a subset of the Framingham cohort that received knee radiographs, Guccione (34) showed only a modest association between osteoarthritis and a summary measure of functional status. As expected, stronger relationships were seen between osteoarthritis of the knee and specific tasks that included stair climbing, walking a mile, and housekeeping. This study also concluded that a generic classification of arthritis was less useful in identifying strong disease-disability relationships than a more refined definition that was limited to a specific joint and included classification information on both symptoms and radiographic grade. Similar types of specific relationships were also found in the study by Ettinger and colleagues (19).

The co-occurrence of multiple chronic conditions, or comorbidity, is common in the older population. In a nationally representative sample of persons who were asked about physician-diagnosed chronic conditions, nearly half of those aged 60 years and older reported two or more chronic conditions out of a list of the nine most commonly reported chronic conditions. In general, the prevalence of comorbidity for specific combinations of conditions was strongly related to the prevalence of each condition itself. For example, the two most commonly reported chronic conditions, high blood pressure and arthritis, co-occurred in 24% of this older population (41). Multiple impairments have also been found to co-occur in persons with disability. In community-dwelling disabled persons who received a clinical evaluation, over half had impairments in more than one physiological system, including cognitive, sensory, neurological, musculoskeletal, and cardiorespiratory (11).

The association of comorbidity with disability has been clearly demonstrated. Cross-sectional studies have demonstrated that with an increasing number of chronic diseases there is a stepwise increase in disability in ADLs (41), IADLs (25), and mobility (89). A prospective analysis of data from the EPESE study evaluated the impact of comorbidity in persons who, at the study baseline, reported being mobile, defined as the ability to walk 1/2 mile and climb stairs without help. Among these initially nondisabled individuals, those with two conditions were more than 1.5 times as likely to develop mobility disability compared to those with no chronic conditions, those with three conditions were 2.5 times more likely to become disabled, and those with four or more conditions were nearly 3 times as likely to become disabled during the four-year follow-up period (40). In a study that evaluated the impact of four specific chronic conditions (cerebrovascular disease, arthritis, coronary artery disease, and diabetes) on ADL and IADL disability and death, it was found that those with none of these conditions had a 3% chance of becoming disabled and a 4% chance of dying over the four-year follow-up period, compared to those with all four conditions, who had a 13% chance of becoming disabled and a 23% chance of dying (5).

Although the relationship between the number of chronic diseases and disability occurrence is quite striking, further progress in this field will require the study of specific combinations of diseases and their effect on disability. Arthritis has been studied in relation to other diseases in causing disability. In one study, arthritis was found to cause substantially greater risk of mobility difficulty when it was associated with other comorbid conditions than when it was found alone (90). More specific interactions between arthritis and other diseases were evaluated by Ettinger and colleagues using data from the National Health and Nutrition Epidemiologic Follow-up Study (18). In comparison with subjects with no knee osteoarthritis or heart disease, the relative risk for onset of difficulty with ambulation was over 4 for those with knee osteoarthritis alone, 2.3 for people with heart disease alone, but 13.6 for subjects with both knee osteoarthritis and heart disease. In contrast, the synergistic effect was not seen for the combination of knee osteoarthritis and hypertension. Those with hypertension alone had a relative risk of 1.3 compared to those without hypertension or osteoarthritis, and those with knee osteoarthritis plus hypertension had a relative risk of 2.5. From the standpoint of prevention of disability, targeting particular diseases that act synergistically with other diseases in causing disability could be very important in reducing overall population risk of disability.

In addition to disease status, a number of demographic characteristics and behavioral risk factors have also been found to be predictors of disability onset (5). Many of these factors are strongly related to disease status, but they have also been found to be independent predictors of disability onset after adjustment for the presence of specific diseases. For example, in the study from the EPESE populations discussed above (40), incident loss of mobility was 1.5 times as common in those in the lowest versus the highest income bracket, after adjustment for a long list of chronic conditions. Additionally, after adjusting for these chronic conditions and income, men were at a significantly increased risk of disability if they had less than a high school education, although this increased risk was not present in women.

Behavioral risk factors consistently associated with disability onset include smoking, lack of exercise, and excess weight. In the EPESE study on mobility loss, among persons who were not disabled at baseline those who currently smoked were at significantly increased risk of losing mobility over the four-year follow-up period, even after adjusting for the presence of chronic conditions (61). In men, former smokers were at no greater risk of mobility loss than nonsmokers, suggesting that smoking cessation may have benefits that go beyond disease prevention to the prevention of functional decline. Lack of exercise has been demonstrated to place individuals at increased risk of disability, whereas decreased risk has been shown in those who are physically active (61, 83). The risk of mobility loss in individuals who are overweight has been clearly demonstrated (61, 63). Furthermore, Launer and colleagues (63) demonstrated that change in weight status was a strong predictor of loss of mobility. Persons who had been in the highest tertile of body mass index (BMI) in the past who then lost weight were eight times as likely to develop disability compared to those with stable low BMI. This was a substantially greater risk than for those with high BMI who remained stable or gained weight. In those who were in the middle tertile of BMI in the past, significantly increased risks for disability were found for those who both gained weight and lost weight, but not for those who remained stable. Finally, in persons in the lowest tertile of past BMI, those who gained weight were not at increased risk, but those who lost weight were three times as likely to develop disability.

PHYSICAL PERFORMANCE MEASURES

A recent innovation in assessing functional status in older persons has been the development of physical performance measures. These are assessment instruments that objectively evaluate a specific aspect of physical functioning by having the individual perform a standardized task that is evaluated using objective, predetermined criteria (36). In many of these tasks the level of performance is evaluated by timing the task, whereas in others the evaluation is simply of the subject's ability to complete the task.

The assessment of disability in older persons has traditionally relied on self-report or proxy report, and the use of objective physical performance measures is appealing because it allows for direct, standardized assessment. This approach is analogous to assessment methods in other domains of functional status. For example, in the domains of cognitive functioning, hearing, and vision, comprehensive evaluation includes both self- or proxy report of functional difficulties and standardized testing to objectively document functional decrements, such as the use of a mental status questionnaire, visual acuity testing, and audiometry.

A growing body of research has demonstrated that physical performance measures add important information in the assessment of older persons. Performance measures identify functional problems that were not reported by the individual or family (16, 78). They have been demonstrated to be strong predictors of outcomes such as mortality (43, 75), falls (71, 76, 87), institutionalization (43, 75, 95), and other health services utilization (60, 95). Specific performance measures have been demonstrated to show improvement in response to interventions such as exercise (22) and cataract surgery (2), and to decline after hospitalization and with the onset of new health problems (82). Evidence has also been developed that performance measures can validly define a gradient of functioning even at the upper end of the functional spectrum (42, 43, 37, 82), and are therefore able to assess the full range of functional status better than self-report measures, which mainly identify the presence of overt disability.

Batteries of physical performance measures, which combine a group of related tasks, have been developed for a variety of purposes. An early performance battery, the Performance Activities of Daily Living, assesses 16 activities such as drinking from a cup, combing the hair, and turning a key in a lock. This battery was designed to assess moderately to severely disabled older persons (59). A more recent, comprehensive battery developed for very frail or nursing home patients assesses range of motion, strength, balance, and mobility (32). A battery of timed manual performance tasks has been extensively evaluated and utilized in comprehensive geriatric assessment settings (81, 95, 96). Lower extremity functioning was evaluated in the EPESE study in participants' homes, using a short battery that assessed balance and the times for participants to rise from a chair five times and walk eight feet (43). Lower extremity functioning is also the focus of the Physical Performance Mobility Examination, a comprehensive evaluation of transfer mobility and lower extremity function developed for use in hospitalized patients (97). Performance measures developed specifically to assess gait and balance (3, 88) have been extensively used. The Physical Performance Test (74) is a battery that assesses multiple categories of physical functioning, such as writing a sentence, simulated eating, putting on a jacket, walking 50 feet, and climbing stairs.

Methodologic work that has evaluated physical performance measures has shown them to have excellent reliability and validity. Test-retest and interobserver reliability, internal consistency reliability for summary scales, and a variety of assessments of validity, including predictive validity for important and relevant outcomes, have been demonstrated for many of these measures. Investigations continue into the use of these measures to evaluate change over time.

Despite the excellent psychometric properties of physical performance measures, a number of issues related to actual application remain to be resolved. Self-reported disability has stood the test of time as an important evaluation tool for the older population, both because of ease of administration and face validity, and it remains an open question as to the circumstances in which objective physical performance measures add useful information to a research study or clinical evaluation. Use of these measures certainly adds cost in terms of training of assessors, maintenance of quality control, and imposing of burden on participants.

A further issue to be clarified is the potential role of physical performance measures outside the research setting. Although these measures have already been employed in comprehensive geriatric assessment protocols and for evaluation of eligibility for support services and long-term care, formal studies have not yet demonstrated that physical performance measures provide useful additional information beyond that currently obtained by self-report. In the clinical setting, these measures may work well to establish the link between specific diseases and specific disabilities, whereas in persons with little or no disability, they may serve as indicators of early functional decline when used to screen patients over a period of time.

IDENTIFYING A PRECLINICAL STATE OF DISABILITY

It has been hypothesized that there is a "preclinical" state of functional loss, in which the individual perceives and reports no difficulties in traditional activities such as ADLs and IADLs, but has functional decrements that can be otherwise documented (29). In these cases, individuals may have impairments or physiological decrements that affect their functional level, but they can compensate in ways that maintain their ability to function in daily life. This compensation may include doing an activity less often or changing the method of performing it, and the individual may not report any difficulty when gradually making these kinds of changes over time. In the Women's Health and Aging Study, among women who reported no difficulty in walking up ten steps without resting, 37% said they did this task less often and 46% said they did it differently from how they did it in the past. As expected, nearly all individuals who reported difficulty in doing this task also said they did it less often or differently. Among those women reporting no difficulty with shopping for personal items, 22% said that they did it differently, compared to women who reported difficulty shopping, of whom over 80% reported that they did this task differently than they did in the past (38).

Performance measures of functioning have proven particularly useful in identifying a hierarchy of functioning in the nondisabled older population. Data from the MacArthur Study of Successful Aging demonstrated, in a population of high-functioning older adults, that performance measures were related to other measures of health status (42) and that lower performance at baseline was predictive of further decline in performance (82). Prospective data from the EPESE study also support the validity of performance measures in assessing functional status at the healthy end of the spectrum. In the total population, a gradient of risk for both mortality and nursing home admission was seen across the full spectrum of physical performance, including nondisabled individuals at the high end of the range of performance (43). In further analyses restricted to individuals who reported no disability in ADLs or items assessing mobility, it was demonstrated that performance, in terms of gait velocity, balance, and ability to rise from a chair, was highly predictive of the subsequent onset, one and four years later, of both ADL disability and disability in mobility (37). Nondisabled individuals who had lower scores on these performance tests were four to five times more likely to have disability four years later than those with the best scores. The performance measures therefore identify a subset of nondisabled individuals who may be thought of as having preclinical disability because they are at high risk of progressing to frank disability over the next several years. The ability to identify nondisabled persons who are at increased risk of disability may prove valuable in targeting preventive interventions to a group that is vulnerable but may have a great deal of capacity to respond to these interventions.

COMPRESSION OF MORBIDITY AND THE MEASUREMENT OF ACTIVE LIFE EXPECTANCY

An important public health issue is the relationship between length of life and the amount of time spent in the disabled state. Life expectancy has increased very substantially in this century. One consequence that has recently been recognized, however, is that escaping death during the early years from infectious diseases and other causes may mean that many more people survive to ages where they suffer from chronic diseases, which can lead to long-term disability and loss of independence. An important goal for the future is to increase longevity without increasing the number of years spent in the disabled or dependent state. Although the recent increase in longevity is well documented, it is not now clear whether these added years of life have been accompanied by years of health and vigor or of disease and disability. This question is of particular concern in the coming century, when continued life expectancy increases and unprecedented numbers of old and very old persons are projected. The theory of compression of morbidity predicts a future decrease in the number of years with severe disease and disability (30).

An important outcome measure that integrates disability onset with vital statistics data has been termed active life expectancy or disability-free life expectancy (54). Active life expectancy, which can be used to evaluate compression of morbidity, is defined as the average number of years an individual at a given age will survive and remain in the active, or nondisabled state. Most analyses of active life expectancy have employed the ADLs to define disability, with active life expectancy calculated using life table techniques that consider transitions from the active, nondisabled state to both death and disability. The original analysis of active life expectancy considered the transitions to both death and disability as irreversible (54). Since recent longitudinal studies have revealed that some disabled older persons make the transition back to the nondisabled state, alternate methods to calculate active life expectancy that incorporate these kinds of changes, using multistate life tables, have been developed (77).

The relationship over time between life expectancy and active life expectancy can be used to evaluate compression of morbidity. Three possible scenarios for population morbidity in women are illustrated schematically in Figure 2. The total length of the bars in this figure represents average life expectancy for women in 1990 and as projected by the Census Bureau for 2040. The length of the unshaded segments of the bars represents active or disability-free life expectancy, and the shaded areas of the bars represent average number of years in the disabled state. In scenario 1, the onset of disability has been postponed the same number of years as life expectancy has increased, and the number of years spent in the disabled state is unchanged

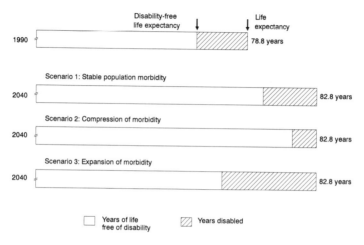

Figure 2   Scenarios for change in average burden of population disability level from 1990 to 2040. Compression of morbidity and alternatives.

from 1990. In scenario 2, there has been a compression of morbidity. Finally, in scenario 3, although disability-free life expectancy in 2040 has increased compared to 1990, it has not kept pace with increases in life expectancy and there is an expansion of population morbidity.

A vigorous debate over the prospects for a compression of morbidity began with a landmark paper by Fries in which he claimed that the compression of morbidity was inevitable in the coming years (30). He argued that in all species the maximum life span is fixed, that human beings are quickly approaching this limit, and that with a stable life expectancy any postponement of disability would result in a compression of morbidity. Although this logic is correct, others have pointed out that life expectancy is probably not going to reach its maximum level for at least the next half century, and we must consider that any of the alternate scenarios depicted in Figure 2 are possible in the face of increasing life expectancy.

PREVENTION OF DISABILITY IN THE OLDER POPULATION

With the rapid growth of the older population expected in the next century, the prevention or postponement of disability is of major public health importance. Prevention is appropriate at all three levels, primary, secondary, and tertiary. Ultimately, the best way to prevent disability from a disease is to prevent the disease itself. However, it is unrealistic to think that all major chronic conditions of aging will be completely prevented in the old and very old population. Tertiary prevention, the prevention of adverse outcomes of disease, is particularly relevant in those with longstanding chronic diseases and comorbidity. Interventions range from the use of medical care for existing diseases through a variety of other strategies, including behavioral changes such as exercise and technological interventions to help the individual compensate for existing impairments. Ongoing observational studies that shed new light on factors important in the pathway from disease to disability will help in the development of potential intervention strategies that can be evaluated in randomized controlled trials.

In addition to interventions that treat a single disease or the functional consequences of a single disease, a new approach uses broad-based interventions oriented to impairments or functional declines that may be the result of multiple diseases, disuse, or the aging process itself. These interventions are applied in areas such as muscular weakness, poor balance, and low exercise tolerance. For example, resistance training has been shown to significantly improve strength in very old, frail, nursing home residents (22) and in community-dwelling ambulatory older persons (50, 51). Exercise regimens and behavioral interventions have also been demonstrated to improve postural stability (86).

As described above, an observational study using performance measures in the EPESE population demonstrated that intermediate endpoints, including balance and gait speed, are highly predictive of onset of disability in initially nondisabled individuals (37). There is thus evidence that interventions can affect intermediate endpoints and these intermediate endpoints are associated with the subsequent onset of disability. What remains to be studied is whether the kinds of interventions that improve aspects of functioning such as gait, strength, and balance can ultimately prevent or delay the onset of disability and other more distal outcomes.

Some success has been demonstrated in community intervention projects in preventing disability and falls. These projects have used multiple interventions targeted to specific problems identified in a medical and functional screening assessment. In a study based in a health maintenance organization, a nurse performed a home-based screening to identify problems that could be targeted with interventions for improving inadequate exercise, excessive alcohol use, increased fall risk, high-risk medication use, and vision and hearing impairments (91). Those receiving one or more of these interventions had a lower incidence of decline in functional status than controls after one year, although this difference had disappeared by the end of the second year. However, interventions in this trial were neither ongoing nor long-term, and greater effects might be seen with more intensive interventions. Another intervention that studied men and women 70 years of age and older who had one or more risk factors for falls found that multiple interventions aimed at an individual's specific risk factors significantly reduced the rate of falls (86). These studies, in which multiple, potentially modifiable risk factors are assessed and targeted with specific interventions, may serve as models for future interventions.

As the size of the older population grows and life expectancy continues to increase, treatment and prevention strategies that address the functional consequences of disease and the burden of disability in a population living to older and older ages will become increasingly important. As demonstrated in this review, we are gaining increased appreciation for the methods that can lead to an understanding of the impact of disability in the population, risk factors along the pathway from disease to disability, and the consequences of disability. Ultimately, the goal of this effort must be to reduce the overall prevalence of disability in the population and increase the number of years in which older people lead highly functional, independent lives.

Literature Cited

1. Applegate WB, Blass JP, Williams TF. 1990. Instruments for the functional assessment of older patients. *N. Engl. J. Med.* 322:1207–14
2. Applegate WB, Miller ST, Elam JT, Freeman JM, Wood TO, et al. 1987. Impact of cataract surgery with lens implantation on vision and physical function in elderly patients. *JAMA* 257:1064–66
3. Berg KO, Wood-Dauphinee SL, Williams JI, Maki B. 1992. Measuring balance in the elderly: validation of an instrument. *Can. J. Public Health* Suppl. 2:S7–S11
4. Bergner M, Bobbitt RA, Pollard WE, Martin DP, Gilson BS. 1976. The Sickness Impact Profile: validation of a health status measure. *Med. Care* 14:57–67
5. Boult C, Kane RL, Louis TA, Boult L, McCaffrey D. 1994. Chronic conditions that lead to functional limitation in the elderly. *J. Gerontol. Med. Sci.* 49:M28–M36
6. Branch LG. 1980. Functional abilities of the elderly: An update on the Massachusetts Health Care Panel Study. In *Second Conference on the Epidemiology of Aging*, ed. SG Haynes, M Feinleib. NIH Publ. No. 80–969. Bethesda, MD: US DHHS
7. Branch LG, Jette AM. 1982. A prospective study of long-term care institutionalization among the aged. *Am. J. Public Health* 72:1373–79
8. Branch LG, Katz S, Kniepmann K, Papsidero JA. 1984. A prospective study of functional status among community elders. *Am. J. Public Health* 74:266–68
9. Branch LG, Meyers AR. 1987. Assessing physical function in the elderly. *Clin. Geriatr. Med.* 3:29–51
10. Branch LG, Wetle TT, Scherr PA, Cook NR, Evans DA, et al. 1988. A prospective study of incident comprehensive medical home care use among the elderly. *Am. J. Public Health* 78:255–59
11. Campbell AJ, Busby WJ, Roberston MC, Lum CL, Langlois JA, et al. 1994. Disease, impairment, disability and social handicap: a community based study people aged 70 years and over. *Disabil. Rehabil.* 16:72–79
12. Cornoni-Huntley J, Blazer DG, Brock DB, Farmer ME, eds. 1990. *Established Populations for Epidemiologic Studies of the Elderly*, Vol. 2. NIH Publ. No. 90–495. Washington, DC: PHS
13. Cornoni-Huntley J, Brock DB, Ostfeld A, Taylor JO, Wallace RB, eds. 1986. *Established Populations for Epidemio-*

logic Studies of the Elderly. Resource Data Book. NIH Publ. No. 86–2443

14. Corti MC, Guralnik JM, Salive ME, Sorkin JD. 1994. Serum albumin and physical disability as predictors of mortality in older persons. JAMA 272:1036–42

15. Donaldson LJ, Clayton DG, Clarke M. 1980. The elderly in residential care: mortality in relation to functional capacity. J. Epidemiol. Community Health 34:96–101

16. Elam JT, Graney MJ, Beaver T, El Derwi D, Applegate WB, et al. 1991. Comparison of subjective ratings of function with observed functional ability of frail older persons. Am. J. Public Health 81:1127–30

17. Ensrud KE, Nevitt MC, Yunis C, Cauley JA, Seeley DG, et al. 1994. Correlates of impaired function in older women. J. Am. Geriatr. Soc. 42:481–89

18. Ettinger WH, Davis MA, Neuhaus JM, Mallon KP. 1994. Long-term physical functioning in persons with knee osteoarthritis from NHANES I: Effects of comorbid medical conditions. J. Clin. Epidemiol. 47:809–15

19. Ettinger WH, Fried LP, Harris T, Shemanski L, Schulz R, Robbins J, for the CHS Collaborative Res. Group. 1994. Self-reported causes of physical disability in older people. The Cardiovascular Health Study. J. Am. Geriatr. Soc. 42: 1035–44

20. Feinleib MF, ed. 1991. Proc. 1988 Int. Symp. Data Aging. Natl. Cent. Health Stat. Vital Health Stat. Ser. 5, No. 6. DHHS Publ. No. (PHS) 91–1482

21. Feinleib S, Cunningham P, Short P. 1994. Use of nursing and personal care homes by the civilian population, 1987. Natl. Med. Exp. Surv. Res. Find. 23. (AHCPR)94–006. Rockville, MD: PHS

22. Fiatarone MA, O'Neill EF, Ryan ND, Clement KM, Solares GR, et al. 1994. Exercise training and nutritional supplementation for physical frailty in very elderly people. N. Engl. J. Med. 330: 1769–75

23. Foley DJ, Ostfeld AM, Branch LG, Wallace RB, McGloin J, et al. 1992. The risk of nursing home admission in three communities. J. Aging Health 4: 155–73

24. Ford AB, Folmar SJ, Salmon RB, Medalie JH, Roy AW, et al. 1988. Health and function in the old and very old. J. Am. Geriatr. Soc. 36:187–97

25. Fried LP. 1995. Health status and related care-seeking behavior of older women. In Commonwealth Fund Survey: Women's Health and Care-Seeking Behav-

iors, ed. KS Collins, M Falik. Baltimore, MD: Johns Hopkins Univ. Press. In press

26. Fried LP, Bush TL. 1988. Morbidity as a focus of preventive health care in the elderly. Epidemiol. Rev. 10:48–64

27. Fried LP, Ettinger WH, Hermanson B, Newman AB, Gardin J, for the Cardiovascular Health Study (CHS) Collaborative Res. Group. 1994. Physical disability in older adults: a physiologic approach. J. Clin. Epidemiol. 42:895–904

28. Deleted in proof

29. Fried LP, Herdman SJ, Kuhn K, Rubin G, Turano K. 1991. Preclinical disability: hypotheses about the bottom of the iceberg. J. Aging Health 3:285–300

30. Fries JF. 1980. Aging, natural death and the compression of morbidity. N. Engl. J. Med. 303:130–35

31. Fulton JP, Katz S, Jack SS, Hendershot GE. 1989. Physical functioning of the aged: United States, 1984. Natl. Cent. Health Stat. Vital Health Stat., Ser. 10, No. 167. DHHS Publ. No. (PHS)89–1595. Hyattsville, MD

32. Gerety MB, Mulrow CD, Tuley MR, Hazuda HP, Lichtenstein MJ, et al. 1993. Development and validation of a physical performance instrument for the functionally impaired elderly: The physical disability index (PDI). J. Gerontol. Med. Sci. 48:M33–M38

33. Greenberg JN, Ginn A. 1979. A multivariate analysis of the predictors of long-term care placement. Home Health Care Serv. Q. 1:75–99

34. Guccione AA, Felson DT, Anderson JJ. 1990. Defining arthritis and measuring functional status in elders: Methodological issues in the study of disease and physical disability. Am. J. Public Health 80:945–49

35. Guccione AA, Felson DT, Anderson JJ, Anthony JM, Zhang Y, et al. 1994. The effects of specific medical conditions on the functional limitations of elders in the Framingham Study. Am. J. Public Health 84:351–58

36. Guralnik JM, Branch LG, Cummings SR, Curb JD. 1989. Physical performance measures in aging research. J. Gerontol. 44:M141–46

37. Guralnik JM, Ferrucci L, Simonsick EM, Salive ME, Wallace RB. 1995. Lower extremity function in persons over the age of 70 years as a predictor of subsequent disability. N. Engl. J. Med. 332:556–61

38. Guralnik JM, Fried LP, Simonsick EM, Kasper J, Lafferty M, eds. 1995. The Women's Health and Aging Study:

Health and Social Characteristics of Older Women with Disability. Bethesda, MD: NIA. NIH Publ. No. 95–4009

39. Guralnik JM, Kaplan GA. 1989. Predictors of healthy aging: prospective evidence from the Alameda County study. *Am. J. Public Health* 79:703–8

40. Guralnik JM, LaCroix AZ, Abbott RD, Berkman LF, Satterfield S, et al. 1993. Maintaining mobility in late life. I. Demographic characteristics and chronic conditions. *Am. J. Epidemiol.* 137:845–57

41. Guralnik JM, LaCroix AZ, Everett DF, Kovar MG. 1989. *Aging in the eighties: the prevalence of co-morbidity and its association with disability.* Advance data from *Vital Health Stat.* No. 170. Hyattsville, MD: Natl. Cent. Health Stat.

42. Guralnik JM, Seeman TE, Tinetti ME, Nevitt MC, Berkman LF. 1994. Validation and use of performance measures of functioning in a non-disabled older population: MacArthur Studies of Successful Aging. *Aging, Clin. Exp. Res.* 6:410–19

43. Guralnik JM, Simonsick EM, Ferruci L, Glynn RJ, Berkman LF, et al. 1994. A short physical performance battery assessing lower extremity function: association with self-reported disability and prediction of mortality and nursing home admission. *J. Gerontol. Med. Sci.* 49:M85–M94

44. Harris T, Kovar MG, Suzman R, Kleinman JC, Feldman JJ. 1989. Longitudinal study of physical ability in the oldest-old. *Am. J. Public Health* 79: 698–702

45. Hing E, Bloom B. 1990. *Long-term care for the functionally dependent elderly.* Natl. Cent. Health Stat. Vital Health Stat. Ser. 13, No. 104

46. Hing E, Sekscenski E, Strahan G. 1989. *Summary for the United States. The National Nursing Home Survey 1985.* Vital Health Stat. Ser. 13, No. 97. DHHS Publ. (PHS) 89–1758

47. Inst. Med. 1991. Committee on a National Agenda for Prevention of Disabilities. *Disability in America: Toward a National Agenda for Prevention,* ed. M Pope, AR Taylor, pp. 76–108. Washington, DC: Natl. Acad. Press

48. Jette AM, Cleary PD. 1987. Functional disability assessment. *Phys. Ther.* 67: 1854–59

49. Jette AM, Pinsky JL, Branch LG, Wolf PA, Feinleib M. 1988. The Framingham Disability Study: Physical disability among community-dwelling survivors of stroke. *J. Clin. Epidemiol.* 41:719–26

50. Judge JO, Underwood M, Gennosa T. 1993. Exercise to improve gait velocity in older persons. *Arch. Phys. Med. Rehabil.* 74:400–6

51. Judge JO, Whipple RH, Wolfson LI. 1994. Effects of resistive and balance exercises on isokinetic strength in older persons. *J. Am. Geriatr. Soc.* 42:937–46

52. Kane RA, Kane RL. 1981. *Assessing the Elderly: A Practical Guide to Measurement.* Lexington, MA: Lexington Books

53. Karnofsky DA, Abelmann WH, Craver LF, Burchenal JH. 1948. The use of nitrogen mustards in the palliative treatment of carcinoma. *Cancer* 1:634–56

54. Katz S, Branch LG, Branson MH, Papsidero JA, Beck JC, et al. 1983. Active life expectancy. *N. Engl. J. Med.* 309: 1218–24

55. Katz S, Ford AB, Moskowitz RW, Jackson BA, Jaffe MW. 1963. Studies of illness in the aged. The index of ADL: A standardized measure of biological and psychosocial function. *JAMA* 185: 914–19

56. Kochanek KD, Hudson BL. 1995. Advance report of final mortality statistics, 1992. *Mon. Vital Stat. Rep.* Vol. 43, No. 6 (Suppl.)

57. Kosorok MR, Omenn GS, Diehr P, Koepsell TD, Patrick DL. 1992. Restricted activity days among older adults. *Am. J. Public Health* 82:1263–67

58. Koyano W, Shibata H, Haga H, Suyama Y. 1986. Prevalence and outcome of low ADL and incontinence among the elderly: five years follow-up in a Japanese urban community. *Arch. Gerontol. Geriatr.* 5:197–206

59. Kuriansky J, Gurland B. 1976. The performance test of activities of daily living. *Int. J. Aging Hum. Dev.* 7:343–52

60. Kuriansky JB, Gurland BJ, Fleiss JL. 1976. The assessment of self-care capacity in geriatric psychiatric patients by objective and subjective methods. *J. Clin. Psychol.* 32:95–102

61. LaCroix AZ, Guralnik JM, Berkman LF, Wallace RB, Satterfield S. 1993. Maintaining mobility in late life. II. Smoking, alcohol consumption, physical activity, and body mass index. *Am. J. Epidemiol.* 137:858–69

62. LaPlante MP. 1993. Prevalence of mobility and self-care disability—United States, 1990. *Morbid. Mortal Wkly. Rep.* 42:760–68

63. Launer LJ, Harris T, Rumpel C, Madans J. 1994. Body mass index, weight change, and risk of mobility disability in middle-aged and older women. *JAMA* 271:1093–98

64. Lawton MP, Brody EM. 1969. Assessment of older people: Self-maintaining and instrumental activities of daily living. *Gerontologist* 9:179–86
65. Manton KG. 1988. A longitudinal study of functional change and mortality in the United States. *J. Gerontol. Med. Sci.* 43:5153–61
66. Manton KG, Corder LS, Stallard E. 1993. Estimates of change in chronic disability and institutional incidence and prevalence rates in the U.S. elderly population from the 1982, 1984, and 1989 National Long Term Care Survey. *J. Gerontol. Soc. Sci.* 48:S153–66
67. Mor V, Murphy J, Masterson-Allen S, Willey C, Razmpour A, et al. 1989. Risk of functional decline among well elders. *J. Clin. Epidemiol.* 42:895–904
68. Mor V, Wilcox V, Rakowski W, Hiris J. 1994. Functional transitions among the elderly: Patterns, predictors and related hospital use. *Am. J. Public Health* 84:1274–80
69. Nagi SZ. 1976. An epidemiology of disability among adults in the United States. *Milbank Mem. Fund Q.* 6:493–508
70. Natl. Cent. Health Stat. 1992. *Vital statistics of the United States, 1989*, Vol. 2, Sect. 6, Life Tables. Washington, DC: PHS
71. Nevitt MC, Cummings SR, Kidd S, Black D. 1989. Risk factors for recurrent nonsyncopal falls: a prospective study. *JAMA* 261:2663–68
72. Pinsky JL, Leaverton PE, Stokes J III. 1987. Predictors of good function: The Framingham Study. *J. Chron. Dis.* 40 (Suppl. 1):S159–67
73. Reuben DB, Laliberte L, Hiris J, Mor V. 1990. A hierarchical exercise scale to measure function at the Advanced Activities of Daily Living level. *J. Am. Geriatr. Soc.* 38:855–61
74. Reuben DB, Siu AL. 1990. An objective measure of physical function of elderly patients. The physical performance test. *J. Am. Geriatr. Soc.* 38:1105–12
75. Reuben DB, Siu AL, Kimpau S. 1992. The predictive validity of self-report and performance-based measures of function and health. *J. Gerontol. Med. Sci.* 47:M106–10
76. Robbins AS, Rubenstein LZ, Josephson KR, Schulman BL, Osterweil D, et al. 1989. Predictors of falls among elderly people: results of two population-based studies. *Arch. Intern. Med.* 149:1628–33
77. Rogers A, Rogers RG, Belanger A. 1990. Longer life but worse health? Measurement and dynamics. *Gerontologist* 30:640–49
78. Sager MA, Dunham NC, Schwantes A, Mecum L, Halverson K, Harlowe D. 1992. Measurement of activities of daily living in hospitalized elderly: a comparison of self-report and performance-based methods. *J. Am. Geriatr. Soc.* 40:457–62
79. Salive ME, Collins KS, Foley DJ, George LK. 1993. Predictors of nursing home admission in a biracial population. *Am. J. Public Health* 83:1765–67
80. Schneider EL, Guralnik JM. 1990. The aging of America. Impact on health care costs. *JAMA* 263:2335–40
81. Scholer SG, Potter JF, Burke WJ. 1990. Does the Williams manual test predict service use among subjects undergoing geriatric assessment? *J. Am. Geriatr. Soc.* 38:767–72
82. Seeman TE, Charpentier PA, Berkman LF, Tinetti ME, Guralnik JM, et al. 1994. Predicting changes in physical performance in a high functioning cohort: MacArthur Studies of Successful Aging. *J. Gerontol. Med. Sci.* 49:M97–108
83. Simonsick E, Lafferty ME, Phillips CL, Mendes de Leon CF, Kasl SV, et al. 1993. Risk due to inactivity in physically capable older adults. *Am. J. Public Health* 83:1443–50
84. Soldo BJ, Manton KG. 1985. Health status and service needs of the oldest old: current patterns and future trends. *Milbank Q.* 63:286–323
85. Strawbridge WJ, Kaplan GA, Camacho T, Cohen RD. 1992. The dynamics of disability and functional change in an elderly cohort: results from the Alameda County Study. *J. Am. Geriatr. Soc.* 40:799–806
86. Tinetti ME, Baker DI, McAvay G, Claus EB, Garrett P, et al. 1994. A multifactorial intervention to reduce the risk of falling among elderly people living in the community. *N. Engl. J. Med.* 331:821–27
87. Tinetti ME, Speechley M, Ginter SF. 1990. Risk factors for falls among elderly persons living in the community. *N. Engl. J. Med.* 322:286–90
88. Tinetti ME, Williams TF, Mayewski R. 1986. Fall risk index for elderly patients based on number of chronic disabilities. *Am. J. Med.* 80:429–34
89. Verbrugge LM, Lepkowski JM, Imanaka Y. 1989. Comorbidity and its impact on disability. *Milbank Q.* 67:450–84
90. Verbrugge LM, Lepkowski JM, Konkol LL. 1991. Levels of disability among U.S. adults with arthritis. *J. Ger. Soc. Sci.* 46:S71–S83

91. Wagner EH, LaCroix AZ, Grothaus L, Leveille SG, Hecht JA, et al. 1994. Preventing disability and falls in older adults: A population-based randomized trial. *Am. J. Public Health* 84:1800–6

92. Wan TTH, Odell BG. 1981. Factors affecting the use of social and health services among the elderly. *Aging Soc.* 1:95–115

93. Warren MD, Knight R. 1982. Mortality in relation to the functional capacities of people with disabilities living at home. *J. Epidemiol. Community Health* 36:220–23

94. Wiener JM, Hanley RJ, Clark R, Van Nostrand JR. 1990. Measuring the activities of daily living: comparisons across national surveys. *J. Gerontol. Soc. Sci.* 45:S229–37

95. Williams ME. 1987. Identifying the older person likely to require long-term care services. *J. Am. Geriatr. Soc.* 35: 761–66

96. Williams ME, Hornberger JC. 1984. A quantitative method of identifying older persons at risk for increasing long term care services. *J. Chron. Dis.* 37:705–11

97. Winograd CH, Lemsky CM, Nevitt MC, Nordstrom TM, Stewart AL, et al. 1994. Development of a physical performance and mobility examination. *J. Am. Geriatr. Soc.* 42:743–49

98. WHO. 1980. *International Classification of Impairments, Disabilities and Handicaps.* Geneva: WHO

Annu. Rev. Public Health. 1996. 17:47–67

EPIDEMIOLOGY AND PREVENTION OF BREAST CANCER

Jennifer L. Kelsey and Leslie Bernstein

Department of Health Research and Policy, Stanford University, Stanford, California 94305; Department of Preventive Medicine, University of Southern California, Los Angeles, California 90033

KEY WORDS: breast cancer, epidemiology, prevention

ABSTRACT

Breast cancer is the most common cancer in women, accounting for 32% of all newly diagnosed cancers. Demographic characteristics associated with an increased risk include increasing age, birth in North America or northern Europe, high socioeconomic status, never having been married, and, for breast cancer diagnosed after 45 years of age, the white race. Early age at menarche, late age at menopause, late age at first full-term pregnancy, and low parity increase risk, while removal of the ovaries at an early age is protective. Obesity increases risk in postmenopausal women. Having a first degree relative with breast cancer confers an increased risk, especially if both a mother and a sister have had breast cancer at an early age. Mutations in the BRCA1 and BRCA2 genes are associated with an inherited susceptibility to breast cancer at an early age. Other markers of increased risk include atypical and hyperplastic epithelial cells in nipple aspirate fluid, nodular densities on mammogram, and biopsy-confirmed benign proliferative breast disease. Little can be done at present to reduce breast cancer risk through primary prevention, but secondary prevention by mammographic screening in women of age 50 and older reduces mortality from breast cancer.

MAGNITUDE OF PROBLEM AND DESCRIPTIVE EPIDEMIOLOGY

Breast cancer is the most common cancer in women in the United States, accounting for 32% of all newly diagnosed cancers (61). On the basis of current incidence rates, the American Cancer Society estimates that one of every eight women in the United States will develop breast cancer at some time during her life (15). As a cause of cancer deaths, breast cancer ranks second to lung cancer. In 1995, an estimated 182,000 new cases of breast cancer and 46,000

47

0163-7525/96/0510-0047$08.00

deaths from breast cancer occurred in the United States. Five-year survival rates over the period 1983–90 were 82% for white women and 66% for Black women. Age-adjusted mortality rates have been relatively constant for many years. Age-adjusted incidence rates increased gradually for several decades until 1980, then increased more steeply from 1980–1987, but have leveled off during 1987–1992 (30; Northern California Cancer Center, unpublished data). The extent to which the increase in incidence rates during most of the 1980s is attributable to early detection through mammography screening programs and to changes in diagnostic criteria is uncertain.

About 95% of breast cancers are adenocarcinomas. The vast majority of these are infiltrating duct carcinomas. In about 1% of breast cancer cases, simultaneous primary tumors in both breasts are noted. If routine biopsies of the opposite breast are taken at the time of mastectomy, however, about 12–15% of tumors are classified as simultaneous bilateral primary tumors (30).

For many years incidence rates have been highest in North America and northern Europe, intermediate in southern Europe and South America, and lowest in Asia and Africa. However, one of the most notable descriptive features of breast cancer epidemiology is the recent marked increases in incidence and mortality rates in several Asian and central European countries (30). In Japan, for instance, the incidence rates more than doubled during the period 1970–1985. Accordingly, although the differences in incidence rates between high-risk countries such as the United States and low-risk countries such as Japan are still present, the differences have decreased in recent years. The rapid increase in incidence rates in countries such as Japan indicates that environmental factors are important. Reasons for the international variation in incidence rates are uncertain, but possibilities include differences in body weight, some aspect of diet, endogenous hormone levels, and reproductive characteristics such as age at menarche, menstrual cycle length, parity, and lactation.

Studies of migrants to the United States also indicate that environmental factors are mainly responsible for the differences in incidence rates among countries. Generally, the incidence rates in migrants from low-risk countries and the second- and third-generation offspring of the migrants approach those of the United States, although the speed with which the incidence rates increase has varied from one study to another and from one ethnic group to another (30, 65).

Among women in high-risk areas, incidence rates increase with age, but the upward slope of the age-specific incidence curve becomes less after about 45–50 years of age. Areas in which incidence rates are lower show smaller or no increases in incidence rates after age 45–50. The shapes of the age-specific incidence curves are becoming more similar as breast cancer rates increase in the low- and intermediate-risk countries. The change in the slope of breast cancer incidence rates around age 45–50 is consistent with the involvement of reproductive hormones in the etiology of breast cancer. Only organ systems directly controlled by female hormones show this change in incidence rates around the time of menopause (47).

Within the United States, overall incidence rates are highest among white women, followed by Black, Hispanic, and Asian American women (21). However, below age 40–45 years, Blacks have the highest rates. Incidence rates in Black, Hispanic, and Asian women have continued to increase, even as the rates in whites appear to have leveled off (Northern California Cancer Center, unpublished data). Women of high socioeconomic class have about twice the risk for breast cancer as women of low socioeconomic status. Other groups at higher-than-average risk include women who have never married, residents of urban areas, Jewish women, and residents of the northern (as compared with southern) United States (30).

ESTABLISHED AND POSSIBLE ETIOLOGIC FACTORS

Reproductive Characteristics

It has been recognized for many years that a woman's reproductive characteristics affect her risk for breast cancer (see Tables 1 and 2 in section on Primary Prevention). Modest elevations in risk are associated with early age at menarche, late age at menopause, and late age at first full-term pregnancy. For breast cancer diagnosed after 40 years of age, nulliparity and a small number of full-term pregnancies are also associated with small increases in risk. The immediate effect of a full-term pregnancy, however, appears to be to increase risk. Oophorectomy before menopause reduces the risk of breast cancer. Some recent studies suggest that late age at any full-term pregnancy, regardless of whether it is the first, is associated with an increased risk. Although the evidence is not entirely consistent, studies suggest that long-term breast-feeding, especially if it occurs at a young age, is protective (43). Also, most studies (29) find that a small number of days between menstrual periods is associated with an increased risk, although one recent study (60) found that both small and large numbers of days between cycles elevate risk. Still less certain are the etiologic roles of spacing of births, spontaneous and induced abortion (12, 52), characteristics of the menstrual cycle other than number of days between cycles, infertility, and multiple births at the last birth (29).

Weight and Height

Heavy body weight increases the risk for breast cancer in postmenopausal women (25). Most studies report relative risks of 2.0 or less for the heaviest group compared with the lightest group. In contrast, heavy body weight appears to be associated with a slightly decreased risk in premenopausal women, with relative risk estimates of about 0.7–0.9 (59). The increased risk in heavy postmenopausal women is probably attributable to the higher levels of circulating estrogen in heavy postmenopausal women, since the main source of endogenous estrogen after menopause is the conversion of the androgen precursor androstenedione to estrone in adipose tissue. In several studies, tallness has been associated with a modest elevation in risk, particularly in postmenopausal women. One hypothesis is that high caloric intake during childhood and adolescence is associated with both tallness and increased breast cancer risk (25).

Endogenous Hormones

There is evidence that the reproductive and weight characteristics described above are associated with breast cancer risk because they represent measures of the cumulative exposure of the breast to estrogen and, perhaps, progesterone. Exogenous estrone, estradiol, and, under some conditions, estriol increase the incidence of mammary tumors in mice and rats, increase tumor yield, and decrease the time to induction following administration of a carcinogen. Removing the ovaries or administering an antiestrogenic drug has the opposite effect (13).

Three interrelated hypotheses regarding the relationship of estrogens to breast cancer in women have been most often proposed. These hypotheses are that risk is related to (a) total estrogen exposure, (b) exposure to bioavailable or free estrogen, and (c) exposure to the combination of estrogen and progesterone. All three hypotheses are based on the concept that cell division plays a critical role in the pathogenesis of human breast cancer; that is, any factor (such as some component of these ovarian hormones) that increases mitotic activity in breast epithelium will increase risk (51). Studies of epithelial cell division rates show that proliferation rates are lower during the follicular phase of the menstrual cycle when estradiol and progesterone levels are low than during the luteal phase when they are high (47).

Several recent carefully designed case-control studies, and studies comparing women at high and at low risk of breast cancer, provide evidence that differences in estrogen profiles may account for differences in breast cancer risk (4). The results are least clear for studies of premenopausal breast cancer cases and controls. These studies are complicated by the practical necessity of using only one or a few samples to represent the overall hormonal milieu in the face of extreme cyclic hormonal variation occurring during the menstrual cycle. Among postmenopausal cases and controls, study results are more consistent in showing higher estrogen levels among breast cancer cases than among controls. The higher breast cancer risk associated with an early age at menarche is probably not only a function of more years of ovarian activity, but also represents greater cumulative exposure to estrogen and progesterone through more regular ovulatory menstrual cycles during adolescence and possibly through higher estradiol exposure in early adulthood (4). Furthermore, estrogen as well as prolactin levels appear to be permanently altered after a full-term pregnancy. Studies comparing Asian women to Caucasian women consistently show that estrogen levels are substantially lower among Asians, both during the premenopausal years and postmenopausally. As noted in the section above, postmenopausal obesity may increase breast cancer risk because estrone production is increased through the aromatization of androstenedione by enzymes in fat cells. Heavier women also have higher levels of bioavailable estrogens because of a reduction in binding protein.

The available evidence regarding case-control differences in endogenous progesterone levels is confusing and inconsistent. Studies of differences in progesterone levels of premenopausal breast cancer cases and controls have in general not reported whether women in both groups were measured during an ovulatory cycle. Furthermore, it is impossible in practice in epidemiologic studies to make sure that progesterone measurement occurs on the day of progesterone peak within a menstrual cycle. Thus, the role of progesterone is uncertain.

Exogenous Hormones

Evidence is quite consistent that long-term use of oral contraceptives increases the risk for breast cancer diagnosed before age 35 and possibly up to age 45, ages at which breast cancer is relatively uncommon. The relative risk appears to be less than 2.0 (38). To date, the risk for breast cancer diagnosed after age 45 does not appear to be affected by oral contraceptive use, but this situation needs to be closely monitored as substantial numbers of women with a history of long-term use enter this age group. Progestin-only oral contraceptives and the long-acting injectable progestogen contraceptive, depot-medroxyprogesterone acetate (DMPA), do not appear to affect breast cancer risk (56).

Most studies that have included sufficiently large numbers of long-term users of estrogen replacement therapy indicate a modest (less than twofold) increase in risk among women who have used the estrogen for 15 years or more (9). Short-term use does not appear to affect risk. Data are just beginning to become available on whether replacement therapy with both estrogen and progestin affects risk. To date no firm conclusions can be reached.

Use of diethylstilbestrol (DES) by pregnant women in the late 1940s to the 1960s to reduce risk of fetal loss has been found in most studies to be associated with relative risk for breast cancer of about 1.5 relative to unexposed women (37).

Family History and Genetics

A family history of breast cancer confers a somewhat increased risk. The risk is particularly high if both the mother and sister have been affected at a young age (11). A mutation in the BRCA1 gene on the long arm of chromosome 17 is associated with an inherited susceptibility to breast cancer in some families with early onset disease (17). BRCA1 mutations appear to account for cancer in most families with both early onset breast and ovarian cancers. Other breast cancer susceptibility genes are being sought, and one, BRCA2, has been localized to the long arm of chromosome 13 (63). A few cases probably also arise from mutations in the p53 gene on the short arm of chromosome 17, and heterozygosity for the ataxia telangiectasis (AT) gene on the long arm of chromosome 11 may also be associated with an increased risk. It is likely that less than 10% of all breast cancer in Western countries is attributable to genetic predisposition (39), but, at younger ages, this percentage is much higher. It has been estimated that about 25% of breast cancers diagnosed before age 40 years are attributable to BRCA1 mutations (24).

Research is being undertaken to try to identify the products of BRCA1 mutations that contribute to the development of breast cancer. This research may lead to a better understanding of the pathogenesis of nonhereditary forms of breast cancer as well. The ability to identify breast cancer susceptibility genes raises significant questions about what advice should be given to women with these genes (33). Options for these women include increased surveillance through frequent mammography and physical examination, use of the thera- peutic agent tamoxifen as a prophylactic agent (see discussion below), pro- phylactic mastectomy, and prophylactic oophorectomy. Oophorectomy has the additional important advantage of affording protection against ovarian cancer for women with BRCA1 mutations. None of these is a proven preventive strategy, and women known to be at high risk because of genetic attributes should be thoroughly informed of the various choices. Research is needed to delineate more clearly what options may be best for specific subgroups of women.

Diet

The role of diet in the etiology of breast cancer is controversial. For many years it has been hypothesized, largely on the basis of international variation in incidence rates and animal experiments, that a diet high in fat increases the risk for breast cancer. Although results have been somewhat conflicting, most cohort studies do not indicate that a high-fat diet in adulthood increases the risk for breast cancer. However, the possibility remains that a high-fat diet in childhood and adolescence could affect risk. It has also been suggested (25) that low total energy intake during growth and adolescence may reduce risk, but to date evidence is only circumstantial. Some studies suggest that vitamin A and other antioxidant vitamins slightly decrease risk, but data on this issue are at present sparse. Finally, it has been suggested that consumption of phytoestrogens (estrogens in plants) from such foods as soybean products reduces risk. Phytoestrogens are weakly estrogenic and could compete with stronger human endogenous estrogens at binding sites and thereby reduce the possibly carcinogenic effects of these stronger estrogens. They may affect the uptake and metabolism of sex hormones by contributing to the regulation of sex hormone binding globulin (1), and also appear to have antioxidant properties (40). Research on the effects of phytoestrogen consumption is currently being undertaken by several groups.

Alcohol Consumption

Alcohol consumption has been associated with an increased risk of breast cancer in most studies of this relationship. A meta-analysis of 38 epidemiologic studies concluded that a modest, linear, statistically significant dose-response relationship exists (35). In relation to nondrinkers, the breast cancer risks of women consuming one, two, and three alcoholic drinks daily were increased 11, 24, and 38%, respectively. No particular type of alcoholic beverage was more predictive of increased risk than any other. However, a combined analysis of six breast cancer case-control studies that controlled for dietary factors did not support a linear relationship between daily consumption of alcohol and breast cancer risk. A positive effect was observed for three or more drinks daily, but daily consumption of fewer drinks did not increase risk (23). Some, but not all, studies suggest that intake prior to age 30 years is more predictive of breast cancer risk than consumption at later ages (35). No completely satisfactory biologic explanation of the alcohol-breast cancer relationship has been identified, although several possible mechanisms have been proposed (53). The most plausible of these is a possible mediating effect of reproductive steroid hormones. Other possible mechanisms include direct cytotoxic effects of alcohol and alterations in breast cell proliferation rates, cell membrane integrity, liver microsomal enzymes, DNA repair, and immunologic surveillance. Although a causal relationship is possible, confounding cannot be ruled out as an explanation for the association. Many questions regarding the alcohol-breast cancer relationship remain.

Cigarette Smoking

Most evidence indicates that cigarette smoking does not affect breast cancer risk, although the possibility that women who begin smoking at a young age have an increased risk has not been ruled out (45). One study (2) has reported an increased risk for breast cancer among cigarette smokers who are genetically predisposed to be slow acetylators of aromatic amines, which are present in cigarette smoke. This association needs to be examined in other studies.

Radiation

Exposure of the chest of women below the age of 40 years to ionizing radiation in moderate to high doses is known to increase risk for breast cancer. The higher the dose, the greater the risk. Estimates of relative risk have ranged from 1.4 to 2.2 and of excess risk from 5.5 to 10.7 cases per 10,000 woman-years per Gray (27). A variety of sources of radiation have been implicated, including the atomic bomb explosions in Japan in 1945, and repeated exposure in the course of medical treatment for such conditions as tuberculosis, post-partum mastitis, benign breast conditions, Hodgkin's disease, ankylosing spondylitis, scoliosis, tinea capitis, enlarged thymus, skin hemangioma, and childhood cancer. The effect of very low doses such as might occur during certain diagnostic procedures or occupational exposures, however, is uncertain.

Other Environmental Exposures

Among other environmental exposures, considerable interest has recently been focused on the possible effects of exposure to electromagnetic fields and light at night on breast cancer risk. The proposed mechanism (57) is that exposure to 60-Hz electric fields or light at night reduces production of melatonin in the pineal gland; melatonin suppresses the production of estrogen and prolactin. Reduced melatonin production could result in higher levels of estrogen and prolactin, thus bringing about greater turnover of breast epithelial cells. This greater rate of turnover could make the cells more susceptible to the effects of carcinogens. Epidemiologic data on this issue are limited, but so far provide little evidence of an increased risk in females from residential exposure to electromagnetic fields. The few studies relating breast cancer risk in males to occupational exposure to electromagnetic fields, however, are suggestive of a positive association (18). Several studies in women are currently under way to examine this issue further.

It has been hypothesized (19) that exposure to solar radiation, which brings about vitamin D synthesis in the skin, could protect against breast cancer. The increased vitamin D synthesis could result in increased levels of vitamin D metabolites in the body, which in turn might protect against breast cancer. In the United States, breast cancer rates are lower in the south than the north, an observation consistent with this hypothesis. However, at present few other data are available to support or refute this hypothesis.

It has been speculated (14) that certain chemicals in the environment mimic the action of estrogen or alter the activity of estrogen such that the production of 16-alpha-hydroxyestrone, which may enhance breast cell proliferation and perhaps damage DNA, is increased. One study (62) reported a positive association between organochlorine pesticides and breast cancer risk, but a second study by some of the same investigators (34) provided little support for this finding. Additional epidemiologic studies of this relationship are currently being undertaken.

In Utero Exposures

Another hypothesis that needs further study is that in utero exposures, such as to high levels of maternal estrogens during pregnancy, increase breast cancer risk in daughters (58). Possible positive associations between maternal and paternal ages and breast cancer risk and a report of a negative association of breast cancer risk with preeclampsia during pregnancy provide some support for the relevance of in utero exposures (18).

Physical Activity

Few studies have assessed the effects of physical activity on breast cancer risk. Nearly all that have evaluated this relationship have used surrogate measures of activity levels, such as occupation or participation in college sports (6, 16). Despite the indirect measurement of activity, most of these studies have shown a decreased risk of breast cancer among women who were more active. One case-control study of women 40 years of age or younger collected lifetime histories of exercise activities, and showed a marked reduction in breast cancer risk with increasing number of hours of exercise per week during the women's reproductive years (3). In another case-control study whose participants were primarily postmenopausal women, daily strenuous physical activity during adolescence and early adulthood was associated with a reduced breast cancer risk (41). A protective effect of physical activity is biologically plausible because of its potential influence on menstrual cycle patterns and ovulatory frequency (6). Because exercise offers a feasible opportunity for breast cancer risk reduction, more research is needed to evaluate the relationship and to establish the mechanisms by which the possible protection might occur.

Benign Breast Diseases

For many years it has been known that women with benign breast disease confirmed by biopsy are at a somewhat elevated risk for subsequent breast cancer. It is now known that certain subtypes of benign breast disease are mainly responsible for the overall elevated risk (7). Relative risks of 3–5 are associated with benign proliferative disease with atypical hyperplasia, and relative risks of around 2 for proliferative disease without atypia. Little or no elevation in risk is seen in the absence of proliferative disease, although some studies suggest that sclerosing adenosis and gross cystic disease increase risk.

Women with ductal carcinoma in situ and lobular carcinoma in situ are at very high risk. Invasive breast cancer tends to develop near the site of the previous ductal carcinoma in situ, whereas invasive disease following lobular carcinoma in situ is about as likely to develop in the contralateral breast as in the breast where the lobular carcinoma in situ was diagnosed.

Nipple Aspirates

Fluid aspirated from nipples can also provide information about breast cancer risk (46). About 30–50% of women in the age range 30–55 years produce fluid upon aspiration from nipples. Relative to women from whom no breast fluid can be obtained, women with atypical epithelial cells in their fluid have about five times the risk of subsequent breast cancer. Women with hyperplasia but no atypia have a relative risk of about 2.5 compared to women from whom no fluid can be obtained. Nipple aspirates containing cholesterol epoxides, which are established mutagens and carcinogens in animals, have been found to be associated with histologically diagnosed hyperplasia and especially atypical hyperplasia (64). Further studies of constituents of nipple aspirate fluid in relation to breast cancer risk are warranted.

Mammographic Parenchymal Patterns

The usefulness of mammography to screen for early breast cancer will be discussed below. Certain attributes seen on mammogram are also useful as markers of future breast cancer risk. Women with breasts in which the parenchyma seen on the mammogram contains a relatively large amount of diffuse or nodular densities are at elevated risk for breast cancer, and so, to a lesser extent, are women with prominent ducts seen on mammogram. Women in whom more than 75% of the breast volume is occupied by mammographic densities have a risk 3–4 times that of women whose parenchyma is composed mostly of fat (44). Whether densities are classified by radiologists or by a computer-assisted method, increasing mammographic density is associated with an increased risk for breast cancer (8).

Multiple Primary Cancers Involving the Breast

About 5% of women who have cancer in one breast will develop it in the other breast. Breast cancer cases also appear to be at slightly increased risk for cancers of the endometrium, ovary, colon, thyroid, and salivary glands, and for malignant melanoma. Conversely, women with tumors at these sites appear to be at increased risk for breast cancer (22). Shared hormonal, dietary, or genetic risk factors may explain some of these associations, while increased medical surveillance and the effect of cancer treatment may contribute to others.

PRIMARY PREVENTION

Table 1 shows the established risk factors for breast cancer that were discussed above. Most of these risk factors are associated with only moderate elevations in risk, and few can be easily modified either by environmental or behavior changes. Postmenopausal obesity is probably the only established risk factor that could be affected by behavior modification, but a decrease in the amount of postmenopausal obesity would have only a small effect on breast cancer incidence. If some of the probable (Table 2) and possible risk factors, such as alcohol, hormone replacement therapy, certain dietary constituents, and pesticide exposure are found in fact to be involved in the causation of breast cancer, and if physical activity is established as protective, then the prospects for primary prevention would be enhanced, although other risks and benefits of some of these agents (e.g. hormone replacement therapy), and the difficulty of modifying life-style characteristics (e.g. physical activity patterns and diet) somewhat dampen optimism about population-wide reductions in breast cancer incidence.

Despite these uncertainties, two large randomized trials concerned with the prevention of breast cancer have been started in the United States, as well as a small pilot study in Los Angeles, California.

The Women's Health Initiative

The overall goal of the Women's Health Initiative is to test strategies to reduce the risk for cardiovascular disease, breast cancer, colorectal cancer, and osteoporotic fractures. It is the largest research study ever funded by the National Institutes of Health, and it is intended to include a randomized trial, an observational study, and a community prevention study. The randomized trial is by far the most expensive component of the Women's Health Initiative, and it has received the most attention to date. It is to include 63,000 women in at least one of its three branches that test hypotheses regarding (a) dietary modification, (b) hormone replacement, and (c) calcium/vitamin D. Its large sample size is driven primarily by the intent to test the hypothesis that dietary modification can reduce the incidence of breast cancer.

In the dietary modification branch of the trial, 48,000 women are to be enrolled by 45 clinical centers, with 40% in the intervention group, and 60% in the control group. The goal for the women in the intervention group is to attain a low fat dietary pattern consisting of (a) total fat no more than 20% of daily calories, (b) saturated fat less than 7% of daily calories, (c) at least five daily servings of fruits and vegetables, and (d) at least six daily servings of grain products. Both control and intervention groups are being provided with a standard packet of health promotion materials, including information on a

Table 1 Established risk factors for breast cancer in women

Factor	High-risk group	Low-risk group
Relative risk greater than 4.0		
Age	Old	Young
Country of birth	North America, Northern Europe	Asia, Africa
Mother *and* sister with history of breast cancer, especially if diagnosed at an early age	Yes	No
Atypical epithelial cells in niple aspirate fluid	Yes	No fluid produced
Mutations in BRCA1 or BRCA2, breast cancer at early age	Yes	No
Relative risk of 2.1–4.0		
Nodular densities on mammogram	Densities occupy- ing >75% of breast volume	Parenchyma composed entirely of fat
History of cancer in one breast	Yes	No
Mother *or* sister with history of breast cancer	Yes	No
Biopsy-confirmed benign proliferative breast disease	Yes	No
Hyperplastic epithelial cells without atypia in nipple aspirate fluid	Yes	No fluid produced
Radiation to chest in moderate to high doses	Yes	No
Relative risk of 1.1–2.0		
Socioeconomic status	High	Low
Marital status	Never married	Ever married
Place of residence	Urban	Rural
Place of residence (within United States)	Northern	Southern
Race/ethnicity, breast cancer ≥45 years of age	White	Hispanic, Asian
Race/ethnicity, breast cancer <40 years of age	Black	Hispanic, Asian
Religion	Jewish	Seventh Day Adventist, Mormon
Removal of ovaries before age 40	No	Yes
Parity, breast cancer ≥40 years of age	Nulliparous	≥4
Parity, breast cancer <40 years of age	Parous	Nulliparous
Age at first full-term pregnancy	≥30	<20
Age at menarche	≤11	≥15
Age at menopause	≥55	<45
History of primary cancer in endometrium, ovary	Yes	No
Weight, breast cancer ≥50 years of age	Obese	Thin

Table 2 Risk factors for breast cancer in women found in many studies, but for which some uncertainty exists[a]

Factor	High-risk group	Low-risk group
Time between menstrual periods	≤21 days	≥30 days
Breast-feeding, breast cancer <50 years of age	None	≥10 years
Age at any full-term pregnancy	≥30	<20
Long-term use of oral contraceptives, breast cancer <35–45 years of age	Yes	No
Long-term use of estrogen replacement therapy	Yes	No
Diethylstilbestrol use during pregnancy	Yes	No
Weight; breast cancer <50 years of age	Thin	Obese
Height	Tall	Short
Alcohol consumption	Yes	No
Physical activity level	Inactive	Active

aAll relative risks appear to be less than 2.0, with the possible exception of time between menstrual periods.

healthy diet. Various additional techniques are being used to try to persuade the intervention group to reach and maintain a low fat dietary pattern, including group meetings with a nutritionist and self-monitoring tools. The average intervention period is anticipated to be nine years. Although breast cancer is also an endpoint of interest to the hormone replacement therapy branch of the trial, it is an increased risk for breast cancer that is of concern in that branch, not a reduction in risk. In this branch women are being randomized to receive either a placebo or estrogen plus a continuous low-dose progestin.

Although this level of national interest in the prevention of breast cancer is clearly warranted in view of the magnitude of the problem, serious reservations have been expressed as to whether this large trial should be carried out at this time (26). First, as discussed above, there is at most only weak evidence that a diet high in fat increases the risk for breast cancer, or that a diet high in fruits and vegetables decreases breast cancer risk. Furthermore, should there be any effect, it is likely to be small. Therefore, it does not seem worth investing such an enormous amount of resources in a study that has such a low probability of yielding any dividends. Second, in the unlikely event that a change in risk is seen, it will not be possible to attribute it to any one specific dietary constituent, such as fat, fruits and vegetables, or fibers. Third, a continued trend towards decreasing fat content in the US diet will make it difficult to detect differences between the low fat dietary pattern and control groups. Fourth, optimistic assumptions were made about recruitment, retention, and adherence, especially for the many older women and minority women who are to be in the trial. Finally, despite the high cost of the study, it is the opinion of most people experienced with large prevention trials that the Women's Health Initiative is severely underfunded for what it proposes to accomplish.

In fact, many of the clinical centers are having difficulty recruiting the proposed number of women with the limited resources available.

Thus, it seems unlikely that the dietary modification branch of the Women's Health Initiative will be able to provide much information about the prevention of breast cancer. If the hormone replacement therapy branch is able to recruit enough women and to continue for a long enough period of time, it is possible that information would be obtained as to whether use of conjugated estrogen combined with low-dose progestin increases the risk for breast cancer. However, whether the number of women recruited and the trial duration will be sufficient is not clear at this time. It is also uncertain that the hormone regimen being used in this trial will be the regimen of choice a few years from now.

The Breast Cancer Prevention Trial

Tamoxifen, a synthetic, nonsteroidal antiestrogen to breast tissue, has proved effective in the treatment of breast cancer. Tamoxifen apparently blocks estrogen receptors at the level of the tumor by competitively inhibiting estradiol binding; it has been labeled as an "antiestrogen" on this basis (28). It also may act as an antitumor agent on the hypothalamic-pituitary axis, where it affects the release of growth hormone, thereby reducing the amount of circulating insulin-like growth factor, which stimulates growth of breast tissue (50). Thus, tamoxifen appears to provide a model of direct and indirect endocrine control of estrogen-regulated breast tumor growth. Because it reduces the incidence of contralateral breast tumors and delays breast cancer recurrence, tamoxifen has been considered as a potential chemopreventive agent to reduce the risk of developing breast cancer in "high risk" apparently healthy women.

The Breast Cancer Prevention Trial, a randomized controlled clinical trial to test the efficacy of tamoxifen as a breast cancer chemopreventive agent, was begun in April 1992 in 270 centers in the United States and Canada. Eligible women are those who are at least 35 years of age and whose risk of breast cancer is at least that of an average 60-year old woman. A secondary aim of the trial is to determine whether tamoxifen reduces the risk of cardiovascular disease. The trial investigators will recruit 16,000 eligible women as participants, randomizing half to receive tamoxifen on a daily basis for at least five years and half to receive a placebo. Although accrual of participants was to have been completed during the first two years, recruitment has been slower than expected, and accrual was halted briefly during 1994.

A number of concerns have been expressed with regard to the conduct of the Breast Cancer Prevention Trial (5, 10, 36). One major issue is whether large numbers of healthy women should be treated with a potentially toxic drug for the primary prevention of a rare event. As designed, 645 women would be treated annually in the trial to prevent one case of breast cancer.

Tamoxifen is associated with an increased risk of endometrial cancer and pulmonary embolism in cancer patients, and may increase the risk of retinopathy and other ocular conditions. Breast cancer patients taking tamoxifen are also more likely to experience vasomotor symptoms such as hot flashes that are serious enough to raise the question of whether apparently healthy women would comply with the required daily regimen over a five-year period. The risk-benefit equation for tamoxifen use by healthy women to be employed in assessing the results of the trial has also been questioned because it equates events that have different implications for health and ignores certain outcomes. The appropriateness of including premenopausal women is another major issue of contention, since available evidence suggests that its effects may to some extent differ in premenopausal and postmenopausal women. An argument in favor of proceeding with the trail is the concern that physicians may prescribe tamoxifen to women to prevent breast cancer because of its efficacy in the treatment of breast cancer and that this will become a standard practice without a clinical trial to establish whether tamoxifen is actually beneficial in healthy women.

Possible Prevention Through Use of Luteinizing-Hormone-Releasing Hormone Agonists

As discussed above, oral contraceptives appear to increase modestly the risk of breast cancer among young premenopausal women, but they also substantially reduce the risk of ovarian and endometrial cancer (31). Luteinizing-hormone-releasing hormone (LHRH) agonists can be used as a contraceptive regimen, as they inhibit ovulation and eliminate ovarian estrogen and progesterone production. Pike and colleagues (49) have proposed using LHRH agonists as a contraceptive agent. Their regimen would retain the beneficial effects of oral contraceptives on the ovary and uterus, yet exploit the fact that LHRH agonists inhibit ovulation without replacing estrogen and progesterone, thereby lowering breast cancer risk. The rationale behind this proposal is that LHRH agonists induce a reversible "bilateral oophorectomy" that serves to reduce a woman's breast-tissue aging rate (48) at a time when breast cancer risk increases most dramatically. It is predicted that such a regimen taken for 5 years during the premenopausal years would lead to a reduction in breast cancer risk of 38% and that such a regimen taken for 15 years might reduce risk by as much as 80% (49).

The proposed regimen was found to be associated with adverse side effects, primarily those related to a hypoestrogenic state and elimination of ovarian function (54). Of particular concern were hot flashes, bone loss, and probably a significant increased risk for cardiovascular disease, attributable at least in part to an increase in low-density lipoprotein cholesterol. Therefore, the regimen was modified. Estrogen replacement therapy was added at a dose low enough to retain the major beneficial component of this regimen on breast cancer risk, yet sufficient to eliminate hot flashes and produce a beneficial lipid profile. Periodic progestogen was added to the regimen to avoid any increased risk for endometrial hyperplasia or carcinoma associated with low-dose estrogen replacement therapy. A small amount of testosterone to replace that normally produced by the ovary, in conjunction with the estrogen, was added to reduce the risk of bone loss.

The original and then the modified regimens have been tested in a small, two-year, pilot clinical trial among premenopausal women with an extremely high risk of breast cancer. At the end of the first year relatively few side effects were noted (54) and potentially beneficial mammographic changes, measured as reductions in mammographic densities, were observed (55).

SECONDARY PREVENTION

In light of the present paucity of prospects for the primary prevention of breast cancer, the possibility of secondary prevention through screening assumes considerable importance. The effectiveness of mammography, with or without professional physical examination of the breast, has been the object of a great deal of study. Breast self-examination has been studied to a lesser extent.

Mammography

Evidence from randomized trials clearly indicates that screening for breast cancer by mammography reduces mortality from breast cancer in women in the age range 50–74 years. The evidence is sufficiently strong to justify organized efforts at early detection by mammography as a public health measure (42). Estimates of the percentage reduction in breast cancer mortality from mammography have ranged from 17 to 33%. Programs employing two-view mammography combined with physical examination, as well as those using single-view or two-view mammography alone, have been shown to decrease mortality. The screening intervals that have been shown to be effective have varied from approximately yearly to approximately every three years.

Little information is available on the effectiveness of screening by mammography in women over 74 years of age. However, it is believed likely that women somewhat older than 74 years will show a beneficial effect similar to that seen in women in the 60–74 year age group. The age at which a benefit from screening would become too small to be useful is unknown (42).

Whether mammography screening programs in women in the age range 40–49 are worthwhile is controversial. In 1987, the American Cancer Society, the National Cancer Institute, and other organizations together issued guidelines recommending that women in the age range 40–49 years have mammography performed every 1–2 years, and that women of age 50 years and older have mammography every year. However, based in part on new data and in part on reconsideration of existing data, an International Workshop on Screening for Breast Cancer convened by the National Cancer Institute in 1993 concluded that for women in the age range 40–49 randomized trials showed no benefit from mammography during the first 5–7 years following initiation of screening, though possibly some benefit after 10–12 years of follow-up. Since 1993, the National Cancer Institute has no longer recommended routine mammography screening for all women in the age range 40–49 years, although other organizations such as the American College of Radiology and the American Cancer Society have still recommended screening for women in their forties.

Possible reasons that screening may not be effective in women under age 50 are that (*a*) the benefit is delayed in younger women, (*b*) mammograms are more difficult to read and cancers easier to miss in younger women because their breast tissue is more dense than in older women, and (*c*) breast cancers may be more aggressive in younger women and are thus more likely to occur between screening examinations or are too far advanced when detected (VL Ernster, personal communication). Also, mammography should not be considered a procedure without risks. It involves exposure to radiation, although in very low doses. False positive mammograms are especially common among the younger women, resulting in more expensive diagnostic follow-up with biopsies, and considerable anxiety and inconvenience (32). In addition, mammography detects many in situ cancers that might never progress to breast cancer if left untreated. Although the current standard of care for in situ lesions appears to be lumpectomy with radiation, almost half of in situ cases in the United States in 1991 were treated by mastectomy. These data suggest that mammography is probably leading to many more surgical removals of breasts than are warranted (VL Ernster, personal communication).

An argument in favor of routine screening for women in the age range 40–49 is that some evidence suggests a benefit after 10–12 years of follow-up that was not seen with shorter periods of follow-up. However, if the benefit is not apparent until after 10–12 years have elapsed, it is likely that if the screening were started at age 50 instead of before age 50, these lesions would still be detected soon enough for treatment to be started early. Finally, it has been pointed out (20) that because breast cancer is much less common at younger ages, the number of lives saved by mammographic screening at younger ages will be relatively small.

Breast Self-Examination and Physical Examination

Although breast self-examination at frequent intervals has considerable intuitive appeal as an inexpensive way of detecting breast lesions at an early stage, the limited available data do not find it to be an effective screening method (42). Two major problems appear to be compliance and the frequent lack of proficiency of the woman doing the self-examination. The effectiveness of physical examination alone by a health professional has not been evaluated. Further work in these areas is warranted, however, since these screening methods may be particularly useful in geographic areas in which mammography is not available.

CONCLUSION

Knowledge of the epidemiology of breast cancer continues to evolve, but much remains to be learned. Unfortunately, on the basis of the currently established risk factors, there is little practical advice that can be given to most women about how to reduce their risk through primary prevention. Secondary prevention through mammographic screening is at present the most effective means of reducing the impact of breast cancer.

Nevertheless, ongoing and future epidemiologic research may change the prospects for primary prevention. For instance, research is being undertaken to try to establish with more certainty the etiologic risks of certain potentially modifiable life-style characteristics, such as physical activity, diet, and use of hormone replacement therapy and oral contraceptives (Table 2). Studies of the mechanisms by which endogenous hormones have their effects may lead to increased understanding of risk factors and preventive measures. As breast cancer susceptibility genes are identified, gene-environment interactions can be studied. It is possible that subtypes of breast cancer will be identified for which associations with the various risk factors are stronger than for breast cancer as a whole. New ideas about possible etiologic agents will undoubtedly be put forth. With these various approaches, it is hoped that knowledge will be gained that can be used to reduce the incidence of breast cancer.

Literature Cited

1. Aldercreutz H, Mousavi Y, Clark J, Hockerstedt K, Hamalainen E, et al. 1992. Dietary phytoestrogens and cancer: in vitro and in vivo studies. *J. Steroid Biochem. Mol. Biol.* 41:331–37
2. Ambrosone CB, Freudenheim JL, Marshall JR, Graham S, Vena JE, et al. 1995. N-acetyltransferase (NAT), ciga-rette smoking, and breast cancer risk. *Proc. Am. Assoc. Cancer Res.* 36:283 (Abstr.)
3. Bernstein L, Henderson BE, Hanisch R, Sullivan-Halley J, Ross RK. 1994. Physical exercise and reduced risk of breast cancer in young women. *J. Natl. Cancer Inst.* 86:1403–8

4. Bernstein L, Ross RK. 1993. Endogenous hormones and breast cancer risk. *Epidemiol. Rev.* 15:48–65

5. Bernstein L, Ross RK, Henderson BE. 1992. Prospects for the primary prevention of breast cancer. *Am. J. Epidemiol.* 135:142–52

6. Bernstein L, Ross RK, Lobo R, Hanisch R, Krailo MD, Henderson BE. 1987. The effects of moderate physical activity on menstrual cycle patterns in adolescence: implications for breast cancer prevention. *Br. J. Cancer* 55: 681–85

7. Bodian CA. 1993. Benign breast diseases, carcinoma in situ, and breast cancer risk. *Epidemiol. Rev.* 15:177–87

8. Boyd NF, Byng JW, Jong RA, Fishell EK, Little LE, et al. 1995. Quantitative classification of mammographic densities and breast cancer risk: results from the Canadian National Breast Screening Study. *J. Nat Cancer Inst.* 87:670–75

9. Brinton LA, Schairer C. 1993. Estrogen replacement therapy and breast cancer risk. *Epidemiol. Rev.* 15:66–79

10. Bush TL, Helzlsouer KJ. 1993. Tamoxifen for the primary prevention of breast cancer: a review and critique of the concept and trial. *Epidemiol. Rev.* 15: 233–43

11. Claus EB, Risch NJ, Thompson WD. 1990. Age at onset as an indicator of familial risk of breast cancer. *Am. J. Epidemiol.* 131:961–72

12. Daling JR, Malone KE, Voigt LF, White E, Weiss N. 1994. Risk of breast cancer among young women: relationship to induced abortion. *J. Natl. Cancer Inst.* 86:1584–92

13. Dao TL. 1981. The role of ovarian steroid hormones in mammary carcinogenesis. In *Hormones and Breast Cancer (Bradbury Rep. no. 8)*, ed. MC Pike, PK Siiteri, CW Welsch, pp. 281–95. Cold Spring Harbor, NY: Cold Spring Harbor Lab.

14. Davis DL, Bradlow HL. 1995. Can environmental estrogens cause breast cancer? *Sci. Am.* 273:166–72

15. Feuer EJ, Wun LM, Boring CC, Flanders WD, Timmel MJ, Tong T. 1993. The life-time risk of developing breast cancer. *J. Natl. Cancer Inst.* 85:892–97

16. Friedenreich CM, Rohan TE. 1995. A review of physical activity and breast cancer. *Epidemiology* 6:311–17

17. Futreal PA, Liu Q, Shattuck-Eidens D, Cochran C, Harshman K, et al. 1994. BRCA1 mutations in primary breast cancer and ovarian carcinomas. *Science* 266:120–22

18. Gammon MD, John EM. 1993. Recent etiologic hypotheses concerning breast cancer. *Epidemiol. Rev.* 15:163–68

19. Garland FC, Garland CF, Gorham ED, Young JF. 1990. Geographic variation in breast cancer mortality in the United States: a hypothesis involving exposure to solar radiation. *Prev. Med.* 19:614–22

20. Harris R, Leininger L. 1995. Clinical strategies for breast cancer screening: weighing and using the evidence. *Ann. Intern. Med.* 122:539–47

21. Hoegh H, McKendry CJ, Wright WE, Young JL Jr. 1992. *Cancer Incidence by Race/Ethnicity California, 1988–1989*. Calif. DHS, Sacramento

22. Horn-Ross PL. 1993. Multiple primary cancers involving the breast. *Epidemiol. Rev.* 15:169–76

23. Howe G, Rohan T, Decarli A, Iscovich J, Kaldor J, et al. 1991. The association between alcohol and breast cancer risk: evidence from the combined analysis of six dietary case-control studies. *Int. J. Cancer* 47:707–10

24. Hulka BS, Stark AT. 1995. Breast cancer: cause and prevention. *Lancet* 346: 883–87

25. Hunter DJ, Willett WC. 1993. Diet, body size, and breast cancer. *Epidemiol. Rev.* 15:110–32

26. Institute of Medicine, Committee to Review the Women's Health Initiative. 1993. *An Assessment of the NIH Women's Health Initiative*. Washington, DC: Natl. Acad.

27. John EM, Kelsey JL. 1993. Radiation and other environmental exposures and breast cancer. *Epidemiol. Rev.* 15:157–62

28. Jordan VC. 1990. Estrogen receptor-mediated direct and indirect antitumor effects of tamoxifen. *J. Natl. Cancer Inst.* 82:1662–63

29. Kelsey JL, Gammon MD, John EM. 1993. Reproductive factors and breast cancer. *Epidemiol. Rev.* 15:36–47

30. Kelsey JL, Horn-Ross PL. 1993. Breast cancer: magnitude of the problem and descriptive epidemiology. *Epidemiol. Rev.* 15:7–16

31. Kelsey JL, Whittemore AS. 1994. Epidemiology and primary prevention of cancers of the breast, endometrium, and ovary. A brief overview. *Ann. Epidemiol.* 4:89–95

32. Kerlikowske K, Grady D, Barclay J, Sickles EA, Eaton A, Ernster V. 1993. Positive predictive value of screening mammography by age and family history of breast cancer. *JAMA* 270:2444–50

33. King MC, Rowell S, Love SM. 1993.

Inherited breast and ovarian cancer. *JAMA* 269:1975–80

34. Krieger N, Wolff MS, Hiatt RA, Rivera M, Vogelman J, Orentreich N. 1994. Breast cancer and serum organochlorines: a prospective study among white, black, and Asian women. *J. Natl. Cancer Inst.* 86:589–99

35. Longnecker MP. 1994. Alcoholic beverage consumption in relation to risk of breast cancer: meta-analysis and review. *Cancer Causes Control* 5:73–82

36. Love RR. 1993. The National Surgical Adjuvant Breast Project (NSABP) Breast Cancer Prevention Trial revisited. *Cancer Epidemiol. Biomarkers Prev.* 2:403–7

37. Malone KE. 1993. Diethylstilbestrol (DES) and breast cancer. *Epidemiol. Rev.* 15:108–9

38. Malone KE, Daling JR, Weiss NS. 1993. Oral contraceptives and breast cancer. *Epidemiol. Rev.* 15:80–97

39. McPherson K, Steel CM, Dixon JM. 1994. Breast cancer—epidemiology, risk factors, and genetics. *Br. Med J.* 309:1003–6

40. Messina M, Messina V. 1991. Increasing use of soyfoods and their potential role in cancer prevention. *J. Am. Diet. Assoc.* 91:836–40

41. Mittendorf R, Longnecker MP, Newcomb PA, Dietz AT, Greenbert ER, et al. 1995. Strenuous physical activity in young adulthood and risk of breast cancer. *Cancer Causes Control.* In press

42. Morrison AS. 1993. Screening for cancer of the breast. *Epidemiol. Rev.* 15: 244–55

43. Newcomb PA, Storer BE, Longnecker MP, Mittendorf R, Greenberg R, et al. 1994. Lactation and a reduced risk of premenopausal breast cancer. *N. Engl. J. Med.* 330:81–87

44. Oza AM, Boyd NF. 1993. Mammographic parenchymal patterns: a marker of breast cancer risk. *Epidemiol. Rev.* 15:196–208

45. Palmer JR, Rosenberg L. 1993. Cigarette smoking and the risk of breast cancer. *Epidemiol. Rev.* 15:145–56

46. Petrakis NL. 1993. Nipple aspirate fluid in epidemiologic studies of breast disease. *Epidemiol. Rev.* 15:188–95

47. Pike MC, Spicer DV, Dahmoush L, Press MF. 1993. Estrogens, progestogens, normal breast cell proliferation, and breast cancer risk. *Epidemiol. Rev.* 15:17–35

48. Pike MC, Krailo MD, Henderson BE, Casagrande JT, Hoel DG. 1983. "Hormonal" risk factors, "breast tissue age"

and the age incidence of breast cancer. *Nature* 303:767–70

49. Pike MC, Ross RK, Lobo RA, Key TJA, Potts M, Henderson BE. 1989. LHRH agonists and the prevention of breast and ovarian cancer. *Br. J. Cancer* 60: 142–48

50. Pollak M, Constantino J, Polychronakos C, Blauer SA, Guyda H, et al. 1990. Effects of tamoxifen on serum insulin-like growth factor I levels in stage I breast cancer patients. *J. Natl. Cancer Inst.* 82:1693–97

51. Preston-Martin S, Pike MC, Ross RK, Jones PA, Henderson BE. 1990. Increased cell division as a cause of human cancer. *Cancer Res.* 50:7415–21

52. Rosenberg L. 1994. Induced abortion and breast cancer: more scientific data are needed. (Editorial) *J. Natl. Cancer Inst.* 86:1569–70

53. Schatzkin A, Longnecker MP. 1994. Alcohol and breast cancer: Where are we now and where do we go from here? *Cancer* 74:1101–10

54. Spicer DV, Pike MC, Pike A, Rude R, Shoupe D, Richardson J. 1993. Pilot trial of a gonadotropin hormone agonist with replacement hormones as a prototype contraceptive to prevent breast cancer. *Contraception* 47:427–44

55. Spicer DV, Ursin G, Parinsky YR, Pearce JG, Shoupe D, et al. 1994. Changes in mammographic densities induced by a hormonal contraceptive designed to reduce breast cancer risk. *J. Natl. Cancer Inst.* 86:431–36

56. Stanford JL, Thomas DB. 1993. Exogenous progestins and breast cancer. *Epidemiol. Rev.* 15:98–107

57. Stevens RG. 1987. Electric power use and breast cancer: a hypothesis. *Am. J. Epidemiol.* 125:556–61

58. Trichopoulos D. 1990. Hypothesis: Does breast cancer originate in utero? *Lancet* 335:939–40

59. Ursin G, Longnecker MP, Haile RW, Greenland S. 1995. A meta-analysis of body mass index and risk of premenopausal breast cancer. *Epidemiology* 6: 137–41

60. Whelan EA, Sandler DP, Root J, Smith KR, Weinberg CR. 1994. Menstrual cycle patterns and risk of breast cancer. *Am. J. Epidemiol.* 140:1081–90

61. Wingo PA, Tong T, Bolden S. 1995. Cancer Statistics, 1995. *CA Cancer J. Clin.* 45:8–30

62. Wolff MS, Toniolo PG, Lee EW, Rivera M, Dubin N. 1993. Blood levels of organochlorine residues and risk of breast cancer. *J. Natl. Cancer Inst.* 85: 648–52

63. Wooster R, Neuhausen SL, Mangion J, Quirk Y, Ford D, et al. 1994. Localization of a breast cancer susceptibility gene, BRCA2, to chromosome 13q12–13. *Science* 265:2088–90

64. Wrensch MR, Petrakis NL, Gruenke LD, Miike R, Ernster VL, et al. 1989. Breast fluid cholesterol and cholesterol β-epoxide concentrations in women with benign breast disease. *Cancer Res.* 49:2168–74

65. Ziegler RG, Hoover RN, Pike MC, Hildesheim A, Nomura AM, et al. 1993. Migration patterns and breast cancer risk in Asian-American women. *J. Natl. Cancer Inst.* 85:1819–27

Annu. Rev. Public Health. 1996. 17:69–84

CERVICAL INTRAEPITHELIAL NEOPLASIA, CERVICAL CANCER, AND HPV

Elizabeth A. Holly

Department of Epidemiology and Biostatistics, School of Medicine, University of California San Francisco, San Francisco, California 94143 and Department of Health Research and Policy, Stanford University School of Medicine, Stanford, California 94305

KEY WORDS: cervical intraepithelial neoplasia, CIN, cervical cancer, human papillomavirus, HPV, risk factors

ABSTRACT

Major progress has been made to control cervical cancer in the United States and Europe using screening programs, although it remains a major cause of morbidity and mortality in the developing world. The association between cervical cancer and a sexually transmissible etiologic agent was hypothesized long before identification of human papillomaviruses (HPV) as agents that infected the genital tract. HPVs are among the most common sexually transmitted agents and have been shown to induce several squamous anogenital cancers, including squamous cell cancer of the cervix. After an etiologic role for HPV was identified in cervical cancer and CIN, efforts to understand the molecular biology of HPV were greatly expanded, enhanced by the advent of deoxyribonucleic acid (DNA) probes to identify HPV infection. Recent research has focused on specific types of HPV in relation to other recognized risk factors in the pathogenesis of CIN and invasive cervical cancer.

MAGNITUDE OF THE PROBLEM AND GENERAL DESCRIPTIVE EPIDEMIOLOGY

In the United States in 1995, an estimated 55,000 women will be diagnosed with carcinoma in situ of the cervix, and an additional 15,800 with invasive cancer (7, 92). An estimated 4800 women will die from this disease in 1995 in the United States (92). Incidence rates vary from fewer than 4/100,000 (after correction for hysterectomy prevalence in the USA) (2) to more than 100/100,000 in some countries. Major progress has been made to control cervical cancer in the United States and Europe using screening programs (57), although

69

it remains a major cause of morbidity and mortality in the developing world with about 440,000 invasive cases each year worldwide (40). Recent work indicates that incidence rates for cervical cancer are increasing among young white women in some populations in the USA (90). Reports on black and white differences from the US National Center for Health Statistics death tapes show age-specific mortality rates for cervical cancer among older blacks generally to be more than twice those of older whites, with very little differences at younger ages (1, 46).

The association between cervical cancer and a sexually transmissible etiologic agent has been hypothesized for more than a century (6, 15, 77). Several lines of epidemiologic evidence provided support for this concept long before current molecular laboratory methods were able to identify the responsible agents. In 1842, Rigoni-Stern reported on the marked difference between the occurrence of cervical cancer in married women compared with nuns, who had no appreciable cervical cancer (77). More recently, higher cervical and penile cancer rates have been shown to cluster in several different geographic regions (21, 51, 58); men who were diagnosed with penile cancer have wives with elevated rates of cervical cancer (30, 59); higher number of male sexual partners and earlier age at first sexual intercourse are primary risk factors for this disease (6, 9, 15, 19, 45, 82); and women with cervical cancer with only one sexual partner have husbands who have had a greater number of sexual partners (18), more extramarital affairs, and more extensive histories of sexually transmitted diseases when compared with control subjects' husbands (19). Several excellent reviews discuss the relationships among invasive cervical cancer, its precursor lesion cervical intraepithelial neoplasia (CIN), sexually transmissible etiologic agents, and other risk factors (8, 14, 15, 26, 39, 40, 42, 64, 74, 79, 88). This paper summarizes recent developments in epidemiologic studies that link human papillomaviruses (HPV) to CIN and invasive cervical cancer with only brief reference made to other risk factors for cervical disease as they relate to HPV. Cigarette smoking and oral contraceptive use will be considered in some detail in relation to HPV because stratified analyses have been conducted by presence or absence of HPV in multiple studies.

ROLE OF HPV IN RELATION TO CIN AND CERVICAL CANCER

The observation that cervical cancer is a sexually transmitted disease long predated our understanding of HPV as an agent that infected the genital tract. HPVs are among the most common of sexually transmitted agents and induce several squamous anogenital cancers, the most common being squamous cell cancer of the cervix. HPVs also induce proliferative genital lesions such as condylomata acuminata (genital warts). Recent research efforts have focused on specific types of HPV in relation to other recognized epidemiologic risk factors in the pathogenesis of CIN and invasive cervical cancer. By stratifying questionnaire risk factor data according to the presence or absence of onco-genic HPV types, a better understanding has been obtained of mechanisms relating HPV to classic risk factors for cervical disease.

After an etiologic role for HPV was identified in cervical cancer and CIN, efforts to understand the molecular biology of HPV were greatly expanded. This effort was enhanced substantially by the advent of deoxyribonucleic acid (DNA) probes to identify HPV infection. The past decade has seen a broad expansion in our understanding of the functions of HPV genes, patterns of HPV gene expression in cervical tissues, and how these genes contribute to the development of malignancy (recently reviewed in (67)). New forms of molecular probes and new methods such as polymerase chain reaction (PCR) were applied to the study of cervical tissues.

Current understanding of the pathogenesis of cervical cancer reflects a complicated interplay between epidemiology and basic molecular biology. With the advent of molecular studies using PCR to enhance classic studies based only on interview data, epidemiologists have reached more precise conclusions regarding the relationship between CIN and invasive cervical cancer and sexually transmissible etiologic agents. Historically, substantial disagreement among laboratories has been reported for HPV diagnosis (11, 83). However, in recent years, serious cross-reactivity among HPV types and other laboratory problems have been overcome using carefully controlled techniques (31, 46). It is crucial to the success of future molecular epidemiol-ogy studies that tests for HPV be sensitive and reliable (83, 84). Odds ratios and relative risks for the association between HPV and cervical disease vary tremendously depending upon the HPV types considered, the laboratory meth-ods used to test for HPV, and the severity of cervical disease. However, when the most sensitive laboratory methods are used to test for HPV 16/18 among women with high-grade CIN or invasive cervical cancer, odds ratios occasion-ally are more than 100. Because of these extremes in risk estimates, and extensive variation among studies, odds ratios for the HPV-cervical disease association are only occasionally reported here and then only for the most recent studies.

Although the concept of sexual transmission has been known for more than a century, HPV was suggested as a sexually transmitted etiological agent associated with cervical cancer only two decades ago (95). A summary pre-sented following the Second International Workshop on the Epidemiology of Cervical Cancer and HPV (10) provided a clear rationale for causality with principal arguments as follows: 1. agreement among many studies that HPV DNA is present in 85 to 100% of high-grade CIN and cervical cancer speci-mens (when using PCR or high-quality Southern hybridization methods); 2.

Table 1   Risk factors associated with cervical cancer prior to and after adjustment for presence of HPV infection*

Factor	High risk group	Low risk group	Effect of adjustment for HPV**
Age	Older	Younger	Correlate of HPV infection and cofactor for progression
Number of sexual partners	Many	One or few	Correlate of HPV infection
Husband's/Partner's number of sexual partners	Many	One or few	Correlate of HPV infection
Age at first intercourse	Young	Older	Correlate of HPV infection and cofactor for progression
Cigarette smoking	Yes	None	Weak cofactor for progression (?)
Use of oral contraceptives	Current; recent use; long-term use	None	Cofactor for progression (?)
Barrier contraceptive use	Never/seldom	Often/always	Negative correlate of HPV infection
Pap smear screening	Never	Routine	Cofactor for progression
Immune function	Suppressed	Normal	Cofactor for viral persistence and progression
Number of live births	Many	None	Cofactor for progression
HSV2 status, chlamydia, other sexually transmitted diseases	Positive	Negative	Correlate of infection, weak cofactor (?)
Socioeconomic status	Low	High	Correlate of infection, weak cofactor (?)

*After consideration of HPV (many risk factors for HPV and for cervical cancer are the same (73), the independent effects of most risk factors for cervical cancer are substantially diminished.

**Correlate—effect diminished after consideration of HPV. Cofactor—remains a risk factor in HPV+ women

consistent and strong association between HPV DNA detection and cervical cancer in case-control studies; 3. a limited number of HPV types commonly found in the genital tract providing specificity of the association; and, 4. dose-response relationship between estimates of viral load and the risk of cervical cancer (10). More recent work from the International Agency for Research on Cancer has found sufficient evidence to declare HPV types 16 and 18 as carcinogens and HPV types 31 and 33 as probable carcinogens in humans (40).

Determining a distinction between the Bethesda Classification of low-grade squamous intraepithelial lesions (LSIL) of the cervix (includes koilocytotic atypia and CIN 1) and high-grade squamous intraepithelial lesions (HSIL) (includes CIN 2 and 3) is relevant because different HPV types are related to different lesion grades. Strongest evidence exists for a link between the more oncogenic high-risk HPV types 16 or 18 and high-grade CIN and cervical cancer lesions that are less likely to regress spontaneously (4, 8, 23, 43, 54, 75, 82). While allowing for variation among studies, HPV types 6, 11, 42, 43, and 44 primarily are associated with more benign cervical disease such as koilocytotic atypia and CIN 1 with the low-grade lesions being more likely to regress than high-grade lesions (4, 23, 54, 75, 82). HPV types 31, 33, 35, 39, 45, 51, 52, and 58 are associated with an intermediate risk of progression to malignancy (23, 52–54). The rarity of several of these intermediate HPV-types has precluded proper evaluation of their true risk. Nevertheless, similar conclusions regarding some HPV types have been reported in many geographic regions of the world (47, 50, 54, 62, 71, 82, 89). Recent work investigating geographical variation of HPV prevalence among women with cervical cancer has detected HPV DNA in 93% of the tumors with no significant variation by HPV positivity in South East Asia, North America, Central and South America, Europe, and Africa (8). Geographical variation existed in the prevalence of some of the less common types of HPV. However, there was little geographic variation in HPV 16. Regarding the tumor morphology, HPV 16 predominated in squamous-cell tumors and HPV 18 (as well as HPV 16) predominated in adenocarcinomas and adenosquamous tumors (8).

Molecular Biology

Why some HPV types are more strongly associated with invasive cancer is not yet fully understood. However, in the HPV types 16 and 18 that frequently are associated with cervical cancer, the E6 and E7 oncoproteins of these viruses interfere particularly strongly with the normal tumor suppressor function of p53 and pRB (56). Furthermore, the level of HPV E7 expression is greater in tissues infected with HPV types associated with higher risks of malignancy (86, 87). Because HPV viral E6 and E7 oncoproteins are selectively expressed and maintained in HPV-related tumors, they are likely to be targets for therapeutic vaccines (56). More detail on the molecular biology of HPV and cervical cancer may be found in a recent review (67). Recent work shows progress in the development of serological tests to detect specific types of HPV antibodies (29, 41), but DNA testing of cervical specimens currently is the more sensitive detection technique.

Cervical HPV infection is relatively common among young women who are sexually active. Early cytologic manifestations of HPV, koilocytotic atypia and CIN 1, also are relatively common, while CIN 3 and invasive cervical cancer are somewhat rare in the United States and occur more often among older than among younger women (80, 81). CIN 2 or 3 are thought to be precursor lesions to invasive cervical cancer, with the risk of invasive disease increasing in the more serious forms of CIN (66, 76). In contrast, HPV infections and CIN 1 often are detectable transiently: They may be cleared by the individual, possibly through immunologic control mechanisms, or they may become dormant. It is currently unknown whether an initial infection with a specific HPV type confers immunity against reinfection with the same or other HPV types (81). Which HPV types persist in their expression over time and which are more transient also is uncertain. HPV DNA may become undetectable within one to two years of infection, although these preliminary time estimates have been reported as not yet trustworthy (35, 81).

RISK FACTORS FOR CERVICAL DISEASE

A large multicenter case-control study with 759 cervical cancer patients and 1467 controls was conducted in four countries in Latin America to evaluate an association between HPV infection and invasive cervical cancer. HPV DNA was detected in 62% of the cases and only 32% of the controls, using filter in situ hybridization; this assay is now judged to be neither sensitive nor specific. The adjusted risk of cancer increased substantially (up to OR = 13) with hybridization reactions of increasing strength for HPV 6/11 and 16/18. The elevated risk associated with HPV 16/18 was not affected by statistical adjustment for other more traditional risk factors for cervical cancer (71). A recent hospital-based case-control study in Brazil used the more sensitive polymerase chain reaction (PCR) method to detect HPV and found that 66% of the 199 cases were positive for HPV types 16, 18, 31, and 33 as compared with only 6% of the 225 age-frequency matched controls. The adjusted odds ratios for the association between cervical cancer and HPV 16, 18, 31, and 33 was nearly 70 (95% CI 29–170) (28).

A cohort study of 241 women conducted in a sexually transmitted disease clinic in Washington State, using dot-filter hybridization and Southern transfer hybridization to detect HPV DNA, determined the temporal relationship between infection with HPV, incidence of high-grade squamous intraepithelial lesions—HSIL (CIN 2 or 3) and the temporal influence of other risk factors associated with CIN. After two years of follow-up among women who began the study with negative PAP smears, the cumulative incidence of CIN 2 or 3 was 28% among women who tested positive for HPV versus 3% among those who had tested negative (47). The authors noted that CIN 2 or 3 was an early and common manifestation of HPV infection in this high-risk group of women. They also reported that all of the HPV-associated cases were observed within two years of the initial detection of HPV DNA. The risk of HSIL was highest for the more malignant types of HPV (types 16 and 18, adjusted relative risk = 11) when compared with women with no detectable HPV. From a clinical viewpoint, it is worth noting that 36% of women (10 of 28) had a smear that showed CIN 1 prior to the first smear that showed CIN 2 or 3. Detection of antibodies to herpes simplex virus type 2 (HSV-2) or isolation of HSV-2 from the cervix were associated with development of CIN 2 or 3 (47). After adjustment for presence of HPV infection, common risk factors (e.g. cigarette smoking, number of sexual partners, and age at first intercourse) no longer were independently associated with CIN 2 or 3. Only gonococcal infection and antibodies to chlamydia remained independent risk factors for CIN. Among the women in this cohort study, the authors estimated that 78% of biopsy-confirmed CIN could be attributed to one or more types of HPV DNA, with 52% attributable to types 16 or 18 (47). In a separate cross-sectional study that used the same detection methods to test for HPV, presence of types 42 through 45 added another 15% to the number of HPV infections detected in these women (44). Powerful new tests such as PCR are more sensitive but the clinical relevance of detecting HPV using PCR as it relates to the ultimate risk of CIN grades 2 or 3 or cervical cancer currently is unknown.

PCR used to detect HPV DNA in cervicovaginal lavage specimens in Oregon provided compelling epidemiologic evidence linking specific HPV types as etiologic agents for CIN (82). Common risk factors for CIN and for invasive cervical cancer (greater number of sexual partners, earlier age at first sexual intercourse, less education, lower family income, and cigarette smoking) also were studied in conjunction with HPV infection in the Oregon report on CIN (82). After adjustment for common risk factors for CIN, elevated risks for HPV types associated with low, medium, and high risk for CIN were unchanged. Conversely, after statistical adjustment for HPV type-groups (HPV 16 and 18 were most commonly associated with high-grade CIN and cervical cancer), the risk estimates for the classic risk factors diminished substantially and were no longer significant, indicating the importance HPV plays in the etiology of CIN and the strong association between risk factors for HPV and cervical cancer.

Work conducted at a California student health center, using Virapap to test for HPV among young women with and without CIN, confirmed HPV as a major risk factor for CIN. Elevated risks for HPV remained unchanged after adjustment for age, number of sexual partners, and oral contraceptives (49). In the Oregon study, women with multiple HPV types were more likely to have been in the case group than women with single types (82). The authors estimated that 76% of the entire CIN case group could be attributed to HPV infection. Further, with classification by abnormality, 70% of condylomatous atypia, 90% of CIN 1, and 88% of CIN 2 and 3 could be attributed to HPV (82).

Smoking

The original hypothesis linking smoking and cervical cancer (93) and the numerous subsequent studies that have confirmed this association have been reviewed (94). However, when HPV also was considered, an inconsistent association between cervical disease and cigarette smoking has been reported. Many of the early studies did not have the most powerful laboratory techniques available for definitive HPV-work among patients with cervical cytological abnormalities. In the Oregon study, the association between smoking and risk of CIN was explained by adjusting for lifetime number of sexual partners (82). Further adjustment provided no evidence that smoking remained associated with risk for CIN when all CIN levels and all HPV types were considered together. However, in the same study, HPV-positive current smokers had estimated risk ratios of 2.7 for CIN 2 or 3 when compared to HPV-positive women who did not smoke, indicating that current smoking may be linked to the more advanced forms of CIN in ways that are not currently understood (82). Among current smokers in the cohort study conducted in Washington State, smoking was not found to be a risk factor for CIN grades 2 and 3 after adjustment for HPV infection (47). Smoking was correlated with HPV infection in crude analyses in California, but the association diminished after adjustment for number of male sexual partners (50). Cigarette smoking showed no consistent or significant association with CIN in Spain and Colombia after careful adjustment for PCR-determined HPV and other risk factors (63). Smoking was associated with cervical cancer in Latin America but was not associated with HPV infection (72). Later detailed analysis in this population suggested that smoking has a limited effect on cervical cancer risk, perhaps only among women with specific types of HPV (33). In recent work conducted in New Mexico, a modestly elevated risk was reported between smoking and high-grade CIN (OR = 1.7) after adjustment for the effects of HPV (5). A dose-response relationship also was reported with number of cigarettes smoked per day and for pack-years of use, whereas no association was noted for former cigarette use.

Other types of evidence without consideration of HPV have provided support for the association between smoking and CIN and cervical cancer. In one clinical study, women who were seen for various levels of CIN or cervical cancer and who smoked were more likely than nonsmokers with these conditions to have mutagenic cervical fluids (37), although this effect was attenuated using different laboratory techniques (36). In addition, nicotine and cotinine were found in the mucous secretions of the uterine cervix of women who smoked (60, 78).

Tobacco by-products may produce a decrease in the concentration of antigen-presenting Langerhans cells in the normal cervical epithelium causing a smoking-mediated immunological defect (3) that allows HPV to infect and persist in the cervical epithelium (20). Further, tobacco by-products also may enhance chromosomal instability with or without the effects of HPV. More work is needed to ascertain the effects of smoking on the Langerhans cells and how these cells are affected by HPV. Whether the immunosuppressive effects of smoking enhance the possible hormonal effects of oral contraceptive use also should be explored. More work is required to determine whether smoking induces chromosomal mutations, what role smoking plays in the susceptibility of HPV infection, and whether the effects of smoking are potentiated by the presence of HPV. Simulation modeling done to examine whether the effects of confounding have been adequately controlled in relation to cigarette smoking and cervical cancer have shown that some of the effect may be due to residual confounding (70), even though there are possible biological mechanisms to account for the association.

Oral Contraceptives

An association between oral contraceptives (OCs), CIN, and cervical cancer that is not related to confounding is somewhat controversial, and comprehensive reviews have been published on the possible association (13, 27). Most of the earlier studies on this topic have had little or no information on presence of HPV, leaving unresolved the relevance of the OC-CIN association after adjustment for HPV. In four Latin American countries, ever use of OCs after control for HPV was shown to be related to adenocarcinomas of the cervix (adjusted OR = 2.4) but not to squamous cell tumors (adjusted OR = 1.1) (16), which provides support for earlier descriptive studies that have shown increasing incidence rates for adenocarcinomas among young women (85). The overall results for OC use in the Latin American study were not related to ever use, duration of use, or years since first or last use (16). The authors concluded that the effect of OC use on cervical neoplasia could not be excluded entirely, although it is likely to be limited only to a small proportion of all cases (16). However, there was some indication of an elevated risk for invasive cervical cancer among women who had used injectable contraceptives for five or more years. Although numbers were small, prolonged use confirmed higher risk for women who reported first use ten or more years previously (32). A slightly elevated risk for CIN 3 with use of OCs among women who were HPV positive was reported in Colombia and Spain, although the association could have been due to chance and there was an inconsistent dose-response relationship (63). Among HPV-positive women, hormonal factors such as ever use of oral contraceptives and high parity possibly conferred additional risk for progression from chronic HPV infection to cancer (61). However, there was no linear relationship with parity in this group.

When HPV-positive and HPV-negative women were analyzed separately in Oregon, odds ratios for risk of CIN among women who were HPV positive were 0.5 for current use and 0.7 for past use of OCs, and 2.1 for current use and 2.0 for past use among those who were HPV negative, although confidence limits for all values overlapped unity (82). In Washington State (47), after adjustment for HPV infection, no association of risk for CIN 2 and 3 was found for use of OCs in their cohort study, nor were OCs a risk factor for CIN in a cohort study conducted in Washington, D.C. after a similar adjustment for HPV (55). Other work at the molecular level that explored the reputed relationship between OC use and CIN found no support for OCs affecting gene expression of HPV (38). However, others have found that HPV can interact with hormone-reponse elements in the viral genes, enhancing transcription and ultimately transforming cervical cells (68, 69). This work suggests that if OCs play a role in HPV-mediated carcinogenesis, it may not be through quantitative changes in gene expression in vivo. Further, it is important to remember that women who take OCs usually are not using barrier contraceptives, which would prevent the transmission of sexually transmitted diseases. A large WHO-sponsored multinational study in nine countries reported an association with invasive cervical cancer and long-term use of OCs within the past eight years. Unfortunately, no laboratory data were available on HPV prevalence so the role of HPV as a confounding factor cannot be ruled out (91).

Other Risk Factors

Factors less well studied in relation to HPV are mentioned here with little detail. Number of sexual partners and early sexual intercourse have been reported consistently as risk factors for cervical disease and were mentioned as cofactors for HPV acquisition in many of the studies already cited. The period of sexual maturation is a time of high regenerative activity and rapid proliferation of cells infected with HPV (96). This rapid expansion of cells that harbor the HPV viral genome may partially account for early sexual intercourse as one of the common risk factors for the development of CIN and cervical cancer.

Parity has been investigated in numerous studies as a potential risk factor for cervical cancer. Increased parity was found to be significantly related to cervical cancer with risk estimates of greater than threefold associated with multiple births in both the HPV-positive and in the HPV-negative strata (17). Parity also was reported to be an independent prognostic factor for survival: Women with six or more pregnancies had more than a twofold excess risk of dying of cervical cancer compared with women who had three or fewer pregnancies (24). More recent data from Brazil indicate that, after adjustment for HPV, parity remained an independent risk factor with fourfold risks for women who have had numerous children (28).

The role that sexually transmitted diseases (STDs), other than HPV, play as cofactors in CIN and cervical cancer has been reviewed (48), and some STDs were considered briefly in the other studies discussed above. Work conducted in Latin America showed an interaction between the presence of both HSV-2 and HPV 16/18. Those who tested positive for the presence of HSV-2 alone showed no increased risk of invasive cervical cancer (34). Subsequent case-control studies conducted in Colombia and Spain that used serological assays found weak and inconsistent associations between HSV-2 (and subclasses) and HPV (25, 65). These results suggest that HSV-2 infection is not an important factor in cervical neoplasia. Infection with the human immunodeficiency virus (HIV) is a relatively recently recognized cofactor for development of CIN and cervical cancer. In 1992, the Centers for Disease Control included invasive cervical cancer as an AIDS-defining illness in women because several studies reported increased cervical cancer morbidity in women infected with HIV (22). The degree of the relationship between HIV, HPV, and cervical cancer currently is unclear although several studies have considered this association with varying results. Two primary means by which HIV infection may influence the pathogenesis of HPV-associated cervical pathology are through effects on the function of the immune system in HIV-positive women, or through molecular interactions between HIV and HPV genes (see 12). More work is required to understand the possible role of sexually transmitted infections other than HPV, as well as the role that parity and nutritional factors may play in the incidence of CIN and cervical cancer. These and other cofactors need to be studied in relation to the presence or absence of specific HPV types using sensitive molecular techniques.

Cervical disease generally takes several years to progress from benign to malignant (76). Recent studies using techniques such as PCR suggest that only a small proportion of HPV-infected individuals develop clinically detectable disease (79). Because HPV infection alone may be insufficient for development of disease, cofactors most likely play a role. The mechanism currently is unclear for the role of cofactors such as smoking, other sexually transmitted diseases, use of oral contraceptives, and HIV. The table provides a list of the major risk factors thought to be associated with cervical cancer and CIN and the women likely to be at high and low risk for these conditions. The fourth column provides an assessment of how each risk factor is affected by adjustment for HPV.

CONCLUSION

A dominant role for HPV in the pathogenesis of cervical cancer is supported by exceedingly strong evidence. Much information exists on the molecular mechanisms employed by the virus and the host. HPV may be the best understood of any human carcinogen at the mechanistic level (40). This evidence includes detection of HPV DNA in most cases of cervical cancer and high-grade CIN;

transcriptional activity documented in the tissues; and the evidence that viral genes HPV E6 and E7 have transforming ability and can generate tumors in animal models [reviewed in (67)]. Because only a small proportion of HPV-infected individuals develop HPV-associated cervical disease, and some women without HPV develop cervical disease, the role of cofactors must be considered. Some of these cofactors and their relationship with cervical disease have been described here. Whereas some studies have considered the biological interaction of these cofactors with HPV in the pathogenesis of cervical disease, others have not. Other cofactors, for example sexually transmitted infections other than HPV and oral contraceptive use, must be considered in studies designed to observe them in the presence or absence of specific HPV types. These studies must be based on detection methods with adequate sensitivity, such as PCR, and need to be conducted with excellent laboratory assays (81, 84).

Acquisition and persistence of HPV infection, and development and progression of cervical disease are the result of complex interactions. A better understanding of the mechanistic action of the HPV virus, the epidemiologic risk factors, and the effects of these factors on the molecular biology of the cell have led to substantial progress in comprehending the pathogenesis of cervical disease. This new knowledge of mechanisms will provide further insight into methods for vaccine development that may help prevent or control HPV. Current prevention strategies would include use of condoms and routine Pap-smear screening. Efficient public health measures are needed to diagnose HPV infection effectively, to encourage those at highest risk to attend screening clinics, to determine factors associated with progression of HPV-associated cervical lesions to malignancy and to devise effective preventive interventions.

ACKNOWLEDGMENTS

The author is grateful to Drs. MH Schiffman and FX Bosch for their comments and careful review of the manuscript.

Literature Cited

1. Black-White differences in cervical cancer mortality—United States, 1980–1987. *Morbid. Mortal. Wkly. Rep.* 1990. 39:245–48
2. Hysterectomy prevalence and death rates for cervical cancer—United States, 1965–1988. *Morbid. Mortal. Wkly. Rep.* 1990. 41:17–20
3. Barton SE, Jenkins D, Cuzick J, Maddox

PH, Edwards R, Singer A. 1988. Effect of cigarette smoking on cervical epithelial immunity: a mechanism for neoplastic change? *Lancet* II:652–54
4. Beaudenon S, Kremsdorf D, Croissant O, Jablonska S, Wain-Hobson S, Orth G. 1986. A novel type of human papillomavirus associated with genital neoplasias. *Nature* 321:246–49

5. Becker TM, Wheeler CM, McGough NS, Parmenter CA, Stidley CA, et al. 1994. Cigarette smoking and other risk factors for cervical dysplasia in southwestern Hispanic and non-Hispanic white women. *Cancer Epidemiol. Biomarkers Prev.* 3:113–19

6. Beral V. 1974. Cancer of the cervix: a sexually-transmitted infection? *Lancet* 1:1037–40

7. Boring CC, Squires TS, Tong T, Montgomery S. 1994. Cancer statistics, 1994. *CA Cancer J. Clin.* 44:7–26

8. Bosch FX, Manos MM, Munoz N, Sherman M, Jansen AM, et al. 1995. Prevalence of human papillomavirus in cervical cancer: a worldwide perspective. *J. Natl. Cancer Inst.* 87:796–802

9. Bosch FX, Munoz N, de Sanjose S, Izarzugaza I, Gili M, et al. 1992. Risk factors for cervical cancer in Colombia and Spain. *Int. J. Cancer* 52:750–8

10. Bosch FX, Munoz N, Shah KV, Meheus A. 1992. Second international workshop on the epidemiology of cervical cancer and human papillomavirus. *Int. J. Cancer* 52:171–73

11. Brandsma J, Burk RD, Lancaster WD, Pfister H, Schiffman MH. 1989. Interlaboratory variation as an explanation for varying prevalence estimates of human papillomavirus infection. *Int. J. Cancer* 43:260–62

12. Braun L. 1994. Role of human immunodeficiency virus infection in the pathogenesis of human papillomavirus-associated cervical neoplasia. *Am. J. Pathol.* 144:209–14

13. Brinton LA. 1991. Oral contraceptives and cervical neoplasia. *Contraception* 43:581–95

14. Brinton LA. 1992. Epidemiology of cervical cancer—overview. See Ref. 64, pp. 3–23

15. Brinton LA, Fraumeni JF Jr. 1986. Epidemiology of uterine cervical cancer. *J. Chronic Dis.* 39:1051–65

16. Brinton LA, Reeves WC, Brenes MM, Herrero R, de Britton RC, et al. 1990. Oral contraceptive use and risk of invasive cervical cancer. *Int. J. Epidemiol* 19:4–11

17. Brinton LA, Reeves WC, Brenes MM, Herrero R, de Britton RC, et al. 1989. Parity as a risk factor for cervical cancer. *Am. J. Epidemiol.* 130:486–96

18. Brinton LA, Reeves WC, Brenes MM, Herrero R, Gaitan E, et al. 1989. The male factor in the etiology of cervical cancer among sexually monogamous women. *Int. J. Cancer* 44:199–203

19. Buckley JD, Harris RWC, Doll R, Vessey MP, Williams PT. 1981. Case-control study of the husbands of women with dysplasia or carcinoma of the cervix uteri. *Lancet* II:1010–15

20. Burger MPM, Hollema H, Gouw ASH, Pieters WJL, Quint WGV. 1993. Cigarette smoking and human papillomavirus in patients with reported cervical cytological abnormality. *Br. Med. J.* 306:749–52

21. Cartwright RA, Sinson JD. 1980. Carcinoma of penis and cervix. *Lancet* 1:97

22. Cent. Dis. Control. 1992. 1993 revised classification system for HIV infection and expanded surveillance case definition for AIDS among adolescents and adults. *Morb. Mortal. Wkly. Rep.* 41:1–19

23. Crum C, Mitao M, Levine MR, Silverstein S. 1985. Cervical papillomaviruses segregate within morphologically distinct precancerous lesions. *J. Virol.* 54:675–81

24. de Britton RC, Hildesheim A, de Lao SL, Brinton LA, Sathya P, Reeves WC. 1993. Human papillomaviruses and other influences on survival from cervical cancer in Panama. *Obstet. Gynecol.* 81:19–24

25. de Sanjose S, Munoz N, Bosch FX, Reimann K, Pedersen NS, et al. 1994. Sexually transmitted agents and cervical neoplasia in Colombia and Spain. *Int. J. Cancer* 56:353–63

26. de Sanjose S, Santamaria M, Alonso de Ruiz P, Aristizabal N, Guerrero E, et al. 1992. HPV types in women with normal cervical cytology. See Ref. 64, pp. 75–84

27. Delgado-Rodriguez M, Sillero-Arenas M, Martin-Moreno JM, Galvez-Vargas R. 1992. Oral contraceptives and cancer of the cervix uteri—a meta-analysis. *Acta Obstet. Gynecol. Scand.* 71:368–76

28. Eluf-Neto J, Booth M, Munoz N, Bosch FX, Meijer CJLM, Walboomers JMM. 1994. Human papillomavirus and invasive cervical cancer in Brazil. *Br. J. Cancer* 69:114–19

29. Galloway DA. 1994. Papillomavirus capsids: a new approach to identify serological markers of HPV infection. *J. Natl. Cancer Inst.* 86:474–75

30. Graham S, Priore R, Graham M, Browne R, Burnett W, West D. 1979. Genital cancer in wives of penile cancer patients. *Cancer* 44:1870–74

31. Gravitt PE, Manos MM. 1992. Polymerase chain reaction-based methods for the detection of human papillomavirus DNA. See Ref. 64, pp. 121–33

32. Herrero R, Brinton LA, Reeves WC, Brenes MM, deBritton RC, et al. 1990. Injectable contraceptives and risk of in-

vasive cervical cancer: evidence of an association. *Int. J. Cancer* 46:5–7

33. Herrero R, Brinton LA, Reeves WC, Brenes MM, Tenorio F, et al. 1989. Invasive cervical cancer and smoking in Latin America. *J. Natl. Cancer Inst.* 81:205–11

34. Hildesheim A, Mann V, Brinton LA, Szklo M, Reeves WC, Rawls WE. 1991. Herpes simplex virus type 2: a possible interaction with human papillomavirus types 16/18 in the development of invasive cervical cancer. *Int. J. Cancer* 49: 335–40

35. Ho GYF, Burk RD, Klein S, Kadish AS, Chang CJ, et al. 1995. Persistent genital human papillomavirus infection as a risk factor for persistent cervical dysplasia. *J. Natl. Cancer Inst.* 87:1365–71

36. Holly EA, Cress RD, Ahn DK, Aston DA, Kristiansen JJ, et al. 1993. Detection of mutagens in cervical mucus in smokers and nonsmokers. *Cancer Epidemiol. Biomarkers Prev.* 2:223–28

37. Holly EA, Petrakis NL, Friend NF, Sarles DL, Lee RE, Flander LB. 1986. Mutagenic mucus in the cervix of smokers. *J. Natl. Cancer Inst.* 76:983–86

38. Hsu EM, McNicol PJ, Guijon FB, Paraskevas M. 1993. Quantification of HPV-16 E6-E7 transcription in cervical intraepithelial neoplasia by reverse transcriptase polymerase chain reaction. *Int. J. Cancer* 55:397–401

39. Hulka BS. 1982. Risk factors for cervical cancer. *J. Chronic Dis.* 35:3–11

40. Int. Agency Res. Cancer. 1995. *IARC Monographs on the Evaluation of Carcinogenic Risks to Humans. Vol. 64. Human Papillomavirus.* Lyon: IARC

41. Kirnbauer R, Hubbert NL, Wheeler CM, Becker TM, Lowy DR, Schiller JT. 1994. A virus-like particle enzyme-linked immunosorbent assay detects serum antibodies in a majority of women infected with human papillomavirus type 16. *J. Natl. Cancer Inst.* 86:494–99

42. Kiviat NB, Critchlow CW, Kurman RJ. 1992. Reassessment of the morphological continuum of cervical intraepithelial lesions: Does it reflect different stages in the progression to cervical carcinoma? See Ref. 64, pp. 59–66

43. Kiviat NB, Koutsky LA. 1993. Specific human papillomavirus types as the causal agents of most cervical intraepithelial neoplasia: implications for current views and treatment. *J. Natl. Cancer Inst.* 85:934–35

44. Kiviat NB, Koutsky LA, Critchlow CW, Lorincz AT, Cullen AP, et al. 1992. Prevalence and cytologic manifestations of human papilloma virus (HPV) types 6, 11, 16, 18, 31, 33, 35, 42, 43, 44, 45, 51, 52, and 56 among 500 consecutive women. *Int. J. Gynecol. Pathol.* 11:197–203

45. Kjaer SK, Dahl C, Engholm G, Bock JE, Lynge E, Jensen OM. 1992. Case-control study of risk factors for cervical neoplasia in Denmark. II. Role of sexual activity, reproductive factors, and venereal infections. *Cancer Causes Control* 3:339–48

46. Kosary C, Schiffman MH, Trimble EL. 1993. Cervix uteri. In *SEER Cancer Statistics Review*, ed. B Miller, et al. Bethesda: NCI, NIH Publ. #93.2789

47. Koutsky LA, Holmes KK, Critchlow CW, Stevens CE, Paavonen J, et al. 1992. A cohort study of the risk of cervical intraepithelial neoplasia grade 2 or 3 in relation to papillomavirus infection. *N. Engl. J. Med.* 327:1272–78

48. Lacey CJN. 1992. Assessment of exposure to sexually transmitted agents other than human papillomavirus. See Ref. 64, pp. 93–105

49. Levine AJ, Harper J, Hilborne L, Rosenthal DL, Weismeier E, Haile RW. 1993. HPV DNA and the risk of squamous intraepithelial lesions of the uterine cervix in young women. *Am. J. Clin. Pathol.* 100:6–11

50. Ley C, Bauer HM, Reingold A, Schiffman MH, Chambers JC, et al. 1991. Determinants of genital human papillomavirus infection in young women [see comments]. *J. Natl. Cancer Inst.* 83:997–1003

51. Li JY, Li FP, Blot WJ, Miller RW, Fraumeni JF Jr. 1982. Correlation between cancers of the uterine cervix and penis in China. *J. Natl. Cancer Inst.* 69:1063–65

52. Lorincz AT, Lancaster W, Temple G. 1986. Cloning and characterization of the DNA of a new human papillomavirus from a woman with dysplasia of the uterine cervix. *J. Virol.* 58:225–29

53. Lorincz AT, Quinn A, Lancaster W, Temple GF. 1987. A new type of papillomavirus associated with cancer of the uterine cervix. *Virology* 159:187–90

54. Lorincz AT, Reid R, Jenson AB, Greenberg MD, Lancaster W, Kurman RJ. 1992. Human papillomavirus infection of the cervix: relative risk associations of 15 common anogenital types. *Obstet. Gynecol.* 79:328–37

55. Lorincz AT, Schiffman MH, Jaffurs WJ, Marlow J, Quinn AP, Temple GF. 1990. Temporal associations of human papillomavirus infection with cervical cy-

tologic abnormalities. *Am. J. Obstet. Gynecol.* 162:645–51

56. Lowy DR, Kirnbauer R, Schiller JT. 1994. Genital human papillomavirus infection. *Proc. Nat. Acad. Sci. USA* 91: 2436–40

57. MacGregor JE, Campbell MK, Mann EM, Swanson KY. 1994. Screening for cervical intraepithelial neoplasia in north east Scotland shows fall in incidence and mortality from invasive cancer with concomitant rise in preinvasive disease. *Br. Med. J.* 308:1407–11

58. MacGregor JE, Innes G. 1980. Carcinoma of penis and cervix (letter). *Lancet* 1:1246–47

59. Martinez I. 1969. Relationship of squamous cell carcinoma of the cervix uteri to squamous cell carcinoma of the penis: among Puerto Rican women married to men with penile carcinoma. *Cancer* 24:777–80

60. McCann MF, Irwin DE, Walton LA, Hulka BS, Morton JL, Axelrad CM. 1992. Nicotine and cotinine in the cervical mucus of smokers, passive smokers, and nonsmokers. *Cancer Epidemiol. Biomarkers Prev.* 1:125–29

61. Munoz N, Bosch FX, de Sanjose S, Shah KV. 1994. The role of HPV in the etiology of cervical cancer. *Mutat. Res.* 305:293–301

62. Munoz N, Bosch FX, De Sanjose S, Tafur L, Izarzugaza I, et al. 1992. The causal link between human papillomavirus and invasive cervical cancer: a population-based case-control study in Colombia and Spain. *Int. J. Cancer* 52: 743–49

63. Munoz N, Bosch FX, de Sanjose S, Vergara A, del Moral A, et al. 1993. Risk factors for cervical intraepithelial neoplasia grade III/carcinoma in situ in Spain and Colombia. *Cancer Epidemiol. Biomarkers Prev.* 2:423–31

64. Munoz N, Bosch FX, Shah KV, Meheus A. 1992. *The Epidemiology of Cervical Cancer and Human Papillomavirus.* IARC Sci. Publi. No. 119. Lyon: IARC

65. Munoz N, Kato I, Bosch FX, de Sanjose S, Sundquist V-A, et al. 1995. Cervical cancer and herpes simplex virus type 2: case-control studies in Spain and Colombia, with special reference to immunoglobulin-G sub-classes. *Int. J. Cancer* 60:438–42

66. Nasiell K, Nasiell M, Vaclavinkova V. 1983. Behavior of moderate cervical dysplasia during long-term follow-up. *Obstet. Gynecol.* 61:609–14

67. Palefsky JM, Holly EA. 1995. Molecular virology and epidemiology of human papillomavirus and cervical cancer. *Cancer Epidemiol. Biomarkers Prev.* 4: 415–28

68. Pater A, Bayatpour M, Pater M. 1990. Oncogenic transformation by human papillomavirus type 16 deoxyribonucleic acid in the presence of progesterone or progestins from oral contraceptives. *Am. J. Obstet. Gynecol.* 162: 1099–103

69. Pater MM, Mittal R, Pater A. 1994. Role of steroid hormones in potentiating transformation of cervical cells by human papillomaviruses. *Trends Microbiol.* 2:229–34

70. Phillips AN, Smith GD. 1994. Cigarette smoking as a potential cause of cervical cancer: Has confounding been controlled? *Int. J. Epidemiol.* 23:42–49

71. Reeves WC, Brinton LA, Garcia M, Brenes MM, Herrero R, et al. 1989. Human papillomavirus infection and cervical cancer in Latin America. *N. Engl. J. Med.* 320:1437–41

72. Reeves WC, Caussy D, Brinton LA, Brenes MM, Montalvan P, et al. 1987. Case-control study of human papillomaviruses and cervical cancer in Latin America. *Int. J. Cancer* 40:450–54

73. Reeves WC, Gary HE Jr, Johnson PR, Icenogle JP, Brenes MM, et al. 1994. Risk factors for genital papillomavirus infection in populations at high and low risk for cervical cancer. *J. Infect. Dis.* 170:753–58

74. Reeves WC, Rawls WE, Brinton LA. 1989. Epidemiology of genital papillomaviruses and cervical cancer. *Rev. Infect. Dis.* 11:426–39

75. Reid R, Greenberg M, Jenson AB, Husain M, Willett J, et al. 1987. Sexually transmitted papillomavirus infections. 1. The anatomic distribution and pathologic grade of neoplastic diseases associated with different viral types. *Am. J. Obstet. Gynecol.* 156:212–22

76. Richart RM, Barron BA. 1969. A follow-up study of patients with cervical dysplasia. *Am. J. Obstet. Gynecol.* 105: 383–93

77. Rigoni-Stern D. 1842. Fatti statistici relativi alle mallattie cancrose che servirono di base alle poche cose dette dal dott. *G. Servire Progr. Pathol. Terap. Ser.* 2 2:507–17

78. Sasson IM, Haley NJ, Hoffmann D, Wynder EL, Hellberg D, Nilsson S. 1985. Cigarette smoking and neoplasia of the uterine cervix: smoke constituents in cervical mucus (letter). *N. Engl. J. Med.* 312:315–16

79. Schiffman MH. 1992. Recent progress in defining the epidemiology of human papillomavirus infection and cervical

neoplasia. *J. Natl. Cancer Inst.* 84:394–98

80. Schiffman MH. 1993. Latest HPV findings: some clinical implications. *Contemp. Obstet. Gynecol.* pp. 27–40

81. Schiffman MH. 1995. New epidemiology of human papillomavirus infection and cervical neoplasia. *J. Natl. Cancer Inst.* 87:1345–47

82. Schiffman MH, Bauer HM, Hoover RN, Glass AG, Cadell DM, et al. 1993. Epidemiologic evidence showing that human papillomavirus infection causes most cervical intraepithelial neoplasia. *J. Natl. Cancer Inst.* 85:958–64

83. Schiffman MH, Kiviat N, Bork RD, Shah K, Daniel R, et al. 1995. Accuracy and interlaboratory reliability of HPV DNA testing using hybrid capture. *J. Clin. Microbiol.* 33:545–50

84. Schiffman MH, Schatzkin A. 1994. Test reliability is critically important to molecular epidemiology: an example from studies of human papillomavirus infection and cervical neoplasia. *Cancer Res.* 54:1944s–47s

85. Schwartz SM, Weiss NS. 1986. Increased incidence of adenocarcinoma of the cervix in young women in the United States. *Am. J. Epidemiol.* 124:1045–47

86. Sedman SA, Barbosa MS, Vass WC, Hubbert NL, Haas JA, et al. 1991. The full-length E6 protein of human papillomavirus type 16 has transforming and trans-activating activities and cooperates with E7 to immortalize keratinocytes in culture. *J. Virol.* 65:4860–66

87. Smotkin D, Prokoph H, Wettstein FO. 1989. Oncogenic and nononcogenic human genital papillomaviruses generate the E7 mRNA by different mechanisms. *J. Virol.* 63:1441–47

88. Tindle RW, Frazer IH. 1990. Immunology of anogenital human papillomavirus (HPV) infection. Australian and New Zealand. *J. Obstet. Gynaecol.* 30:370–75

89. Vandenvelde C, Van Beers D. 1993. High-risk genital papillomaviruses and degree of dysplastic changes in the cervix: a prospective study by fast multiplex polymerase chain reaction in Belgium. *J. Med. Virol.* 39:273–77

90. Weiss LK, Kau T-Y, Sparks BT, Swanson GM. 1994. Trends in cervical cancer incidence among young black and white women in metropolitan Detroit. *Cancer* 73:1849–54

91. WHO Collaborative Study of Neoplasia and Steroid Contraceptives. 1993. Invasive squamous-cell cervical carcinoma and combined oral contraceptives: results from a multinational study. *Int. J. Cancer* 55:228–36

92. Wingo PA, Tong T, Bolden S. 1995. Cancer Statistics, 1995. *CA. Cancer J. Clin.* 45:8–30

93. Winkelstein W Jr. 1977. Smoking and cancer of the uterine cervix: hypothesis. *Am. J. Epidemiol.* 10:257–59

94. Winkelstein W Jr. 1990. Smoking and cervical cancer—current status: a review. *Am. J. Epidemiol.* 131:945–57

95. zur Hausen H. 1974. Attempts to detect detect virus specific DNA in human tumors. *Int. J. Cancer* 13:650–56

96. zur Hausen H. 1988. Papillomaviruses in human cancers. *Mol. Carcinog.* 1: 147–50.

Annu. Rev. Public Health. 1996. 17:85–96

OVARIAN CANCER

C. Westhoff

Department of Obstetrics and Gynecology and School of Public Health, College of
Physicians and Surgeons, Columbia University, New York, New York 10032

KEY WORDS: ovarian neoplasms, oral contraceptives, familial diseases, infertility

ABSTRACT

Ovarian cancer incidence rates are highest and stable in white populations; in
Asia previously low incidence rates may be increasing. Most cases present with
disseminated disease, and mortality rates remain high despite the use of aggressive polychemotherapy. Mortality among younger women has decreased, which
has been attributed to widespread use of oral contraceptives. Studies consistently
show a protective effect of oral contraceptives that increases with duration of
use; no dose effect has been identified to date. Risk decreases substantially with
increasing numbers of pregnancies; periods of lactation are relatively less protective. Periods of oral contraceptive use are less protective than equal periods
of pregnancy. These factors may protect against ovarian cancer due to inhibition
of ovulation or due to suppression of another aspect of ovarian function. Hysterectomy and tubal ligation are both protective, perhaps by preventing the ascent
of environmental carcinogens that are as yet unidentified. A positive family
history substantially increases risk; mutations in the BRCA1 gene may be responsible for about 5% of cases. No other exposures have been consistently
associated with disease risk. Whether risk is modified by ovarian damage mediated by dietary galactose is being evaluated; studies to date have conflicting
results. The effect of infertility and its treatments on ovarian cancer risk is
controversial; two studies suggest that infertility treatments increase risk.

DISEASE BURDEN

Incidence

Invasive ovarian cancer annual incidence rates of about 12–15 cases per
100,000 white women are seen in the United States (53) and also among
women in Europe, Scandinavia, Israel, Australia and New Zealand (45). Incidence in the U.S. among population groups with non-European ancestry is
about 8–10 cases per 100,000. Incidence in countries populated by few or no
people of European ancestry is about 2–6 cases per 100,000 women per year.
Age-specific incidence rates are low in young women, with the most common
epithelial cancers being essentially absent prior to puberty. Incidence rates

85

increase logarithmically during young adulthood; rates reach about 40 cases per 100,000 women by age 50 and increase more slowly thereafter to an incidence near 50 cases per 100,000 by age 65. Most data sets suggest a decrease or a plateau in incidence rates after age 75, but this may represent a decrease in the accuracy of diagnosis. Ovarian cancer incidence rates do not take into account what portion of the population has intact ovaries and is therefore at risk of the disease. Incidence rates at older ages may consequently be underestimated in countries such as the U.S. where bilateral oophorectomy is prevalent. Secular changes in frequency of oophorectomy may also distort changes in cancer incidence rates (52, 68). Nevertheless, the shape of the age incidence curve for epithelial ovarian cancers appears to be similar in various populations. The nonepithelial cancers are so rare that stable estimates of their incidence are difficult.

A subtype of ovarian cancer called low-malignant potential or borderline cancer has been described; this good prognosis subgroup may be analogous to in-situ cancers of other organs. Until recently, low malignant potential cases were not reportable to most cancer registries; therefore, data regarding the incidence of this subgroup are limited. Analyses of data from the SEER registry in western Washington State from 1975–83 indicate that borderline ovarian cancers are diagnosed in about 4 per 100,000 women per year, and that they may be increasing (28).

Although increasing numbers of epithelial ovarian cancer cases are predicted in the U.S. and in European countries due to the changing age structure of the population, there is no evidence of increasing age-specific incidence rates in the high-incidence countries (15, 16, 45, 53, 70, 71). In Japan, which is a low-incidence country, mortality, an acceptable surrogate for incidence, has increased in recent decades from 2.2 per 100,000 in 1958–62 to 4.2 per 100,000 in 1978–82 (38). Incidence rates in Singapore and China have increased from 3.2 per 100,000 to 8.6 per 100,000 during the same time periods (50). Few data are available regarding incidence in other low-incidence countries (50). Worldwide, it remains difficult to distinguish improved accuracy of diagnosis and more complete registration of these cancers from small increases in the true incidence of the disease. Relative incidence of various histological subtypes of the invasive epithelial cancers may be changing (9).

Mortality

Ovarian cancer mortality remains high despite the introduction of new chemotherapeutic drugs and polychemotherapy regimens in recent decades. In the United States, overall mortality for invasive ovarian cancers is about 10 per 100,000 women per year, and overall five-year survival among cases has improved very slightly to about 37%, with most fatalities occurring within three years of diagnosis. About 65% of cases are diagnosed with regional or distant spread of the disease, and survival remains dismal in this large group (77). Even women with localized disease die from ovarian cancer, and understaging due to limited surgery or occult metastases may explain the bad outcomes in apparently favorable cases. Nearly all borderline cases are localized; their mortality is lower than that observed for localized cases with true invasive features. Stage at diagnosis is the strongest predictor of disease-specific mortality, but age is also important. Younger women are more likely to be diagnosed at early stages, and they also experience better stage-specific survival rates. This may, at least in part, be due to less aggressive care provided to older cases (33).

Data from England and Wales (69) and from the U.S. (1) show that ovarian cancer mortality has dropped since the late 1970s among women younger than 55 years. Villard-Mackintosh et al (69) show that most of the improvement in England has occurred among women born since 1930 who have been widely exposed to combined oral contraceptives (see below). Not enough data exist in either country to confirm these long-term mortality trends with incidence data over the same period.

PROTECTIVE FACTORS

Parity

An ecologic analysis by Beral showed a tight linear inverse relationship between total fertility rates and ovarian cancer mortality rates for birth cohorts of English and American women (3; see also Table 1). Since then, case-control analyses have consistently shown a strong protective effect of parity against epithelial ovarian cancer. In a collaborative analysis of data from 12 US case-control studies Whittemore and colleagues found a monotonic decrease in risk associated with each additional term pregnancy in analyses, including more than 2000 cases of invasive cancer and almost 9000 controls (75, 76). In analyses of data from white subjects in the population-based studies, the relative risk of epithelial ovarian cancer was 0.47 for women with any term pregnancy compared to women with none. The protective effect of parity was almost identical (RR = 0.54) in subjects with borderline epithelial tumors (30). Analyses of 110 black cases with invasive or borderline ovarian cancers compared to 365 black controls showed a similar protective effect of term pregnancy (37).

In a combined analysis of three European studies (U.K., Greece, and Italy) with 1140 cases and 2724 controls, Negri and colleagues also identified a monotonic decrease in risk with each additional pregnancy (49). Smaller case-control studies from Japan (44), Shanghai (61), and Beijing (7) all identified

Table 1 Established risk factors for ovarian cancer (relative risks of at least 2.0)

Factor	High-risk group	Low-risk group
Age	60+ years	<50 years
Locations	Europe, North America, Israel	Africa, Asia
Parity	Nulliparous	Parous
Oral contraceptive use	Never users	Ever users
Family history	2+ affected relatives	No affected relatives

a decrease in risk of ovarian cancer with increasing numbers of births. A Norwegian cohort with 445 cases of ovarian cancer found a protective effect of parity that agrees with the findings from case-control studies (40).

Data regarding other pregnancy related factors are less extensive. All of the case-control analyses cited above showed a decrease in risk associated with incomplete pregnancies, but the effect was not as strong or as consistent as the effect of a term pregnancy. Age at first live birth had no consistent effect in the US collaborative analyses, in Shanghai, or in Beijing, but risk increased with age at first live birth in the collaborative European analyses. Lactation was slightly protective in the collaborative US analyses, but not in the analyses from Japan and Beijing. Analyses of the WHO Collaborative Study, which included subjects from seven countries (56), did identify a significantly reduced risk associated with lactation. All of the studies that found an independent protective effect of lactation showed a stronger effect of parity itself. Analyses from the Cancer and Steroid Hormone study showed that a month of pregnancy was more protective than a month of lactation (24). A case-control study of borderline tumors from western Washington State identified similar risks for these reproductive variables (29).

Oral Contraceptives

The collaborative US analyses identified decreased risk of both invasive and borderline ovarian cancers in both black and white oral contraceptive (OC) users (30, 37, 76). In the comparisons with the largest numbers of subjects, those where the cases were white women with invasive epithelial cancers, there was a monotonically decreasing risk of cancer with increasing duration of oral contraceptive use (for ever use OR = 0.70 in hospital-based studies, and 0.66 in population-based studies). Little additional protection was observed after six years of use. The collaborative European analyses showed a similar decrease in risk with increasing duration of use, even among women with five or more years of use (RR = 0.60 for ever use) (22). The WHO collaborative study compared 367 cases and 2397 controls from nine centers in seven countries. In the overall analysis there was decreasing risk of epithelial ovarian cancer with increasing duration of oral contraceptive use (65). The magnitude of protection was similar among centers in developed and developing countries (RR = 0.75 for ever use). The individual case-control studies from Japan (44) and Beijing (7) do not report on this association because of no oral contraceptive use in those populations; however, the Shanghai study is the sole report in the literature that identifies an increased risk of ovarian cancer associated with OC use (61). In that study ever-use of OCs among controls was 7%; the overall risk of 1.8 associated with ever use had 95% confidence intervals of 0.8–4.1.

Hankinson and colleagues performed a meta-analysis of the results of the studies described above, using original results from the individual studies that contributed to the collaborative analyses (36), and several other case-control studies. She also included the results from Oxford-Family Planning Association, Royal College of General Practitioners, and Walnut Creek cohort studies. These cohorts followed-up over 50,000 women who had been enrolled during the 1960s. The summary relative risk for ever-use from the nine hospital-based case-control studies was 0.70; for the eight population-based case-control studies the summary relative risk was 0.63; for the three cohort studies the relative risk was 0.43. All of these summary relative risks had tight 95% confidence intervals that did not include 1.0. They found no evidence that this protective effect was modified by parity or age. Their regression model predicts 11% reduction in risk with each year of OC use.

Because most ovarian cancer is diagnosed long after the reproductive years, nearly all of the oral contraceptive use reported in the above studies occurred during the early years of OC availability when the hormone content was several times greater than that of currently used OCs. Of all of the above studies only the Cancer and Steroid Hormone (CASH) study had sufficient information to look at risk by OC formulation. It is reassuring that they found similar levels of protection among subjects who reported use of low-dose and high-dose oral contraceptives; however, their power to look at this was limited. Because OC formulations continue to change, inferences from epidemiologic studies regarding newer exposures will need to be made cautiously (74).

Hysterectomy and Tubal Ligation

American studies are the most useful to examine the effect of hysterectomy on ovarian cancer risk because this operation is much more common in the USA than elsewhere (68). The collaborative US case-control analyses identified a decreased risk of invasive epithelial ovarian cancer among women who had either a tubal ligation (adjusted OR = 0.59 in hospital-based studies, and

0.87 in population-based studies) or a hysterectomy (OR = 0.66, and 0.88), with no evidence of an effect of time since surgery (76). Data from the Nurses' Health Study (25) showed a strong protective effect of tubal ligation (multivariate RR = 0.33) and hysterectomy (multivariate RR = 0.67). A decreased risk associated with tubal ligation (OR = 0.4) was reported from Japan (44), and a decreased risk associated with hysterectomy (OR = 0.7) was reported from Italy (51); other studies have not reported on these exposures. That these operations protect by preventing access of carcinogens to the upper genital tract is hypothesized, but existing data are too sparse to evaluate this idea rigorously.

RISK FACTORS

Diet

The main dietary factors of current interest are animal fat and galactose, a mono-saccharide portion of lactose that is a major constituent of dairy products. Increased risk of ovarian cancer has been associated with consumption of meat (42), whole milk (43), or animal fat (12, 62, 64) in several studies with various approaches to defining nutrient intake. However, many other published studies report no association between ovarian cancer and fats or dairy products (5, 18, 63, 67). None of these reports considers how fat consumption might influence ovarian cancer risk. Effects of other nutrients are even more limited.

The hypothesis that galactose-induced ovarian damage might lead to increased gonadotropin secretion and consequent increased ovarian cancer risk has stimulated interest in lactose consumption and metabolism (14). Ecological analyses provide support for this hypothesis, and one case-control study reported increased ovarian cancer risk among women who consumed more lactose and also had less activity of the enzyme galactose-1-phosphate uridyltransferase, which is needed to metabolize the galactose molecule (13, 27). Two subsequent case-control studies have not found associations that support this hypothesis (32, 54). Large studies that are under way may resolve this issue.

Infertility and Its Treatments

Essentially all analyses have noted that childless women have higher rates of ovarian cancer than parous women; however, distinguishing the effects of childlessness or low parity itself on ovarian cancer risk from any effects due to the causes of low parity is not yet settled (72). Four cohort studies of infertile women have calculated risk ratios, comparing observed cases in the cohort to expected cases based on age-specific population rates of ovarian cancer. Reports from two cohorts indicated no effect (8, 55) and one identified a weak, nonsignificant effect (4), but all of these cohorts had limited woman-years of observation, and thus had little statistical power to identify even strong associations. The fourth study (57), using a case-cohort analysis, identified an overall ovarian cancer risk 2.5 times greater than expected. The excess risk was concentrated among those infertile women who had used clomiphene, an ovulation induction drug, for 12 or more cycles. Only 4 of the 11 ovarian tumors identified in that study were invasive epithelial cancers that have high case fatality; the other cases included two granulosa cell tumors and five epithelial tumors of low malignant potential, which all tend to be curable. That study is being extended to a larger cohort.

The meta-analysis of US case-control studies identified an increased risk among infertile women (76) that was essentially limited to the subgroup of nulliparous women who used fertility drugs; that subgroup had a relative risk of 27.0 based on 12 exposed cases and one exposed control. The meaning of this finding has been controversial primarily because the treatments used were not identified or verified, and also because the timing of these treatments preceded the introduction of any of the fertility drugs in current use (2, 35, 39). In Italy, fertility drug use was not associated with ovarian cancer risk in a small case-control study (21). Because ovulation induction drugs increase ovarian activity, it is plausible that their effect on ovarian cancer risk might be opposite to the protective effect of oral contraceptives that decrease ovarian activity; however, the baseline ovarian cancer risk of oligo-ovulatory women is unknown (and might be low), so the net effect of infertility plus fertility drugs is difficult to predict.

Family History

Nearly all case-control studies that have evaluated ovarian cancer risk in terms of family history have identified increased risk in women whose relatives have been diagnosed with ovarian cancer (6, 10, 34, 48, 66). To date, no studies have verified the reported family histories. The most detailed and precise analyses come from the Cancer and Steroid Hormone study (59) in which the adjusted relative risk in first and second degree relatives was 3.6; this risk was similar for different histological types of invasive epithelial cancers, but no increased risk was identified for borderline cancers.

Due to the results of case-control studies and to the clinical recognition of familial clusters of this cancer, numerous registries soliciting affected women and family members have been established in the U.S. and the U.K. (73). These registries are involved in pedigree analysis, collection of blood for molecular genetic analyses, and clinical programs aimed at early detection of incident cases among family members. Case reports and pedigree analyses indicate the occurrence of site-specific ovarian cancer families, breast-ovarian cancer families, and increased ovarian cancer risk in other cancer family syndromes such as the hereditary nonpolyposis colorectal cancer (HNPCC) syndrome. These syndromes may be caused by a highly penetrant autosomal dominant mutation (23, 46, 58); however, this mechanism may be responsible for only about 5% of all ovarian cancer. Mutations in the BRCA1 gene are responsible for the disease in some portion of the site-specific ovarian and breast-ovarian cancer families (17, 60). Other autosomal dominant genes, such as BRCA2, may also prove to be involved (47).

The evidence that other inherited characteristics influence ovarian cancer risk is still limited. Cramer has proposed that susceptibility is influenced by variants in a gene that regulates galactose metabolism, and has identified an increased frequency of these variants in women who have first degree relatives with ovarian cancer compared to women with no such family history (11). Blood group type "A" has been frequently reported to be more common in women with ovarian cancer, and is hypothesized to influence risk due to diminished immunologic surveillance of those tumors that present antigens similar to the "A" antigen (31). These inherited characteristics are common and appear to have at most a small influence on cancer risk.

The recognition that there are some families at high risk of ovarian cancer due to a mutation in the gene known as BRCA1 has cause widespread interest. The extremely high risks among women who are members of families known to carry these mutations apply to a very small portion of the population. Identification of families that may be affected and quantification of risk within those families needs to continue in research settings in order to identify the most relevant specific mutations.

PATHOGENESIS

In 1971, Fathalla (19) proposed that the risk of epithelial ovarian cancer in the human female—and the domestic fowl—may be a consequence of incessant ovulation. This hypothesis is supported by the consistently observed protective effect of pregnancy, breast-feeding, and oral contraceptive use, all of which inhibit ovulation. In 1979, Casagrande and colleagues (6) extended this concept by calculating ovarian cancer risk according to ovulatory age. They found that the total time spent ovulating between menarche and menarche was more closely associated with risk than either parity or oral contraceptive use alone. The ovulation hypothesis predicts that a month of anovulation for any reason should provide equal protection against ovarian cancer. Analyses from the CASH study (24), however, showed that a month of pregnancy is more protective than a month of lactation or a month of oral contraceptive use. In addition, both the US collaborative (76) and the European (20, 41) analyses are inconsistent regarding the effect of age at menarche and menopause (both separately and as components of ovulatory age) on ovarian cancer risk. The observation of menstrual bleeding at the extremes of reproductive life may not be a good indicator of ovulation itself, and the calculation of ovulatory age based on recollection of these events may be incorrect.

Cramer (10a) also extended the ovulation hypothesis by observing that gonadotropin stimulation of the ovary, which is associated with ovulatory function, may increase ovarian cancer risk separate from the mechanical damage of ovulation itself. This hypothesis would allow for protection to vary with different causes of anovulation, and also can accommodate other factors that influence ovarian cancer risk. Based on the US Collaborative analyses, Whittemore and colleagues (74) state that present data appear to partly support and partly refute both of these hypotheses. Existing data and both hypotheses generally indicate that suppression of ovarian activity leads toward prevention of ovarian cancer.

FUTURE DIRECTIONS AND SCREENING

Several US case-control studies are currently under way with goals of providing more refined risk estimates for the factors discussed above. In addition, historical cohort studies are attempting to assess more precisely the risks of ovarian cancer that may be associated with treatment of infertility. Several investigators, both in the U.S. and U.K., are actively recruiting women with a family history of ovarian cancer in order to study risk and to provide early diagnosis.

The notion of early diagnosis has enormous appeal to clinicians and the public due to hopes that ovarian cancer mortality might be diminished. Both circulating tumor antigens and ultrasound imaging of the ovaries have been proposed as screening modalities (73). It is possible to identify early stage disease in some women by using these tests, but studies of screening have so far been either small or short term; therefore, there is no evidence regarding ovarian cancer mortality in screened populations. To remedy this ignorance, the National Cancer Institute is carrying out a cancer screening trial that will enroll some 70,000 women, and that may provide some indication whether ovarian cancer screening can decrease mortality from this disease. At present, there is no reason for women at average risk of ovarian cancer to seek out the tests that are being studied.

Literature Cited

1. Aoki, Kunio. 1992. *Death Rates for Malignant Neoplasms for Selected Sites by Sex and Five-Year Age Group in 33 Countries.* Int. Union Against Cancer
2. Balasch J, Barri PN. 1993. Follicular stimulation and ovarian cancer? *Hum. Reprod.* 8:990–96
3. Beral V, Fraser P, Chilvers C. 1978. Does pregnancy protect against ovarian cancer? *Lancet* (May 20):1083–87
4. Brinton LA, Melton LJ, Malkasian GD. Bond A, Hoover R. 1989. Cancer risk after evaluation for infertility. *Am. J. Epidemiol.* 129:712–22
5. Byers T, Marshall J, Graham S, Mettlin C, Swanson M. 1983. A case-controlled study of dietary and nondietary factors in ovarian cancer. *J. Natl. Cancer Inst.* 71:681–86
6. Casagrande J, Pike MC, Ross RK. 1979. Incessant ovulation and ovarian cancer. *Lancet* 2:170–73
7. Chen Y, Wu P, Lang J, Ge W, Hartge P, Brinton LA. 1992. Risk factors for epithelial ovarian cancer in Beijing, China. *Int. J. Epidemiol.* 21:23–29
8. Coulam CB, Annegers JF, Kranz JS. 1983. Chronic anovulation syndrome and associated neoplasia. *Obstet. Gynecol.* 61:403–7
9. Cramer DW, Devesa SS, Welch WR. 1981. Trends in the incidence of endometrioid and clear cell cancers of the ovary in the United States. *Am. J. Epidemiol.* 114:201–8
10. Cramer DW, Hutchison GB, Welch WR, Scully RE, Ryan KJ. 1983. Determinants of ovarian cancer risk. I. Reproductive experiences and family history. *J. Natl. Cancer Inst.* 71:711–16
10a. Cramer DW, Welch WR, 1983. Determinants of ovarian cancer risk. II. Inferences regarding pathogenesis. *J. Natl. Cancer Inst.* 71:717–21
11. Cramer DW, Muto MG, Reichardt JKV, Xu H, Welch WR, et al. 1994. Characteristics of women with a family history of ovarian cancer. I. Galactose consumption and metabolism. *Cancer* 74:1309–17
12. Cramer DW, Welch WR, Hutchison GB, Willett W, Scully RE. 1984. Dietary animal fat in relation to ovarian cancer risk. *Obstet. Gynecol.* 63:833–38
13. Cramer DW, Willett WC, Bell DA, Ng WG, Harlow BL, et al. 1989. Galactose consumption and metabolism in relation to the risk of ovarian cancer. *Lancet* (July 8):66–71
14. Cramer DW, Xu H, Sahi T. 1994. Adult hypolactasia, milk consumption, and age-specific fertility. *Am. J. Epidemiol.* 139:282–89
15. Doll R, Muir C, Waterhouse J. 1976. *Cancer Incidence in Five Continents, II.* IARC Sci. Publ. 15
16. Doll R, Payne P, Waterhouse J. 1966. *Cancer Incidence in Five Continents. I, A Technical Report.* Berlin: Springer-Verlag
17. Easton DF, Ford D, Bishop DT, and the Breast Cancer Linkage Consortium. 1995. Breast and ovarian cancer incidence in BRCA1-mutation carriers. *Am. J. Hum. Genet.* 56:265–71
18. Engle A, Muscat JE, Harris RE. 1991. Nutritional risk factors and ovarian cancer. *Nutr. Cancer* 15:240–47
19. Fathalla MF. 1971. Incessant ovulation—a factor in ovarian neoplasia. *Lancet* (July 17):163
20. Franceschi S, LaVecchia C, Booth M, Tzonou A, Negri E, et al. 1991. Pooled analysis of 3 European case-control studies of ovarian cancer: II. Age at menarche and at menopause. *Int. J. Cancer* 49:57–60
21. Franceschi S, LaVecchia C, Negri E, Guarneri S, Montella M, et al. 1994. Fertility drugs and risk of epithelial ovarian cancer in Italy. *Hum. Reprod.* 9:1673–75
22. Franceschi S, Parazzini F, Negri E, Booth M, LaVecchia C, et al. 1991. Pooled analysis of 3 European case-control studies of epithelial ovarian cancer: III. Oral contraceptive use. *Int. J. Cancer* 49:61–65
23. Gallion HH, Smith SA. 1994. Hereditary ovarian carcinoma. *Semin. Surg. Oncol.* 10:249–54
24. Gwinn ML, Lee NC, Rhodes PH, Layde PM, Rubin GL. 1990. Pregnancy, breast feeding, and oral contraceptives and the risk of epithelial ovarian cancer. *J. Clin. Epidemiol.* 43:559–68
25. Hankinson SE, Hunter DJ, Colditz GA, Willett WC, Stampfer MJ, et al. 1993. Tubal ligation, hysterectomy, and risk of ovarian cancer. *JAMA* 270:2813–18
26. Hankinson SE, Colditz GA, Hunter DJ, Spencer TL, Rosner B, Stampfer MJ. 1992. A quantitative assessment of oral contraceptive use and risk of ovarian cancer. *Obstet. Gynecol.* 80:708–14
27. Harlow BL, Cramer DW, Geller J, Willett WC, Bell DA, Welch WR. 1991. The influence of lactose consumption on the association of oral contraceptive

use and ovarian cancer risk. *Am. J. Epidemiol.* 134:445–61

28. Harlow BL, Weiss NS, Lofton S. 1987. Epidemiology of borderline ovarian tumors. *J. Natl. Cancer Inst.* 78:71–74

29. Harlow BL, Weiss NS, Roth GJ, Chu J, Daling JR. 1988. Case-control study of borderline ovarian tumors: reproductive history and exposure to exogenous female hormones. *Cancer Res.* 48:5849–52

30. Harris R, Whittemore Itnyre J, and the Collaborative Ovarian Cancer Group. 1992. Characteristics relating to ovarian cancer risk: collaborative analysis of 12 US case-control studies. III. Epithelial tumors of low malignant potential in white women. *Am. J. Epidemiol.* 136:1204–11

31. Henderson J, Seagrroatt V, Goldacre M. 1993. Ovarian cancer and ABO blood groups. *J. Epidemiol. Comm. Health* 47:287–89

32. Herrinton LJ, Weiss NS, Beresford SAA, Stanford JL, Wolrla DM, et al. 1995. Lactose and galactose intake and metabolism in relation to the risk of epithelial ovarian cancer. *Am. J. Epidemiol.* 141:407–16

33. Hightower RD, Nguyen HN, Averette HE, Hoskins W, Harrison T, Steren A. 1994. National survey of ovarian carcinoma IV: patterns of care and related survival for older patients. *Cancer* 73:377–83

34. Hildreth NG, Kelsey JL, LiVolsi VA, Fischer DB, Holford TR, et al. 1981. An epidemiologic study of epithelial carcinoma of the ovary. *Am. J. Epidemiol.* 114:398–405

35. International Federation of Fertility Societies. 1993. Fertility drugs and ovarian cancer. *Fertil. Steril.* 60:406–8

36. Irwin KL, Wiess NS, Lee NC, Peterson HB. 1991. Tubal sterilization, hysterectomy, and the subsequent occurrence of epithelial ovarian cancer. *Am. J. Epidemiol.* 134:362–69

37. John EM, Whittemore AS, Harris R, Itnyre J and the Collaborative Ovarian Cancer Group. 1993. Characteristics relating to ovarian cancer risk: collaborative analysis of seven U.S. case-controlled studies. Epithelial ovarian cancer in black women. *J. Natl. Cancer Inst.* 85:142–47

38. Kato I, Tominaga S, Duroishi T. 1987. Relationship between Westernization of dietary habits and mortality from breast and ovarian cancers in Japan. *Jpn. J. Cancer Res.* 78:349–57

39. Kaufman SC, Spirtas R, Alexander NJ.

1995. Do fertility drugs cause ovarian tumors? *J. Women's Health* 4:247–59

40. Kvale G, Heuch I, Nilssen S, Beral V. 1988. Reproductive factors and risk of ovarian cancer: a prospective study. *Int. J. Cancer* 42:246–51

41. LaVecchia C, Franceschi S, Gallus G, DeCarli A, Liberati A, Tognoni G. 1983. Incessant ovulation and ovarian cancer: a critical approach. *Int. J. Epidemiol.* 12:161–64

42. LaVecchia C, Decarli A, Negri E, Parazzini F, Gentile A, et al. 1987. Dietary factors and the risk of epithelial ovarian cancer. *J. Natl. Cancer Inst.* 79:663–69

43. Mettlin CJ, Piver MS. 1990. A case-control study of milk-drinking and ovarian cancer risk. *Am. J. Epidemiol.* 132:871–76

44. Mori M, Harabuchi I, Miyake H, Casagrande JT, Henderson BE, Ross RK. 1988. Reproductive, genetic, and dietary risk factors for ovarian cancer. *Am. J. Epidemiol.* 128:771–77

45. Muir CS, Waterhouse J, Mack T, Powell J, Whelan S. 1987. *Cancer Incidence in Five Continents, V.* IARC Sci. Publ. 88

46. Narod SA. 1994. Genetics of breast and ovarian cancer. *Br. Med. Bull.* 50:656–76

47. Narod SA, Ford D, Deville P, Barkardottir RB, Lynch HT, et al. 1995. An evaluation of genetic heterogeneity in 145 breast-ovarian cancer families. *Am. J. Hum. Genet.* 56:254–64

48. Narod SA, Madlensky L, Bradley L, Cole D, Tonin P, et al. 1994. Hereditary and familial ovarian cancer in southern Ontario. *Cancer* 74:2341–46

49. Negri E, Franceschi S, Tzonou A, Booth M, LaVecchia C, et al. 1991. Pooled analysis of 3 European case-control studies: I. Reproductive factors and risk of epithelial ovarian cancer. *Int. J. Cancer* 49:50–56

50. Parazzini F, Franceschi S, LaVecchia C, Fasoli M. 1991. The epidemiology of ovarian cancer. *Gynecol. Oncol.* 43:9–23

51. Parazzini F, Negri E, LaVecchia C, Luchini L, Mezzopane R. 1993. Hysterectomy, oophorectomy, and subsequent ovarian cancer risk. *Obstet. Gynecol.* 81:363–66

52. Persky V, Davis F, Barrett R, Ruby E, Sailer C, Levy P. 1990. Recent time trends in uterine cancer. *Am. J. Public Health* 80:935–39

53. Ries LAG, Hankey BF, Edwards BK, et al. 1990. *Cancer Statistics Review 1973–1987.* DHHS Publ No. (NIH) 90–2789. Bethesda, MD

54. Risch HA, Jain M, Marrett LD, Howe GR. 1994. Dietary lactose intake, lactose intolerance, and the risk of epithelial ovarian cancer in southern Ontario (Canada). *Cancer Caus. Cont.* 5:540–48

55. Ron E, Lunenfeld B, Menczer J, Blumstein T, Katz L, et al. 1987. Cancer incidence in a cohort of infertile women. *Am. J. Epidemiol.* 125:780–90

56. Rosenblatt KA, Thomas DB and the WHO Collaborative Study of Neoplasia and Steroid Contraceptives. 1993. Lactation and the risk of epithelial ovarian cancer. *Int. J. Epidemiol.* 22:192–97

57. Rossing MA, Daling JR, Weiss NS, Moore DE, Self SG. 1994. Ovarian tumors in a cohort of infertile women. *N. Engl. J. Med.* 331:771–76

58. Rowell S, Newman B, Boyd J, King M-C. 1994. Inherited predisposition to breast and ovarian cancer. *Am. J. Hum. Genet.* 55:861–65

59. Schildkraut JM, Thompson WD. 1988. Familial ovarian cancer: a population-based case-control study. *Am. J. Epidemiol.* 128:456–66

60. Shattuck-Eidens D, McClure M, Simard J, Labrie F, Narod S, et al. 1995. A collaborative survey of 80 mutations in the BRCA1 breast and ovarian cancer susceptibility gene. Implications for presymptomatic testing and screening. *JAMA* 273:535–41

61. Shu XO, Brinton LA, Gao YT, Yuan JM. 1989. Population-based case-control study of ovarian cancer in Shanghai. *Cancer Res.* 49:3670–74

62. Shu XO, Gao YT, Yuan JM, Ziegler RG, Brinton LA. 1989. Dietary factors and epithelial ovarian cancer. *Br. J. Cancer* 59:92–96

63. Slattery ML, Schuman KL, West DW, French TK, Robison LM. 1989. Nutrient intake and ovarian cancer. *Am. J. Epidemiol.* 130:497–502

64. Snowdon D, Phillips R. 1983. The relationship between fatal ovarian cancer and diet and reproductive factors. *Am. J. Epidemiol.* 118:439

65. Stanford JL, Thomas DB, Ray RM, Noonan EA and the WHO Collaborative Study of Neoplasia and Steroid Contraceptives. 1989. Epithelial ovarian cancer and combined oral contraceptives. *Int. J. Epidemiol.* 18:538–45

66. Tavani A, Negri E, Franceschi S, Parazzini F, LaVecchia C. 1993. Risk factors for epithelial ovarian cancer in women under age 45. *Eur. J. Cancer* 29A:1297–301

67. Tzonou A, Hsieh C, Polychronopoulou A, Kaprinis G, Toupadaki N, et al. 1993. Diet and ovarian cancer: a case-control study in Greece. *Int. J. Cancer* 55:411–14

68. US Department of Health and Human Services. 1987. *Hysterectomies in United States, 1965–84. Data from the Natl. Health Survey*, Ser. No. 92. DHHS Publ. No. (PHS) 88–1753. Washington, DC: GPO

69. Villard-Mackintosh L, Vessey MP, Jones L. 1989. The effects of oral contraceptives and parity on ovarian cancer trends in women under 55 years of age. *Br. J. Obstet. Gynecol.* 96:783–88

70. Waterhouse J, Muir C, Correa P, Powell J. 1976. *Cancer Incidence in Five Continents, III.* IARC Sci. Publ. 15

71. Waterhouse J, Muir C, Shanmugaratnam K, Powell J, Peacham D, Whelan S. 1982. *Cancer Incidence in Five Continents, IV.* IARC Sci. Publ. 42

72. Weiss NS. 1988. Measuring the separate effects of low parity and its antecedents on the incidence of ovarian cancer. *Am. J. Epidemiol.* 128:451–55

73. Westhoff C. 1994. Current status of screening for ovarian cancer. *Gynecol. Oncol.* 55:S34–37

74. Whittemore AS, Harris R, Itnyre J and the Collaborative Ovarian Cancer Group. 1992. Characteristics relating to ovarian cancer risk: collaborative analysis of 12 US case-control studies: IV. The pathogenesis of epithelial ovarian cancer. *Am. J. Epidemiol.* 136:1212–20

75. Whittemore AS, Harris R, Itnyre J, Halpern J and the Collaborative Ovarian Cancer Group. 1992. Characteristics relating to ovarian cancer risk: collaborative analysis of 12 US case-control studies: I. Methods. *Am. J. Epidemiol.* 136:1175–83

76. Whittemore AS, Harris R, Itnyre J and the Collaborative Ovarian Cancer Group. 1992. Characteristics relating to ovarian cancer risk: collaborative analysis of 12 US case-control studies: II. Invasive epithelial ovarian cancers in white women. *Am. J. Epidemiol.* 136:1184–203

77. Wynder EI, Dodo H, Barber HRK. 1969. Epidemiology of cancer of the ovary. *Cancer* 23:352–70

78. Yancik R, Gloeckler Ries L, Yates J. 1986. Ovarian cancer in the elderly: an analysis of surveillance, epidemiology, and end results program data. *Am. J. Obstet. Gynecol.* 154:639–47

Annu. Rev. Public Health. 1996. 17:97–114

FEMALE LUNG CANCER

Virginia L. Ernster

Department of Epidemiology and Biostatistics, School of Medicine, University of California, San Francisco, California 94143-0560

KEY WORDS: smoking, epidemiology, environmental tobacco smoke, radiation, occupation, diet, family history

ABSTRACT

Female lung cancer death rates increased by more than 550 percent between 1950 and 1991. In 1986 lung cancer surpassed breast cancer to become the leading cause of cancer death in women in the United States. The lung cancer epidemic is primarily attributable to cigarette smoking, which is responsible for at least 80% of the disease in women. There are gender differences in the distribution of lung cancer by histologic type, even controlling for smoking, and some data suggest greater female than male susceptibility to lung cancer at a given level of smoking. Exposure to environmental tobacco smoke increases risk of lung cancer in nonsmoking women. Family history of lung cancer, personal history of lung disease (e.g. asthma, chronic bronchitis, pneumonia, or tuberculosis), and a history of radiotherapy also appear to be associated with increased risk. Data specific to women on the role of household radon exposures or of specific occupational or environmental exposures are relatively sparse and inconsistent. Finally, many studies have reported a decreased risk of lung cancer in individuals who consume high levels of fruits and vegetables; however, clinical trials fail to support a beneficial effect of beta-carotene supplementation. Since cigarette smoking accounts for the vast majority of lung cancer cases in women, efforts to prevent adolescent girls from starting to smoke and to encourage cessation among established smokers have the greatest potential for reducing the female lung cancer burden.

LUNG CANCER STATISTICS

Introduction: A 20th Century Epidemic

During the first half of this century, lung cancer was a rare disease in women. However, between 1950 and 1991, lung cancer mortality rates in women in the United States increased by over 550% (1). Whereas lung cancer accounted for only 3% of all female cancer deaths in 1950, by 1995 it accounted for an estimated 24% (85a). Age-adjusted death rates for lung cancer surpassed those of breast cancer in white women in 1986 and in black women in 1990, and it

97

0163-7525/96/0510-0097$08.00

is now the leading cause of cancer death in U.S. women (1). There were an estimated 62,000 female deaths due to lung cancer in 1995, compared to 46,000 breast cancer deaths (85a). Were lung cancer not included, age-adjusted overall cancer death rates among U.S. women would have actually declined by 7.3% between 1973 and 1991. As discussed below, the lung cancer epidemic is primarily attributable to cigarette smoking, and therefore most cases are preventable.

Incidence and Mortality Rates by Race and Age

Age-adjusted lung cancer mortality rates have been similar in U.S. white and black women for decades. Age-adjusted mortality rates were 4.9 and 3.8 per 100,000 population for white and black women, respectively, in 1950 and 32.6 and 32.0, respectively, in 1991 (1, 59). However, when age-specific rates for recent years are examined, white women have higher rates in the age groups 65 years and older, while black women have higher rates under age 65. This suggests that, as the younger cohorts age, overall age-adjusted rates might be higher among black than white women in the future. On the other hand, smoking prevalence rates have recently plummeted in black female teens, which would portend lower lung cancer rates among black compared to white women in the more distant future. Lung cancer rates among women of other racial/ethnic groups in the U.S. are considerably lower than among whites and blacks. In California, for example, age-adjusted lung cancer death rates among Hispanic and Asian women are less than half those of whites and blacks (58), and smoking prevalence rates in the U.S. continue to be considerably lower in Hispanic and Asian women compared to white and black women (2). It should also be noted that there is a strong inverse relation between educational level and smoking prevalence in the U.S. today (2), which means that lung cancer will disproportionately affect individuals of lower socioeconomic status in the future.

The rate of the increase in overall age-adjusted lung cancer incidence rates among U.S. women appears to be slowing. Whereas age-adjusted rates increased 24.2% from 1977 to 1981, they increased only 9.1% from 1987 to 1991. The birth cohorts of women characterized by the highest smoking prevalence are still passing through the age groups when lung cancer risk is highest, so that overall female lung cancer rates are projected to continue to rise until around the year 2000 to 2010. About that time female lung cancer rates should converge with male rates, which have already begun to plateau (9, 14). Smoking prevalence among U.S. adult females declined from 31.9% in 1965 (24) to 22.5% in 1993 (3), although progress has been slow or nonexistent among white female teens since the early 1980s (62) and in white women of reproductive age in the early 1990s (3). Assuming continuing declines, the epidemic of lung cancer may be expected to wane substantially in the 21st century.

Although it is beyond the scope of this review to cover the global epidemiology of lung cancer, suffice to say that there are ominous signs of an international epidemic of the disease in women. Just as widespread adoption of cigarette smoking by women in the U.S. trailed that of men by about a quarter of a century, tobacco use is now common in men and gaining in popularity among women in many other parts of the world. As a result, the increases in lung cancer death rates already seen among men are being followed by increases in rates among women (42). In the late 1980s, the standardized ratios of male to female lung cancer rates in the United Kingdom and Scandinavian countries had declined to only 2 or 3, although they were still 10 or more in France, Italy, and Spain (40). Of major concern are the cigarette marketing campaigns targeted to women in Asia, Eastern Europe, Latin America, and other areas where tobacco prevalence among women has traditionally been low. Already in 1985 lung cancer was the sixth ranking cause of cancer death among women worldwide (70).

Survival Rates

Survival rates for lung cancer are among the poorest of all cancer sites. Five-year relative survival for U.S. women diagnosed with lung cancer between 1983–90 relative to that of women in the general population was only 15.8% for all races combined, 16.2% for whites, and 12.3% for blacks. Even two-year relative survival is relatively poor, 25.4% for women diagnosed in 1989. Women with localized lung cancer have much better five-year relative survival rates (52.5%) than women with regional (17.4%) or distant (2%) disease, but only 16% of all female cases diagnosed between 1983–90 were localized cases. Women under the age of 45 also appear to have better five-year relative survival (26.9%) than older women (13.2% for ages 65 years and older), although these data are not controlled for stage (59). To date, clinical trials to screen for early stage lung cancer have not demonstrated efficacy in reducing lung cancer mortality, at least among males, and the U.S. Preventive Services Task Force concluded that "screening asymptomatic persons for lung cancer by performing routine chest radiography or sputum cytology is not recommended" (81).

SMOKING: THE MAJOR RISK FACTOR FOR LUNG CANCER

Highlights of a Well-Established Causal Association

Lung cancer was rare in women before the adoption of cigarette smoking earlier in this century, and women in subgroups of the population that proscribe smoking continue to have much lower than average lung cancer rates. For example, lung cancer death rates during 1971–85 were about 55% lower among

Mormon women than among non-Mormon women in the state of Utah (48). About 80% of female lung cancer in the U.S. is currently thought to be attributable to cigarette smoking (68).

The well-established evidence that cigarette smoking is a strong causal risk factor for female lung cancer has been reviewed elsewhere (19, 78, 83). Risk of lung cancer increases with number of cigarettes smoked daily and particularly with years of cigarette smoking, and risk decreases with time since cessation. Data from the American Cancer Society's Cancer Prevention II prospective study reported the overall relative risk of lung cancer in female smokers to be 10.8, ranging from 5.5 among women who smoked 1–10 cigarettes per day to 22.0 among smokers of 31 or more cigarettes daily (67). Most studies have demonstrated that risk is reduced in female smokers of lower compared to higher tar cigarettes and in those who smoke filtered compared to unfiltered cigarettes (25, 44, 93); these studies were recently reviewed (69). All histologic types of lung cancer show strong dose-response relationships to smoking, but relative risks appear to be much greater for small-cell carcinoma and squamous cell carcinoma than for adenocarcinoma (19). The issue of whether age at initiation has an effect on lung cancer risk that is independent of lifetime amount of smoking has received relatively little attention. Hegman et al recently reported that, controlling for pack-years of smoking, women who began smoking at or before age 25 had a relative risk of lung cancer of 10 (95% CI: 4.7–21.2) compared to nonsmokers but that women who began smoking after age 25 had a relative risk of only 2.6 (95% CI: 0.53–12.4) compared to nonsmokers (31); the effect of age at smoking initiation on lung cancer risk was stronger for women than men. This area warrants further investigation, particularly in light of the young ages at which most smoking is initiated today.

Three issues that have received considerable attention in recent years are discussed below. Two issues have to do with possible gender differences in the relationship between smoking and lung cancer: Does the same pattern of smoking result in a greater risk of lung cancer for women than men, and are there gender differences among smokers in risk of developing specific histologic types of lung cancer? Another question is the effect of exposure to environmental tobacco smoke on lung cancer risk among nonsmokers.

Gender Differences in Risk of Lung Cancer Associated with Smoking

An area of great interest in the epidemiology of lung cancer is whether women are more susceptible than men to the effects of cigarette smoking. When data on smoking and lung cancer first began to emerge, studies were based largely on men, because widespread smoking among men predated that among women by about two decades. The first report of the U.S. Surgeon General on smoking and health concluded that the evidence for a causal link between smoking and lung cancer was strong for men but only "pointed in the same direction" for women (82). Within a decade or so, sufficient evidence had accumulated from cohort and case-control studies to conclude that a causal association existed in women as well (83), although it appeared that the relative risks of lung cancer for women smokers were considerably lower than for male smokers. For example, the American Cancer Society's Cancer Prevention I prospective study, which was based on adults enrolled around 1960, reported relative risks of 2.0 and 9.4 for females and males, respectively. However, the average male smoker in that study had started smoking earlier and had smoked much more than the average female smoker. About twenty years later, when the results for the ACS's Cancer Prevention II study, based on adults enrolled in the early 1980s, became available, the relative risk for female smokers had increased to 10.8. It was reported that female smokers in CPS II had begun smoking an average of 7.2 years earlier than those in CPS I and were much more likely to smoke 20 or more cigarettes daily (24). The relative risk for male smokers had also increased between CPS I and CPS II (to 17.4); historic gender differences in smoking patterns may well have been responsible for the continuing gender differences in lung cancer risk.

Some studies suggest that if degree of smoking (duration or amount smoked per day) is controlled, women smokers may actually be at greater risk of lung cancer than male smokers. In a large case-control study conducted in Western Europe, Lubin & Blot found that the increase in relative risk with increasing years of smoking and number of cigarettes smoked per day tended to be greater for women than men (44), and this finding held up across histologic types of lung cancer (43). In a registry-based case-control study, stratified by level of smoking (less than 20 cigarettes per day vs 20 or more cigarettes per day), Brownson et al reported higher odds ratios in women compared to men for all histologic types of lung cancer except adenocarcinoma. The gender difference was greatest for small cell carcinoma; for example, compared to nonsmokers, the odds ratio for smokers of 20 or more cigarettes per day was 53.1 in women and 19.2 in men (12). In a comparison of lung cancer cases with nonsmoking-associated cancer cases drawn from a population-based tumor registry, Osann et al found that women and men who smoked two or more packs per day had similar overall lung cancer odds ratios but that the odds ratio for small-cell carcinoma was much higher in females (57). Based on a comparison of results from one case-control study of white males and another of white females and stratifying smokers by years smoked (less than 35 years or 35 or more years) and amount smoked (less than 20 cigarettes per day or 20 or more cigarettes per day), Schoenberg et al also reported higher female than male odds ratios for small cell carcinoma but slightly higher male odds ratios for squamous cell carcinoma (64). In a hospital-based case-control study, Harris et al reported that for any given level of cumulative tar exposure, the odds ratios for developing either Kreyberg type I lung cancer (which includes squamous cell and small-cell carcinomas) were higher for white and black women than for their male counterparts, and odds ratios for Kreyberg type II lung cancer (which includes adenocarcinoma) were higher for women than men among whites but not blacks (29); the combined odds ratio across all levels of tar exposure for women compared to men was 1.7 (95% CI: 1.2–2.2). Finally, in another hospital-based case-control study, Risch et al reported higher odds ratios for females compared to males at all levels of packyears of lifetime cigarette consumption, taking years since quitting into account, for all major histologic types of lung cancer. The overall odds ratio associated with 40 pack-years of smoking compared to nonsmoking was 27.9 (95% CI: 14.9–52.0) for women and 9.6 (95% CI: 5.64–16.3) for men, and higher odds ratios were observed in women for every histologic type of lung cancer, with the excess being most pronounced for the category small-cell or oat-cell carcinoma (61). Concerns were raised that the higher odds ratios in women might simply reflect lower baseline risks of lung cancer in female compared to male nonsmokers (33). In response, Risch and colleagues noted that across nine studies with baseline data on lung cancer rates for male and female nonsmokers, the combined weighted estimate of the ratio of female to male age-adjusted rates is 0.78 (95% CI: 0.71–0.86), which could not account for the magnitude of the differences in the odds ratios between men and women observed in their study (60). However, they noted that a number of studies that have examined male-female differences in risk by number of cigarettes smoked per day or by pack-years smoked have reported opposite findings, namely higher odds ratios in males, or no clear differences between males and females (61). This issue requires further study, with more precise categorization of amount and duration of smoking, as well as standardized pathology review for classifying histologic types of lung cancer.

Gender Differences in Histologic Types of Lung Cancer Among Smokers

Data on histologic type of lung cancer from tumor registries, large case series, and epidemiologic studies all demonstrate gender differences in the distribution of cases by histologic type (15, 17, 73, 77, 88), which persist after controlling for smoking status. A review of approximately 35,000 cases of microscopically confirmed lung cancers diagnosed among Florida residents between 1981–85 reported that among *smokers*, 36.8% of male cases and 24.3% of female cases were squamous cell carcinomas, 25.2% of male and 32.7% of female cases were adenocarcinomas, and 16.7% of male and 23.4% of female cases were small-cell carcinomas. Among male and female *nonsmokers*, 29.0% and 18.2%

of cases, respectively, were squamous cell carcinomas, 31.1% and 49.0% were adenocarcinomas, and 14.2% and 11.2% were small-cell carcinomas (73). As these and other data (5) show, among smokers who develop lung cancer, males are more likely than females to be diagnosed with squamous cell carcinoma, whereas females are more likely to be diagnosed with adenocarcinoma or small-cell carcinoma; among nonsmokers who develop lung cancer, females are more likely than males to be diagnosed with adenocarcinoma.

More research is needed to determine the extent to which the observed differences in histologic type may reflect differential smoking patterns by males and females (e.g. differences in age at initiation, pack-years of smoking, or types of cigarettes smoked) as opposed to true gender differences in the effect of smoking and possibly other factors on lung cancer type. As noted above, several studies have reported strikingly higher relative risks for small-cell carcinoma in female compared to male smokers, taking amount smoked into account (12, 57, 64), and several papers have noted relative increases in adenocarcinoma and small-cell carcinoma over time (6, 17, 18, 77, 88).

Environmental Tobacco Smoke

In 1993, the Environmental Protection Agency issued a report summarizing the effects on respiratory health of exposure to environmental tobacco smoke (51), which resulted in the classification of environmental tobacco smoke as a Group A carcinogen (along with indoor radon gas, asbestos, benzene, and arsenic, among others). Most studies to date have focused on nonsmoking women with lung cancer. Based on the combined results of 11 epidemiologic studies conducted in the United States, the EPA report concluded that risk of lung cancer in nonsmokers ever exposed to smoking by a spouse was 1.19 (95% CI: 1.04–1.35) and, for the highest level of spousal smoke exposure, it was 1.38 (95% CI: 1.13–1.7). Since that report was prepared, two additional studies and the final report of a multicenter case-control study that had contributed preliminary results to the EPA report have been published. One of the two new studies found no increased risk with ever exposure to spousal smoke but an estimated relative risk of 1.3 (95% CI: 1.0–1.7) for greater than 40 pack-years of exposure (11), while the second new study reported higher relative risks, 1.6 (95% CI: 0.8–3.0) for ever exposed women and 2.4 (95% CI: 1.1–5.3) for those with 40 or more adult smoke-years of exposure (72). The final report of the multicenter study, a population-based case-control study that is the largest study to date on this subject, with 653 nonsmoking female lung cancer cases and 1253 controls, generally confirmed its earlier findings (22). The adjusted odds ratio for lung cancer among women whose spouses used tobacco was 1.29 (95% CI: 1.04–1.6). Among those exposed to 40–79 and those exposed to 80 or more pack-years of tobacco smoke, the odds ratios were 1.36 (95% CI:0.97–1.91) and 1.79 (95% CI: 0.99–3.25), respectively. The Environmental Protection Agency estimated that 3.9% of lung cancer deaths among female nonsmokers in the U.S. in 1985 was attributable to ETS (51).

OTHER LUNG CANCER RISK FACTORS

Radiation: Radon and Radiotherapy

Radon has been shown to be a lung carcinogen in studies of both underground miners and laboratory animals (46). However, whether indoor exposure to the levels of radon found in some residential dwellings increases risk of female lung cancer is not clear from the relatively limited data on the subject to date. The results of three case-control studies that together included 966 female lung cancer cases and 1158 controls were recently examined in a combined analysis (47). Controlling for smoking and other factors, two of the studies, one conducted in New Jersey (63) and the other in Stockholm (75), found weak nonsignificant excess relative risks associated with radon exposure. The third study, conducted in Shenyang, China, where female lung cancer rates are very high (presumably due to cooking practices or other environmental exposures) and the majority of cases are not explained by smoking, did not find increased risk with radon exposure (7). The overall excess relative risk per pCi/l (picocurie per liter) across the three studies was 0.00 (95% CI: −.05 to −.07). In all three of the studies, smoking was a strong and significant risk factor for lung cancer, but the results for radon in relation to lung cancer risk by smoking status were not consistent across studies. Based on the very broad confidence limits and the methodologic difficulties of conducting studies of indoor radon in humans, the authors concluded that the observed results could alternately be interpreted as consistent with one another, consistent with extrapolation from studies in miners, or consistent with no effect of exposure. A later case-control study from Winnipeg, Canada, reporting results for 738 male and female lung cancer cases combined and their matched controls, found no increased risk in relation to cumulative household radon exposure, controlling for cigarette smoking and education (39).

Ionizing radiation is known to be a lung carcinogen, based on effects in A-bomb survivors, uranium miners, and Hodgkin's disease patients treated with radiation. Two cohort studies (30, 50) found that breast cancer patients treated with radiotherapy have a two- to threefold greater risk of subsequently developing primary lung cancer than breast cancer patients who do not receive radiation therapy. A case-control study that included information on smoking status confirmed the increased risk associated with radiotherapy and found that the effect was much greater in smokers than nonsmokers (49). In these studies, the radiation effect was not observed until ten or more years after the breast cancer diagnosis and, in two of the studies at least, the effect was limited to the ipsilateral lung. It should be noted that modern radiotherapy for breast cancer delivers significantly lower radiation doses to the lung than was true at the time the study patients were treated (49).

Occupational and Environmental Exposures

Most studies of occupation in relation to lung cancer are based largely or entirely on men, in whom such exposures as asbestos, arsenic, uranium, and polycyclic aromatic hydrocarbons have been shown to be lung carcinogens. A large case-control study conducted in areas of China found that, controlling for smoking, risk of female lung cancer was elevated for employment in the manufacture of transportation equipment, especially automobiles, occupations involved in sewing, metal smelting and treatment, especially current foundry work, and workplace exposures to coal dust and smoke from burning fuel, while decreased risks were found among textile industry employees and state and party leaders (91). The authors caution that many occupations were examined, that numbers in many groups were small, and that not all exposures demonstrated dose-response relationships, so that some of the observed associations may have been chance findings. A population-based case-control study of occupation in relation to female lung cancer in nonsmokers and ex-smokers conducted in Missouri reported significantly increased risks for exposure to asbestos, pesticides, and work in dry cleaning, after adjustment for age, history of previous lung disease, and previous smoking (10). Further studies of occupational risk factors for female lung cancer are warranted, particularly studies of whether there are differential effects in smokers compared to nonsmokers.

In addition to the studies of environmental tobacco smoke and radon exposure discussed above, there are several studies of air pollution in relation to female lung cancer, most of which have been conducted outside of the United States. Studies in China have reported higher risks for women living in homes without a separate kitchen or with poor air circulation (41) and for women exposed to "kang" (beds warmed by heated smoke from various fuel sources or under which the fuel is actually burned) (90, 92) or who perceive their outdoor (92) or cooking (23, 90) environments to be smoky. A case-control study among white women in Los Angeles reported an increased risk for childhood exposure to coal burning (87). With respect to outdoor air pollution, a case-control study in Athens, Greece, reported a significant effect among female smokers in the highest quartile of pollution exposure but no effect among nonsmokers (36). A recent ecologic study examined the relation between various measures of air pollution and mortality in six US cities and reported a positive association for lung cancer, but that finding was not statistically significant and results for female lung cancer were not presented separately (16).

Thus, although not well studied in women, particularly in the United States, certain occupational and environmental exposures do appear to increase risk of female lung cancer. However, given the relatively low prevalence of such exposures for women in the USA, the relatively weak relative risks at the levels of exposure characteristic of most women, and the much higher prevalence of cigarette smoking with its much higher relative risk, it is safe to conclude that occupational and environmental exposures account for only a small fraction of female lung cancer in the United States today.

Diet

Numerous case-control and cohort studies have examined the relationship of various dietary factors to lung cancer. The strongest and most common finding is that of a protective effect for fruit and vegetable consumption, although this effect has been observed more consistently for men than women (94) and the detailed results are far from consistent and may reflect covariance with other relevant exposures (54). Fruits and vegetables are the sources of the provitamin A carotenoids, including beta-carotene. Many studies (13, 37, 87, 89) but not all (34, 35, 71, 90) suggest that beta-carotene, which has known antioxidant properties, may be partially or largely responsible for the protective effect. Several studies suggest that the effect may be stronger in smokers than nonsmokers, although the exact relationship of smoking and carotenoid consumption is unclear; smokers have lower plasma total carotenoid and plasma beta-carotene levels than nonsmokers, even at similar levels of carotenoid intake (74). However, the results of a recently published large randomized controlled trial of Finnish male smokers do not support a beneficial effect of beta-carotene or vitamin E supplementation, at least among male middle-aged heavy smokers; more than 29,000 such men were randomly assigned to receive daily supplementation over six years with beta-carotene, alpha-tocopherol (Vitamin E), both, or neither, and there was no protective effect seen for men in either of the vitamin groups (76). In fact, there was a statistically significant increase in lung cancer in the beta-carotene group. Whether this is a chance finding, whether it is appropriate to extrapolate the study's results to interventions that might begin much earlier in life, and whether its findings apply to women are all open questions. Preliminary results from the Physicians Health Study (22,000 male physicians receiving beta-carotene versus placebo), and from the Carotene and Retinol Efficacy Trial (CARET, comparing beta-carotene plus vitamin A versus placebo) also show no benefit in terms of lung cancer mortality. CARET has 18,314 participants, smokers and former smokers and asbestos-exposed workers; 6289 are women smokers or former smokers;

the study was designed to have 80% power to detect a 49% reduction in lung cancer incidence in the female subgroup, as well as 35% reduction in the former smoker subgroup but was terminated 21 months early because of the preliminary (not significant) results in the opposite direction (53, 54). The results of these clinical trials suggest that if there is a lung cancer benefit from vegetable and fruit consumption, beta-carotene acting alone is not responsible.

Although total vitamin A has been associated with a reduced risk of lung cancer, studies that have separately examined preformed vitamin A (retinol, retinyl esters, and retinal—found in animal products, supplements, and fortified foods)—have not found it to be associated with lower risk. This suggests that if the carotenoids in fruits and vegetables are responsible for the protective effect observed with consumption of such foods, they do not have to be metabolized to the physiologically active form of vitamin A to exert their protective effect. Although some studies suggest a decreased risk of lung cancer associated with consumption of vitamins C or E (66) or increased risk for dietary fat or cholesterol (26), data are currently insufficient to draw conclusions. Quite a few studies have reported an inverse association between serum selenium levels and overall cancer risk, although numbers of lung cancer cases, especially in women, have been small and rarely have the results been statistically significant. A large, recently published Danish cohort study reported an inverse association between toenail selenium levels in both sexes, although only in men were the findings statistically significant (84).

Family History/Genetic Susceptibility

Some pedigree studies suggest that lung cancer may cluster in certain families, and several epidemiologic studies have found that relatives of lung cancer cases are more likely than relatives of controls to have a family history of the disease (55, 65, 89), although the extent to which smoking was taken into account and reports of familial cancer verified is not entirely clear. At least one study of female lung cancer suggests that smoking may act synergistically with family history to increase risk (56). There may also be ethnic differences in the impact of smoking on lung cancer risk; a recent report from Hawaii found that, controlling for pack-years of smoking and other variables, the relative risk of lung cancer associated with smoking was greater for ethnic Hawaiians, Caucasians, and Filipinos of both sexes than for Japanese, although these findings were statistically significant only in males (38). Such differences could reflect either differential genetic susceptibility or other factors, such as diet, that vary across ethnic groups. Not all epidemiologic studies support a role for inherited genetic predispostion. A recently reported study based on 15,924 male twin pairs found no difference between monozygotic and dizygotic twin pairs in lung cancer death rates, even though the monozygotic twins in the study population were more likely to be concordant for smoking; although numbers were small, no lung cancer deaths were found during 300 person-years of follow-up among 47 monozygotic twin smokers whose smoking twins had died of lung cancer, despite similar smoking histories within the pairs (8).

Several metabolic traits and their associated genetic markers have been identified that are more common in lung cancer patients than controls, including increased aryl hydrocarbon hydroxylase (AHH) activity, extensive metabolism of the antihypertensive drug debrisoquine sulfate, and deficiences in the μ isozyme of the glutathione-S-transferases, enzymes that are involved in the inactivation of toxins and electrophilic substrates (20). Positive results, however, have not been found in all studies. Compared to most other cancers, the prevalence of mutations in the p53 tumor suppressor gene in lung cancers is high (>50%), ranging from about a third of lung adenocarcinomas to about two thirds of small cell lung carcinomas. The p53 mutational spectrum differs for tumors in smokers compared to those in nonsmokers, and it will be of interest to learn whether lung cancers in nonsmokers associated with environmental tobacco smoke exposure show mutations similar to those in smokers (27).

Previous Lung Disease

Several studies suggest that women with a history of nonmalignant lung disease are at increased risk of developing lung cancer, although the studies vary in how smoking was taken into account (4, 56, 86, 87, 89, 90). Most of the studies that controlled for smoking found a history of previous lung disease (especially chronic bronchitis, pneumonia, emphysema, or tuberculosis) to be associated with increased risk. Although asthma and hay fever were associated with decreased risk in one study of female lung cancer (4), other studies suggest that risk in asthmatic patients may be increased by more than 50% (85). A large multicenter case-control study of lung cancer in nonsmoking women (86) found a significant increase in risk for a history of any previous lung disease (odds ratio of 1.56; 95% CI=1.2–2.0) and concluded that approximately 15% of lung cancer in nonsmoking women might be attributable to preexisting lung disease, similar to an estimate of 16% based on another case-control study published earlier (4).

PREVENTION AND CESSATION

Given the poor prognosis for the vast majority of individuals who develop lung cancer and the fact that an effective screening test for the disease has not yet been demonstrated, the greatest opportunity to reduce incidence and mortality from lung cancer lies with primary prevention. School-based smoking prevention programs that include the teaching of skills to resist influences to use tobacco have shown reductions in adolescent smoking prevalence, and the effects appear to be augmented when combined with programs that involve parents, mass media, or other aspects of the adolescent social environment (80). Young women who smoke are more likely to have parents of lower educational attainment, to have peers, parents, or siblings who smoke, to engage in other risk-taking behaviors, and may be more likely to believe in the efficacy of cigarette smoking for weight control than nonsmokers; these and other factors need to be taken into account in the design of prevention programs.

Numerous studies have demonstrated that smoking cessation reduces risk of lung cancer and that relative risk declines with years of cessation, although it may never entirely revert to that of never smokers (24, 45, 52, 79). Controlling for time since quitting, greatest benefits accrue from quitting at younger compared to older ages, but reductions in risk for those who quit even very late in life compared to continuing smokers have been demonstrated (32). A recent analysis of data from the American Cancer Society's Cancer Prevention Study II showed, for example, that 75-year old women who had quit at ages 30–39 had only 10% the risk of lung cancer of continuing smokers, compared to 23% for those who quit when aged 50–54 and 49% for those who quit when aged 60–64 (28). For established smokers, a variety of formal cessation approaches have been described, although most smokers who quit do so on their own (21). In controlled trials, physician counseling, coupled with follow-up, and nicotine replacement therapy for the more addicted smoker, have been shown to increase quit rates in intervention groups compared to controls. It is of continuing interest to develop programs targeted to specific subgroups of female smokers, including teens, pregnant women, older women, heavy smokers, and women of lower socioeconomic status, all of whom may have unique needs.

Since cigarette smoking currently accounts for the vast majority of lung cancer cases in women, efforts to prevent adolescent and teenage girls from starting to smoke and to encourage smokers to quit have the greatest potential to impact the disease. A combination of efforts targeted to high-risk individuals as well as policies that serve to change social norms regarding smoking and limit youth access to tobacco are needed. Exposure to environmental tobacco smoke should also be added. While of much less relative importance, minimizing exposure to radiation, and certain occupational and environmental exposures, as well as encouraging consumption of fruits and vegetables, may also be beneficial.

CONCLUSIONS AND FUTURE RESEARCH ISSUES

Female lung cancer death rates increased by more than 550% between 1950 and 1991. In 1986, lung cancer surpassed breast cancer to become the leading cause of cancer death in U.S. women. The lung cancer epidemic is primarily attributable to cigarette smoking, which is responsible for at least 80% of the disease in women. There are gender differences in the distribution of lung cancer by histologic type that persist after controlling for smoking. Some data suggest greater female than male susceptibility to lung cancer at a given level of smoking. Exposure to environmental tobacco smoke is associated with an increased risk of lung cancer in nonsmoking women, and evidence is mounting that a personal history of lung disease (e.g. asthma, chronic bronchitis, pneumonia, or tuberculosis) or previous exposure to radiotherapy are also associated with increased risk. Data specific to women on the role of household exposures to radon or of specific occupational or environmental exposures are relatively sparse and inconsistent. However, various measures of household pollution are associated with increased risk in China, where lung cancer rates are relatively high and female smoking prevalence relatively low. Many studies have reported a decreased risk of lung cancer in individuals who consume high levels of fruits and vegetables, although, contrary to expectation, large-scale clinical trials have failed to demonstrate a beneficial effect of beta-carotene supplementation on lung-cancer mortality.

Future research should attempt to clarify whether gender differences in smoking-related lung cancer susceptibility exist and to better understand how smoking patterns relate to the variation in histologic type of lung cancers seen in women compared to men. Given the young ages of smoking initiation characteristic of recent generations of women, it will also be important to confirm whether early age at initiation is an independent risk factor after careful control for amount and duration of smoking. Perhaps most importantly, we need to learn why smoking rates have declined so little among young women in recent years, in the face of the overwhelming evidence of the health hazards of smoking for women. Since cigarette smoking accounts for the vast majority of lung cancer cases in women, efforts to prevent adolescent girls from starting to smoke and to encourage cessation among established smokers have the greatest potential for reducing the female lung cancer burden.

ACKNOWLEDGMENTS

This was written while the author was supported in part by a grant from the Tobacco-Related Disease Research Program administered by the University of California (grant #3RT-0036).

Literature Cited

1. 1993. Mortality trends for selected smoking-related cancers and breast cancer—United States, 1950–1990. *Morbid. Mortal. Wkly. Rep.* 42:857, 863–66

2. 1994. Cigarette smoking among adults—United States, 1993. *Morbid. Mortal. Wkly. Rep.* 43:925–30

3. 1994. Cigarette smoking among women of reproductive age—United States, 1987–1992. *Morbid. Mortal. Wkly. Rep.* 43:789–91, 797

4. Alavanja MC, Brownson RC, Boice JD Jr, Hock E. 1992. Preexisting lung disease and lung cancer among nonsmoking women. *Am. J. Epidemiol.* 136: 623–32

5. Anton-Culver H, Culver BD, Kurosaki T, Osann Kathryn E, Lee JB. 1988. Incidence of lung cancer by histological type from a population-based registry. *Cancer Res.* 48:6580–83

6. Beard CM, Jedd MB, Woolner LB, Richardson RL, Bergstralh EJ, Melton LJ III. 1988. Fifty-year trend in incidence rates of bronchogenic carcinoma by cell type in Olmsted County, Minnesota. *J. Natl. Cancer Inst.* 80:1494–7

7. Blot WJ, Xu Z-Y, Boice J, John D, Zhao D-Z, Stone BJ, et al. 1990. Indoor radon and lung cancer in China. *J. Natl. Cancer Inst.* 82:1025–30

8. Braun MM, Caporaso NE, Page WF, Hoover RN. 1994. Genetic component of lung cancer: cohort study of twins. *Lancet* 344:440–43

9. Brown CC, Kessler LG. 1988. Projections of lung cancer mortality in the United States: 1985–2025. *J. Natl. Cancer Inst.* 80:43–51

10. Brownson RC, Alavanja MC, Chang JC. 1993. Occupational risk factors for lung cancer among nonsmoking women: a case-control study in Missouri (United States). *Cancer Causes Control* 4:449–54

11. Brownson RC, Alavanja MC, Hock ET, Loy TS. 1992. Passive smoking and lung cancer in nonsmoking women. *Am. J. Public Health* 82:1525–30

12. Brownson RC, Chang JC, Davis JR. 1992. Gender and histologic type variations in smoking-related risk of lung cancer. *Epidemiology* 3:61–64

13. Candelora EC, Stockwell HG, Armstrong AW, Pinkham PA. 1992. Dietary intake and risk of lung cancer in women who never smoked. *Nutri. Cancer* 17: 263–70

14. Devesa SS, Blot WJ, Fraumeni JF. 1989. Declining lung cancer rates among young men and women in the United States: a cohort analysis. *J. Natl. Cancer Inst.* 81:1568–71

15. Devesa SS, Shaw GL, Blot WJ. 1991. Changing patterns of lung cancer incidence by histological type. *Cancer Epidemiol. Biomarkers Prev.* 1:29–34

16. Dockery D, Pope A III, Xu X, Spengler JD, Ware JH, et al. 1993. An association between air pollution and mortality in six U.S. cities. *N. Engl. J. Med.* 329: 1753–59

17. Dodds L, Davis S, Polissar L. 1986. A population-based study of lung cancer incidence trends by histologic type 1974–1981. *J. Natl. Cancer Inst.* 77:53–56

18. el-Torky M, el-Zeky F, Hall JC. 1990. Significant changes in the distribution of histologic types of lung cancer. A review of 4928 cases. *Cancer* 65:2361–67

19. Ernster VL. 1994. The epidemiology of lung cancer in women. *Ann. Epidemiol.* 4:102–10

20. Ernster VL, Mustacchi P, Osann KE. 1994. Epidemiology of Lung Cancer. In *Textbook of Respiratory Medicine,* ed. J Murray, J Nadel, pp. 1504–27. Philadelphia: WB Saunders

21. Fiore MC, Novotny TE, Pierce JP, Giovino GA, Hatziandreu EJ, et al. 1990. Methods used to quit smoking in the United States: Do cessation programs help? *JAMA* 263:2760–65

22. Fontham, ET, Correa, P, Reynolds, P, Wu-Williams, A, Buffler, PA, et al. 1994. Environmental tobacco smoke and lung cancer in nonsmoking women. A multicenter study. *JAMA* 271:1752–59

23. Gao Y-T, Blot WJ, Zheng W, Ershow AG, Hsu CW, et al. 1987. Lung cancer among Chinese women. *Int. J. Cancer* 40:604–9

24. Garfinkel L, Silverberg E. 1991. Lung cancer and smoking trends in the United States over the past 25 Years. *CA Cancer J. Clin.* 41:137–45

25. Garfinkel L, Stellman SD. 1988. Smoking and lung cancer in women: findings in a prospective study. *Cancer Res.* 48: 6951–55

26. Goodman MT, Hankin JH, Wilkens LR, Kolonel LN. 1992. High-fat foods and the risk of lung cancer. *Epidemiology* 3:288–99

27. Greenblatt MS, Bennett WP, Hollstein M, Harris CC. 1994. Mutations in the p53 tumor suppressor gene: clues to

cancer etiology and molecular pathogenesis. *Cancer Res.* 54:4855–78

28. Halpern MT, Gillespie BW, Warner KE. 1993. Patterns of absolute risk of lung cancer mortality in former smokers. *J. Natl. Cancer Inst.* 85:457–64

29. Harris RE, Zang EA, Anderson JI, Wynder EL. 1993. Race and sex differences in lung cancer risk associated with cigarette smoking. *Int. J. Epidemiol.* 22: 592–99

30. Harvey EB, Brinton LA. 1985. Second cancer following cancer of the breast in Connecticut, 1935–82. *Natl. Cancer Inst. Monogr.* 68:99–112

31. Hegmann KT, Fraser AM, Keaney RP, Moser SE, Nilasena DS, et al. 1993. The effect of age at smoking initiation on lung cancer risk. *Epidemiology* 4: 444–48

32. Hermanson, B, Omenn, GS, Kronmal, RA and Gersh, BJ. 1988. Beneficial six-year outcomes of smoking cessation in older men and women with coronary artery disease: Results from the CASS registry. *N. Engl. J. Med.* 319:1365–69

33. Hoover DR. 1994. Re: "Are female smokers at higher risk for lung cancer than male smokers?" A case-control analysis by histologic type. *Am. J. Epidemiol.* 140:186–87

34. Jain M, Burch JD, Howe GR, Risch HA, Miller AB. 1990. Dietary factors and risk of lung cancer: results from a case-control study, Toronto, 1981–1985. *Int. J. Cancer* 45:287–93

35. Kalandidi A, Katsouyanni K, Voropoulou N, Bastas G, Saracci R, Trichopoulous D. 1990. Passive smoking and diet in the etiology of lung cancer among non-smokers. *Cancer Causes Control* 1:15–21

36. Katsouyanni K, Trichopoulos D, Kalandidi A, Tomos P, Riboli E. 1991. A case-control study of air pollution and tobacco smoking in lung cancer among women in Athens. *Prev. Med.* 20:271–78

37. Le Marchand L, Hankin JH, Kolonel LN, Beecher GR, Wilkens LR, Zhao LP. 1993. Intake of specific carotenoids and lung cancer risk. *Cancer Epidemiol. Biomarkers Prev.* 2:183–87

38. Le Marchand L, Wilkens LR, Kolonel LN. 1992. Ethnic differences in the lung cancer risk associated with smoking. *Cancer Epidemiol. Biomarkers Prev.* 1: 103–7

39. Letourneau E, Krewski D, Choi N, Goddard M, McGregor R, et al. 1994. Case-control study of residential radon and lung cancer in Winnipeg, Manitoba, Canada. *Am. J. Epidemiol.* 140:310–22

40. Levi F, La Vecchia C, Lucchini F, Negri E. 1992. Trends in cancer mortality sex ratios in Europe, 1950–1989. *World Health Stat. Q.* 45:117–64

41. Liu Q, Sasco AJ, Riboli E, Hu MX. 1993. Indoor air pollution and lung cancer in Guangzhou, People's Republic of China. *Am. J. Epidemiol.* 137:145–54

42. Lopez AD. 1990. Changes in tobacco consumption and lung cancer risk: evidence from national statistics. In *Evaluating Effectiveness of Primary Prevention of Cancer*, ed. M Hakama, V Beral, JW Cullen, DM Parkin, pp. 57–76. Lyon: Int. Agency Res. Cancer

43. Lubin JH, Blot WJ. 1984. Assessment of lung cancer risk factors by histologic category. *J. Natl. Cancer Inst.* 73:383–89

44. Lubin JH, Blot W, Berrino F, Flamant R, Gillis CR, et al. 1984. Patterns of lung cancer risk according to type of cigarette smoked. *Int. J. Cancer* 33:569–76

45. Lubin JH, Blot WJ, Berrino F, Flamant R, Gillis CR, et al. 1984. Modifying risk of developing lung cancer by changing habits of cigarette smoking. *Br. Med. J.* 288:1953–56

46. Lubin JH, Boice J JD, Edling C, Hornung RW, How G, et al. 1994. *Radon and Lung Cancer Risk: A Joint Analyses of 11 Underground Miners Studies.* US DHHS, Public Health Serv., NIH

47. Lubin JH, Liang Z, Hrubec Z, Pershagen G, Schoenberg JB, et al. 1994. Radon exposure in residences and lung cancer among women: combined analysis of three studies. *Cancer Causes Control* 5:114–28

48. Lyon JL, Gardner K, Gress RE. 1994. Cancer incidence among Mormons and non-Mormons in Utah (United States) 1971–85. *Cancer Causes Control* 5: 149–56

49. Neugut AI, Murray T, Santos J, Amols H, Hayes MK, et al. 1994. Increased risk of lung cancer after breast cancer radiation therapy in cigarette smokers. *Cancer* 73:1615–20

50. Neugut AI, Robinson E, Lee WC, Murray T, Karwoski K, Kutcher GJ. 1993. Lung cancer after radiation therapy for breast cancer. *Cancer* 71:3054–57

51. Off. Health Environ. Assess. 1992. *Respiratory Health Effects of Passive Smoking: Lung Cancer and Other Disorders.* Washington, DC: US EPA

52. Omenn GS, Anderson KW, Kronmal RA, Vlietstra MB. 1990. The temporal pattern of reduction of mortality risk after smoking cessation. *Am. J. Prev. Med.* 6:251–57

53. Omenn GS, Goodman G, Thornquist M, Barnhart S, Balmes J, et al. 1995. Chemoprevention in cancer control: the B-carotene and retinol efficacy trial (CARET) in high-risk smokers and asbestos-exposed workers. In *Chemoprevention in Cancer Control,* ed. M Hakama, V Beral, E Buiatti, J Faivre, DM Parkins, Lyon: IARC. In press

54. Omenn GS, Goodman G, Thornquist M, Grizzle J, Rosenstock L, et al. 1994. The B-carotene and retinol efficacy trial (CARET) for chemoprevention of lung cancer in high-risk populations: smokers and asbestos-exposed workers. *Cancer Res.* 54:2038s–43s

55. Ooi WL, Elston RC, Chen VW, Bailey-Wilson JE, Rothschild H. 1986. Increased familial risk for lung cancer. *J. Natl. Cancer Inst.* 76:217–22

56. Osann KE. 1991. Lung cancer in women: the importance of smoking, family history of cancer, and medical history of respiratory disease. *Cancer Res.* 51:4893–97

57. Osann KE, Anton-Culver H, Kurosaki T, Taylor T. 1993. Sex differences in lung-cancer risk associated with cigarette smoking. *Int. J. Cancer* 54:44–48

58. Perkins CI, Morris CR, Wright WE, Young JL. 1995. *Cancer Incidence and Mortality in California by Detailed Race/Ethnicity, 1988–1992.* Calif. Dep. Health Serv.

59. Ries LAG, Miller BA, Hankey BF, Kosary CL, Harras A, Edwards BK. 1994. *SEER Cancer Statistics, 1973– 1991: Tables and Graphs.* Bethesda, MD: Natl. Cancer Inst., NIH Publ. No. 94–2789

60. Risch HA, Howe GR, Holowaty EJ, Miller AB. 1994. The authors reply. *Am. J. Epidemiol.* 140:187–88

61. Risch HA, Howe GR, Jain M, Burch JD, Holowaty EJ, Miller AB. 1993. Are female smokers at higher risk for lung cancer than male smokers? A case-control analysis by histologic type. *Am. J. Epidemiol.* 138:281–93

62. Satcher D, Eriksen M. 1994. The paradox of tobacco control. *JAMA* 271:627–28

63. Schoenberg JB, Klotz JB, Wilcox HB, Nicholls GP, Gil-del-Real MT, et al. 1990. Case-control study of residential radon and lung cancer among New Jersey women. *Cancer Res.* 50:6520–24

64. Schoenberg JB, Wilcox HB, Mason TJ, Bill J, Stemhagen A. 1989. Variation in smoking-related lung cancer risk among New Jersey women. *Am. J. Epidemiol.* 130:688–95

65. Sellers TA, Elston RC, Atwood LD, Rothschild H. 1992. Lung cancer histologic type and family history of cancer. *Cancer* 69:86–91

66. Shibata A, Paganini-Hill A, Ross RK, Henderson BE. 1992. Intake of vegetables, fruits, beta-carotene, vitamin C and vitamin supplements and cancer incidence among the elderly: a prospective study. *Br. J. Cancer* 66:673–79

67. Shopland DR. 1990. Changes in tobacco consumption and lung cancer risk: evidence from studies of individuals. In *Evaluating Effectiveness of Primary Prevention of Cancer,* ed. M Hakama V Beral JW Cullen, DM Parkin, pp. 77–91. Lyon: Int. Agency Res. Cancer

68. Shopland DR, Eyre HJ, Pechacek TF. 1991. Smoking-attributable cancer mortality in 1991: Is lung cancer now the leading cause of death among smokers in the United States? *J. Natl. Cancer Inst.* 83:1142–48

69. Sidney S, Tekawa IS, Friedman GD. 1993. A prospective study of cigarette tar yield and lung cancer. *Cancer Causes Control* 4:3–10

70. Stanley K, Stjernsward J. 1989. Lung cancer in developed and developing countries. In *Basic and Clinical Concepts of Lung Cancer,* ed. HH Hansen, pp. 1–14. Boston: Kluwer

71. Steinmetz KA, Potter JD, Folsom AR. 1993. Vegetables, fruit, and lung cancer in the Iowa Women's Health Study. *Cancer Res.* 53:536–43

72. Stockwell H, Goldman A, Lyman G, Noss CI, Armstrong AW, et al. 1992. Environmental tobacco smoke and lung cancer risk in nonsmoking women. *J. Natl. Cancer Inst.* 84:1417–22

73. Stockwell HG, Armstrong AW, Leaverton PE. 1990. Histopathology of lung cancers among smokers and nonsmokers in Florida. *Int. J. Epidemiol.* 19 (Suppl. 1):S48–52

74. Stryker WS, Kaplan LA, Stein EA, Stampfer MJ, Sober A, Willett WC. 1988. The relation of diet, cigarette smoking, and alcohol consumption to plasma beta-carotene and alpha-tocopherol levels. *Am. J. Epidemiol.* 127: 283–96

75. Svensson C, Pershagen G, Klominek J. 1989. Lung cancer in women and type of dwelling in relation to radon exposure. *Cancer Res.* 49:1861–65

76. The Alpha-Tocopherol Beta Carotene Cancer Prevention Study Group. 1994. The effect of vitamin E and beta carotene on the incidence of lung cancer and other cancers in male smokers. *N. Engl. J. Med.* 330:1029–35

77. Travis WD, Travis LB, Devesa SS. 1995. Lung cancer. *Cancer* 75:191–202

78. US Dep. Health Hum. Serv. 1989. *Reducing the Health Consequences of Smoking: 25 Years of Progress: A Report of the Surgeon General.* Rockville MD: US DHHS, Public Health Serv., CDC, Cent. Chronic Dis. Prev. Health Promot.

79. US Dep. Health Hum. Serv. 1990. *The Health Benefits of Smoking Cessation.* Rockville MD: US DHHS, Public Health Service, CDC, Cent. Chronic Dis. Prev. Health Promot., Off. Smoking Health

80. US Dep. Health Hum. Serv. 1994. *Preventing Tobacco Use Among Young People: A Report of the Surgeon General.* Atlanta, GA: US DHHS, Public Health Ser., CDC, Natl. Cent. Chronic Dis. Prev. Health Promot.

81. US Prev. Serv. Task Force. 1989. *Guide to Clinical Preventive Services: An Assessment of the Effectiveness of 169 Interventions.* Baltimore: Williams & Wilkins

82. US Public Health Serv. 1964. *Smoking and Health. Report of the Advisory Committee to the Surgeon General of the Public Health Service.* Rockville MD: US DHEW

83. US Public Health Serv. 1980. *The Health Consequences of Smoking for Women. A Report of the Surgeon General.* Rockville MD: US DHHS, Off. Smoking Health

84. van den Brandt PA, Goldbohm RA, van't Veer P, Bode P, Dorant E, et al. 1993. A prospective cohort study on selenium status and the risk of lung cancer. *Cancer Res.* 53:4860–65

85. Vesterinen E, Pukkala E, Timonen T, Aromaa A. 1993. Cancer incidence among 78,000 asthmatic patients. *Int. J. Epidemiol.* 22:976–82

85a. Wing PA, Tong T, Bolden S. 1995. Cancer statistics, 1995. *CA Cancer J. Clin.* 45:8–30

86. Wu AH, Fontham ETH, Reynolds P, Greenberg RS, Buffler P, et al. 1995. Previous lung disease and risk of lung cancer among lifetime nonsmoking women in the United States. *Am. J. Epidemiol.* 141:1023–32

87. Wu AH, Henderson BE, Pike MC, Yu MC. 1985. Smoking and other risk factors for lung cancer in women. *J. Natl. Cancer Inst.* 74:747–51

88. Wu AH, Henderson BE, Thomas DC, Mack TM. 1986. Secular trends in histologic types of lung cancer. *J. Natl. Cancer Inst.* 77:53–56

89. Wu AH, Yu MC, Thomas DC, Pike MC, Henderson BE. 1988. Personal and family history of lung disease as risk factors for adenocarcinoma of the lung. *Cancer Res.* 48:7279–84

90. Wu-Williams AH, Dai XD, Blot W, Xu ZY, Sun XW, et al. 1990. Lung cancer among women in north-east China. *Br. J. Cancer* 62:982–87

91. Wu-Williams AH, Xu ZY, Blot WJ, Dai XD, Louie R, et al. 1993. Occupation and lung cancer risk among women in northern China. *Am. J. Ind. Med.* 24:67–79

92. Xu Z-Y, Blot WJ, Xiao H-P, Wu A, Feng Y-P, et al. 1989. Smoking, air pollution, and the high rates of lung cancer in Shenyang, China. *J. Natl. Cancer Inst.* 81:1800–6

93. Zang EA, Wynder EL. 1992. Cumulative tar exposure. A new index for estimating lung cancer risk among cigarette smokers. *Cancer* 70:69–76

94. Ziegler RG. 1991. Vegetables, fruits, and carotenoids and the risk of cancer. *Am. J. Clin. Nutr.* 53:251S-9S

Annu. Rev. Public Health. 1996. 17:115–19

PUBLIC HEALTH ASPECTS OF OPHTHALMIC DISEASE: Introduction

Alfred Sommer

Johns Hopkins School of Hygiene and Public Health, 615 North Wolfe Street, Suite 1041, Baltimore, Maryland 21205–2179

Visually disabling diseases are particularly topical as we grapple with new ways to deliver health services, recognize the imperative of functional status and its impact on quality of life, and seek new opportunities for prevention. It is also timely. Rigorous population-based studies in the U.S. and elsewhere are, for the first time, revealing the magnitude, causes, and impact of disabling ocular disease.

The impacts of visual impairment and blindness were emphasized by the World Bank's landmark publication, *World Development Report 1993: Investing in Health* (26). It introduced the Disability Adjusted Life Year (DALY) as a basis for quantifying the global burden of disease and the relative cost-effectiveness of alternative interventions. The most cost-effective is $1 per DALY gained from vitamin A distribution to prevent blindness.

In the United States and other developed countries, a considerable proportion of visual impairment can be corrected with appropriate spectacles. Blindness, at either the U.S. (20/200 or worse) or WHO (worse than 20/400) definitions, inevitably represents established pathology (23). Prevalence rates of blindness increase with age, particularly among the elderly (9, 23), secondary to a small number of chronic degenerative conditions: cataract, age-related macular degeneration (AMD), primary open angle glaucoma, and diabetic retinopathy (15). Blindness rates among nursing home patients are 15 times as common as among age-matched noninstitutionalized subjects (21).

Cataract, an entirely remedial condition, is paradoxically the commonest single cause of blindness around the world, from India, Nepal, and Cairo, to East Baltimore (13). It accounts for roughly half the 40 million blind people in the world. Cataract surgery, almost inevitably combined (in wealthy countries) with implantation of an intraocular lens, is extraordinarily safe and highly effective, providing complete rehabilitation. It led the movement to safe, cost-effective outpatient surgery that has dramatically reduced costs per case, com-

115

0163-7525/96/0510-0115$08.00

pared with in-hospital surgery and postoperative recovery. Cataract remains an important cause of blindness in developing countries, responsible for a "backlog" of 10 million blind in India alone, from the lack of adequately trained, suitably supported and geographically distributed surgical expertise, as well as inefficiencies of practice. The incidence of new cases in India is estimated at 3 million annually (11); the number treated at roughly 1 million. Why cataract should remain a leading cause of blindness in East Baltimore, where patients have financial access (most were over 65) and geographic access (all live within a few miles of the Johns Hopkins Hospital) remains unknown. The comprehensive cataract PORT demonstrated the importance of patient-based functional status as a superior indication for the need for surgery than simple Snellen acuity (17). While it has been estimated that delaying the onset of visually disabling cataract by 10 years would reduce the need for surgery by half, and a variety of studies support that UV exposure, smoking, and diet may alter the risk and rate of cataract formation, their contributions seem relatively small, and the findings remain in need of corroboration.

Primary open angle glaucoma raises its own challenges. We now have incontrovertible evidence that blacks are far more susceptible to both the disease (22) and its blinding optic nerve destruction (15) than are whites; however, we do not know why. Traditionally, attention has focused almost exclusively on the role of intraocular pressure (IOP). While the risk of glaucomatous optic nerve damage clearly increases with increased pressure (12), we now recognize there is no particular level that is invariably safe, nor do we understand why some patients with a high IOP never suffer glaucomatous damage while others with much lower pressures, often considerably below 21 mm Hg, do (14). Recent data provide some clues, yet suggest that IOP may account for as little as 10% of the risk (1). Other factors probably include the structural organization of the optic nerve and lamina cribrosa, the vascular supply, and related factors (14). Unlike the horde of prior studies that failed to demonstrate that reducing IOP actually slowed or halted progression of optic nerve damage, a recently reported, carefully controlled trial suggests it can (9), but only through dramatic, sustained reductions in IOP associated with surgical intervention (14). Traditional management, utilizing an additive series of topical medications may, in fact, be more harmful than beneficial (3). Finally, we have yet to find an appropriately sensitive and specific approach to screening, an urgent issue as patients are generally unaware of the condition until it impinges on everyday visual functions, by which time 80% or more of the optic nerve has been destroyed (14).

Recent developments have provided effective means for both primary and secondary prevention of diabetic retinopathy; the first through tight diabetic control (5) and the latter through laser photocoagulation (6, 8). In both instances, however, the challenge remains compliance by patient and physician alike. Only a small proportion of diabetics have embraced the inconvenience of tight control, while their physicians have been remarkably lax in referring them for periodic ophthalmologic examination (or even checking their hemoglobin A_{1C}) (24).

Because of space limitations and the absence of important, known, modifiable factors, or of effective therapeutic options, we have omitted a detailed discussion of age-related macular degeneration (AMD) from this mini-symposium.

Also worthy of note are the major preventable causes of blindness largely limited to poor countries of the developing world: xerophthalmia (vitamin A deficiency), measles, onchocerciasis (river blindness), and trachoma. Alone or combined with cataract, they blind half of all adults in some areas of the world, despite being entirely preventable or reversible (13). What is lacking is money, infrastructure, and political will. Fortunately, this once dismal situation is improving.

With the recognition that vitamin A deficiency is responsible for a third or more of all preschool-age deaths (16), both WHO and UNICEF have spurred worldwide efforts for its control. Alternative strategies for improving vitamin A status include periodic supplementation with high-dose capsules (e.g. 200,000 IU every 3 to 6 months), fortification of an appropriate dietary staple used by the population at greatest risk, or increased intake of foods rich in vitamin A. Programs to reduce childhood mortality from vitamin A deficiency will also reduce blindness from xerophthalmia (16), whether uncomplicated or precipitated by measles (7). Increased levels of measles immunization should prevent the half of measles-related blindness not prevented by vitamin A prophylaxis or treatment (2, 16).

Onchocerciasis has yielded to the World Bank/WHO vector control program that totally eliminated transmission of *Onchocerca volvulus*, and more recently, once or twice yearly prophylaxis with the microfilaricide mectizan (ivermectin) (25). However, distribution of mectizan to dispersed populations in poor sub-Saharan countries with rudimentary health infrastructures poses severe obstacles to long-range sustainability.

Trachoma is entirely a disease of unsanitary conditions, which enhances repeated reinfection with chlamydia (especially among young children and their caretakers). It is repeated reinfection, and the attendant inflammation, that ultimately results in tarsal scarring, trichiasis, and corneal opacification. Observational studies (4, 18, 25) and intervention trials (24) indicate that simple face washing can significantly reduce the rate of infection and the incidence and severity of inflammation. The practicality of these approaches is now being tested on a larger scale, as is the added value of mass treatment and prophylaxis with the systemic antibiotic, azithromycin.

The articles that follow explore the nuances of age-old disabling conditions of the western world. More important, they highlight the dramatic advances that recent applications of epidemiologic techniques have made in our understanding of the magnitude and determinants of these conditions, and in delineating the public health challenges they pose.

Literature Cited

1. Airaksinen PJ, Tuulonen A, Alanko HI. 1992. Rate and pattern of neuroretinal rim area decrease in ocular hypertension and glaucoma. *Arch. Ophthalmol.* 110: 206–10
2. Barclay AJG, Foster A, Sommer A. 1987. Vitamin A supplements and mortality related to measles: a randomised clinical trial. *Br. Med. J.* 294:294–96
3. Broadway DC, Grierson I, O'Brien C, Hitchings RA. 1994. Adverse effects of topical antiglaucoma medication. II. The outcome of filtration surgery. *Arch. Ophthalmol.* 112:1446–54
4. Courtright P, Sheppard J, Lane S, Sadek A, Schachter J, Dawson CR. 1991. Latrine ownership as a protective factor in inflammatory trachoma in Egypt. *Br. J. Ophthalmol.* 75:322–25
5. Diabetes Control and Complications Trial Research Group. 1995. The effect of intensive diabetes treatment on the progression of diabetic retinopathy in insulin-dependent diabetes mellitus. The Diabetes Control and Complications Trial.*Arch. Ophthalmol.* 113:36–51
6. Early Treatment Diabetic Retinopathy Study Research Group. 1985. Photocoagulation for diabetic macular edema. *Arch. Ophthalmol.* 103:1796–806
7. Foster A, Sommer A. 1987. Corneal ulceration, measles, and childhood blindness in Tanzania. *Br. J. Ophthalmol.* 71:331–43
8. Kauffman SC, Ferris FL, Seigel DG, Davis MD, DeMets DL, DRS Research Group. 1989. Factors associated with visual outcome after photocoagulation for diabetic retinopathy. *Invest. Ophthalmol. Vis. Sci.* 30:23–28
9. Klein R, Klein BEK, Linton KLP, DeMets DL. 1991. The Beaver Dam eye study: visual acuity. *Ophthalmology* 98: 1310–15
10. Migdal C, Gregory W, Hitchings R. 1994. Long-term functional outcome af-

ter early surgery compared with laser and medicine in open-angle glaucoma. *Ophthalmology* 101:1651–57
11. Minassian DC, Mehra V, Johnson GJ. 1992. Mortality and cataract: findings from a population-based longitudinal study. *Bull. WHO* 70:219–23
12. Sommer A. 1989. Intraocular pressure and glaucoma. *Am. J. Ophthalmol.* 107: 186–88
13. Sommer A. 1995. Toward affordable, sustainable eye care. *Int. Ophthalmol.* 18:287–92
14. Sommer A. 1996. Glaucoma: facts and fancies. The Doyne Memorial Lecture. *Eye.* In press
15. Sommer A, Tielsch JM, Katz J, Quigley HA, Gottsch JD, et al. 1991. Racial differences in the cause-specific prevalence of blindness in East Baltimore. *N. Engl. J. Med.* 325:1412–17
16. Sommer A, West KW Jr. 1996. *Vitamin A Deficiency: Health, Survival, and Vision.* New York: Oxford Univ. Press. In press
17. Steinberg EP, Tielsch JM, Schein OD, Javitt JC, Sharkey P, et al. 1994. The VF-14. An index of functional impairment in patients with cataract. *Arch. Ophthalmol.*112:630–38
18. Taylor HR, Velasco FM, Sommer A. 1985. The ecology of trachoma: an epidemiological study in southern Mexico. *Bull. WHO* 63:559–67
19. Tielsch JM, Javitt JC, Coleman A, Katz J, Sommer A. 1995. The prevalence of blindness and visual impairment among nursing home residents in Baltimore. *N. Engl. J. Med.* 332:1205–9
20. Tielsch JM, Sommer A, Katz J, Royall RM, Quigley HA, Javitt J. 1991. Racial variations in the prevalence of primary open-angle glaucoma: the Baltimore Eye Survey. *JAMA* 266:369–74
21. Tielsch JM, Sommer A, Witt K, Katz J, Royall RM. 1990. Blindness and vis-

ual impairment in an American urban population. The Baltimore Eye Survey. *Arch. Ophthalmol.* 108:286–90

22. Weiner JP, Parente ST, Garnick DW, Fowles J, Lawthers AG, Palmer H. 1995. Variation on office-based quality. A claims-based profile of care provided to Medicare patients with diabetes. *JAMA* 273:1503–8

23. West SK, Congdon N, Katala S, Mele L. 1991. Facial cleanliness and risk of trachoma in families. *Arch. Ophthalmol.* 109:855–57

24. West SK, Muñoz B, Lynch M, Kayongoya A, Chilangwa Z, et al. 1995. Impact of face-washing on trachoma in Kongwa, Tanzania. *Lancet* 345:155–58

25. *WHO Programme Advisory Group on the Prevention of Blindness, 10th Meet.* 1993. Geneva: WHO PBL/AG/93

26. World Development Report. 1993: *Investing in Health.* Washington, DC: World Bank, New York: Oxford Univ. Press

Annu. Rev. Public Health. 1996. 17:121–36

THE EPIDEMIOLOGY AND CONTROL OF OPEN ANGLE GLAUCOMA: A
Population-Based Perspective

James M. Tielsch

Department of International Health, Johns Hopkins University School of Hygiene and Public Health, Baltimore, Maryland 21205

KEY WORDS: prevalence, risk factors, screening, cost

ABSTRACT

Chronic open angle glaucoma is an etiologically heterogeneous group of diseases characterized by damage to the optic nerve, resulting in peripheral visual loss that can progress to involve the fovea and central vision. Open angle glaucoma can be divided into primary conditions and conditions which are secondary to another ocular or systemic disease. Causes of secondary glaucoma include uveitis, cataract, trauma, and disorders affecting the developmental structure of the angle. This review focuses on primary open angle glaucoma (POAG), since it accounts for the vast majority of the disease burden in the US population and its etiology remains unknown.

INTRODUCTION

Chronic open angle glaucoma is an etiologically heterogeneous group of diseases characterized by damage to the optic nerve, resulting in peripheral visual loss that can progress to involve the fovea and central vision. Open angle glaucoma can be divided into primary conditions and conditions which are secondary to another ocular or systemic disease. Causes of secondary glaucoma include uveitis, cataract, trauma, and disorders affecting the developmental structure of the angle. This review focuses on primary open angle glaucoma (POAG), since it accounts for the vast majority of the disease burden in the US population and its etiology remains unknown.

The pathophysiologic mechanism by which damage occurs in POAG is the subject of much debate. Two major hypotheses have been proposed to account for the observed optic nerve damage. The first focuses on reductions in vascular

121

perfusion of the optic nerve and nerve fiber layer; the second centers on mechanical damage occurring at the level of the lamina cribrosa. For both, the damage to the optic nerve is thought to be mediated through a combination of inherent susceptibility of the optic nerve head and elevation in the intraocular pressure (IOP) beyond what the susceptible eye can tolerate. It is likely that both mechanisms operate to produce damage and that their relative importance may depend on a variety of factors, including the level of the IOP. Unfortunately, whatever mechanism plays the leading role in producing glaucomatous optic nerve damage, there is little good information about what initiates this process or about the subgroups of the population who are at high risk for the onset of such damage.

ISSUES OF MEASUREMENT AND DEFINITION

Prior to reviewing the literature on the epidemiology of POAG, it is critical to understand the evolution of diagnostic methods and definitions used for this disorder. It is widely accepted now that POAG is fundamentally an optic neuropathy with the defining clinical sign being damage to the axons of retinal ganglion cells. This damage is evidenced clinically by abnormalities in the visual field, excavation of the optic nerve, or thinning of the nerve fiber layer (78).

A major issue in the epidemiology of POAG continues to be the definition of the disease. For many years, the definition of glaucoma was synonymous with elevated intraocular pressure. As a result, early studies often included groups of cases dominated by patients who had elevated IOP only and neither optic nerve excavation nor visual field loss (25, 81). This confusion was reinforced by a statistical classification of the distribution of IOP that equated infrequent observations with abnormality [personal communication from W Leydhecker to FC Hollows & PA Graham (25)]. In response, two different conditions are now described, glaucoma and ocular hypertension, separating those with optic nerve damage from those with only statistically defined elevated IOP.

There remain, however, large differences in the definitions used for glaucoma. Differences exist in the criteria for glaucomatous optic nerve damage, the techniques used to measure such damage, who is qualified to make such assessments, and whether elevated IOP is a necessary component of the disease definition. Dilated examinations of the optic nerve head are critical to making full use of the dimensional clues to the status of the optic nerve. Despite the relative safety of pupillary dilation [risk of dilating a potentially occludable angle using appropriate screening criteria is less than 3/1000 (51)], few non-ophthalmologists are able to adequately examine the optic nerve for signs of glaucomatous optic nerve damage. The last issue, regarding the role of elevated

IOP in the definition of POAG, has resulted in the further categorization of POAG into classical POAG, which has elevated IOP as well as optic nerve damage, and low-tension glaucoma, which has IOP in the "normal" range, but damage to the optic nerve. While a number of investigators have claimed to demonstrate differences in the clinical presentation of low tension glaucoma as compared with classical POAG (14, 16), a growing body of evidence suggests that most cases are part of the expected distribution of POAG (2, 43, 60, 64). Nevertheless, it is likely that there is heterogeneity in the etiology of POAG in both the classical form as well as those with "normal" IOP. An extremely important problem regarding the definition of POAG from an epidemiologic perspective is the realization that objective structural criteria such as cup:disc ratio or other characteristics of the optic nerve are poorly sensitive to detecting glaucomatous optic nerve damage (28, 73). Examination of the visual field is necessary, as up to one third of cases will be missed when using structural criteria alone.

MAGNITUDE AND SEVERITY OF THE PROBLEM

There is a significant amount of recent data on the prevalence of POAG in the United States and around the world. As can be seen in Table 1, estimates range from 0.42% in Wales to over 14% among blacks on St. Lucia. Two main factors account for the observed variation in rates (excluding sampling error): race of the study population and the definition of glaucoma used. Persons of African heritage have higher rates than whites (see section below on Race). In whites, studies that conducted visual field testing on all subjects and did not require elevated IOP as a criterion for diagnosis suggest that the prevalence is between 1.5% and 2.0% for those 40 years or older.

While good data on the prevalence of glaucoma are now available, adequate information on the incidence of POAG is not. Statistical models that incorporate age-specific cross-sectional prevalence data and general population survival rates (41) as well as longitudinal studies that were not population-based (5, 6, 52) have been used to estimate incidence rates for various populations, primarily white residents of the United States. Such studies indicate that, even in study populations enriched with subjects who are considered high risk for the development of glaucomatous optic nerve damage, the incidence of new cases is quite low, in the range of 1/1000 to 1/100 per year (5, 6, 52). Results from statistical modeling of incidence indicate that, for a general population of whites, rates are even lower, ranging from 0.08/1000 per year for those in their early forties to 1.46/1000 per year for persons in their eighties (41). Direct estimates of incidence will be available over the next few years from longitudinal studies currently under way in Baltimore, Beaver Dam (Wisconsin), and Barbados.

Table 1 Prevalence of open angle glaucoma in various populations

Source	Criteria for defining POAG	N	Age range	Prevalence estimate	Ethnicity
Europe					
Wales, 1966 (25)	Concurrent cupping of the optic disc and visual field loss (visual fields were only done on 1/3 of the sample)	4231	40–75 years	0.42%	White Welsh
Dalby, Sweden, 1981 (10)	Concurrent visual field loss and optic nerve cupping	1511	55–69 years	0.86%	White Swedish
Iceland, 1986 (80)	Pharmacy and physician dispensary records indicating treatment for glaucoma or hospital records indicating surgery for glaucoma	—	≥50 years	1.91%	White Icelandic
Sweden, 1982 (45)	Diagnoses of optic disc cupping and visual field loss as recorded in clinical records	Entire population of Sweden	≥50 years	1.4%	White Swedish
Rotterdam, The Netherlands, 1994 (20)	Visual field loss plus either optic disk cupping or elevated intraocular pressure	3062	≥55 years	1.1%	White Dutch
Ireland, 1993 (17)	At least two of the following: visual field loss, cupping of the optic disc, elevated intraocular pressure	2186	≥50 years	1.9%	White Irish
United States					
Framingham, U.S. 1980 (28)	Visual field loss	2631	52–85 years	2.1%	White Americans
Baltimore, U.S., 1991 (75)	Visual field loss and/or severe optic disc cupping	5308	≥40 years	1.7%	White Americans,
				5.6%	Black Americans
Beaver Dam, Wisconsin, U.S., 1992 (38)	At least two of the following: visual field loss, cupping of the optic disc, elevated intraocular pressure	4926	43–84 years	2.1%	White Americans

Table 1 (*continued*)

Source	Criteria for defining POAG	N	Age range	Prevalence estimate	Ethnicity
Caribbean					
Jamaica, 1969 (81)	Concurrent cupping of the optic disc and visual field loss	574	≥35 years	1.4%	Black Jamaicans
St. Lucia, 1989 (48)	Visual field loss and/or severe optic disc cupping	1679	≥30 years	8.8% –14.7%	Black St. Lucians
Barbados, 1994 (40)	Visual field loss and cupping of the optic nerve	4314	40–84 years	7.0%	Black Barbadians

The degree of functional loss associated with glaucoma is not well understood but is thought to be relatively low except in far advanced disease. Recently, a variety of patient-oriented measures of visual functional status have been developed and applied to patients with cataract (11, 46, 66). Whether such instruments will be useful for a disease like glaucoma, where central vision is spared until the latest stages, is not clear, but modifications will likely be needed in these instruments in order to detect functional loss associated with peripheral vision deficits.

Data are limited on the prevalence of the most severe form of visual functional impairment, blindness due to glaucoma. Most data come from blindness registration systems which are usually incomplete in their ascertainment of blind persons. The Model Reporting Area Study, which last reported results from 1970, used data from 16 states in the U.S. that agreed to a common reporting format and criteria for the definition of blindness (30). Standardization of diagnostic criteria for defining the cause of blindness was not possible, however, nor was there any assurance that ascertainment was equivalent across all participating states. Despite these problems, the Model Reporting Area Study remains a heavily used source of data on the cause-specific rates of blindness in the U.S. In 1970, glaucoma was the third leading cause of blindness (after cataract and age-related macular degeneration) with a prevalence of 16.2/100,000 and an incidence of new blindness registrations of 1.5/100,000 per year (30). Data from other sources suggest that these rates are serious underestimates. The Baltimore Eye Survey estimated the prevalence of glaucomatous blindness at 1.7/1000 in a population with equal numbers of blacks and whites, of which more than 75% was due to POAG (63, 76).

Global estimates of prevalence are particularly difficult, since adequate information is missing from large parts of the world. Thylefors & Negrel used available prevalence data and population models to estimate that there are 13.5 million persons 40 years or older affected with POAG, of whom 3 million are blind (68). Better systems are needed for measuring the burden of disability caused by glaucoma in the population, especially as such data begin to play a major role in evaluating the effectiveness of health care delivery systems.

Another perspective on the size of the glaucoma problem is economic. While cost-of-illness studies often suffer from lack of adequate data, reasonable assumptions can be used to develop a more comprehensive picture of the impact of disease on society than prevalence alone can provide. Such efforts divide total costs into those associated with the direct medical care of persons with illness (direct costs), indirect costs such as lost wages, and income transfer. In 1991, the best estimate of total direct costs for glaucoma in the U.S. was approximately $1.6 billion (69). This estimate reflects the costs of treating one half the total number of persons with glaucoma, as only 50% of those who have POAG have been diagnosed (17, 38, 75). Treating the additional 50% of cases would more than double this estimate, since costly efforts would be required to identify the undiagnosed group. Another $1.1 billion was paid by the government to support individuals blind from glaucoma, and indirect costs were estimated very conservatively at $235 million (69).

DEMOGRAPHIC RISK FACTORS

Age

Glaucoma is strongly associated with age (Figure 1). An increased prevalence with older age has been found in every population-based study. The magnitude

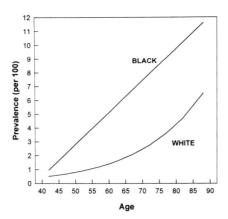

Figure 1 Prevalence of primary open angle glaucoma in whites and blacks based on data from the Baltimore Eye Survey (72).

of this association is large, with prevalence rates between four and ten times higher in the oldest age groups as compared persons in their forties (25, 38, 39, 75). Similarly, the 13-year incidence of glaucomatous visual field defects rose from 0.7% among those less than 40 years of age at baseline to 4.8% among those 60 years or older at baseline in the Collaborative Glaucoma Study (6). Leske et al's statistical projections for white populations show a rise from 0.08/1000 per year to 1.46/1000 per year with increasing age (41), as noted above.

Gender

The relationship of gender to risk of POAG is inconsistent. The Framingham and Barbados Eye Studies found that men had a significantly higher prevalence of POAG than women (39, 40), whereas the opposite was found in Sweden (9, 10), and no association was found in Wales (25), Baltimore (56, 75), Beaver Dam (38), or the Collaborative Glaucoma Study (6). Thus, gender is unlikely to be a major risk factor for POAG.

Race

Racial variations in the risk of POAG are an important part of the epidemiology of this disease. Persons of West African ancestry, including black populations in the Caribbean and the U.S., have significantly higher prevalence of POAG than do caucasians. The evidence for this excess risk in blacks comes from a wide variety of sources. Clinic-based studies have shown that blacks comprise a higher proportion of glaucoma clinic attendees than among general eye clinic populations (47, 83). Blacks also have glaucoma surgery at higher rates than whites (18), and among those who self present to glaucoma screening programs, blacks are more likely to be diagnosed as having glaucoma (23). Prevalence surveys conducted in primarily black populations have shown higher rates of glaucoma than those using similar methods in white populations. Using similar diagnostic criteria, Jamaican blacks had a rate three times higher than that found among the Welsh (25, 81). More recent studies in St. Lucia and Barbados have found extremely high rates, 7% to 16% among those 40 or older, among the black populations of these islands (40, 48). In the United States, the only direct comparison of prevalence between blacks and whites comes from the Baltimore Eye Survey, which found an age-adjusted 4.3-fold excess prevalence of POAG in blacks as compared with their white neighbors (75).

POAG also may be a more severe disease among blacks as they have a younger onset, have more advanced disease at the time of first diagnosis, and are more often refractory to medical therapy (24, 75, 85). It is unclear whether this reflects a more rapid progression of disease or whether it is a combination of a higher age-specific incidence and poor access to or utilization of appropriate eye care services. Clinical trials and longitudinal population studies of POAG in blacks and whites are currently under way and should provide the information necessary to determine if progression and treatment efficacy vary by race.

The reason for the excess risk among blacks is not well understood, but is likely related to an underlying predisposition (75). The association of other conditions such as sickle cell disease, systemic hypertension, and diabetes with race led to suggestions that the racial variation in POAG risk may be a function of this excess comorbidity. However, this hypothesis has not been supported for sickle cell trait, systemic hypertension, or diabetes (67, 70, 71); these factors act independently, if at all, on the risk of POAG.

OCULAR RISK FACTORS

Intraocular Pressure

The relationship between IOP and POAG is strong and consistent even when elevated IOP is excluded as a diagnostic criterion (5, 6, 38, 39, 40, 56, 60, 64). Especially convincing evidence for an etiologic role of increased IOP in development of glaucomatous optic nerve damage comes from the monotonic increase in risk of POAG with increasing IOP (Figure 2), from studies that show asymmetric optic nerve damage in persons with ipsilateral asymmetric elevations in intraocular pressure (15, 19), and from studies that demonstrate a reduction in risk of optic nerve damage among high-risk populations in whom the IOP was lowered (31). While elevated IOP is one of the strongest predictors of who will develop glaucomatous optic neuropathy, even at levels considered

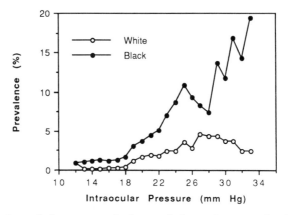

Figure 2   Prevalence of primary open angle glaucoma by intraocular pressure based on data from the Baltimore Eye Survey. Taken from Sommer et al, *Arch. Ophthalmol.* 1991. 109:1090–95 (62), Copyright 1991/95, American Medical Association

dangerously high a significant proportion of persons will never be affected (5). In addition, because of the dramatic overlap of intraocular pressure distributions between those with and without POAG, a large proportion of cases have IOP well within the "normal" range (25, 39, 60, 64). The sensitivity of the classical cut-off for IOP of greater than 21mm Hg is less than 50%, and there is no level at which a reasonable balance of sensitivity and specificity is achieved (39, 60, 64, 73). The implications of these results for the use of tonometry in glaucoma screening are well known; this approach is now generally discouraged (22, 73).

Optic Disc Parameters

Characteristics of the optic nerve head have been used over the years both to identify groups of the population with high risk for glaucomatous optic nerve damage and as criteria for the definition of disease. Such parameters include the cup:disc ratio, the narrowest neuroretinal rim width, rim area, cup volume, and a variety of others, often based on sophisticated three-dimensional imaging of the optic disc. As these parameters are often used to define POAG or determine whether progression has occurred, they are not risk factors in an etiologic sense, but actual markers of damage. In spite of this direct measurement of optic nerve status, the ability of these parameters to accurately classify people into diseased and nondiseased states is poor. As with tonometry, there is no cut-off point in the distribution of cup:disc ratios that achieves adequate balance in terms of sensitivity and specificity (39, 73). Similarly, the narrowest width of the neuroretinal rim, cup volume, and rim area are poor discriminators of disease status and rely on more sophisticated techniques for their measurement (72, 73; unpublished data from the Baltimore Eye Survey).

The integrity of the nerve fiber layer (the axons of retinal ganglion cells) as assessed by clinical examination or fundus photography is a more direct measure of damage to the optic nerve (26) and has been shown to be both sensitive and specific in its ability to classify persons into diseased and non-diseased states (1, 62) and to predict who will develop glaucomatous visual field loss (61). Significant issues remain, however, regarding the transfer of this technology into the general practice of ophthalmology, let alone population screening.

More recently, sophisticated hardware and software systems have been developed to three-dimensionally image the optic nerve head and measure the thickness of the nerve fiber layer. A variety of imaging technologies have been used for this purpose, including stereo-photography, stereo-video imaging, and scanning laser tomography and polarimetry (13, 79, 82). As yet, there is limited information on how these various technologies perform both for classification of persons with and without disease and for detection of progression. This technology is still early in its development, especially of algorithms that can summarize the vast quantities of raw data in a meaningful fashion.

Myopia

Myopia has been associated with glaucoma in a number of studies. Wilson et al found a twofold excess prevalence of myopia among cases of POAG as compared with clinic-based controls (84). Perkins & Phelps reported an odds ratio of almost five when clinic-based cases were compared to age-specific national norms (53). The potential for selection bias when using clinic-based ascertainment for cases is strong for a variable such as myopia, because those with refractive error are more likely to seek eye care and have a higher probability of being diagnosed with glaucoma. However, a small population-based study from Sicily showed a fivefold excess risk associated with myopia of 1.5 diopters or greater (55).

NONOCULAR RISK FACTORS

Diabetes

While it is well known that complications of diabetes can produce secondary glaucoma, the association of diabetes with POAG has been less clear. Case-control studies, all of which ascertained their cases of glaucoma and controls from a clinic or private practice setting, have reported odds ratios ranging from 1.6 to 4.7 (33, 50, 57, 84). Controls were ascertained from similar sources as were cases, but selection cannot be completely ruled out as the source of the observed association in these situations. Population-based prevalence studies in Framingham, Sweden, and Baltimore, and the Collaborative Glaucoma Study have found no association between diabetes and POAG (5, 6, 9, 27, 70). In contrast, the Beaver Dam study found a twofold excess risk of diabetes in persons with POAG as compared with controls (36). This conflict with other population-based studies may be due to the lack of a direct clinical assessment by an ophthalmologist in the Beaver Dam study. Retinal complications of diabetes can produce visual field loss similar in appearance to that of POAG but without its underlying pathology. Such false positive visual field findings could account for this discrepancy.

Systemic Hypertension

The association of systemic hypertension with POAG is controversial and likely to be complicated. Much of the confusion is due to reports that have associated intraocular pressure with systemic blood pressure (27, 35, 42, 49). However, within many of these same investigations, no association was found

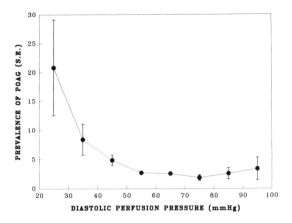

Figure 3   Prevalence of primary open angle glaucoma by diastolic perfusion pressure based on data from the Baltimore Eye Survey. Taken from Tielsch et al, *Arch. Ophthalmol.* 1995. 113:216–21 (68), Copyright 1991/95, American Medical Association.

between POAG and systemic hypertension (27, 42). Other case-control studies also have shown no association with POAG (33, 50), though one has demonstrated a strong and statistically significant association between untreated systolic hypertension and POAG (84).

More recent evidence from the Baltimore Eye Survey suggests that the relationship between POAG and systemic blood pressure is complex and related to a variety of other hemo- and oculo-dynamic factors (71). Age modified the effect of systemic hypertension on risk of POAG. Those below age 60 were protected, while those older than 70 showed a positive association. Such a pattern would be expected if, early in the course of systemic hypertension, the elevated blood pressure resulted in increased perfusion, while later, after significant microvascular damage had occurred, blood flow to the optic nerve head was reduced. An additional important finding was that perfusion pressure was significantly associated with the risk of POAG in a way that would be predicted from autoregulation of blood flow. The prevalence of POAG remained constant across a wide range of perfusion pressure; when perfusion pressure was below 50mm Hg, the prevalence rose dramatically (Figure 3). Unfortunately, because of the cross-sectional nature of these data, we cannot determine the directionality of this observed association, nor do we understand the duration of low perfusion pressure necessary to produce an elevated risk of glaucomatous optic nerve damage. These data support the hypothetical role for vascular factors in the etiology of POAG.

Another mechanism by which glaucomatous optic nerve damage may occur involves vascular spasm, which can result in an acute disruption in blood flow to the retinal nerve fiber layer and optic nerve. This idea is supported by studies showing an association of migraine and Raynaud's syndrome with low tension glaucoma (21, 54), although the one population-based study which examined this matter found no association between migraine-like headache and POAG (37).

Family History of Glaucoma

A number of studies have suggested that between 13 and 25% of patients with glaucoma have a positive family history (8, 34). Epidemiologic studies have estimated that a positive family history of glaucoma is associated with between a two- and fivefold excess risk of POAG (5, 34, 74, 77). In addition, it is well accepted that a number of ocular parameters associated with POAG are influenced by heredity (3, 4,7) and that certain forms of juvenile glaucoma have a genetic basis (44). The search for genetic markers associated with POAG or a common mode of inheritance, however, has not been successful. Early reports of strong associations between selected HLA antigens and glaucoma (58, 59) have not been confirmed (32) and have no value in defining high-risk groups for this disease. While there is little doubt that familial factors play an important role in the underlying susceptibility to the development of POAG through population variations in the mechanical support of the optic nerve head, methodologic weaknesses in previous studies have made it difficult to study familial associations well. Specifically, since POAG is strongly age-related, complete family studies that apply uniform criteria for diagnosis and staging are very difficult.

SCREENING

Glaucoma has long been regarded as a disease that fits well the criteria for screening; it has a long asymptomatic period; it is highly prevalent in the population; and treatment begun early in its course is probably more effective at preventing significant loss of vision. As a result, glaucoma screening has been a popular activity for health and community service organizations based primarily on the use of tonometry (12, 23). Over the past 20 years, however, tonometry has been discredited as an effective screening technique for glaucoma because of a poor balance between sensitivity and specificity (22, 73). Similarly, poor results are produced when classical optic nerve findings are used (73). As a result, screening with tonometry or ophthalmoscopy alone is discouraged by most agencies active in the blindness prevention field, including Prevent Blindness America, and there is general acknowledgement that visual field testing is needed. Unfortunately, even visual field testing has significant error rates, especially among those with early damage.

More recently, it was suggested by Douglas Anderson, University of Miami, that screening using a modified visual field approach be limited to detecting those with moderate-to-severe optic nerve damage who needed to be treated as soon as possible to prevent further loss of vision. Using two different visual field testing strategies, the sensitivity of this approach is estimated between 92% and 97% and the specificity between 94% and 96% (65). In response to these findings, it now seems reasonable to again conduct population screening for glaucoma using trained lay personnel, especially on high-risk populations such as elderly African Americans.

SUMMARY

Epidemiologic studies have provided us with more accurate measures of the magnitude and severity of the disease burden caused by primary open angle glaucoma (POAG). Recent investigations that have included visual field measurements on all subjects have demonstrated that previous estimates of the prevalence of this disorder were too low, by as much as 30 to 50%. Population-based studies also have confirmed the markedly elevated risk of POAG among blacks, although the basis for this excess risk remains unclear. Age and intraocular pressure are the strongest risk factors for POAG across all population groups. There is an exponential rise in rate of POAG with increasing age and intraocular pressure. Family history of glaucoma is also a major risk factor for this disease; however, the genetic and/or environmental source of this association has yet to be elucidated. Other risk factors for this disease include myopia and vascular disorders that result in lowered perfusion pressure to the optic nerve and retina.

Future research on the epidemiology of primary open angle glaucoma will quantify the incidence of this disorder and evaluate the interaction of heredity and environmental factors in producing excess risk.

Literature Cited

1. Airaksinen PJ, Drance SM, Douglas GR, Mawson DK, Nieminen H. 1984. Diffuse and localized nerve fiber layer loss in glaucoma. *Am. J. Ophthalmol.* 98:566–71
2. Anderson DR. 1989. Glaucoma: the damage caused by pressure. XLVI Edward Jackson Memorial Lecture. *Am. J. Ophthalmol.* 108:485–95
3. Armaly MF. 1967. Genetic determination of cup/disc ratio of the optic nerve. *Arch. Ophthalmol.* 78:35–43
4. Armaly MF. 1967. The genetic determinants of ocular pressure in the normal eye. *Arch. Ophthalmol.* 78:187–92
5. Armaly MF. 1980. Lessons to be learned from the Collaborative Glaucoma Study. *Surv. Ophthalmol.* 25:139–44
6. Armaly MF, Krueger DE, Maunder L, Becker B, Hetherington J Jr, et al. 1980. Biostatistical analysis of the Collaborative Glaucoma Study. I. Summary report of the risk factors for glaucomatous visual field defects. *Arch. Ophthalmol.* 98:2163–71
7. Armaly MF, Monstavicius BF, Sayegh

RE. 1968. Ocular pressure and aqueous outflow facility in siblings. *Arch. Ophthalmol.* 80:354–60

8. Becker B, Kolker AE, Roth FD. 1960. Glaucoma family study. *Am. J. Ophthalmol.* 50:557–67

9. Bengtsson B. 1981. Aspects of the epidemiology of chronic glaucoma. *Acta Ophthalmol.* 146(Suppl.):4–26

10. Bengtsson B. 1981. The prevalence of glaucoma. *Br. J. Ophthalmol.* 65: 46–49

11. Bernth-Peterson P. 1982. Outcomes of cataract surgery. II. Visual functioning in aphakic patients. *Acta Ophthalmol.* 60:243–51

12. Brav SS, Kirber HP. 1951. Mass screening for glaucoma. *JAMA* 147:1127–8

13. Caprioli J, Miller JM. 1988. Videographic measurements of optic nerve topography in glaucoma. *Invest. Ophthalmol. Vis. Sci.* 29:1294–98

14. Caprioli J, Spaeth GL. 1984. Comparison of visual field defects in low-tension and high-tension glaucoma. *Am. J. Ophthalmol.* 97:730–37

15. Cartwright MJ, Anderson DR. 1988. Correlation of asymmetric damage with asymmetric intraocular pressure in normal tension glaucoma. *Arch. Ophthalmol.* 106:898–900

16. Chauhan BC, Drance SM, Douglas GR, Johnson CA. 1989. Visual field damage in normal-tension and high-tension glaucoma. *Am. J. Ophthalmol.* 108: 636–42

17. Coffey M, Reidy A, Wormold R, Xian WX, Wright L, Courtney P. 1993. Prevalence of glaucoma in the west of Ireland. *Br. J. Ophthalmol.* 77:17–21

18. Coulehan JL, Helzlsouer KJ, Rodgers KD, Brown SI. 1980. Racial differences in intraocular tension and glaucoma surgery. *Am. J. Epidemiol.* 111:759–68

19. Crichton A, Drance SM, Douglas GR, Schulzer M. 1989. Unequal intraocular pressure and its relation to asymmetric visual field defects in low tension glaucoma. *Ophthalmology* 96:1312–14

20. Dielemans I, Vingerling JR, Wolfs RCW, Hofman A, Grabbee DE, de Jong PTVM. 1994. The prevalence of primary open-angle glaucoma in a population based study in the Netherlands. *Ophthalmology* 101:1851–55

21. Drance SM, Douglas GR, Wijsman K, Schulzer M, Britton RJ. 1988. Response of blood flow to warm and cold in normal and low-tension glaucoma patients. *Am. J. Ophthalmol.* 105: 35–39

22. Eddy DM, Sanders LE, Eddy JF. 1983. The value of screening for glaucoma with tonometry. *Surv. Ophthalmol.* 28: 194–205

23. Frydman JE, Clower JW, Fulghum JE, Hester MW. 1966. Glaucoma detection in Florida. *JAMA* 198:1237–40

24. Grant WM, Burke JF. 1982. Why do some people go blind from glaucoma? *Ophthalmology* 89:991–98

25. Hollows FC, Graham PA. 1966. Intraocular pressure, glaucoma and glaucoma suspects in a defined population. *Br. J. Ophthalmol.* 50:570–86

26. Hoyt WF, Frisen L, Newman NM. 1973. Fundoscopy of nerve fiber layer defects in glaucoma. *Invest. Ophthalmol. Vis. Sci.* 12:814–29

27. Kahn HA, Leibowitz HM, Ganley JP, Kini MM, Colton T, et al. 1977. The Framingham Eye Study II. Association of ophthalmic pathology with single variables previously measured in the Framingham Heart Study. *Am. J. Epidemiol.* 106:33–41

28. Kahn HA, Milton RC. 1980. Alternative definitions of open-angle glaucoma. Effect on prevalence and associations in the Framingham Eye Study. *Arch. Ophthalmol.* 98:2172–79

29. Kahn HA, Milton RC. 1980. Revised Framingham Eye Study prevalence of glaucoma and diabetic retinopathy. *Am. J. Epidemiol.* 111:769–76

30. Kahn HA, Moorhead HB. 1973. *Statistics on Blindness in the Model Reporting Area 1969–1970.* US DHEW Publ. No. (NIH) 73–427

31. Kass MA, Gordon MO, Hoff MR, Parkinson JM, Kolker AE, et al. 1989. Topical Timolol administration reduces the incidence of glaucomatous damage in ocular hypertensive individuals. A randomized, double-masked, long-term clinical trial. *Arch. Ophthalmol.* 107: 1590–98

32. Kass MA, Palmberg P, Becker B, Miller JP. 1978. Histocompatibility antigens and primary open-angle glaucoma. A reassessment. *Arch. Ophthalmol.* 96: 2207–8

33. Katz J, Sommer A. 1988. Risk factors for primary open angle glaucoma. *Am. J. Prev. Med.* 4:110–14

34. Kellerman L, Posner A. 1955. The value of heredity in the detection and study of glaucoma. *Am. J. Ophthalmol.* 40: 681–85

35. Klein BE, Klein R. 1981. Intraocular pressure and cardiovascular risk factors. *Arch. Ophthalmol.* 99:837–39

36. Klein BEK, Klein R, Jensen SC. 1994. Open-angle glaucoma and older-onset diabetes: the Beaver Dam Eye Study. *Ophthalmology* 101:1173–77

37. Klein BEK, Klein R, Mever SM, Goetz LA. 1993.. Migraine headache and its association with open-angle glaucoma: the Beaver Dam Eye Study. *Invest. Ophthalmol. Vis. Sci.* 34:3024–27

38. Klein BEK, Klein R, Sponsel WE, Franke T, Cantor LB, et al. 1992. Prevalence of glaucoma. The Beaver Dam Eye Study. *Ophthalmology* 99:1499–504

39. Leibowitz HM, Krueger DE, Maunder LR, Milton RC, Kini MM, et al. 1980. The Framingham Eye Study Monograph. *Surv. Ophthalmol.* 24(Suppl.): 335–610

40. Leske MC, Connell AMS, Schachat RP, Hyman L, and the Barbados Eye Study Group. 1994. The Barbados Eye Study. Prevalence of open angle glaucoma. *Arch. Ophthalmol.* 112:821–29

41. Leske MC, Ederer F, Podgor M. 1981. Estimating incidence from age-specific prevalence in glaucoma. *Am. J. Epidemiol.* 113:606–13

42. Leske MC, Podgor MJ. 1983. Intraocular pressure, cardiovascular risk variables and visual field defects. *Am. J. Epidemiol.* 118:280–87

43. Lewis RA, Heyreh SS, Phelps CD. 1983. Optic disc and visual field correlations in primary open angle and low tension glaucoma. *Am. J. Ophthalmol.* 96:148–52

44. Lichter PR. 1994. Genetic clues to glaucoma's secrets. The L. Edward Jackson Memorial Lecture. Part 2. *Am. J. Ophthalmol.* 117:706–27

45. Lindblom B, Thorborn W. 1982. Prevalence of visual field defects due to capsular and simple glaucoma in Halsingland, Sweden. *Acta Ophthalmol.* 60: 353–61

46. Mangione CM, Phillips RS, Seddon JM, Lawrence MG, Cook EF, et al. 1992. Development of the Activities of Daily Vision Scale: a measure of visual functional status. *Med. Care* 30:1111–26

47. Martin MJ, Sommer A, Gold EB, Diamond EL. 1985. Race and primary open angle glaucoma. *Am. J. Ophthalmol.* 99:383–87

48. Mason RP, Kosoko O, Wilson MR, Martone JF, Cowan CL Jr, et al. 1989. National survey of the prevalence and risk factors of glaucoma in St. Lucia, West Indies. Part I: prevalence findings. *Ophthalmology* 96:1363–68

49. McLeod SD, West SK, Quigley HA, Fozard JL. 1990. A longitudinal study of the relationship between intraocular and blood pressures. *Invest. Ophthalmol. Vis. Sci.* 31:2361–66

50. Morgan RW, Drance SM. 1975. Chronic open-angle glaucoma and ocular hypertension: an epidemiological study. *Br. J. Ophthalmol.* 59:211–15

51. Patel KH, Javitt JC, Tielsch JM, Street DA, Katz J, et al. 1995. Incidence of acute angle-closure glaucoma after pharmacologic mydriasis. *Am. J. Ophthalmol.* In press

52. Perkins ES. 1973. The Bedford glaucoma survey. I. Long-term follow-up of borderline cases. *Br. J. Ophthalmol.* 57: 179–85

53. Perkins ES, Phelps CD. 1982. Open angle glaucoma, ocular hypertension, low tension glaucoma, and refraction. *Arch. Ophthalmol.* 100:1464–67

54. Phelps CD, Corbett JJ. 1985. Migraine and low-tension glaucoma. A case-control study. *Invest. Ophthalmol. Vis. Sci.* 26:1105–8

55. Ponte F, Giuffre G, Giammanco R, Dardononi G. 1994. Risk factors of ocular hypertension and glaucoma. The Casteldaccia Eye Study. *Doc. Ophthalmol.* 85:203–10

56. Quigley HA, Enger C, Katz J, Sommer A, Scott R, Gilbert D. 1994. Risk factors for the developoment of glaucomatous visual field loss in ocular hypertension. *Arch. Ophthalmol.* 112:644–49

57. Reynolds DC. 1977. Relative risk factors in chronic open angle glaucoma: an epidemiological study. *Am. J. Optom. Physiol. Optics* 54:116–20

58. Shin DH, Becker B. 1977. HLA-A11 and HLA-Bw35 and resistance to glaucoma in white patients with ocular hypertension. *Arch. Ophthalmol.* 95: 423–24

59. Shin DH, Becker B, Waltman SR, Palmberg PF, Bell E Jr. 1977. The prevalence of HLA-B12 and HLA-B7 antigens in primary open-angle glaucoma. *Arch. Ophthalmol.* 95:224–25

60. Sommer A. 1989. Intraocular pressure and glaucoma. *Am. J. Ophthalmol.* 107: 186–88

61. Sommer A, Katz J, Quigley HA, Miller NR, Robin AL, et al. 1991. Clinically detectable nerve fiber layer atrophy precedes the onset of glaucomatous field loss. *Arch. Ophthalmol.* 109:77–83

62. Sommer A, Quigley HA, Robin AL, Miller NR, Katz J, Arkell S. 1984. Evaluation of nerve fiber layer assessment. *Arch. Ophthalmol.* 102:1766–71

63. Sommer A, Tielsch JM, Katz J, Quigley HA, Gottsch JD, et al. 1991. Racial differences in the cause-specific prevalence of blindness in east Baltimore. *N. Engl. J. Med.* 325:1412–17

64. Sommer A, Tielsch JM, Katz J, Quigley HA, Gottsch JD, et al. 1991. Relation-

ship between intraocular pressure and primary open angle glaucoma among white and black Americans: the Baltimore Eye Survey. *Arch. Ophthalmol.* 109:1090–95

65. Sponsel WE, Ritch R, Stamper R, Higginbotham EJ, Anderson D, et al. 1995. Prevent Blindness America visual field screening study. *Am. J. Ophthalmol.* In press

66. Steinberg EP, Tielsch JM, Schein OD, Javitt JC, Sharkey P, et al. 1994. The VF-14. An index of functional impairment in patients with cataract. *Arch. Ophthalmol.* 112:630–38

67. Steinmann W, Stone R, Nichols C, Werner E, Schweitzer J, et al. 1983. A case-control study of the association of sickle cell trait and chronic open-angle glaucoma. *Am. J. Epidemiol.* 118:288–93

68. Thylefors F, Negrel A-D. 1994. The global impact of glaucoma. *Bull WHO* 72:323–26

69. Tielsch JM. 1993. Therapy for glaucoma: costs and consequences. In *Glaucoma: Diagnosis and Therapy. Trans. New Orleans Acad. Ophthalmol.*, ed. SF Ball, RM Franklin, pp. 61–68. Amsterdam: Kugler

70. Tielsch JM, Katz J, Quigley HA, Javitt JC, Sommer A. 1995. Diabetes and primary open-angle glaucoma in the Baltimore Eye Survey. *Ophthalmology* 102:48–53

71. Tielsch JM, Katz J, Quigley HA, Javitt JC, Sommer A. 1995. Hypertension, perfusion pressure and primary open angle glaucoma: a population-based assessment. *Arch. Ophthalmol.* 113:216–21

72. Tielsch JM, Katz J, Quigley HA, Miller NR, Sommer A. 1988. Intraobserver and interobserver agreement in measurement of optic disc characteristics. *Ophthalmology* 95:350–56

73. Tielsch JM, Katz J, Singh K, Quigley HA, Gottsch JD, et al. 1991. A population-based evaluation of glaucoma screening: the Baltimore Eye Survey. *Am. J. Epidemiol.* 134:1102–10

74. Tielsch JM, Katz J, Sommer A, Quigley HA, Javitt JC. 1994. Family history and risk of primary open angle glaucoma: the Baltimore Eye Survey. *Arch. Ophthalmol.* 112:69–73

75. Tielsch JM, Sommer A, Katz J, Royall RM, Quigley HA, Javitt J. 1991. Racial variations in the prevalence of primary open angle glaucoma: the Baltimore Eye Survey. *JAMA* 266:369–74

76. Tielsch JM, Sommer A, Witt K, Katz J, Royall RM. 1990. Blindness and visual impairment in an American urban population: the Baltimore Eye Survey. *Arch. Ophthalmol.* 108:286–90

77. Uhm KB, Shin DH. 1992. Positive family history of glaucoma is a risk factor for increased IOP rather than glaucomatous optic nerve damage (POAG vs OH vs Normal Control). *Korean J. Ophthalmol.* 6:100–4

78. Van Buskirk EM. 1994. Glaucomatous optic neuropathy. *J. Glaucoma* 3:S2–S3

79. Varma R, Spaeth GL. 1988. The PARIS 2000: a new system for retinal digital image analysis. *Ophthal. Surg.* 19:183–92

80. Viggosson G, Bjornsson G, Ingvason JG. 1986. The prevalence of open-angle glaucoma in Iceland. *Acta Ophthalmol.* 64:138–41

81. Wallace J, Lovell HG. 1969. Glaucoma and intraocular pressure in Jamaica. *Am. J. Ophthalmol.* 67:93–100

82. Weinreb RN, Dreher AW, Bille JF. 1989. Quantitative assessment of the optic nerve head with the laser tomographic scanner. *Int. Ophthalmol.* 13:25–29

83. Wilensky JT, Gandhi N, Pan T. 1978. Racial influences in open angle glaucoma. *Am. J. Ophthalmol.* 10:1398–402

84. Wilson MR, Hertzmark E, Walker AM, Childs-Shaw K, Epstein DL. 1987. A case-control study of risk factors in open angle glaucoma. *Arch. Ophthalmol.* 105:1066–71

85. Wilson R, Richardson TM, Hertzmark E, Grant WM. 1985. Race as a risk factor for progressive glaucomatous damage. *Ann. Ophthalmol.* 17:653–59

Annu. Rev. Public Health. 1996. 17:137–58

DIABETIC RETINOPATHY

R. Klein

Department of Ophthalmology and Visual Sciences, University of
Wisconsin-Madison Medical School, Madison, Wisconsin 53705

KEY WORDS: epidemiology, glycemic control, risk factors, screening

ABSTRACT

Diabetic retinopathy is a leading cause of loss of vision in the United States (74).
Results of recent population-based studies and randomized controlled clinical
trials suggest that glycemic control can lower the incidence and prevent the
progression of retinopathy and loss of vision associated with diabetes (16, 17,
45, 50, 79). In addition, data from clinical trials showed that timely photocoagulation treatment of severe proliferative retinopathy or clinically significant macular edema prevents loss of vision (18, 21). This report reviews the epidemiology
of diabetic retinopathy and highlights areas in need of further epidemiologic
research.

BRIEF BACKGROUND REGARDING THE NATURAL HISTORY AND PATHOGENESIS OF DIABETIC RETINOPATHY

Introduction

Diabetic retinopathy is a leading cause of loss of vision in the United States
(74). Results of recent population-based studies and randomized controlled
clinical trials suggest that glycemic control can lower the incidence and prevent
the progression of retinopathy and loss of vision associated with diabetes (16,
17, 45, 50, 79). In addition, data from clinical trials showed that timely photocoagulation treatment of severe proliferative retinopathy or clinically significant macular edema prevents loss of vision (18, 21). This report reviews the
epidemiology of diabetic retinopathy and highlights areas in need of further
epidemiologic research.

Diabetic retinopathy is characterized by the development of various lesions
involving the blood vessels in the back layer of the eye, the retina. The initial
clinical manifestations of retinopathy are retinal microaneurysms, outpouch-
ings of the capillary bed (9). Soft exudates, large intraretinal hemorrhages,
intraretinal microvascular abnormalities, and venous dilation and beading re-

137

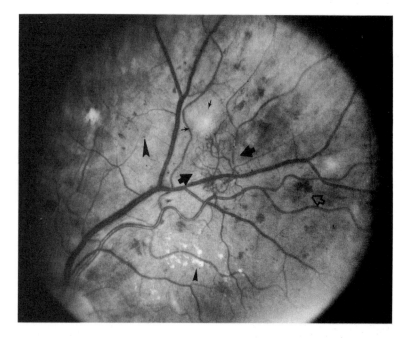

Figure 1 Black and white fundus photograph of the left eye of a patient with diabetes showing nonproliferative and proliferative retinal changes. At the lower left corner the margin of the optic nerve head is seen. The darker larger vein is beaded. There are retinal microaneurysms (*long black arrowhead*), blot hemorrhages (*open arrow*), hard exudate (*short black arrowhead*), intraretinal microvascular abnormalities and soft exudates (signs of nonproliferative retinopathy; *small black arrows*), and retinal new blood vessels (proliferative retinopathy; *larger black arrows*) present.

sult from ischemic changes in the retina (Figure 1). Breakdown in the retinal-blood-brain barrier may result in exudation of lipids and proteinaceous material and thickening of the retinal tissue, or macular edema. This edematous process is an important cause of loss of vision in people with diabetes (41, 67). These retinal changes are called nonproliferative retinopathy.

Severe retinal ischemia may result in the development of abnormal retinal new vessels associated with fibrous tissue (9). This is called proliferative retinopathy. Initially, these new vessels are not associated with symptoms. However, contraction of the abnormal new retinal blood vessels may result in hemorrhage into the vitreous cavity of the eye, tractional detachment of the retina, and significant decreases in visual acuity. In one study assigning causes of visual impairment, proliferative diabetic retinopathy and/or macula edema was the sole or contributing cause of visual acuity of 20/200 or worse in about 86% of eyes in younger-onset persons and in 33% of eyes of older-onset persons (41).

While the natural history of diabetic retinopathy has been well described since the end of the nineteenth century, its pathogenesis remains uncertain. Hyperglycemia is associated with changes in blood flow, viscosity, aggregation and deformability characteristics of red blood cells and platelets, release of various growth factors (such as vascular endothelial growth factor and insulin-like growth factors), and biochemical changes involving glycosylation, aldose reductase and protein kinase activity, and nitrous oxide metabolism (39). Some of these pathogenetic mechanisms may be more important only at specific stages in the evolution of diabetic retinopathy. Significant variability across individuals regarding specific physiologic and biochemical responses to hyperglycemia is also likely.

PREVALENCE AND INCIDENCE OF DIABETIC RETINOPATHY

Data from recent population-based epidemiologic studies have permitted estimates of prevalence and incidence of diabetic retinopathy (5, 12, 13, 19, 20, 22, 24, 25, 27, 28, 31, 32, 34, 46–48, 52, 53, 61–63, 65, 66, 75–77, 80, 81, 84, 89; Table 1). In one such study, composed largely of non-Hispanic whites living in and receiving their primary care in an 11-county area of southcentral Wisconsin, the Wisconsin Epidemiologic Study of Diabetic Retinopathy (WESDR), estimates of retinopathy were based on masked gradings of 30° stereoscopic fundus color photographs (46–48, 52, 53). In that study, the highest frequencies of any retinopathy, proliferative retinopathy, and macular edema were in younger-onset persons diagnosed before 30 years of age; the lowest frequencies were in older-onset persons not taking (not requiring) insulin who were diagnosed at 30 years of age or older (47, 48; Table 2). The higher prevalence of proliferative retinopathy in those taking insulin compared to those not taking insulin has been shown to be related to poorer glycemic control associated with the "severity" of the disease and not the use of insulin (44).

Based on the observations from the WESDR, it has been estimated that of the 5.8 million people in the United States known to have diabetes in 1980–82, 700,000 had proliferative retinopathy and 325,000 had clinically significant macular edema (40), of whom 390,000 had both complications. These may be underestimates, as recent data from the National Health and Nutrition Examination Survey III suggest that rates of retinopathy and proliferative retinopathy are higher in non-Hispanic blacks and Mexican Americans than in non-Hispanic whites (27).

The incidence of diabetic retinopathy, progression of retinopathy, and progression to proliferative retinopathy over a ten-year period also have been estimated in the WESDR (46). Consistent with the prevalence data, the highest

Table 1 Selected list of population-based studies describing the prevalence and/or incidence of diabetic retinopathy in patients with diabetes

Reference	Site	Type of diabetes	No. studied	Duration of diabetes (years)	Retinopathy detection[a]	Crude prevalence (%)	Crude incidence
19	Pima Indians, AZ	NIDDM	399	0–10+	O	18	
5,75	Pima Indians, AZ	NIDDM	279		O		4 years = 2.6%
32	Framingham, MA	NIDDM	229		O	18	
62,63,89	Oklahoma Indians	NIDDM	973	0–20+	O,P	24	
28	Poole, England	IDDM	714	0–30+	O,P	Not reported	10–16 years = 72.3%
		NIDDM				Severe Ret. 8.3	
34	Nauru, Central Pacific	NIDDM	343	0–10+	O	24	
20	Rochester, MN	IDDM	75				45.8/1000 person-years
	Rochester, MN	NIDDM	1060		O		15.6/1000 person-years
13	Iceland	IDDM	212	0–20+	P	34	
12	Perth, Australia	IDDM	179	0–20+	O,P	33	
		NIDDM	904	0–20+	O,P	27	
81	County of Fynn, Denmark	IDDM	718	0–30+	O	48	
76,77	Falster, Denmark	IDDM	215	0–58	P	66	1 year = 3.7%
		NIDDM	333	0–42	P	41	1 year = 3.7%
84	Switzerland	IDDM	105	0–30+	O	51	8 years = 39%
		NIDDM	94			9	8 years = 15%
24	San Antonio, TX	NIDDM	257	0–10+	O,P	45	
31	Gotland, Sweden	IDDM	160	0–20+	P	56–65	
		NIDDM	140			17	

Table 1 (Continued)

Reference	Site	Type of diabetes	No. studied	Duration of diabetes (years)	Retinopathy detection[a]	Crude prevalence (%)	Crude incidence
25	San Luis Valley, CO (Hispanics)	NIDDM	166	0–5+	P	19	
66	Leicester, England	IDDM	350	15+		88	
				0–30+	O,P	41	
46,47,48, 52,53	South Central, WI	IDDM	996	0–30+	O,P	71	4 years = 59%
		NIDDM	1370	0–30+	O,P	39	10 years = 89% 4 years = 34% 10 years = 79%
61,65	Allegheny County, PA	IDDM	657	6–38	O,P	86	
22	Seattle, WA (2nd generation Japanese-American men)	IDDM	78	0–10+	O,P	11.5	2 years = 33%
		NIDDM					
80[b]	Alberta, Canada	IDDM	2300	0–60+	O,P	59.9	
		NIDDM	1346	0–35+	O,P	29.9	
27	United States	NIDDM	457	0–15+	P		
	(White)					13.1	
	(Non-Hispanic Black)					27.7	
	(Mexican American)					35.1	

[a] O = Ophthalmoscopy, P = Photography
[b] Unpublished data

SOURCE: Klein R, Klein BEK, Moss SE. 1989. The Wisconsin Epidemiologic Study of Diabetic Retinopathy: A review. *Diabetes Metab. Rev.* 5:559–70. Copyright 1989, John Wiley & Sons Ltd. Reprinted by permission.

Table 2 Prevalence of Retinopathy in the Wisconsin Epidemiologic Study of Diabetic Retinopathy

Retinopathy Status	Younger-onset taking insulin (No. at risk = 996) %	Older-onset taking insulin (No. at risk = 673) %	Older-onset not taking insulin (No. at risk = 692) %
None	29.3	29.9	61.3
Early nonproliferative	30.4	30.6	27.3
Moderate to severe nonproliferative	17.6	25.7	8.5
Proliferative			
without high risk of visual loss	13.2	9.1	1.4
with high risk of visual loss or worse	9.5	4.8	1.4
Clinically significant macular edema	5.9[a]	11.6[b]	3.7[c]

[a, b, c] No. at risk = 953, 631, 672, respectively

rates of incidence and of progression of retinopathy were found in the younger-onset group, and the lowest rates were in the older-onset group not using insulin (Table 3). Based on the WESDR data, we estimated that each year, of the 7.3 million Americans with known diabetes in 1990, about 80,000 will develop proliferative retinopathy and 95,000 will develop macular edema. While the ten-year incidence of proliferative retinopathy was higher in the younger-onset group in the WESDR, the estimated number of incident cases of proliferative

Table 3 Ten-year incidence of any retinopathy, progression of retinopathy, progression to proliferative retinopathy, or incidence of macular edema in the Wisconsin Epidemiologic Study of Diabetic Retinopathy

	Younger-onset taking insulin		Older-onset taking insulin		Older-onset not taking insulin	
	No. at risk	%	No. at risk	%	No. at risk	%
Incidence of any retinopathy	261	89.3	146	79.2	301	66.9
Progression	712	75.8	417	68.7	487	52.9
Progression to proliferative retinopathy	712	29.8	417	23.6	487	9.7
Incidence of macular edema	688	20.1	329	25.4	444	13.9

SOURCE: Klein R, Klein BEK, Moss SE, Cruickshanks KJ. 1994. The Wisconsin Epidemiologic Study of Diabetic Retinopathy. XIV. Ten-year incidence and progression of diabetic retinopathy. *Arch. Ophthalmol.* 112:1217–28. Copyright 1994, American Medical Association.

retinopathy over the ten-year period was higher in the older-onset group (387 vs 226, respectively). Similarly, the number of incident cases of macular edema over the ten-year period is higher in the older-onset group than in the younger-onset group (426 vs 157, respectively). In the WESDR, even after controlling for duration of diabetes or severity of retinopathy at baseline, the estimated yearly incidence of proliferative retinopathy and macular edema in older-onset persons appeared to be increasing during the last six-year interval of the study (1984–1990) compared to the first four years of the study (1980–1984) (46). These data underscore the need for timely referral and appropriate ophthalmologic care for people with older-onset diabetes and also suggest the possible need for additional health care resources to detect and treat these individuals with photocoagulation.

The prevalence of diabetic retinopathy is strongly related to duration of diabetes since diagnosis. In the WESDR, after 20 or more years of diabetes, 99% of the younger-onset group had signs of retinopathy, 53% had proliferative retinopathy, and 29% had macular edema (47, 49; Figure 2). Lower frequencies were found in older-onset people (48, 49; Figure 2). However, in the first three years after diagnosis of diabetes, 23% of the older-onset group not taking insulin had retinopathy and 2% had proliferative retinopathy. Harris et al (26), using data from the WESDR and another population-based study of diabetes in Australia, showed that by extrapolating prevalence of retinopathy at different durations of diabetes back to the time when retinopathy prevalence was estimated to be zero, the onset of noninsulin-dependent diabetes was calculated as likely to have begun at least 5 to 7 years prior to the time of diagnosis. These data support the importance of examination of the retinal fundus in people with older-onset diabetes at the time of diagnosis.

RELATION OF DIABETIC RETINOPATHY TO HYPERGLYCEMIA

Recent epidemiologic studies and clinical trials have demonstrated a strong inverse relationship between good glycemic control and the development and progression of diabetic retinopathy (4, 5, 13, 19, 22, 24, 25, 28, 31, 34, 45, 50, 59, 61–63, 65, 84, 89; Table 4). In the WESDR, we examined the relationship of hyperglycemia, as measured by glycosylated hemoglobin (the unit of measurement is percentage), an indicator of blood sugar over the preceding three months, to the incidence and progression of diabetic retinopathy over the ten-year period of the study (45). Quartiles for baseline glycosylated hemoglobin were calculated after combining the younger- and older-onset groups in that study. Strong trends for increasing ten-year incidence, progression, and progression to proliferative retinopathy were found with increasing quartiles of glycosylated hemoglobin (poorer glycemic con-

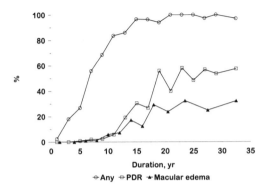

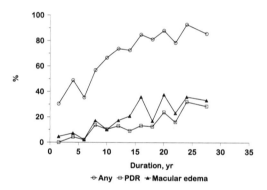

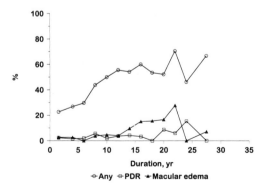

Figure 2 The prevalence of any retinopathy, proliferative retinopathy, and macular edema by duration of diabetes in the younger-onset group (*top*) and the older-onset groups taking (*center*) and not taking (*bottom*) insulin participating in the Wisconsin Epidemiologic Study of Diabetic Retinopathy, 1980–82.

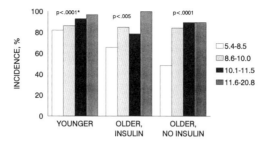

* MANTEL-HAENSZEL TEST OF TREND

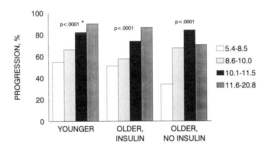

* MANTEL-HAENSZEL TEST OF TREND

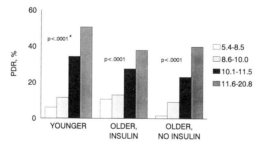

* MANTEL-HAENSZEL TEST OF TREND

Figure 3   The relationship of incidence (*top*), progression (*center*), and progression to proliferative retinopathy (*bottom*) in persons with younger-onset diabetes, persons with older-onset diabetes taking insulin, and persons with older-onset diabetes not taking insulin over a ten-year period to glycosylated hemoglobin levels by quartiles for the whole population at baseline. *P* values are based on the Mantel-Haenszel test of trend. Source: Klein R, Klein BEK, Moss SE, Cruickshanks KJ. 1994. Relationship of hyperglycemia to the long-term incidence and progression of diabetic retinopathy. *Arch. Intern. Med.* 154:2169–78. Copyright 1994, American Medical Association.

trol) at baseline in the younger-onset, older-onset taking insulin, and older-onset not taking insulin groups (Figure 3). These findings remained after controlling for other risk variables and suggested that *glycemic control,* not *type* of diabetes, was more important as a predictor of incidence and progression of retinopathy.

The WESDR data showed that the relationship between level of glycemia and the incidence and progression of retinopathy extended across the whole range of levels of hyperglycemia in people with younger- and older-onset diabetes, with no evidence of a threshold below which lowering blood sugar did not have a beneficial effect (38). In addition, the relation between glycemic control and the incidence and progression of retinopathy remained regardless of the years since diagnosis of diabetes or at any retinopathy severity level. These data suggest that glycemic control anytime during the course of diabetes or at any stage of retinopathy prior to the development of proliferative retinopathy, is related to the long-term incidence and progression of retinopathy.

In the WESDR, after controlling for age, duration of diabetes, baseline retinopathy level, and glycosylated hemoglobin at baseline, it was estimated that a 2% decrease in glycosylated hemoglobin (for example, from 11.5% to 9.5%) from baseline to the four-year follow-up resulted in statistically significant reductions of 42% and 47% in the younger-onset group and 50% and 38% in the older-onset group not taking insulin for the ten-year incidence of proliferative retinopathy and macular edema, respectively (38).

Recently, the Diabetes Control and Complications Trial (DCCT) reported findings comparable to those of the WESDR (16, 17). In that trial, a total of 1441 patients with IDDM (726 persons with no retinopathy at baseline, labeled the primary prevention cohort; and 715 with mild retinopathy, labeled the secondary-intervention cohort) were randomly assigned to intensive therapy (external insulin pump or three or more daily insulin injections and frequent blood glucose monitoring) or to conventional therapy (one or two daily insulin injections). In the DCCT, intensive glycemic control was associated with a dramatic reduction in the incidence and progression of retinopathy in people with IDDM (Figures 4, 5). In addition, intensive insulin therapy resulted in significant reductions in the incidence of severe nonproliferative or proliferative retinopathy (47%), laser photocoagulation (51%), and macular edema (26%), compared with those treated conventionally. The DCCT concluded that "the beneficial effect of intensive treatment in slowing the progression of retinopathy was very substantial, increased with time, was consistent across all outcome measures assessed, and was present across the spectrum of retinopathy severity enrolled in the DCCT."

These findings have important public health implications because of the high prevalence of relatively poor glycemic control in people with insulin-

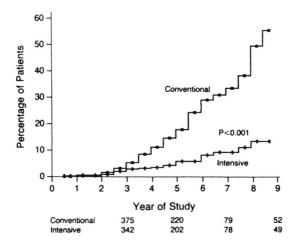

Figure 4 Cumulative incidence of a sustained change in retinopathy in patients with IDDM receiving intensive or conventional therapy in the primary prevention group of the DCCT. Year of study refers to sample sizes at different years of the study. Reprinted by permission of *The New England Journal of Medicine*. The DCCT Research Group, 329:977–86, 1993. Copyright 1993. Massachusetts Medical Society. All rights reserved.

dependent diabetes. In 1980–82, in the WESDR, only 6.7% of people with younger-onset insulin-dependent diabetes mellitus fell within two standard deviations of the mean glycosylated hemoglobin (8.0%) for people without diabetes (54). Although there was some improvement in glycemic control in the following four years in Wisconsin, as well as elsewhere, there remains a significant number of poorly controlled patients with insulin dependent diabetes mellitus who would benefit from intensive glycemic control (56).

In Wisconsin, only 34.8% of the older-onset group not taking insulin fell within two standard deviations of the mean glycosylated hemoglobin (8.0%) for people without diabetes, and there has been little change in levels of glycemia in this group over the ten years of the study (R Klein, unpublished data). An important question is whether the results of the DCCT can be extrapolated to people with NIDDM (43, 71). The American Diabetes Association recently revised their guidelines for glycemic control by making the lowering of the glycosylated hemoglobin A1c to <7% (this value corresponds to 7.5% in the WESDR) (normal, <6%, this value corresponds to 6.4% in the WESDR) a new goal for people with NIDDM (3). In the absence of comparable clinical trial data for people with NIDDM, this decision has led to a debate over whether similar goals of glycemic control, as used in the DCCT, should

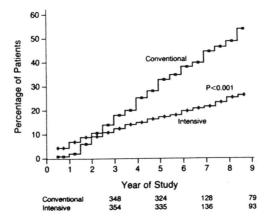

Figure 5 Cumulative incidence of a sustained change in retinopathy in patients with IDDM receiving intensive or conventional therapy in the secondary intervention group of the DCCT. Year of study refers to sample sizes at different years of the study. Reprinted by permission of *The New England Journal of Medicine*. The DCCT Research Group, 329:977–86, 1993. Copyright 1993. Massachusetts Medical Society. All rights reserved.

be pursued in those with NIDDM (71). Epidemiologic data, while suggesting a possible causal relation between hyperglycemia and the incidence and progression of retinopathy in people with NIDDM, do not provide estimates of the risks and benefits of reduction of hyperglycemia in this group. Persons with IDDM who were studied in the DCCT were young, normotensive, non-obese, had normal lipid patterns and had no history of cardiovascular disease at baseline (16). This is in sharp contrast to people with NIDDM who are more likely to be older, obese, dyslipidemic, hypertensive, and have a history of cardiovascular disease. Moreover, intensive insulin treatment in people with NIDDM may result in complications such as weight gain, severe hypoglycemia and possibly increased risk of development or progression of cardiovascular disease. The only large long-term randomized controlled clinical trial in people with NIDDM to date, the University Group Diabetes Program, failed to find a benefit of glycemic control in preventing retinopathy (86). A smaller pilot project of intensive insulin control showed that patients receiving intensive therapy had about twice the incidence of major cardiovascular disease events compared with those who received standard therapy during the two years of the study (1). These differences failed to reach statistical significance after controlling for baseline variables. A larger clinical trial of newly diagnosed people with NIDDM, the United Kingdom Prospective Diabetes Study, may provide data needed to address this important issue (85).

BLOOD PRESSURE

High blood pressure has been hypothesized to damage the retinal blood vessels, contributing to the incidence and progression of diabetic retinopathy (60). Anecdotal observations abound (15), and most epidemiologic data support such a relationship (Table 4). In the WESDR, systolic blood pressure was a significant predictor of the four-year incidence of retinopathy, and diastolic blood pressure was a significant predictor of the four-year progression of retinopathy in only the younger-onset group (51; Figure 6). After controlling for other risk factors such as glycosylated hemoglobin, retinopathy severity, and duration of diabetes at baseline, the relationship between blood pressure and retinopathy remained in the younger-onset group only. Neither systolic or diastolic blood pressure nor hypertension status was found to be related to the four-year incidence or progression of retinopathy in the older-onset groups. Even after controlling for use of antihypertensive medications, no relationship was found in the older-onset group.

The reasons for the differences in the relation between blood pressure and the incidence and progression of retinopathy between younger- and older-onset persons are not known. It is likely that elevated blood pressure in younger-onset persons is due to diabetic nephropathy, a condition associated with changes in platelet, angiotensin-renin, and lipid metabolism (7, 90). The latter have been postulated as factors in the pathogenesis of diabetic retinopathy (39). Thus, elevated blood pressure in the younger-onset group may be serving only as a risk indicator and not a risk factor. In older-onset persons, elevated blood pressure is usually due to essential hypertension and not diabetic nephropathy. Regardless of whether hypertension is causally related to the development of diabetic retinopathy, controlling elevated blood pressure is important to reduce the increased risk of renal disease, stroke, and cardiovascular morbidity and mortality in people with diabetes (23, 33, 58, 78).

The type of blood pressure control may also be important. The WESDR data suggested that use of diuretics may increase the risk of cardiovascular mortality in people with diabetes (36, 58). Similar findings were reported in diabetic patients followed in the Joslin Clinic, but not in other studies (88). Use of diuretics may result in elevations of glucose and lipids, and decreases in electrolytes. Clinical trials have shown that use of other agents such as ACE inhibitors have a beneficial effect in preventing the progression of nephropathy in people with IDDM (64). To date, there are no clinical trial data that support a beneficial effect of these agents in prevention of progression of retinopathy.

OTHER RISK FACTORS

There are less consistent epidemiologic data regarding other systemic and ocular risk factors (Table 4). Data from the WESDR suggest no relation

Table 4 Characteristics associated with the prevalence and/or incidence or progression of diabetic retinopathy from selected population-based studies and clinical trials

Reference	Type of diabetes	Hyper-glycemia	High blood pressure	History of smoking	History of renal disease	High lipids
Incidence						
4	NIDDM	Yes	No	No	No	
84	IDDM	No	Yes			
	NIDDM	Yes	Yes			
37,45,50,51,57,68	IDDM	Yes	Yes	No	Yes	Yes
	NIDDM	Yes	Yes/no[a]	No	No	
16,17	IDDM	Yes				
79	NIDDM	Yes				
Prevalence						
19	NIDDM	Yes	Yes			
5,75	NIDDM	Yes	Yes			
62,63,89	NIDDM	Yes	No/Yes[b]	No	Yes/No[b]	No/Yes[b]
28	IDDM		Yes			
	NIDDM		Yes			
34	NIDDM	Yes	Yes			
13	IDDM	No				
59	IDDM	Yes	Yes		Yes	No
	NIDDM	Yes	Yes		Yes	No
81	IDDM	Yes	No	Yes	No	
24	NIDDM	Yes	Yes	No	Yes	
31	NIDDM	Yes			Yes	
		Yes				
25	NIDDM	Yes	Yes	Yes		No
66	IDDM	No	Yes			
61, 65	IDDM	Yes	Yes	No	Yes	Yes
22	NIDDM	Yes				

[a] Relationship of high blood pressure with prevalence but not four-year incidence of retinopathy is significant.

[b] No relationship of high blood pressure or high cholesterol with prevalence, significant relationship with incidence; relationship of gross proteinuria is significant with prevalence but not incidence of retinopathy.

SOURCE: Klein R, Klein BEK, Moss SE. 1989. The Wisconsin Epidemiologic Study of Diabetic Retinopathy: A review. *Diabetes Metab. Rev.* 5:559-70. Copyright 1989, John Wiley & Sons Ltd. Reprinted by permission.

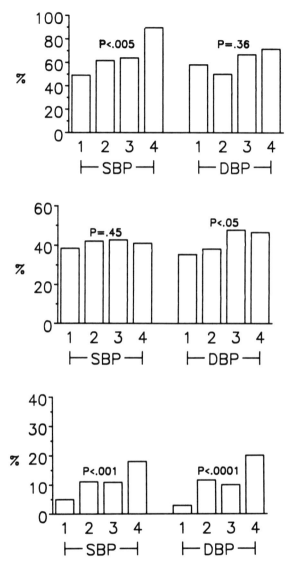

Figure 6   The relationship of incidence (*top*), progression (*center*), and progression to proliferative retinopathy (*bottom*) in persons with younger-onset diabetes over a four-year period to systolic and diastolic blood pressure levels by quartiles at baseline. *P* values are based on the Mantel-Haenszel test of trend. Source: Klein R, Klein BEK, Moss SE, Davis MD, DeMets DL. 1989. Is blood pressure a predictor of the incidence or progression of diabetic retinopathy? *Arch. Intern. Med.* 149:2427–32. Copyright 1989, American Medical Association.

between smoking or alcohol consumption and the incidence and progression of retinopathy (68, 69). Elevated cholesterol or decreased HDL-cholesterol have been associated with the accumulation of lipid exudates in the retina in some studies (11, 37). Fibrinogen was related to the incidence and progression of retinopathy in one study (65). Pregnancy has been shown to increase the risk of progression of retinopathy (35).

HEALTH CARE DELIVERY

Data from a number of epidemiologic studies suggest that many patients with diabetic retinopathy are not receiving optimal care (8, 70, 82, 91). Based on data from the WESDR, in 1980–82, it was estimated that 35,000 Americans at risk of loss of vision due to severe proliferative retinopathy or clinically significant macular edema had not received ophthalmologic care within two years of the study (91). In Wadena, Minnesota, Sprafka et al (82) reported that 32% of diabetic patients living there had never had ophthalmologic care. Nearly half of those without such care required immediate treatment or referral. More recently, using National Health Interview Survey data from 1989, Brechner et al (8) found that only 57% of people with IDDM, 55% of people with NIDDM, and 44% of people with NIDDM not treated with insulin reported a dilated eye examination within a year of the interview.

Poor compliance with recent guidelines suggesting ophthalmologic examinations through dilated pupils may be the result of a number of patient and physician factors. In the WESDR, people with ten or more years of diabetes who had not undergone an eye examination within one year of the study were asked why they had not been examined (70). Seventy-nine and 71% of younger- and older-onset persons, respectively, reported not having been examined because they had no problems with their eyes; 31 and 35% reported not having been told they needed an eye examination; 32 and 11% said they were too busy; and 30 and 12% said they could not afford an eye examination.

In addition, there are several physician-related factors that may be responsible for the lack of dilated eye examinations. First, nonophthalmologists have poor ophthalmoscopic skills and have been shown to have low sensitivity for detecting vision-threatening retinopathy using ophthalmoscopy even through a dilated pupil (72, 83, 87). Second, for fear of inducing angle-closure glaucoma, because of lack of self-confidence, or because of time, nonophthalmologists routinely choose not to dilate the pupils. Even for ophthalmologists, the ability to detect vision-threatening retinopathy through an undilated pupil is less than 50% (55). Third, primary care physicians may not be aware of current guidelines and the results of clinical trials demonstrating the benefits of photocoagulation treatment in preventing visual loss.

Cost-effectiveness of screening to detect and treat eyes at risk of loss of vision due to diabetic retinopathy has been clearly demonstrated (14, 29, 30). Public health strategies have been developed to ensure that diabetic patients receive an annual dilated eye examination by competent eye care professionals (2). These include the National Eye Health Education Program, supported by the National Eye Institute (73). This program involves a coalition of service, industry, professional, and government groups and is designed to educate people with diabetes and their families about the need for dilated eye examinations. Professional groups such as the American Diabetes Association, the American Academy of Ophthalmology, and the American Optometric Society have developed educational programs directed at patients and health care professionals regarding standards of care to prevent loss of vision due to diabetic eye disease.

There are few data available regarding the use of nonophthalmologists in screening diabetic patients for photocoagulation-treatable retinal changes. In one such study in England, the predictive value of a positive finding of serious retinopathy was only 35%, indicating over-referral (6, 10). In addition, a high proportion of patients found by opticians to have serious retinopathy failed to comply with the suggested need for further ophthalmological examination. Another approach to screening of patients in areas where ophthalmologic care or physician availability is limited is the use of nonmydriatic cameras (55). With such a system, trained technicians take photographs of the retina. Photographs are then sent to a retinal specialist at a central location with referral based on finding vision-threatening retinopathy. The cost-effectiveness of this approach is currently being evaluated in England and in the United States.

OTHER CHALLENGES

The most important challenge ahead is to prevent the onset of diabetes itself. Clinical trials are now under way using insulin and other therapeutic modalities to prevent IDDM in those at high risk. Primary prevention trials of weight reduction and increased physical activity are being planned to prevent NIDDM.

In those with diabetes, research is needed to develop more user-friendly methods of delivering insulin to lower blood sugar without significant hypoglycemic side effects and weight gain. Another challenge is finding the resources to support the professional team approach (consisting of health educators, social workers, psychologists, nurses, rehabilitation specialists, etc) necessary to implement the DCCT recommendations and the resources to overcome economic barriers to receiving optimal eye care.

Finally, research is needed (and is under way) to examine other treatment approaches which may block the incidence or progression of diabetic retinopathy. Various strategies designed to block postulated pathogenetic mechanisms, such as aminoguanidine for stopping glycosylation, aldose reductase inhibitors for blocking aldose reductase conversion of blood sugars to sugar alcohols, and agents for blocking vascular neogenesis may provide additional approaches resulting in preventing visual loss due to diabetic retinopathy.

SUMMARY

In summary, public health approaches for prevention of loss of vision through control of hyperglycemia and timely laser photocoagulation are available. Educational programs for physicians and patients and reductions in economic barriers are needed to put these approaches into practice.

ACKNOWLEDGMENTS

This work was supported by National Institute of Health Grant EY-03083 and, in part, by Research to Prevent Blindness (R Klein, Senior Scientific Investigator). I want to acknowledge the collaborative effort of Barbara EK Klein, Scot E Moss, and Karen J Cruickshanks, as well as other staff members.

Literature Cited

1. Abraira C, Johnson N, Colwell J, the VA CSDM Group. 1994. VA Cooperative Study on Glycemic Control and Complications in Type II Diabetes (VA CSDM): results of the complete feasibility trial. *Diabetes* 43:59A (Abstr.)

2. American College of Physicians, American Diabetes Association, and American Academy of Ophthalmology. 1992. Screening guidelines for diabetic retinopathy. *Ann. Intern. Med.* 116:683–85

3. American Diabetes Association. 1995. Standards of medical care for patients with diabetes mellitus. *Diabetes Care* 18:8–13 (Suppl. 1)

4. Ballard DJ, Melton LJ, Dwyer MS, Trautmann JC, O'Fallon WM, Palumbo PJ. 1986. Risk factors for diabetic retinopathy: a population-based study in Rochester, Minnesota. *Diabetes Care* 9:334–42

5. Bennett PH, Rushforth NB, Miller M, LeCompte PM. 1976. Epidemiologic studies of diabetes in the Pima Indians. *Recent Prog. Horm. Res.* 32:333–76

6. Bhopal RS, Hedley AJ. 1985. Screening of diabetics for retinopathy by ophthalmic opticians. *Br. Med. J.* (Letter) 290:1589

7. Borch-Johnsen K, Kreiner S. 1987. Proteinuria: value as predictor of cardiovascular mortality in insulin dependent diabetes mellitus. *Br. Med. J.* 294:1651–54

8. Brechner RJ, Cowie CC, Howie LJ, Herman WH, Will JC, Harris MI. 1993. Ophthalmic examination among adults with diagnosed diabetes mellitus. *JAMA* 270:1714–18

9. Bresnick G. 1977. Diabetic retinopathy. In *Principles and Practice of Ophthalmology*, ed. GA Peyman, DR Sanders, MF Goldberg, pp. 1205–76. Philadelphia: Saunders

10. Burns Cox CJ, Dean Hart JC. 1985. Screening of diabetics for retinopathy by ophthalmic opticians. *Br. Med. J.* 290:1052–54

11. Chantry KH, Klein ML, Chew EY, Ferris FL III. 1989. Early Treatment Retinopathy Study Research Group: asso-

ciation of serum lipids and retinal hard exudates in patients enrolled in the Early Treatment Diabetic Retinopathy Study. *Invest. Ophthalmol. Vis. Sci.* 30:434 (Suppl.)

12. Constable IJ, Knuiman MW, Welborn TA, Cooper RL, Stanton KM, et al. 1984. Assessing the risk of diabetic retinopathy. *Am. J. Ophthalmol.* 97:53–61

13. Danielsen R, Jonasson F, Helgason T. 1982. Prevalence of retinopathy and proteinuria in Type I diabetics in Iceland. *Acta Med. Scand.* 212:277–80

14. Dasbach E, Fryback DG, Newcomb PA, Klein R, Klein BEK. 1991. Cost-effectiveness of strategies for detecting diabetic retinopathy. *Med. Care* 29:20–39

15. Davis MD. 1986. Diabetic retinopathy, diabetic control and blood pressure. *Transplant Proc.* 18:1565–68

16. DCCT Research Group. 1993. The effect of intense diabetes treatment on the development and progression of long-term complications in insulin-dependent diabetes. The Diabetes Control and Complications Trial. *New Engl. J. Med.* 329:977–86

17. DCCT Research Group. 1995. The effect of intensive diabetes treatment on the progression of diabetic retinopathy in insulin-dependent diabetes mellitus. The Diabetes Control and Complications Trial. *Arch. Ophthalmol.* 113:36–51

18. Diabetic Retinopathy Study Group. 1981. Photocoagulation treatment of proliferative diabetic retinopathy: clinical application of Diabetic Retinopathy Study (DRS) findings. DRS Rep. No. 8. *Ophthalmology* 88:583–600

19. Dorf A, Ballintine EJ, Bennett PH, Miller M. 1976. Retinopathy in Pima Indians. Relationships to glucose level, duration of diabetes, age at diagnosis of diabetes, and age at examination in a population with a high prevalence of diabetes mellitus. *Diabetes* 25:554–60

20. Dwyer MS, Melton LJ III, Ballard DJ, Palumbo PJ, Trautmann JC, Chu C-P. 1985. Incidence of diabetic retinopathy and blindness: a population-based study in Rochester, Minnesota. *Diabetes Care* 8:316–22

21. ETDRS Research Group. 1985. Photocoagulation for diabetic macular edema. *Arch. Ophthalmol.* 103:1796–806

22. Fujimoto W, Fukuda M. 1976. Natural history of diabetic retinopathy and its treatment in Japan. In *Diabetes Mellitus in Asia*, ed. S Baba, Y Goto, I Fukui, pp. 225–31. Amsterdam: Excerpta Med

23. Fuller JH, Shipley MJ, Rose G, Jarrett RJ, Keen H. 1983. Coronary heart disease and stroke mortality by degree of glycaemia: The Whitehall Study. *Br. Med. J.* 287:867–70

24. Haffner SM, Fong D, Stern MP, Pugh JA, Hazuda HP, et al. 1988. Diabetic retinopathy in Mexican Americans and non-Hispanic Whites. *Diabetes* 37:878–84

25. Hamman RF, Mayer EJ, Moo-Young GA, Hilldebrandt W, Marshall JA, Baxter J. 1989. Prevalence and risk factors of diabetic retinopathy in non-Hispanic whites and Hispanics with NIDDM. San Luis Valley Diabetes Study. *Diabetes* 38:1231–37

26. Harris MI, Klein R, Welborn TA, Knuiman MW. 1992. Onset of NIDDM occurs at least 4–7 years before clinical diagnosis. *Diabetes Care* 15:815–19

27. Harris MI, Rowland M, Klein R. 1995. Racial differences in the prevalence, severity, and treatment of retinopathy among adults with diabetes in the U.S. population. *JAMA.* In review

28. Houston A. 1982. Retinopathy in the Poole area: an epidemiological inquiry. In *Advances in Diabetes Epidemiology*, ed. E Eschwege, pp. 196–206. Amsterdam: Elsevier

29. Javitt JC, Aiello LP, Chiang Y, Ferris FL III, Canner JK, Greenfield S. 1994. Preventive eye care in people with diabetes is cost-saving to the federal government. Implications for health care reform. *Diabetes Care* 17:909–17

30. Javitt JC, Canner JK, Frank RG, Steinwachs DM, Sommer A. 1990. Detecting and treating retinopathy in Type I diabetics: a health policy model. *Ophthalmology* 97:483–95

31. Jerneld B. 1988. Prevalence of diabetic retinopathy. *Acta Scand. Ophthalmol.* 188:3–32 (Suppl.)

32. Kahn HA, Leibowitz HM, Ganley JP, Kini MM, Colton T, et al. 1977. The Framingham Eye Study. I. Outline and major prevalence findings. *Am. J. Epidemiol.* 106:17–32

33. Kannel WB. 1976. Diabetes and cardiovascular disease: The Framingham Study: 18-year follow-up. *Cardiol. Dig.* 11:11–15

34. King H, Balkau B, Zimmet P, Taylor R, Raper LR, et al. 1983. Diabetic retinopathy in Nauruans. *Am. J. Epidemiol.* 117:659–67

35. Klein BEK, Moss SE, Klein R. 1990. Effect of pregnancy on progression of diabetic retinopathy. *Diabetes Care* 13:34–40

36. Klein BEK, Moss SE, Klein R. 1992. Use of cardiovascular disease medica-

tions and mortality in people with older onset diabetes. *Am. J. Public Health* 82:1142–44

37. Klein BEK, Moss SE, Klein R, Surawicz TS. 1991. The Wisconsin Epidemiologic Study of Diabetic Retinopathy. XIII. Relationship of serum cholesterol to retinopathy and hard exudate. *Ophthalmology* 98:1261–65

38. Klein R. 1995. Hyperglycemia and microvascular and macrovascular disease in diabetes. *Diabetes Care* 18:258–68

39. Klein R. 1995. Retinopathy and other ocular complications in diabetes. In *Ellenberg and Rifkin's Diabetes Mellitus*, ed. D Porte Jr, RS Sherwin. Norfalk, CT: Appleton & Lange. 5th ed. In press

40. Klein R, Klein BEK. 1995. Vision disorders in diabetes. In *Diabetes in America*, ed. MWH Harris, 10:4. Bethesda, MD: US Public Health Serv., NIH Publ. 2nd ed.

41. Klein R, Klein BEK, Moss SE. 1984. Visual impairment in diabetes. *Ophthalmology* 91:1–9

42. Klein R, Klein BEK, Moss SE. 1989. The Wisconsin Epidemiologic Study of Diabetic Retinopathy: a review. *Diabetes Metab. Rev.* 5:559–70

43. Klein R, Klein BEK, Moss SE. 1996. The relationship of glycemic control to diabetic microvascular complications in IDDM and NIDDM. *Ann. Intern. Med.* 124:90–96 (Suppl.)

44. Klein R, Klein BEK, Moss SE. 1995. The Wisconsin Epidemiologic Study of Diabetic Retinopathy. XVI. The relationship of c-peptide to the incidence and progression of diabetic retinopathy. *Diabetes* 44:796–801

45. Klein R, Klein BEK, Moss SE, Cruickshanks KJ. 1994. Relationship of hyperglycemia to the long-term incidence and progression of diabetic retinopathy. *Arch. Intern. Med.* 154:2169–78

46. Klein R, Klein BEK, Moss SE, Cruickshanks KJ. 1994. The Wisconsin Epidemiologic Study of Diabetic Retinopathy. XIV. Ten-year incidence and progression of diabetic retinopathy. *Arch. Ophthalmol.* 112:1217–28

47. Klein R, Klein BEK, Moss SE, Davis MD, DeMets DL. 1984. The Wisconsin Epidemiologic Study of Diabetic Retinopathy. II. Prevalence and risk of diabetic retinopathy when age at diagnosis is less than 30 years. *Arch. Ophthalmol.* 102:520–26

48. Klein R, Klein BEK, Moss SE, Davis MD, DeMets DL. 1984. The Wisconsin Epidemiologic Study of Diabetic Retinopathy. III. Prevalence and risk of diabetic retinopathy when age at diagnosis

is 30 or more years. *Arch. Ophthalmol.* 102:527–32

49. Klein R, Klein BEK, Moss SE, Davis MD, DeMets DL. 1984. The Wisconsin Epidemiologic Study of Diabetic Retinopathy. IV. Diabetic macular edema. *Ophthalmology* 91:1464–74

50. Klein R, Klein BEK, Moss SE, Davis MD, DeMets DL. 1988. Glycosylated hemoglobin predicts the incidence and progression of diabetic retinopathy. *JAMA* 260:2864–71

51. Klein R, Klein BEK, Moss SE, Davis MD, DeMets DL. 1989. Is blood pressure a predictor of the incidence or progression of diabetic retinopathy? *Arch. Intern. Med.* 149:2427–32

52. Klein R, Klein BEK, Moss SE, Davis MD, DeMets DL. 1989. The Wisconsin Epidemiologic Study of Diabetic Retinopathy. IX. Four-year incidence and progression of diabetic retinopathy when age at diagnosis is less than 30 years. *Arch. Ophthalmol.* 107:237–43

53. Klein R, Klein BEK, Moss SE, Davis MD, DeMets DL. 1989. The Wisconsin Epidemiologic Study of Diabetic Retinopathy. X. Four-year incidence and progression of diabetic retinopathy when age at diagnosis is 30 years or more. *Arch. Ophthalmol.* 107:244–49

54. Klein R, Klein BEK, Moss SE, Shrago ES, Spennetta TL. 1987. Glycosylated hemoglobin in a population-based study of diabetes. *Am. J. Epidemiol.* 126:415–27

55. Klein R, Klein BEK, Neider MW, Hubbard LD, Meuer SM, Brothers RJ. 1985. Diabetic retinopathy as detected using ophthalmoscopy, a nonmydriatic camera and a standard fundus camera. *Ophthalmology* 92:485–91

56. Klein R, Moss SE, Klein BEK. 1992. Change in glycemia in a four-year interval in younger-onset insulin-dependent diabetes. *Ann. Epidemiol.* 2:283–94

57. Klein R, Moss SE, Klein BEK. 1993. Is gross proteinuria a risk factor for the incidence of proliferative diabetic retinopathy? *Ophthalmology* 100:1140–46

58. Klein R, Moss SE, Klein BEK, DeMets DL. 1989. Relation of ocular and systemic factors to survival in diabetes. *Arch. Intern. Med.* 149:266–72

59. Knuiman MW, Welborn TA, McCann VJ, Stanton KG, Constable IJ. 1986. Prevalence of diabetic complications in relation to risk factors. *Diabetes* 35:1332–39

60. Kohner EM. 1989. Diabetic retinopathy. *Br. Med. Bull.* 45:148–73

61. Kostraba JN, Klein R, Dorman JS,

Becker DJ, Drash AL, et al. 1991. The Epidemiology of Diabetes Complications Study. IV. Correlates of diabetic background and proliferative retinopathy. *Am. J. Epidemiol.* 133:381–91

62. Lee ET, Lee VS, Kingsley RM, Lu M, Russell D, et al. 1992. Diabetic retinopathy in Oklahoma Indians with NIDDM: incidence and risk factors. *Diabetes Care* 15:1620–27

63. Lee ET, Lee VS, Lu M, Russell D. 1992. Development of proliferative retinopathy in NIDDM, a follow-up study of American Indians in Oklahoma. *Diabetes* 41:359–67

64. Lewis EJ, Hunsicker LG, Bain RP, Rohde RD, the Collaborative Study Group. 1993. The effect of angiotensin-converting enzyme inhibition on diabetic nephropathy. *New Engl. J. Med.* 329:1456–62

65. Lloyd CE, Klein R, Maser RE, Kuller LH, Becker DJ, Orchard TJ. 1995. The progression of retinopathy over two years: The Pittsburgh Epidemiology of Diabetes Complications (EDC) Study. *J. Diabet. Comp.* 9:140–48

66. McLeod BK, Thompson JR, Rosenthal AR. 1988. The prevalence of retinopathy in the insulin-requiring diabetic patients of an English county town. *Eye* 2:424–30

67. Moss SE, Klein R, Klein BEK. 1988. The incidence of vision loss in a diabetic population. *Ophthalmology* 95:1340–48

68. Moss SE, Klein R, Klein BEK. 1991. Association of cigarette smoking with diabetic retinopathy. *Diabetes Care* 14:119–26

69. Moss SE, Klein R, Klein BEK. 1994. The association of alcohol consumption with the incidence and progression of diabetic retinopathy. *Ophthalmology* 101:1962–68

70. Moss SE, Klein R, Klein BEK. 1995. Factors associated with having eye examinations in persons with diabetes. *Arch. Fam. Med.* 4:529–34

71. Nathan DM. 1995. Inferences and implications. Do results from the Diabetes Control and Complications Trial apply in NIDDM? *Diabetes Care* 18:251–57

72. Nathan DM, Fogel HA, Godine JE, Lou PL, D'Amico DJ, et al. 1991. Role of diabetologist in evaluating diabetic retinopathy. *Diabetes Care* 14:26–33

73. National Institutes of Health. 1990. *The National Eye Health Education Program. From Vision Research to Eye Health Education: Planning the Partnership.* Bethesda: NIH

74. National Society to Prevent Blindness. 1980. *Vision Problems in the US: Data Analysis, Definitions, Data Sources, Detailed Data Tables, Analyses, Interpretation.* New York: Natl, Soc. Prev. Blindness

75. Nelson RG, Newman JM, Knowler WC, Sievers ML, Kunzelman CL, et al. 1988. Incidence of end-stage renal disease in Type 2 (non-insulin-dependent) diabetes mellitus in Pima Indians. *Diabetologia* 31:730–36

76. Nielsen NV. 1984. Diabetic retinopathy. I. The course of retinopathy in insulin-treated diabetics. A one-year epidemiological cohort study of diabetes mellitus. The Island of Falster, Denmark. *Acta Ophthalmol.* 62:256–65

77. Nielsen NV. 1984. Diabetic retinopathy. II. The course of retinopathy in diabetics treated with oral hypoglycemic agents and diet regime alone. A one-year epidemiologic cohort study of diabetes mellitus. The Island of Falster, Denmark. *Acta Ophthalmol.* 62:266–73

78. Palumbo PJ, Elveback LR, Whishnaut JP. 1978. Neurologic complications of diabetes mellitus: transient ischaemic attack, stroke, and peripheral neuropathy. *Adv. Neurol.* 19:593–601

79. Reichard P, Nilsson BY, Rosenqvist U. 1993. Retardation of the development of the microvascular complications after long-term intensified insulin treatment: The Stockholm Diabetes Intervention Study. *New Engl. J. Med.* 329:304–9

80. Ross SA, Huchcroft SA. 1989. Hyperlipidemia and vascular risk factors among diabetics in southern Alberta. *Clin. Invest. Med.* 12:B25

81. Sjolie AK. 1985. Ocular complications in insulin treated diabetes mellitus. An epidemiological study. *Acta Ophthalmol.* 172:1–72 (Suppl.)

82. Sprafka JM, Fritsche TL, Baker R, Kurth D, Whipple D. 1990. Prevalence of undiagnosed eye disease in high-risk diabetic individuals. *Arch. Intern. Med.* 150:857–61

83. Sussman EJ, Tsiaras WG, Soper KA. 1982. Diagnosis of diabetic eye disease. *JAMA* 247:3231–34

84. Teuscher A, Schnell H, Wilson PWF. 1988. Incidence of diabetic retinopathy and relationship to baseline plasma glucose and blood pressure. *Diabetes Care* 11:246–51

85. UKPDS Group. 1990. UK Prospective Diabetes Study. Complications in newly diagnosed Type 2 diabetic patients and their association with clinical and bio-

chemical risk factors. *Diabetes Res.* 13: 1–11

86. University Group Diabetes Program. 1982. Effects of hypoglycemic agents on vascular complications in patients with adult-onset diabetes. VIII. Evaluation of insulin therapy; final report. *Diabetes* 31:1–81 (Suppl. 5)

87. Valez R, Haffner S, Stern MP, Van-Heuven WAJ. 1987. Ophthalmologist vs. retinal photographs in screening for diabetic retinopathy. *Clin. Res.* 35:363A (Abstr.)

88. Warram JH, Laffel LMB, Valsania P, Christlieb R, Krolewski AS. 1991. Excess mortality associated with diuretic therapy in diabetes mellitus. *Arch. Intern. Med.* 151:1350–56

89. West KM, Erdreich LJ, Stober JA. 1980. A detailed study of risk factors for retinopathy and nephropathy in diabetes. *Diabetes* 19:501–8

90. Winocour PH, Durrington PN, Ishola M, Anderson DC, Cohen H. 1987. Influence of proteinuria on vascular disease, blood pressure, and lipoproteins in insulin dependent diabetes mellitus. *Br. Med. J.* 294:1648–51

91. Witkin SR, Klein R. 1984. Ophthalmologic care for persons with diabetes. *JAMA* 251:2534–37

Annu. Rev. Public Health. 1996. 17:159–77
Copyright © 1996 by Annual Reviews Inc. All rights reserved

BLINDNESS DUE TO CATARACT: Epidemiology and Prevention

Jonathan C. Javitt and Fang Wang

Worthen Center For Eye Care Research, Center For Sight, Georgetown University Medical Center, Washington, DC 20007

Sheila K. West

Dana Center for Preventive Ophthalmology, Wilmer Eye Institute, The Johns Hopkins School of Medicine, Baltimore, Maryland 21287-9019

KEY WORDS: cataract, blindness, epidemiology, prevention, risk factor, cost

ABSTRACT

Cataract is the leading cause of blindness, accounting for 50% of blindness worldwide. Although significant progress has been made toward identifying risk factors for cataract, there is no proven primary prevention or medical treatment. Surgical removal of cataract remains the only therapy. In this paper, we reviewed (*a*) the prevalence and incidence data of cataract, (*b*) the findings on risk factors for cataract, and (*c*) health service utilization and outcome of cataract surgery in both developed and developing countries.

INTRODUCTION

Cataract is an opacity of the natural, crystalline lens of the eye and remains the most frequent cause of blindness in the world today. The World Health Organization (WHO) estimates that 50% (17 million) of persons currently blind worldwide are blind from cataract (95, 95a). Because of increasing life expectancy and the resulting expansion of the elderly population, prevalent cases of blinding cataract are expected to double by the year 2010 (11).

Although significant progress has been made toward identifying risk factors for cataract, there is no proven primary prevention or medical treatment. Surgical removal of cataract remains the only proven therapy and can be successful in restoring vision in over 94% of persons without other concurrent

159

eye disease. This technology is widely accepted by developed countries and is increasingly available in the developing world. In 1993, the World Bank ranked cataract surgery in the most highly cost-effective category, the only surgical intervention to reach that rank (i.e. less than $25 per disability discounted healthy year of life added) (48, 49).

ASSESSMENT AND CLASSIFICATION OF CATARACT

Typically, cataracts are defined as lens opacities associated with some degree of visual impairment (107). For epidemiologic studies, cataract may be classified, according to anatomic location, into nuclear, cortical, posterior subcapsular (PSC), or mixed types. In advanced or hypermature cataract, the whole lens becomes opaque. Differentiation of the morphologic types is important, as risk factors appear to be different for each type of cataract (107).

Clinically, the lens is examined and graded using a slit-lamp by a trained professional for the presence of cortical, nuclear, and PSC opacities. In epidemiological studies, nuclear cataracts can be documented by slit-lamp photography and graded by assigning ordinal scores according to the degree of opacification based on standard color photographs. Cortical and PSC opacities can be documented by retro-illumination photography and graded according to the percentage area of the lens obscured by the opacity or categorized based on standard photographs. A number of systems have been developed to document lens opacities and are used in epidemiological studies (16, 63, 88, 94, 106).

PREVALENCE OF CATARACT

Blindness from Cataract

In 1987, the WHO estimated that the prevalence of cataract-associated blindness, where the better eye has visual acuity of <20/400, ranged from 14 per 100,000 persons in the most highly developed countries to 2000 per 100,000 in parts of the developing world (Table 1) (108). Cataract accounts for 30–50% of blindness in most African and Asia countries (95a).

Although the prevalence of blinding cataract in the United States is far lower than in the developing world, cataract remains a leading cause of blindness (in the United States, the definition of blindness is visual acuity ≤20/200 in the better eye). In the Framingham Eye Study, 25% of all cases of blindness in a white population aged 52 years or older were attributed to cataract (68). During the 1980s cataract surgery underwent major technological improvement, with the adoption of outpatient, microsurgical techniques and the use of intraocular lens implants. Even so, the Baltimore Eye Survey, performed ten

Table 1 Prevalence of cataract blindness, by country[a]

Country	Prevalence of blindness	Percentage of blindness from cataract	Prevalence of cataract blindness	Population (millions)	Cataract (millions)
AFRICA					
Botswana	1.4	0.45	0.63	1.01	0.01
Chad	2.3	0.48	1.10	4.79	0.05
Egypt	3.3	0.32	1.06	44.50	0.47
Ethiopia	1.3	0.46	0.60	33.68	0.20
Gambia	0.7	0.55	0.385	0.80	0.00
Kenya	1.1	0.67	0.74	18.78	0.14
Liberia	2.1	0.45	0.945	2.06	0.02
Malawi	1.3	0.40	0.52	6.43	0.03
Mali	1.3	0.32	0.42	7.53	0.03
Nigeria	1.5	0.41	0.615	89.02	0.55
Sudan	6.4	0.30	1.92	20.36	0.39
Togo	1.3	0.45	0.585	2.76	0.02
Tunisia	3.9	0.52	2.03	6.89	0.14
Zimbabwe	1.2	0.40	0.48	7.14	0.03
AMERICAS					
United States	0.2	0.13	0.026	233.70	0.06
Brazil	0.3	0.10	0.03	129.70	0.04
Peru	1.0	0.34	0.34	18.70	0.06
ASIA					
Afghanistan	2.0	0.31	0.62	17.22	0.11
Bangladesh	0.9	0.33	0.30	94.65	0.28
China (average)	0.875	0.22	0.14	1040.00	1.41
Yemen	3.6	0.34	1.22	2.16	0.03
Hong Kong	0.2	0.34	0.07	5.31	0.01
India	0.5	0.55	0.27	732.00	2.01
Indonesia	1.2	0.67	0.80	159.00	1.28
Japan	0.3	0.23	0.07	119.00	0.08
Nepal	0.8	0.67	0.54	15.74	0.08
Pakistan	2.3	0.60	1.38	89.00	1.23
Korea	0.1	0.36	0.04	40.00	0.01
Saudi Arabia	1.5	0.55	0.82	10.40	0.09
Vietnam	0.8	0.39	0.31	57.00	0.18
Sri Lanka	2.0	0.46	0.92	15.00	0.14
Syria	0.3	0.35	0.10	9.60	0.01
Thailand	1.1	0.57	0.62	49.00	0.31
EUROPE					
Germany	0.1	0.04	0.004	61.42	0.002
Norway	0.2	0.07	0.014	4.13	0.001
Sweden	0.3	0.05	0.015	8.00	0.001
USSR	0.27	0.16	0.043	27.50	0.12

[a] *Source:* WHO Programme for the Prevention of Blindness, 1987

years after the Framingham study, found that unoperated cataract remained a common cause of blindness, accounting for 13% of blindness among white Americans and 27% of blindness among black Americans (87).

Cataract as a cause of blindness is particularly prevalent among the elderly institutionalized population. A recent study of the nursing home population in East Baltimore determined that blindness was 13 to 15 times higher among nursing home residents than among noninstitutionalized persons of the same age, sex, and race from the same neighborhood. The study detected a 5.6% prevalence of cataract blindness in this population, accounting for 30% of all cases of blindness (97).

Prevalence of Cataract

There is no uniform definition of lens opacity or cataract, making summary estimates across different studies difficult. Different types and severity of lens opacities may have unpredictable effects on visual acuity, rendering loss of visual acuity an insensitive basis for ascertaining prevalence of different cataract type. No standard method has been routinely used in collecting data on cataract prevalence and incidence. Lens opacities have been measured using different grading systems (16, 63, 88, 94, 106), and cataract has been defined using a variety of criteria (40, 57, 60, 70, 89). Development of a uniform method for defining a cataract is crucial for comparison across regions and studies.

Prevalence of cataract and lens opacity has been reported in four population surveys in the United States: the National Health and Nutritional Examination Survey (NHANES) (40, 70), the Framingham Eye Study (FES) (57, 68), the Maryland Watermen Study (1), and the Beaver Dam Eye Study (BDES) (60). "Cataract" required a lens opacity that was associated with, or accompanied by, vision loss. The lens opacity was detected by clinical examination in NHANES and FES and by slit-lamp photography in the Maryland Watermen Study and BDES. The criterion for significant vision loss varied between surveys, with a vision of 20/30 or worse in NHANES, 20/25 or worse in FES, and 20/32 or worse in BDES. As shown in Table 2, the prevalence of cataract (in at least one eye) in these studies ranges from approximately 2% at ages 45–54 years to 45% at ages 75–85. An estimated 12.9 million Americans age 40 and older have cataract today (96).

Cataract (and blinding cataract) is more prevalent in developing countries where it may occur at an earlier age than in developed countries. The data on prevalence of cataract in developing countries, however, have not been well assessed. The Nepal Blindness Survey found a prevalence rate of 2.8% in the overall population (7). The prevalence of cataract accompanied by best visual acuity of 20/60 or worse, or aphakia, was 4.3% for all age groups and 15.3% among persons aged 30 or older in the Punjab, India (12). In a suburban county

Table 2 Prevalence of cataract, the United States

Age	NHANES %	FES %	Watermen %		BDES %
45 – 54	2.6	—	3[a]	—	1.6[c]
55 – 64	10.0	4.5[d]	10[a]	5[b]	7.2
65 – 74	28.5	18.0	38[a]	25[b]	19.6
75 – 85	—	45.9	—	59[b]	43.1

NHANES: National Health and Nutrition Examination Survey (70)
FES: Framingham Eye Study (57)
BDES: Beaver Dam Eye Study (60)
Watermen: Maryland Watermen Study (1)
[a] FES definition of cataract and FES age group applied
[b] NHANES definition of cataract and NHANES age group applied
[c] Age 43– 54 years old
[d] Age 52– 64 years old

of Beijing, China, the prevalence of cataract was 6.0% in the overall population and 18.6% among those aged 40 or older (43). Cataract, in this survey, was defined as lens opacity associated with a vision of 20/30 or worse. Data from India suggested higher rates in younger age groups compared to the Chinese and the US population (Table 3).

Incidence of Cataract

While relatively accurate figures of cataract blindness and prevalence are available, data on cataract incidence are extremely limited. Podgor et al (78) used age-specific prevalence data from the Framingham Eye Study to estimate incidence for "any" lens opacity and for visually significant (i.e. visual acuity

Table 3 Prevalence of cataract, India and China

Age (year)	Prevalence (%)	
	Punjab, India[a]	Shunyi, China[b]
30 – 39	0.2	—
40 – 49	2.2	0.40
50 – 59	14.7	6.83
60 – 69	42.0	25.79
70 – 79	55.7	59.95
80+	87.8	83.02
Total	15.3	18.58

[a] Reference 12
[b] Reference 43

20/30 or worse) cataract. Based on the predicted model, the five-year incidence for any lens opacity was estimated at 10, 16, 31, and 37%, respectively, for ages 55, 60, 65, 70, and 75 years. The corresponding incidence rates for visually significant cataract were 1, 2, 5, 9, and 15%.

The Italian-American Cataract Study provided data on incidence and progression of lens opacity in a group of cataract cases and clinic-based controls (45). Lens status was assessed from photographs taken on 1399 participants at baseline visit and three years later using the Lens Opacities Classification System II. The three-year cumulative incidence for persons 65 to 74 years old were 18, 6, and 6%, respectively, for cortical, nuclear, and PSC cataract. Progression was much higher than incidence for each type of lens opacity. These data are generated from a case-control study and cannot be extrapolated to a population.

The incidence of blinding cataract in India was measured in a population-based study of 19 communities (72). A total of 1655 persons were examined clinically in 1982 and reexamined four years later. Using a person-year method, the annual incidence of blinding cataract (WHO definition) was 0.19 per 100 persons between ages 35–39 and increased to 5.8 per 100 persons for ages 65 and older (Table 4). The findings suggest that an estimated 3.8 million persons lose vision because of cataract each year in India—a figure far higher than previously projected.

PREVENTING BLINDNESS FROM CATARACT

Lowering and Postponing Cataract Incidence

The National Eye Institute estimates that a ten-year delay in the onset of cataract would result in a 50% reduction in the prevalence of cataract (10). Delaying the incidence of cataract depends upon the identification of risk

Table 4   Incidence of blinding cataract, India[a]

Age	Incidence rate/ person-year	Projected number of new cases per year
0 – 34	0.0000	0
35 – 39	0.0019	95,486
40 – 44	0.0025	104,473
45 – 49	0.0059	209,610
50 – 54	0.0134	399,157
55 – 59	0.0239	600,218
60 – 64	0.0373	678,842
65+	0.0581	1,723,399
Total		3,811,185

[a]Adapted from Table 1 in Reference 72

factors for cataractous change. From the public health perspective, risk factors for cataract are readily classified as those that are unmodifiable and those that may be potentially modified (8, 22, 89, 107).

UNMODIFIABLE RISK FACTORS FOR CATARACT   Age is by far the strongest known risk factor for cataract. In addition, a small excess risk of cataract for women compared to men has been found in several studies (39, 40, 44, 58, 60, 69). The sex-specific risk is associated with cortical cataract, which may explain the 10–20% excess risk of cataract diagnosis and surgery among women. In spite of evidence that unoperated cataract is more common among blacks than among whites (87), information is limited on racial differences in cataract prevalence; data from NHANES suggested a slight increased risk of cortical and nuclear cataracts in black persons (40). Two case-control studies examined family history as a risk factor for cataract. The Italian-American Cataract Study Group reported that cases were more likely to report a family history for cortical cataract, PSC cataract, and mixed cataract (44), whereas Leske and coworkers found a significant association for mixed cataract only (69). Two recent, large population-based studies provided further evidence for an association between lens opacity and family history of cataract. In the Framingham Offspring Eye Study (28), data from 1086 parents and 896 off-spring were used to examine familial associations for all types of cataract. For any pair of siblings, the odds of nuclear lens opacity in one sibling were threefold higher if the other sibling had nuclear opacity. No significant association was noted for any form of lens opacity between spouses or between parents and offspring. The BDES assessed lens status of 63 singletons and 1212 people from 501 sibships. These data were analyzed using regression models to examine the possible effect of genetic predisposition for cataract. The findings suggested that a single major gene may account for 58% of variability of cortical cataract presence and 35% of nuclear cataract presence (36, 37) after adjusting for age and sex effect.

MODIFIABLE FACTORS   Life style, nutrition, and environmental factors may well play a role in cataractogenesis, and are factors for which preventive strategies could be targeted.

Smoking   An increased risk of lens opacities in smokers has been demonstrated in cross-sectional (26, 62, 103), case-control (69), and prospective studies (14, 32). These studies documented a significant association of heavy smoking and an even greater association of current heavy smoking with nuclear cataract. In the Maryland Watermen study, the risk of nuclear opacities increased with increasing cigarette dose (odds ratio = 1.11 per increment of 20 pack-years) and decreased if subjects had quit smoking for more than 10 years

(103). An association of smoking and PSC cataract was observed in three studies (14, 32, 62). A dose-response relationship of increasing pack-years and prevalence of PSC opacities was found for men, and, although not significant, for women in the Beaver Dam study (62).

Two clinic-based, case-control studies did not find an association between smoking and senile cataract (44, 73). In the India study, "smokes" referred to cigarettes and other tobacco and nontobacco products common in the subcontinent. The comparability of these products to cigarettes smoked by persons in the United States and Europe is unclear. Similarly, no association was found in the Italian case-control study (44), although the same methodology was used as in the United States (69).

Consistent findings across several different studies strengthen the role of cigarette smoking as a risk factor for nuclear opacities and possibly for PSC opacities. Currently, 26% of the US population smokes cigarettes, suggesting that as much as 20% of the cataract cases are attributable to smoking in the USA (102).

Alcohol   An association between regular alcohol consumption and cataract has been found in two cross-sectional studies (75, 79) and three case-control studies (17, 34, 35, 74). Clayton et al reported a "J-shaped relationship" of alcohol consumption and cataract, with a slightly high risk among total abstainers and an increased risk among heavy drinkers compared to occasional drinkers (17). The high risk of cataract among heavy drinkers has been confirmed by other studies, with an odds ratio ranging from 1.34 to 4.6 (34, 35, 74, 75, 79). Light consumption of alcohol was found to have no association with PSC in one clinic-based study (74) and an association with less severe nuclear opacities in BDES (79).

Nutrition   Early studies, largely animal experiments, initially suggested a possible role of nutritional status in cataract formation (107). In particular, antioxidant status has received the most attention because of the link between oxidative stress and cataractogenesis. Ascorbate is concentrated in the aqueous humor that surrounds the lens. Both glutathione synthetase and glutathione reductase are far more concentrated and more active in lens tissues than elsewhere in the body, suggesting that the tissues of the lens and its surroundings are designed to deal with high levels of oxidative stress. While large numbers of published studies have investigated the association between lens opacities and various antioxidants or micronutrients (31, 44, 46, 47, 67, 69, 73, 80, 90, 101), the findings are inconclusive.

In a case-control study in Boston of different lens opacity types, regular intake of multivitamin supplementation decreased the risk of cortical, nuclear, PSC, and mixed opacities (69). This protective effect of multivitamin use was not observed in the other three studies (31, 44, 101). The BDES found that, in persons without diabetes, regular use of multivitamin in the past ten years was associated with decreased risk for nuclear sclerosis and an increased risk of cortical opacities (71c). In persons with diabetes, past multivitamin use was not associated with nuclear sclerosis but with decreased risk for cortical opacities.

The evidence for association of cataract with specific antioxidants or micronutrients is conflicting. For example, a decreased risk of cataract extraction or cortical opacities was associated with higher level of dietary intake of vitamin A/carotene (31, 69) and plasma carotenoid (46, 47) in some studies. However, vitamin A intake, plasma vitamin A, and serum retinol were not found to be associated with cataract in other studies (44, 67, 101), including one prospective study (101). Blood levels of alpha-tocopherol (67, 101), past intake of vitamin E (69, 71a), or prior vitamin E supplement use (80) have been associated with a decreased risk of nuclear opacities (69, 101), cortical opacities (69), cataract, or cataract extraction (67, 80). Other studies did not find any protective effect (31, 44, 46, 47, 71b, 73). Vitamin C supplement use, high levels of serum vitamin C, or dietary intake of vitamin C were found to be associated with a decreased risk of cataract (31, 47, 69, 71a, 80). Other investigations did not corroborate with these findings (44, 73, 101), and one case-control study, done in India, showed that high serum vitamin C increased the risk of mixed (nuclear and PSC) cataracts (73).

An index of antioxidant status, which combines various measures of antioxidant vitamins and erythrocyte enzymes, was created and examined by several investigators. While four studies documented that high antioxidant index scores were associated with lower risk for all types of cataract (46, 67, 69, 73), three studies did not show a protective effect (44, 71a, 101).

Two large randomized intervention trials were conducted in a rural population in China (90) enrolled in an anti-cancer study. Use of vitamin/mineral and riboflavin/niacin supplements for five to six years were found to be associated with a reduction of 36–44% in the prevalence of nuclear, but not cortical, cataract. Although the findings support a protective effect of these supplements, it is difficult to generalize from these findings to better-nourished populations. Future studies, including clinical trials, may address the question of the role of supplements on cataractogenesis.

Ultraviolet Radiation   Lens opacification has been linked to ocular exposure to ultraviolet radiation, particularly ultraviolet B (UV-B). The question of whether long-term, chronic exposure to UV-B in sunlight might increase the risk of cataract in humans has been stated in a series of epidemiologic investigations. Early studies noted that cataract occurred more frequently in tropical or sunny regions where exposures to solar radiation, including ultraviolet light, might be high (38, 98a, 109). Ecological studies in Australia (42), Nepal (6), China (71), and the United States (39, 40) demonstrated increasing prevalence of cataract and cataract surgery in areas with greater UV-B levels.

Ocular exposure to UV radiation is primarily a function of individual habits rather than the amount of ambient UV radiation and is modified by the wearing of hats, glasses, and time spent outdoors. Studies in which personal exposure to UV has been measured to account for these factors provide evidence for an association between UV exposure and both cortical (18, 20, 44, 93) and PSC (2, 18) cataracts. Specifically, those in the highest stratum of personal UV-B exposure were at threefold greater risk of cortical cataract than those in the lowest (93). The BDES found an association between cortical opacities and UV exposure for men but not for women (20). None of these studies found an association between UV-B exposure and nuclear cataract.

Ordinary plastic spectacles and even the most inexpensive of sunglasses are likely to block 95% of UV-B transmission. Wearing a broad-brimmed hat appears to reduce the ocular dose of UV by up to 50% and simultaneously reduces cutaneous facial exposure (53).

Ionizing Radiation   There are limited data on the association of cataract with other types of radiation, such as X-ray exposure, microwave, and infrared exposure. Ionizing radiation is well known to cause cataract in patients undergoing radiotherapy for ocular and orbital malignancies. In one recently published study, there were significant associations between previous exposure to diagnostic computed tomography (CT) and both nuclear and posterior subcapsular opacities (61). These findings suggest the importance of minimizing even diagnostic levels of radiation exposure to the lens of the eye.

Diabetes Mellitus   Diabetes is a well-recognized risk factor for all forms of lens opacity. Ordinarily, there is minimal oxidative phosphorylation in the lens and the majority of glucose metabolism proceeds via the pentose phosphate shunt. Elevated levels of blood (and aqueous humor) glucose overwhelm this pathway, leading to production of sugar alcohols, which in turn increase osmotic pressure and cause lens swelling and cataract. Studies have demonstrated an association between cataract and duration of diabetes among persons with type-I diabetes, age and use of insulin among persons with type-II diabetes (64, 66), and poor control of glycemia (59). However, unlike diabetes-related retinal vascular changes, no prospective study has yet demonstrated a reduction in the formation of cataract in association with strict diabetic control. Inhibition of aldose reductase inhibits the formation of sugar alcohols in laboratory animals. However, initial formulations of aldose reductase inhibitors for humans have proved toxic, with no evidence that they influence cataractogenesis.

Medications   Many drugs are suspected to increase cataract formation. Included are steroids, phenothiazines, miotic cholinergic compounds, allopurinol, diuretics, major tranquilizers, cholesterol-lowing medications, cancer chemotherapy agents, photosensitizing drugs, and many others. Systematic use of corticosteroids in patients with rheumatoid arthritis, asthma, pemphigus, nephrosis, and lupus are associated with PSC opacities. The evidence is less strong for other drugs (89, 107).

Aspirin and other analgesics, notably prostaglandin inhibitors, have been proposed to protect against cataract formation through aldose reductase inhibition and lowering of plasma tryptophan levels. While some studies report a protective effect for aspirin and similar compounds (19, 33, 34, 73), the majority of epidemiologic studies have failed to find any benefit, including three population-based observational studies (65, 84, 104), two case-control studies (44, 69), two prospective studies (30, 76), and four randomized clinical trials (13, 77, 83, 98).

In summary, age-related cataract is a multifactorial disease, and different risk factors appear to be associated with different types of lens opacity. Smoking is associated with increased risk of nuclear cataract, while sunlight exposure, diabetes, heavy alcohol drinking, and some commonly used pharmaceuticals are more closely associated with cortical and posterior subcapsular lens opacities (107).

Risk factors most highly associated with cataract often have other adverse health effects as well. Therefore delaying cataract incidence is yet another good reason to promote smoking cessation, control glycemia in patients with diabetes mellitus, improve nutritional status, and decrease exposure to UV radiation. Other potential interventions, such as vitamin and aspirin supplementation, are not justified from currently available data and await further studies.

Reducing Blindness From Cataract

The only cure for vision loss due to cataract is surgical removal of the opaque lens and provision of an intraocular lens or aphakic spectacle. There are two primary methods of cataract extraction: extracapsular cataract extraction (ECCE) including phacoemulsification, which has been adopted by nearly all developed countries, and intracapsular cataract extraction (ICCE), which was originally popularized in India half a century ago and is still practiced in many parts of the developing world.

Although millions of cataract surgeries are performed worldwide each year, unoperated cataract continues to be the leading cause of blindness. Approximately 5 million people in India and 2 million in China are blind from cataract

(95a). The cataract backlog is not only a phenomenon of the developing world. Drummond et al estimated that 74,000 patients were on ophthalmology hospital waiting lists in England in the first quarter of 1989 (23). In the United States where over one million cataract surgeries are performed annually, unoperated cataract may account for as much as 20% of total blindness (87).

Access to cataract surgery is distributed unequally among Americans. Black Americans were found to be 30% less likely to have cataract surgery than white Americans in two analyses of national data (51, 85). Men were 20% less likely to have cataract surgery than women (51). Several other factors may explain the variation of cataract surgery. Socioeconomic factors such as income were significantly associated with the likelihood of cataract surgery (25, 51). Care-seeking behavior, that is, whether the patient sees a specialist or a primary care physician for eye care, seemed to contribute to the variation (25). Access to cataract surgery was found to be associated with regional optometrist supply, but not ophthalmologist supply and their practice style (25, 51).

In developing countries, the shortage, maldistribution, and inefficiencies of eye-care manpower and facilities are the major barriers to cataract surgery. Africa, as an example, has only one ophthalmologist per 1 million people (one ophthalmologist for every 4000 blind individuals) (27, 48). In contrast, the ratio of ophthalmologists to population in the US is 1:12,000 and in India is 1:100,000 (99). However, only one third of ophthalmologists are actively involved in providing community cataract surgery in India.

Other barriers to cataract surgery in developing countries include reluctance to undergo cataract surgery, and limited social and economic support (5, 100). In India, more than 80% of persons who were blind from cataracts and referred for surgery did not comply with that advice because of economic or social constraints. In Nepal, nearly half of the blind persons from unoperated cataract did not know that cataract surgery was available to restore vision. Even among those who know about the surgery, many cannot afford it (7). Women and those with limited community resources are more likely to be blind from cataract (4). In the areas where transportation is poorly developed, the longer the distance that patients must travel the lower the rate of participation (41). Increasing awareness of surgery as a cure for cataract blindness and the economic advantage this bestows have proved to be effective in improving patient compliance (5, 29).

Outcomes of cataract surgery in the developed world are generally excellent, with 20/40 or better vision achieved in 94% of cases (50). Over 90% of those who undergo cataract surgery without other eye disease reported functional improvement in both distance and near vision, and improvement in quality of life functions (3, 50). Severe complications of surgery are infrequent as measured in the National Study of Cataract Outcome (9, 52, 54–56, 82, 91, 92; Table 5). However, over 20% of patients undergoing modern, extracapsular

Table 5   Complications following cataract extraction, the United States

Complications	Time after surgery	Rate (%) of complications	
		ICCE	ECCE
Endophthalmitis	3 months	0.14	0.10
	6 months	0.15	0.12
	9 months	0.16	0.12
	12 months	0.17	0.12
Corneal edema/ transplantation	1 year	0.2	0.2
	2 years	0.5	0.3
	3 years	0.9	0.5
	4 years	1.4	0.6
Retinal detachment	1 year	0.7	0.3
	2 years	1.1	0.5
	3 years	1.4	0.7
	4 years	1.6	0.9
Nd: YAG laser capsulotomy	1 year		0.24 – 0.27

cataract surgery will develop opacification of the posterior lens capsule that can interfere with vision (54, 82, 92). Capsular opacification is routinely treated in the United States with a Neodynium:YAG laser, a procedure associated with a complication rate of under 2% (54).

Data on the outcomes for cataract surgery in developing countries are limited. Postoperative infection, the most severe complication of cataract surgery, is relatively infrequent. Christy & Lall (15) reported an infection rate of 0.46% for 54,000 ICCE performed at a carefully conducted mass-surgery center in Pakistan. In a Nepalese hospital, the rate of endophthalmitis following simple ECCE was 0.3% (81). Among patients who were followed-up two years after ECCE, the complication rate was 0.3% for retinal detachment and 0.6 for corneal decompensation (81). In the same study, Ruit and co-workers demonstrated that visual acuity better than 20/200 (the threshold for legal blindness in the U.S.) was maintained for over two years of follow-up in 88% of patients after ECCE. Almost half of the patients had uncorrected visual acuity of 20/50 or better and 77% had best corrected vision of 20/50 or better (81). A study at an outpatient clinic in Ghana reported improvement of vision in 90% of patients after ECCE and IOL implantation. Over 50% of patients had a corrected visual acuity of 20/50 or better and another 22% had corrected visual acuity of 20/50 to 20/100 (24).

However, cataract surgery has limited success in some studies. The Nepal

Eye Study revealed that 17% of eyes operated for cataract became irreversibly blind due to surgical complications (6). Over one half of the eyes were functionally blind, mostly because the spectacles distributed after surgery were not replaced after loss or breakage. Capsular opacification was seen in 21% of eyes in the study by Ruit et al (81), raising questions about the practicality of ECCE in developing countries where lasers are not available. Consideration of treating capsular opacification is a serious issue for countries that want to develop capabilities for doing ECCE (105). If modern cataract surgery is to be delivered in the developing world, either facilities for treating subsequent capsular opacification must be available, or the technique must be modified to include safe and effective primary discission of the posterior lens capsule.

ECONOMIC RETURN ON CATARACT SURGERY

In the United States, a typical episode of cataract surgery costs approximately $2500, which equates to a total of $3.4 billion a year nationwide (92). In addition, over $39 million is spent on preoperative ophthalmologic diagnostic tests and $25 million on postoperative ophthalmologic diagnostic tests and preoperative medical care.

The cost of cataract surgery in developing countries depends on the quality of the facilities. It ranges from $15 for a simple cataract extraction in an eye camp to $60 at a regional hospital. The cost of ECCE plus use of an IOL is likely to be twice that amount (23, 48).

Compared with those costs of care, the economic cost of vision loss from cataract is huge. Loss of sight from cataract often begins in the fifth and sixth decades of life. It causes disability that leaves individuals and their families without means to earn a productive living or confines the individual to custodial care (or that of a relative who is similarly removed from the workforce). Such economic loss can be readily reduced or prevented by cataract extraction. In a study conducted in south India, 85% of men and 58% of women who had lost their jobs as a result of blindness regained those jobs. A number of those who did not return to work relieved other family members from household duties, thereby enabling them to return to work (48). Regaining functional vision through cataract surgery could generate 1500% of the cost of surgery in increased economic productivity during the first year following surgery (48).

Published data demonstrate the cost-effectiveness of cataract surgery in both the developed and developing world (23, 48, 49). In most cases, cataract surgery is expected to improve vision function and quality of life, rather than to prolong life. Therefore, its cost-effectiveness is best evaluated in terms of the cost per quality-adjusted life years (QALY) saved.

As compared with other common public health intervention, cataract surgery was ranked as one of most cost-effective interventions ($18–32 per QALY) that can be offered to adults in the developing world using available technology (48, 49). Other technologies in this category included widely advocated and readily funded public health interventions such as vaccination for measles, polio, and tetanus and treatment of tuberculosis. Cost-effectiveness of cataract extraction in developed countries was assessed by Drummond et al (23). The cost was estimated as (£2750 ($4318) per QALY gained through cataract surgery, assuming an individual survives ten years after the surgery. This value compares favorably with many other interventions, such as breast cancer screening [(£5340 ($8384) per QALY], CABG for mild angina [(£19,250 ($30,223) per QALY), and hospital haemodialysis [(£21,500 ($33,755) per QALY]. In analyzing the cost-effectiveness of cataract surgery from the US perspective, we have estimated that cataract surgery costs between $1750 and $2300 per QALY saved, depending on one's assumption about the rate at which lens opacities progress (49a).

CONCLUSION

Blindness from cataract is clearly avoidable. The most pressing need for elimination of blindness due to cataract is to reduce the backlog of cataract through mass surgical intervention. This requires a commitment of resources along with initiatives in operations research designed to reduce barriers to surgery and increase the effectiveness of public health programs. Establishment of local eye care facilities is crucial for long-term success of blindness prevention.

Primary prevention of cataract, should a technology emerge, is an optimal approach and could be more cost-effective than cataract surgery in blindness prevention. Estimates indicate that delaying the onset of cataract by ten years could reduce the need for surgery by 45%, thus saving millions of dollars (10).

Literature Cited

1. Adamsons I, Munoz B, Enger C, Taylor HR. 1991. Prevalence of lens opacities in surgical and general population. *Arch. Ophthalmol.* 109:993–97
2. Bochow TW, West SK, Azar A, Muñoz B, Sommer A, Taylor HR. 1989. Ultraviolet light exposure and risk of posterior subcapsular cataracts. *Arch. Ophthalmol.* 107:369–72
3. Brenner MH, Curbow B, Javitt JC, Legro MW, Sommer A. 1993. Vision change and quality of life in the elderly. Response to cataract surgery and treatment of other chronic ocular conditions. *Arch. Ophthalmol.* 111:680–85
4. Brilliant GE, Brilliant LB. 1985. Using social epidemiology to understand who stays blind and who gets operated for cataract in a rural setting. *Soc. Sci. Med.* 21:553–58
5. Brilliant GE, Lepkowski JM, Zurita B, Thulasiraj RD. 1991. Social determinants of cataract surgery utilization in South India. *Arch. Ophthalmol.* 109: 584–89
6. Brilliant LB, Grasset NC, Pokhrel RP,

Kolstad A, Lepkowski JM, et al. 1983. Associations among cataract prevalence, sunlight hours, and altitude in the Himalayas. *Am. J. Epidemiol.* 118:250–64

7. Brilliant LB, Pokhrel RP, Grasset NC, Lepkowski JM, Kolstad A, et al. 1985. Epidemiology of blindness in Nepal. *Bull. WHO.* 63:375–86

8. Bunce GE, Kinoshita J, Horwitz J. 1990. Nutritional factors in cataract. *Annu. Rev. Nutr.* 10:233–54

9. Canner JK, Javitt JC, McBean MA. 1992. National outcomes of cataract extraction III. Corneal edema and transplant following inpatient surgery. *Arch. Ophthalmol.* 110:1137–42

10. Cataract Panel. 1983. Report. Vision research: a national plan 1983–87. Part 3. *NIH publ. 83–2473.* Washington, DC: US DHHS

11. Cent. Dis. Control. 1983. Cataract—a major blinding condition. *Morbid. Mortal. Wkly. Rep.* 32:119–20

12. Chatterjee A, Milton RC, Thyle S. 1982. Prevalence and aetiology of cataract in Punjab. *Br. J. Ophthalmol.* 66:35–42

13. Chew EY, Williams GA, Burton TC, Remaley MA, Ferris FL. 1992. Aspirin effects on the development of cataracts in patients with diabetes mellitus. Early Treatment Diabetic Retinopathy Study rep. 16. *Arch. Ophthalmol.* 110:339–42

14. Christen WG, Manson JE, Seddon JM, Glynn RJ, Buring JE, et al. 1992. A prospective study of cigarette smoking and risk of cataract in men. *JAMA* 268:989–93

15. Christy NE, Lall P. 1973. Postoperative endophthalmitis following cataract surgery. *Arch. Ophthalmol.* 90:361–66

16. Chylack LT Jr, Leske MA, Sperduto R, Khu P, McCarthy D, Lens Opacities Case-control Study Group. 1988. Lens opacities classification system. *Arch. Ophthalmol.* 106:330–34

17. Clayton RM, Cuthbert J, Seth J, Phillips CI, Bartholomew RS, et al. 1984. Epidemiological and other studies in the assessment of factors contributing to cataractogenesis. *Ciba Found. Symp.* 106:25–47

18. Collman GW, Shore DL, Shy CM, Checkway H, Luria AS. 1988. Sunlight and other risk factors for cataracts: an epidemiologic study. *Am. J. Public Health* 78:1459–62

19. Cotlier E. 1988. Senile cataracts: evidence for acceleration by diabetes and deceleration by salicylate. *Can. J. Ophthalmol.* 16:113–18

20. Cruickshanks KJ, Klein BEK, Klein R. 1992. Ultraviolet light exposure and lens opacities: the Beaver Dam Eye Study. *Am. J. Public. Health.* 82:1658–62

21. Deleted in proof

22. Dolin PJ. 1994. Ultraviolet radiation and cataract: a review of the epidemiological evidence. *Br. J. Ophthalmol.* 78:478–82

23. Drummond MF. 1992. Economic aspects of cataract blindness. In *World Blindness and Its Prevention,* ed. C Kupfer, T Gillen, pp. 157–70. Int. Agency Prevent. Blindness. Vol. 4.

24. Egbert PR, Buchanan M. 1991. Results of extracapsular cataract surgery and intraocular lens implantation in Ghana. *Arch. Ophthalmol.* 109:1761–63

25. Escarce JJ. 1993. Would eliminating differences in physician practice style reduce geographic variations in cataract survey rates? *Med. Care* 31:1106–18

26. Flaye DE, Sullivan KN, Cullinan TR, Silver JH, Whitelock RA. 1989. Cataracts and cigarette smoking. The City Eye Study. *Eye* 3:379–84

27. Foster A. 1991. Who will operate on African's 3 million curable blind people. *Lancet* 337:1267–69

28. Framingham Offspring Eye Study Group. 1994. Familial aggregation of lens opacities: the Framingham eye study and the Framingham Offspring eye study. *Am. J. Epidemiol.* 140:555–64

29. Deleted in proof

30. Hankinson SE, Seddon JM, Colditz GA, Stampfer MJ, Rosner B, et al. 1993. A prospective study of aspirin use and cataract extraction in women. *Arch. Ophthalmol.* 111:503–8

31. Hankinson SE, Stampfer MJ, Seddon JM, Colditz GA, Rosner B, et al. 1992. Nutrient intake and cataract extraction in women: a prospective study. *Br. Med. J.* 305:335–39

32. Hankinson SE, Willett WC, Colditz GA, Seddon JM, Rosner B, et al. 1992. A prospective study of cigarette smoking and risk of cataract surgery in women. *JAMA.* 268:994–98

33. Harding JJ, Egerton M, Harding RS. 1989. Protection against cataract by aspirin, paracetamol and ibuprofen. *Acta Ophthalmol.* 67:518–24

34. Harding JJ, van Heyningen R. 1988. Drugs, including alcohol, that act as risk factors for cataract, and possible protection against cataract by aspirin-like analgesics and cyclopenthiazide. *Br. J. Ophthalmol.* 72:809–14

35. Harding JJ, van Heyningen R. 1989. Beer, cigarettes and military work as risk factors for cataract. *Dev. Ophthalmol.* 17:13–16

36. Heiba IM, Elston RC, Klein BEK, Klein

R. 1993. Genetic etiology of nuclear cataract: evidence for major gene. *Am. J. Med. Genet.* 47:1208–14

37. Heiba IM, Elston RC, Klein BEK, Klein R. 1995. Evidence for a major gene for cortical cataract. *Invest. Ophthalmol. Vis. Sci.* 36:227–35

38. Hiller R, Giacometti L, Yuen K. 1977. Sunlight and cataract: an epidemiologic investigation. *Am. J. Epidemiol.* 105: 450–59

39. Hiller R, Sperduto RD, Ederer F. 1983. Epidemiologic associations with cataract in the 1971–1972 National Health and Nutrition Examination Survey. *Am. J. Epidemiol.* 118:239–49

40. Hiller R, Sperduto RD, Ederer F. 1986. Epidemiologic associations with nuclear, cortical, and posterior subcapsular cataracts. *Am. J. Epidemiol.* 124:916–25

41. HKI (Helen Keller International). 1985. *Kongwa Primary Health Care Report 1984–85.* New York

42. Hollows F, Moran D. 1981. Cataract—the ultraviolet risk factor. *Lancet* 2: 1249–50

43. Hu Z, Zhao JL, Dong FT, et al. 1989. Survey of cataract in Shunyi County, Beijing. *Chin. J. Ophthalmol.* 25:360–64

44. Italian-American Cataract Study Group. 1991. Risk factors for age-related cortical, nuclear, and posterior subcapsular cataracts. *Am. J. Epidemiol.* 133:541–53

45. Italian-American Cataract Study Group. 1994. Incidence and progression of cortical, nuclear, and posterior subcapsular cataracts. *Am. J. Ophthalmol.* 118:623–31

46. Jacques PF, Chylack LT, McGandy RB, Hartz SC. 1988. Antioxidant status in persons with and without senile cataract. *Arch. Ophthalmol.* 106:337–40

47. Jacques PF, Hartz SC, Chylack LT Jr, McGandy RB, Sadowski JA. 1988. Nutritional status in persons with and without senile cataract: blood vitamin and mineral levels. *Am. J. Clin. Nutr.* 48: 152–58

48. Javitt JC. 1993. Cataract. In *Disease Control Priorities in Developing Countries,* ed. DT Jamison, WH Mosley, AR Measham, JL Bobadilla, pp. 635–45. Oxford: Oxford Med. Publ.

49. Javitt JC. 1993. The cost-effectiveness of restoring sight. *Arch. Ophthalmol.* 111:1615

49a. Javitt JC. 1993. *Cost-effectiveness of cataract surgery.* Oral presentation. Am. Acad. Ophthalmol.

50. Javitt JC, Brenner MH, Curbow B, Legro MW, Street DA. 1993. Outcomes of cataract surgery. Improvement in visual acuity and subjective visual function after surgery in the first, second, and both eyes. *Arch. Ophthalmol.* 111:686–91

51. Javitt JC, Kendix M, Tielsch JM, Steinwachs DM, Schein OD, Kolb MM, et al. 1995. Geographic variation in utilization of cataract surgery. *Med. Care* 33:90–105

52. Javitt JC, Street DA, Tielsh JM, Wang Q, Kolb MM, et al. 1994. National outcomes of cataract extraction. Retinal detachment and endophthalmitis after outpatient cataract surgery. *Ophthalmology* 101:100–5

53. Javitt JC, Taylor HR. 1995. Cataract and latitude. *Doc. Ophthalmol.* 88:307–25

54. Javitt JC, Tielsch JM, Canner JK, Kolb MM, Sommer A, Steinberg EP. 1992. National outcome of cataract extraction I. Increased risk of retinal complications associated with Nd:YAG laser capsulotomy. *Ophthalmology* 99:1487–98

55. Javitt JC, Vitale S, Canner JK, Krakauer H, McBean AM, Sommer A. 1991. National outcomes of cataract extraction. Retinal detachment after inpatient surgery. *Ophthalmology* 98:895–902

56. Javitt JC, Vitale S, Canner JK, Street DA, Krakauer H, et al. 1991. National outcomes of cataract extraction. Endophthalmitis following inpatient surgery. *Arch. Ophthalmol.* 109:1085–89

57. Kahn HA, Leibowitz HM, Ganley JP, et al. 1977. The Framingham Eye Study. I. Outline and major prevalence findings. *Am. J. Epidemiol.* 106:17–32

58. Kahn HA, Leibowitz HM, Ganley JP, Kini MM, Colton T, et al. 1977. The Framingham Eye Study. II. Association of ophthalmic pathology with single variables previously measured in the Framingham Heart Study. *Am. J. Epidemiol.* 106:33–41

59. Karasik A, Modan M, Halkin H, Trister G, Fuchs Z, et al. 1984. Senile cataract and glucose intolerance: the Israel Study of Glucose Intolerance Obesity and Hypertension (The Israel GOH Study). *Diabetes Care* 7:52–56

60. Klein BEK, Klein R, Linton KLP. 1992. Prevalence of age-related lens opacities in a population. *Ophthalmology* 99:546–52

61. Klein BEK, Klein R, Linton KLP, Franke T. 1993. Diagnostic X-ray exposure and lens opacities: the Beaver Dam Eye Study. *Am. J. Public Health* 83:588–90

62. Klein BEK, Klein R, Linton KLP, Franke T. 1993. Cigarette smoking and

lens opacities: the Beaver Dam Eye Study. *Am. J. Prev. Med.* 9:27–30

63. Klein BEK, Klein R, Linton KLP, Magli YL, Neider NW. 1990. Assessment of cataracts from photographs in the Beaver Dam Eye Study. *Ophthalmology* 97:1428–33

64. Klein BEK, Klein R, Moss SE. 1985. Prevalence of cataracts in a population-based study of persons with diabetes mellitus. *Ophthalmology* 92:1191–96

65. Klein BEK, Klein R, Moss SE. 1987. Is aspirin use associated with lower rates of cataracts in diabetic individuals? *Diabetes Care* 10:495–99

66. Klein BEK, Klein R, Moss SE. 1995. Incidence of cataract surgery in the Wisconsin Epidemiologic Study of diabetic retinopathy. *Am. J. Ophthalmol.* 119: 295–300

67. Knekt P, Heliövaara M, Rissanen A, Aromaa A, Aaran RK. 1992. Serum antioxidant vitamins and risk of cataract. *Br. Med. J.* 305:1392–94

68. Leibowitz HM, et al. 1980. The Framingham Eye Study Monograph. *Surv. Ophthalmol.* 24(Suppl.):335–610

69. Leske MC, Chylack LT Jr, Wu S-Y, the Lens Opacities Case-Control Study Group. 1991. The Lens Opacities Case-Control Study. Risk factors for cataract. *Arch. Ophthalmol.* 109:244–51

70. Leske MC, Sperduto RD. 1983. The epidemiology of senile cataracts: a review. *Am. J. Epidemiol.* 118:152–65

71. Mao WS, Hu TS. 1982. An epidemiologic survey of senile cataract in China. *Chin. Med. J.* 95:813–18

71a. Mares-Perlman JA, Brady WE Klein BEK, Klein R, Haus GJ, et al. 1995. Diet and nuclear lens opacities. *Am. J. Epidemiol.* 141:322–34

71b. Mares-Perlman JA, Brady WE, Klein BEK, Klein R, Palta M, et al. 1995. Serum carotenoids and tocopherols and severity of nuclear and cortical opacities. *Invest. Ophthalmol. Vis. Sci.* 36: 276–88

71c. Mares-Perlman JA, Klein BE, Klein R, Ritter LL. 1994. Relation between lens opacitites and vitamin and mineral supplements use. *Ophthalmology* 101:315–25

72. Minassian DC, Mehra V. 1990. 3.8 million blinded by cataract each year: projections from the first epidemiological study of incidence of cataract blindness in India. *Br. J. Ophthalmol.* 74:341–43

73. Mohan M, Sperduto RD, Angra SK, Milton RC, Mathur RL, et al. 1989. India-US case-control study of age-related cataracts. *Arch. Ophthalmol.* 107: 670–76

74. Muñoz B, Tajchman U, Bochow T, West S. 1993. Alcohol use and risk of posterior subcapsular opacities. *Arch. Ophthalmol.* 111:110–12

75. Muñoz B, West S, Vitale S, Schein OD, Maguire M, Taylor HR. 1993. Alcohol use and cataract in a cohort of Chesapeake Bay watermen. (Abstract). *Invest. Ophthalmol. Vis. Sci.* 34(Suppl.): 1066

76. Paganini-Hill A, Chao A, Ross RK, Henderson BE. 1989. Aspirin use and chronic diseases: a cohort study of the elderly. *Br. Med. J.* 299:1247–50

77. Peto R, Gray R, Collins R, Wheatley K, Hennekens C, et al. 1988. Randomised trial of prophylactic daily aspirin in British male doctors. *Br. Med. J.* 296:313–16

78. Podgor MJ, Leske MC, Ederer F. 1983. Incidence estimates for lens changes, macular changes, open angle glaucoma and diabetic retinopathy. *Am. J. Epidemiol.* 118:206–12

79. Ritter LL, Klein BEK, Klein R, Mares-Perlman JA. 1993. Alcohol use and lens opacities in the Beaver Dam Eye Study. *Arch. Ophthalmol.* 111:113–17

80. Robertson JMcD, Donner AP, Trevithick JR. 1991. A possible role for vitamins C and E in cataract prevention. *Am. J. Clin. Nutr.* 53:346S–51S

81. Ruit S, Robin AL, Pokrel RP, Sharma A, Defaller J. 1991. Extracapsular cataract extraction in Nepal: 2-year outcome. *Arch. Ophthalmol.* 109:1761–63

82. Schein OD, Steinberg EP, Javitt JC, Cassard SD, Tielsch JM, et al. 1994. Variation in cataract surgery practice and clinical outcomes. *Ophthalmology* 101:1142–52

83. Seddon JM, Christen WG, Manson JE, Burning JE, Sperduto RD, Hennekens CH. 1991. Low-dose aspirin and risks of cataract in a randomized trial of US physicians. *Arch. Ophthalmol.* 109:252–55

84. Seigel D, Sperduto RD, Ferris FL III. 1982. Aspirin and cataracts. *Ophthalmology* 89:47A–9A

85. Sharkness CM, Hamburger S, Kaczmarek RG, Hamilton PM, Bright RA, Moore RM. 1992. Racial differences in the prevalence of intraocular lens implants in the United States. *Am. J. Ophthalmol.* 114:667–74

86. Deleted in proof

87. Sommer A, Tielsch JM, Katz J, Quigley HA, Gottsch JD. 1991. Racial differences in the cause-specific prevalence of blindness in east Baltimore. *N. Engl. J. Med.* 325:1412–17

88. Sparrow JM, Bron AJ, Brown NAP,

Ayliffe W, Hill AR. 1986. The Oxford Clinical Cataract Classification and Grading System. *Int. Ophthalmol.* 9: 207–25

89. Sperduto RD. 1994. Age-related cataracts: scope of problem and prospects for prevention. *Prev. Med.* 23:735–39

90. Sperduto RD, Hu T-S, Milton RC, Zhao JL, Everett DF, et al. 1993. The Linxian Cataract Studies. Two nutrition intervention trials. *Arch. Ophthalmol.* 111: 1246–53

91. Steinberg EP, Bergner M, Sommer A, et al. 1990. Variations in cataract management: patient and economic outcomes. *Health Serv. Res.* 25:727–31

92. Steinberg EP, Javitt JC, Sharkey PD, Zuckerman A, Legro MW, et al. 1993. The content and cost of cataract surgery. *Arch. Ophthalmol.* 111:1041–48

93. Taylor HR, West SK, Rosenthal FS, Muñoz B, Newland HS, et al. 1988. Effect of ultraviolet radiation on cataract formation. *N. Engl. J. Med.* 319:1429–33

94. Taylor HR, West SK. 1989. The clinical grading of lens opacities. *Aust. NZ J. Ophthalmol.* 17:81–86

95. Thylefors B. 1990. The World Health Organization's programme for the prevention of blindness. *Int. Ophthalmol.* 14:211–19

95a. Thylefors B, Négrel AP, Pararajasegaram R, Dadzie KY. 1995. Global data on blindness. *Bull. WHO* 73:115–21

96. Tielsch JM. 1994. *Vision Problems in the U.S.* Prevent Blindness America, Schaumburg, IL.

97. Tielsch JM, Javitt JC, Coleman A, Katz J, Sommer A. 1995. The prevalence of blindness and visual impairment among nursing home residents in Baltimore. *N. Engl. J. Med.* 332:1205–9

98. UK-TIA Study Group. 1992. Does aspirin affect the rate of cataract formation? Cross-sectional results during a randomised double-blind placebo controlled trial to prevent serious vascular events. *Br. J. Ophthalmol.* 76: 259–61

98a. van Heyingen R. 1972. The human lens. I. A comparison of cataracts extracted in Oxford (England) and Shikapur (W. Pakistan). *Exp. Eye Res.* 13:136–47

99. Venkataswamy G. 1987. Cataract in the Indian subcontinent. *Ophthal. Surg.* 18: 464–66

100. Venkataswamy G, Brilliant G. 1981. Social and economic barriers to cataract surgery in rural south India. *Vis. Impair. Blind.* Dec.:405–68

101. Vitale S, West S, Hallfrisch J, et al. 1993. Plasma antioxidants and risk of cortical and nuclear cataract. *Epidemiology* 4:195–203

102. West S. 1992. Does smoke get in your eyes? *JAMA* 268:1025–26

103. West S, Muñoz B, Emmett EA, Taylor HR. 1989. Cigarette smoking and risk of nuclear cataracts. *Arch. Ophthalmol.* 107:1166–69

104. West SK, Muoz BE, Newland HS, Emmett EA, Taylor HR. 1987. Lack of evidence for aspirin use and prevention of cataracts. *Arch. Ophthalmol.* 105: 1229–31

105. West SK, Quigley HQ. 1991. Cataract blindness: what to do? *Arch. Ophthalmol.* 109:1765–66

106. West SK, Rosenthal F, Newland HS, Taylor HR. 1988. Use of photographic techniques to grade nuclear cataracts. *Invest. Ophthalmol. Vis. Sci.* 29:73–77

107. West SK, Valmadrid CT. 1995. Epidemiology of risk factors for age-related cataract. *Surv. Ophthalmol.* 39: 323–34

108. WHO (World Health Organization). 1987. *Programme for the Prevention of Blindness. Available Data on Blindness.* 87.14:1–23.34, Geneva

109. Zigman S, Datiles M, Torczynski E. 1979. Sunlight and human cataracts. *Invest. Ophthalmol. Vis. Sci.* 18:462–67

Annu. Rev. Public Health. 1996. 17:179–202

PUBLIC HEALTH AND REGULATORY CONSIDERATIONS OF THE SAFE DRINKING WATER ACT

Robert S. Raucher

Hagler Bailly Consulting, Inc., P.O. Drawer O, Boulder, Colorado 80306-1906

KEY WORDS: benefit-cost, MCL, cost-effectiveness, risk assessment

ABSTRACT

This paper provides an overview of the public health and economic issues associated with drinking water quality regulations in the United States. A historic perspective is provided by the use of filtration and chlorine disinfection, and of public health laws from the early 20th century up to passage of the Safe Drinking Water Act (SDWA), in 1974. The contaminants regulated under the Act, and the 1986 Amendments to the SWDA, are evaluated according to health endpoint, related issues in risk assessment, and the cost of complying with associated regulations. Risk-cost and benefit-cost analyses are offered for carcinogens, systemics, and pathogens. The paper describes the evolution of public health issues from the initial focus on waterborne infectious diseases to concerns over chemical contaminants, and the recent reemergence of microbials as the high-priority public health concern.

INTRODUCTION

Credit for establishing the link between drinking water quality and public health is generally attributed to Dr. John Snow, whose observations isolated a specific water source as the cause of London's cholera outbreak in the mid-nineteenth century. However, the link between health and drinking water quality has been broadly recognized for over 4000 years, in what we might refer to today as "guidance," "advisories," and "regulations" for the gathering, storage, and treatment of water used for human consumption.

Two decades after passage of the Safe Drinking Water Act (SDWA) in 1974, in which Congress first mandated a centralized federal regulatory role, both the statute and the manner in which it is implemented by the U.S. Environmental Protection Agency (US EPA) are in flux. Under close scrutiny

179

0163-7525/96/0510-0179$08.00

by legislators, regulators, public health experts, the regulated community of water suppliers, and public interest advocacy groups alike are such fundamental issues as who should decide (and on what basis) which contaminants to regulate, the stringency and form of such regulations, to whom the regulations should apply, and what information to use in considering how (and how stringently) to set regulatory standards. In this paper, we outline the history and nature of the federal role in regulating drinking water quality in the United States, as it pertains to public health. To place the current issues in context, we briefly review the statutory issues and their background, then present and discuss empirical information on the costs and public health benefits of drinking water quality regulation in the United States. Finally, we combine the historical perspective with empirical evidence to shed light on the continuing debate surrounding the future direction of SDWA reauthorization and the federal drinking water regulatory program as a means of protecting public health.

HISTORICAL PERSPECTIVE: DRINKING WATER AND PUBLIC HEALTH

It is directed to heat foul water by boiling and exposing to sunlight and by dipping seven times into it a piece of hot copper in an earthen vessel.
Sanskrit (c. 2000 B.C.)
When one comes into a city to which he is a stranger ... one should consider most attentively the waters which the inhabitants use ....
Hippocrates (c. 400 B.C.) (7)

Concern over the quality of drinking water, and indeed the need to establish standards to ensure its safety, is at least 4000 years old. Pictures of apparatus to clarify both wine and water have been found on Egyptian walls dating to the fifteenth century B.C. Hippocrates (460–354 B.C.), in his writings on hygiene, directed attention principally to the importance of water in the maintenance of health, and he prescribed that rainwater be both boiled and strained prior to consumption (7). And Vitruvius, a bureaucrat during the reign of Augustus Caesar, was unsuccessful in his bid to eliminate lead piping despite his argument that

Water ... conducted through lead pipes ... is found to be harmful for the reason that white lead is derived from it, and this is said to be hurtful to the human system. (18)

The first clear proof that public water supplies could be a source of infection for humans came in 1854 from the careful epidemiological studies of cholera by Dr. John Snow in London. Dr. Snow concluded that the source of water was the variable that best explained the distribution of cholera deaths. However, the causal agent of cholera, *Vibrio cholera*, was not actually isolated until 1884 by Robert Koch. Subsequently, Koch's study of a cholera epidemic in the German cities of Hamburg and Altona in 1892 provided some of the best evidence for the importance of water filtration in protecting against this disease (7).

In the United States, there were comparable efforts to isolate and prevent typhoid fever. By 1884, the causal agent, *Salmonella typhi,* was isolated and identified, and typhoid was recognized as being transmitted, to a significant degree, by drinking water. In 1887, an experimental sand-filtration station was established at Lawrence, Massachusetts; the incidence of typhoid fever fell markedly, and the death rate from the disease dropped by 79%. By 1907, 33 cities in the United States had installed mechanical filters, and 13 others were using sand filters (7).

The efficacy of chlorination as a disinfectant was first illustrated in an urban water supply in Jersey City, NJ. Occasionally, sewage from river communities above the city's reservoir would pollute the water supply. Rather than installing an expensive filtration device or attempting to control the sewage influx, the water supply company decided in 1908 to introduce a chlorination system. The bacterial count dropped markedly. By the beginning of World War I, both filtration and chlorination were widely accepted as worthwhile water purification techniques (7).

A REGULATORY HISTORY OF DRINKING WATER IN THE UNITED STATES

Federal drinking water standards originated with the Interstate Quarantine Act of 1893, authorizing the Surgeon General to make and enforce regulations to prevent the introduction, transmission, or spread of communicable diseases in the United States (5). In 1912, the first water-related regulation was promulgated, prohibiting the use of common drinking water cups on interstate carriers.[1] A 1942 regulation required that bacteriological samples be taken from water distribution systems, and four years later, quality standards were made applicable to all water supplies in the United States. In 1962, the operation of water supply systems by qualified personnel was required, and recommended maximum concentration limits for several inorganics, radioactivity, and carbon chloroform extracts were added (2).

---

[1]This regulation met with stiff opposition. Critics argued that if cups were unavailable for any reason, the health of passengers deprived of water would be endangered, which might tempt them to indulge in alcoholic beverages (2).

The inadequacy of the regulations, promulgated in the 1962 standards, soon became apparent. For example, only 59% of the nation's water systems surveyed by the Public Health Service in 1969 produced water that met the existing standards.

Meanwhile, heightened scientific interest in the study of toxic substances, coupled with technological advances in monitoring the sensitivity of water quality and in chemical analysis, identified the presence of hazardous substances not covered by the existing regulations in the water consumed by many Americans. Subsequently, the emphasis in the type of health-related issues linked to drinking water quality began to shift from epidemic diseases to cancer, lead poisoning, heart disease, and other ailments associated with exposure to toxic substances[2].

Efforts to revise drinking water regulations began in Congress in 1971, but stalled through lack of support. However, in 1973, the presence of carcinogens was identified in the drinking water in New Orleans and the Ohio River Valley. This study by Page et al for the EDF prompted Congressional action. As Representative Paul Rogers recalled

> Between 1971 and 1973 the issue lacked the type of visibility which ensures congressional action ... without a smoking pistol, there was no compelling force ... But then came the surveys of the drinking water in New Orleans, and the Ohio River Valley. Suddenly, with the discovery of possible carcinogens in the drinking water, we had the visibility and sense of urgency which we needed (13).

The Safe Drinking Water Act of 1974

The Safe Drinking Water Act (PL 93–523) was signed into law in December 1974. Its stated purpose was to assure that the public is provided with safe drinking water and that water supply systems meet minimum national standards to protect human health.

Until passage of the 1974 Act, the federal government was authorized to prescribe and enforce drinking water standards only with respect to contaminants capable of causing communicable diseases. PL 93–523 authorized the US EPA to set national standards for protection from all harmful contaminants, and it established a mechanism to assure compliance with these standards. Specifically, US EPA was charged with establishing national drinking water regulations that "... shall protect health to the extent feasible, using technology, treatment techniques, and other means, which the Administrator determines are generally available (taking costs into consideration)" [Section 1412(a)(2)]. The regulations were to consist of

---

[2]For example, Page et al estimated that as much as 10% of the cancer cases in areas served by surface water may be caused by drinking water (9).

Nonmandatory, health-based maximum contaminant levels goals (MCLGs) established for each toxic substance that "... may have an adverse effect on the health of persons ... allow[ing] an adequate margin of safety" [Section 1412 (b)(1)(B)].[3]

Enforceable maximum contaminant levels (MCLs) to be set as close to the recommended health-based goals (MCLGs) "as is feasible" [Section 1412 (b)(1)(B)(3)].

There are several important ramifications of the language in the sections of the 1974 Act quoted above. The phrase "to the extent feasible" pertains to the technological or purely physical ability to deliver water deemed safe, where *safe* is defined primarily by the health-based MCL goal. The phrase "taking costs into consideration" is nebulous, implying that Congress intended the US EPA to overlook water quality problems that would be too expensive to alleviate, even if it were technologically feasible to do so. There has been little clarification as to what measure of cost should be employed, nor at what level such costs would be considered excessive.

Because MCLGs and MCLs are to be established for any substance that "*may* have an adverse effect on the health of persons," the 1974 law calls for regulations not only for known or probable toxins, but also for substances that *may* be detrimental to health. Thus the 1974 statutory language implies that a known carcinogen need not be regulated stringently under the Act if it is either not feasible to purge it from drinking water (given current technology) or if it is "too costly" to do so. However, a substance that only has a remote possibility of causing any health problems, but that may be neutralized or removed through available and relatively inexpensive treatment procedures, should be regulated according to legislation. Thus it would appear as if Congress intended that some notion of balancing public health benefits against regulatory costs and technical feasibility be embodied in the SDWA.

Legislative and Regulatory Developments Since 1974

In the period between passage of the SDWA in 1974 and 1981, US EPA formally established MCLs for 15 inorganic compounds previously included within the voluntary standards established by the Public Health Service in 1962. An MCL was also established for trihalomethanes (THMs), a class of carcinogenic compounds, including chloroform, identified as by-products of chlorination (caused by the reaction of disinfectant with certain organics typi-

---

[3]The SDWA referred to these as Recommended MCLs, or RMCLs. The term was changed in the 1986 SDWA Amendments to MCL Goals (MCLGs). The latter terminology is used here to avoid confusion.

cally present in raw surface waters). Work also began on establishing standards for a host of additional contaminants, but between 1981 and 1986, the Reagan administration effectively stalled the development of additional federal drinking water regulations.

With the reauthorization of the Safe Drinking Water Act in 1986, Congress established specific requirements and deadlines for promulgating standards for 83 listed contaminants. Regulations were to be promulgated for these 83 contaminants (allowing US EPA to offer up to seven substitute contaminants) by June 1989. Furthermore, the statute called for the regulation of 25 additional contaminants by 1992, and every three years thereafter. This aggressive and highly prescriptive legislative stance was a direct response by Congress to US EPA's lack of progress in meeting its statutory obligations under the Act, as originally established 12 years earlier.[4]

US EPA's rulemaking activities under the Safe Drinking Water Act Amendments of 1986 (SDWAA) have lagged behind the demanding schedule established in the Act. Nonetheless, US EPA has promulgated seven significant rulemaking packages to date, covering more than 70 contaminants. The Agency has also been under court-ordered schedules to develop the remaining standards as mandated under the SDWAA.

The SDWAA's authorization expired September 30, 1991, and the Act has been under reauthorization review by the 103rd and the 104th Congress. Just as the 1986 Amendments reflected Congressional backlash against the Agency's lack of regulatory activity in the preceding 6 to 12 years, US EPA's subsequent rulemaking efforts under the SDWAA have raised new concerns over reauthorization—concerns fueled by the high administrative and enforcement costs of state and federal programs, high compliance costs faced by municipal and privately owned water supply systems, and the current limitations on setting risk-based priorities among competing public health aspects of drinking water quality.

Because many of the administrative and compliance costs of the federal regulatory program are borne by state and local governments, they have become targets in the political debate over unfunded mandates and the role of

---

[4]Other environmental statutes reauthorized in this period suffered from a similar set of circumstances, as seen in the highly prescriptive statutory mandates established for waste disposal and hazardous facility management under RCRA and CERCLA. Unlike statutes written or amended in earlier periods, Congress left little opportunity for US EPA discretion in its use of data, expertise, and the public rule-making process to establish priorities and criteria for what to regulate or how stringently to set its standards.

Congress has also had an interest in mandating an aggressive MCL-setting agenda under the SDWA because of the interrelationship between these standards and Superfund site remediation targets. As such, the SWDA became subject to the pressures to streamline and accelerate Superfund site clean-ups.

the federal government in regulating and imposing costs on other public entities. Questions also have been raised about the relatively meager public health benefits received for the increased costs incurred to comply with standards for some of the regulated contaminants.

The high costs of the accelerated federal regulatory program for carcinogens and other chemical compounds associated with chronic exposure health risks, together with the outbreak of cryptosporidiosis in Milwaukee in 1993 and other high-profile events (such as "boil water orders" in Washington, D.C. and other major metropolitan areas), have brought concern over pathogen-related contamination of drinking water to public attention. Episodic acute risks to public health from drinking water contamination have previously received relatively low priority as US EPA struggled to meet its obligations under the SDWAA—obligations that the Amendments clearly focussed on chemical contaminants and associated chronic exposure risks to public health.

This confluence of concerns regarding the SDWA—the high regulatory compliance costs borne by private and municipal drinking water systems, the limited resources at the state and federal level to administer and enforce the program, and the issues of establishing public health priorities within the federal drinking water regulatory program—is reflected in the Congressional debate over reauthorization of the Act. Senators Chafee and Lautenberg, for example, introduced an amendment in the 1993 appropriations bill for the EPA requiring a *Report to Congress* that would evaluate the Agency's success in meeting the public health protection goals mandated by the Act and would calculate the costs and other social impact imposed by the regulations promulgated. These public health and regulatory issues are explored below.

REVIEW OF THE EXISTING REGULATORY RECORD

In this section of paper, we describe (*a*) the health risks associated with the contaminants regulated, (*b*) reductions in health risk attained by the regulations, (*c*) the occurrence of these contaminants in public water supplies, (*d*) compliance costs, and (*e*) the effectiveness of the regulations in terms of the health risk reductions attained relative to the costs incurred.

The analysis is presented according to the adverse health effect endpoint associated with contaminants. The costs and benefits of regulations covering carcinogens are described first, providing an informative empirical basis for assessing the public health and regulatory aspects of the SDWA as currently structured. An analysis of systemics is provided second and, finally, microbials and associated public health issues are presented.

Data and Methods

The evaluation that follows is based almost exclusively on data and reports used by US EPA in developing its regulations, although additional sources of information are used to the extent available and reliable. For example, all the cost figures reflect estimates published by the US EPA, with minor adjustments for factors recently acknowledged by US EPA and its Science Advisory Board (SAB) as appropriate.[5]   However, they do not include possible adjustments that might be applicable to other cost elements such as unit treatment and site-specific costs (e.g. land acquisition), which could be substantial. As such, the cost estimates probably are somewhat conservative (see Reference 10).

Reductions in estimated health risk are principally based on US EPA's estimates of contaminant occurrence, its quantified risk factors, and standard techniques of health risk assessment. Risk assessment techniques and their strengths and limitations are described in detail elsewhere (see References 12, 14) and therefore are not discussed here.

Quantified human health risk reduction estimates, such as estimated reductions in the number of excess cancer cases, differ slightly from those published by US EPA because, lacking all the necessary raw data, some calculations are based on summaries of the data as provided in US EPA documents. For example, because of variability in US EPA's definitions of different water system-size categories, slightly different estimates of exposed individuals per affected water system may be applied. Likewise, the analysis presented may apply different pre- and/or postregulatory contaminant concentrations (and hence, exposures) than those used in the analyses by US EPA. Nonetheless, the results are consistent with US EPA's estimates.

An important issue in assessing the public health benefits (and costs) of federal drinking water regulations is the lack of occurrence data for many of the contaminants regulated. For example, for about half of the 61 contaminants regulated under the Phase II and Phase V rules (covering synthetic organic and inorganic compounds), no data exist upon which to predict national occurrence. The data suggest no occurrence above the Maximum Contaminant Levels (MCLs) for more than half of the remaining contaminants. The regulatory program for contaminants lacking occurrence data, or

---

[5]Specifically, adjustments have been made to better reflect the cost of financing capital investments in treatment facilities (wherever EPA had used a 3% rate of interest, an adjustment has been made to reflect a 7% rate). Likewise, where EPA has assumed that each impacted utility has only one treatment site, an adjustment has been made to reflect the probability that multiple treatment sites exist for water supplies (with the number of sites adjusted to reflect different categories in system size). Both adjustments reflect changes by EPA in updating its cost-of-compliance estimates for the proposed radon MCL in response to independent studies and critiques. Both changes have been reviewed and approved by the SAB.

for which data indicate no occurrence, is portrayed here as having neither health risk reduction benefits nor compliance costs (apart from monitoring requirements). Therefore, the benefit and cost estimates described below pertain only to those standards that apply to contaminants for which data indicate positive occurrence.[6]

Once costs and risk reduction benefits are estimated, then the basic tools of benefit-cost or risk-based cost-effectiveness analysis can be applied. In the former case, quantified risk reductions are assigned an appropriate estimate of monetary value and then compared to costs. Ideally, risk management choices will be selected that maximize net benefits to society (i.e. standards will be set where benefits exceed costs by the greatest margin, which is where marginal benefits equal marginal costs). However, due to uncertainties inherent in both risk assessment and in the economic valuation of changes in risks to human health, the application of benefit-cost techniques is often limited and controversial, although still useful and valid (described in Reference 12).

The application of risk-based cost-effectiveness techniques avoids some of the uncertainties and controversies inherent in benefit-cost analysis because no attempt is made to explicitly assign monetary values to changes in health status or risks. Instead, the technique divides the costs of a management option by the estimated risk reduction that is anticipated. The resulting estimates of "cost per case avoided" (or, more generically, cost per measure of risk reduction) can then be compared across alternative policy options on drinking water, and/or across different contaminants, and/or across alternative public health programs. The intent of such cost-effectiveness comparisons is to identify which risk management alternatives yield the lowest cost per unit of risk reduction; this information can be used to maximize the risk reductions (public health benefits) that can be obtained from a given total expenditure or budget. In other words, the cost-effectiveness analysis identifies how to obtain the greatest benefit for a fixed total cost, or how to minimize the cost of achieving a target level of risk reduction. The application and usefulness of this approach is demonstrated below.

Carcinogens

Reductions in estimated carcinogenic health risks are based principally on US EPA's estimates of contaminant occurrence, the Agency's quantified risk factors, and standard health risk assessment techniques, including several con-

---

[6]The lack of adequate data is due, in part, to the fact that the SDWAA allowed US EPA limited time to develop and promulgate regulations for specified contaminants. This raises the question of whether the potential public health value of establishing regulations (and hence imposing monitoring and regulatory administrative costs on utilities and state primacy agencies) is justified for compounds for which there are no indications of occurrence or exposure.

Table 1   Carcinogens regulated under the SDWA and SDWAA

Rule and contaminant	MCLG (mg/l)	MCL (mg/l)
Phase I rule (volatile organics)		
Benzene	zero	0.005
Carbon tetrachloride	zero	0.005
1,2-dichloroethane	zero	0.005
Trichloroethylene	zero	0.005
Vinyl chloride	zero	0.002
Phase II		
Acrylamide	zero	TT†
Alachlor	zero	0.002
Chlordane	zero	0.002
Dibromochloropropane (DBCP)	zero	0.0002
Tetrachloroethylene	zero	0.005
1,2-Dichloropropane	zero	0.005
Ethylene dibromide (EDB)	zero	0.00005
Epichlorohydrin	zero	TT†
Heptachlor	zero	0.0004
Heptachlor epoxide	zero	0.0002
PCBs	zero	0.0005
Pentachlorophenol	zero	0.0005
Toxaphene	zero	0.003
Phase V		
Dichloromethane	zero	0.005
2,3,7,8-TCDD (dioxin)	zero	0.00000003
Hexachlorobenzene[+]	zero	0.001
PAHs (benzo(a)pyrnene)	zero	0.0002
Di(2-ethylhexyl)phthalate	zero	0.006
Total trihalomethanes	zero	0.10

† TT, Treatment technique requirement
[+] Indicates contaminants with interim (pre SDWAA) standards that have been or will be revised
Source: Reference 1

servative assumptions such as applying the upper 95% confidence estimate of the dose-response function to estimate carcinogenic risks for given levels of exposure. Known or suspected human carcinogens regulated under the SDWA are listed in Table 1.

Quantified human health carcinogenic risk reductions associated with promulgated rules under the federal drinking water regulatory program amount to between 70 and 121 excess cancer cases avoided annually (11, 15) (approximately one million cancers occur in the USA each year). These "excess cancer cases avoided" refer to the estimated number of individuals predicted to contract the disease due to exposure to carcinogens absent the regulations (i.e. the number of individuals expected to be spared from cancer due to regulation-related exposure reductions). The estimate of 70 cancer cases avoided is based on analysis of US EPA data (11), whereas the Agency's Regulatory Impact Analyses (RIAs) estimate 121 cases avoided. [7]

In monetary terms, the value of the estimated reduction in carcinogenic risks can be presented according to the concept of the "value per statistical life saved," which is an approach accepted and used by US EPA and other entities for regulatory analyses. The approach uses hedonic analyses of wage rates (and other data and analytic techniques) to ascertain how much individuals are willing to pay (or accept, as in the form of higher wage rate compensation) to face reduced (or accept higher) fatality risks. The approach is particularly relevant for issues such as environmental regulation where baseline risks tend to be relatively low (e.g. <1 expected fatality per 10,000 persons with lifetime exposures) and are spread across a relatively large group of individuals (see Reference 12). Thus, the willingness-to-pay values for risk reductions can be aggregated across all exposed individuals and compared to the expected number of "statistical fatalities" over the exposed group, to derive a monetary estimate of the value of risk reductions.

Literature reviews of this research area (16, 17) have been used by US EPA to establish a range of roughly $2 million to $10 million per "statistical fatality avoided." Assuming that each estimated cancer case avoided by drinking water regulations is equivalent to a premature fatality avoided, this implies that the cancer risk reductions associated with the SDWA generate social benefits on the order of $140 million (70 cases at $2 million) to $1.21 billion (121 cases at $10 million) per year.[8] The estimated compliance cost for the MCLs for the regulated carcinogens amounts to $249 million annually. Thus these results suggest that the overall benefits of carcinogenic risk reductions achieved by the regulatory program are roughly commensurate with their costs. However, important additional insight can be gained from examining these results on a contaminant-specific basis.

Table 2 shows the cost per estimated excess cancer case avoided for selected individual carcinogens regulated under the 1986 Amendments. The data provided in Table 2 indicate the degree to which the cost-effectiveness of the regulations varies according to which regulated contaminant is evaluated, and also according to the system size category of the population served for the

---

[7]EPA's reports do not provide sufficient detail with which to determine the underlying source of these differences, but as noted above, they probably reflect minor variations in exposure assessments. Regardless of which estimate of cancer case reduction benefits is used, an examination of the risk reductions attained and of the compliance costs indicates clearly that most carcinogenic risk reduction is achieved through the regulation of a small subset of contaminants.

[8]This assumes every excess case is valued by society as equivalent to a premature fatality. Health statistics indicate that roughly half of cancer victims die from the disease.

Table 2 Average cost per cancer case avoided for US regulations (millions of 1992 dollars per case)

Contaminant	System size (population served)					Average cost per case
	25–100	101–500	501–3300	3301–10,000	>10,000	
EDB (with Aldi-carb and DBCP)	$3.0	$1.4	$0.7	$0.6	$0.5	$0.8
1,2-Dichloropro-pane	$129.2	$56.7	$23.0	$20.0	$15.5	$62.9
Pentachlorophenol	$322.2	$141.7	$61.5	$40.1	$26.0	$48.4
Dichloromethane	$1038.8	$430.6	$134.7	$60.6	a	$169.3

[a] No occurrence above MCL anticipated

impacted public water supply. For example, the cost per excess cancer case avoided is as low as $0.5 million [ethylene dibromide (EDB) in systems serving over 10,000 people], which is well below the benchmark benefit values of $2–10 million per statistical case avoided. Likewise, the data indicate that the estimated cost per case avoided exceeds $1 billion for some compounds and systems (dichloromethane, for systems serving between 25 and 100 persons), which is more than 100 times the upper-bound benefits value for a statistical cancer case avoided. A graphical representation of these results is provided in Figure 1.

The calculations reveal that the regulatory program could have been much more cost-effective, i.e. providing greater public health protection benefits per dollar spent, if the statute had allowed and encouraged US EPA to (a) be more

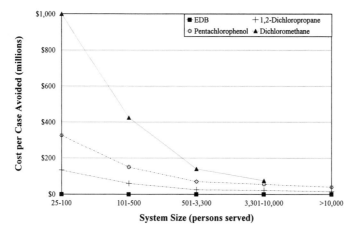

Figure 1 Cost per statistical cancer case avoided.

Table 3 Carcinogenic-specific risk reductions and costs of promulgated rules in the US (millions of 1992 dollars per year)

Rulemaking scenario	Excess cancer cases avoided per year	Total annual compliance costs
Program as implemented[a] (all Phase I, II, and V carcinogens)	69.9 (100%)	$248.7 (100%)
Selected MCLs only[b]	68.9 (98.6%)[c]	$152.2 (61.2%)[d]
Systems serving >100 persons only	68.1 (97.4%)[c]	$215.1 (86.5%)d[c]
Selected MCLs and systems serving >100 persons only[e]	67.1 (95.9%)[c]	$131.8 (53.0%)[d]
Selected MCLs and systems serving >500 persons only	62.8 (89.8%)[c]	$107.8 (43.3%)[d]

[a] All Phase I, II, and V carcinogens

[b] Phase I plus EDB and DBCP only

[c] Percent of total risk reduction of regulatory program as promulgated

[d] Percent of total cost of regulatory program as promulgated

[e] MCLs for Phase I, EDB, and DBCP, applied only in water supply systems serving more than 100 individuals (i.e. excluding community water systems serving 100 or fewer persons).

selective in determining which contaminants are regulated, (b) use cost-effectiveness analysis in considering alternative regulatory limits, and (c) consider setting different standards for different-sized systems (e.g. less stringent standards in systems serving relatively smaller populations, such as <3300 individuals).

Although the average cost per case avoided for all MCLs for carcinogens, averaged across all system size categories, amounts to $3.6 million ($249 million in annual costs, divided by 70 cases avoided per year), which is reasonable relative to the willingness-to-pay estimates ($2–10 million per statistical fatality avoided), the data in Table 2 clearly reveal that specific aspects of the regulatory program are far outside this range. Analysis of risk reduction and cost data is illustrated in Table 3. These data indicate the extent to which a disproportionately large share of the costs, but a disproportionately small share of the benefits, are borne by small systems (SDWA regulations apply to all community water systems, which are defined as supplying 25 or more people—or 15 service connections—for at least 6 months per year). For example, systems serving fewer than 100 people bear 14% of the national costs of the promulgated MCLs for carcinogens, but realize only about 2.5% of the carcinogenic risk reduction. Likewise, individuals using systems that serve fewer than 500 persons bear 29% of the national costs, but receive less than 9% of the carcinogenic risk reduction benefits.

The analysis summarized in Table 3 indicates that most of the program's carcinogenic risk reduction is attained from the regulation of a limited number of contaminants. For example, for the regulated carcinogens (MCLs promulgated under Phases I, II, and V rulemakings), nearly 99% of the program's total carcinogenic risk reduction is attained, for approximately 60% of the total carcinogenic-relevant cost, through the MCLs established for ten contaminants [Phase I volatile organic chemicals (VOCs) [9] EDB, and dibromochloropropane (DBCP)]. Adding the MCLs for additional carcinogen increases annual compliance costs by nearly $100 million per year to achieve one estimated cancer case reduction. Table 3 also indicates, for example, that nearly 90% of the carcinogenic health risk reduction benefits of the current program are realized, with only 43% of the costs of the program as currently implemented, through application of the MCLs for ten contaminants (Phase I, EDB, and DBCP) in systems serving more than 500 persons.

Systemics

Several of the standards issued under the SDWA and SDWAA are expected to reduce risks to health by lowering chronic exposures to noncarcinogenic chemical contaminants. The systemic contaminants covered by the federal regulatory program are summarized in Table 4. Perhaps the most significant of these rules in terms of public health benefits pertains to limiting exposure to lead. The lead and copper rule, promulgated in 1991 and updated in 1992, establishes treatment techniques (in lieu of MCLs) for corrosion control (e.g. via alkalinity and pH levels) and lead service line replacements.

The corrosion control requirements in the lead and copper rule are expected to yield over $24 billion in present value benefits over a 20-year period (approximately $1.5 to $2.0 billion annually). These benefits will be realized by reducing lead exposures for an estimated 60% of the US population (although other benefits besides human health are included in these lead estimates) (20). Public health benefits associated with lower exposures to lead through drinking water include reduced incidence of elevated blood pressure (and hence diminished risk of associated cardiovascular diseases), increased birth weights (and consequent reductions in infant mortality), and reductions in IQ decrements.

---

[9]US EPA reports aggregated data for Phase I contaminants, so it was not feasible to determine how the cost-effectiveness of risk reductions might vary among the eight VOCs regulated under the Phase I rule. Therefore, the results presented here reflect the averages for the group. However, over 90% of the Phase I risk reduction may be attributable to the MCL for vinyl chloride.

Table 4 Noncarcinogens regulated under the SDWA and SDWAA

Rule and contaminant	MCLG (mg/l)	MCL	Potential health effects
Fluoride*	4.0	4.0	Skeletal fluorosis
Phase I			
p-Dichlorobenzene	0.075	0.075	Kidney effects, possible carcinogen
1,1,1-Trichloroethane	0.2	0.2	Liver, nervous system effects
1,1-Dichloroethylene	0.007	0.007	Liver, kidney effects, possible carcinogen
Coliform and Surface Water Treatment			
Giardia lamblia	zero	TT	Gastroenteric disease
Legionella	N/A	TT	Pneumonia-like effects
Standard plate count	N/A	TT	Indicator of treatment effectiveness and water quality
Total coliform*	zero	< 5%[+]	Indicator of gastroenteric infections
Turbidity*	N/A	TT	Interferes with disinfection, indicator of filtration performance
Viruses (enteric)	zero	TT	Gastroenteric disease, respiratory disease and other diseases (e.g. hepatitis, myocarditis)
Phase II			
Aldicarb**	0.001	0.003	Nervous system effects
Aldicarb sulfoxide**	0.001	0.004	Nervous system effects
Aldicarb sulfone**	0.001	0.002	Nervous system effects
Asbestos (fiber > 10 µm/l)	7 MFL	7 MFL	Possible carcinogen by ingestion
Atrazine	0.003	0.003	Liver, kidney, lung, cardiovascular effects, possible carcinogen
Barium*	2	2	Blood pressure effects
Carbofuran	0.04	0.04	Nervous system, reproductive system effects
Cadmium*	0.005	0.005	Kidney effects
Chlorobenzene	0.1	0.1	Nervous system, liver effects
Chromium*(total)	0.1	0.1	Liver, kidney, circulatory system effects
O-Dichlorobenzene	0.6	0.6	Liver, kidney, blood cell effects
cis-1,2-dichloroethylene	0.07	0.07	Liver, kidney, nervous system, circulatory system effects
trans-1,2-dichloroethylene	0.1	0.1	Liver, kidney, nervous system, circulatory system effects
2,4-D*	0.07	0.07	Liver, kidney effects
2,4,5-TP	0.05	0.05	Liver, kidney effects
Ethylbenzene	0.7	0.7	Liver, kidney, nervous system effects
Lindane	0.0002	0.0002	Kidney, central nervous system, immune system, circulatory system effects
Mercury* (inorganic)	0.0002	0.0002	Kidney, central nervous system effects
Methoxychlor	0.04	0.04	Developmental, liver, kidney, nervous system effects
Nitrate*	10	10	Methemoglobinemia (blue baby syndrome)
Nitrite	1.0	1.0	Methemoglobinemia (blue baby syndrome)
Selenium*	0.05	0.05	Nervous system effects
Sytrene	0.1	0.1	Liver, nervous system effects, possible carcinogen

Table 4   (*continued*)

Rule and contaminant	MCLG (mg/l)	MCL	Potential health effects
Toluene	1	1	Liver, kidney, nervous system, circulatory system effects
Xylenes (total)	10	10	Liver, kidney, nervous system effects
Lead and Copper			
Lead*	zero	TT⁺	Kidney, central and peripheral nervous system effects, cancer
Copper	1.3	TT⁺⁺	Gastrointestinal effects
Phase V			
Di(2-ethylhexyl)adipate	0.4	0.4	Reproductive effects
Antimony	0.006	0.006	Decreased longevity, blood effects
Beryllium	0.004	0.004	Bone, lung effects, possible carcinogen
Cyanide	0.2	0.2	Thyroid, central nervous system effects
Dalapon	0.2	0.2	Kidney, liver effects
1,1,2-Trichloroethane	0.003	0.005	Kidney, liver effects, possible carcinogen
Dinoseb	0.007	0.007	Thyroid, reproductive effects
Diquat	0.02	0.01	Ocular, liver, kidney effects
Endothall	0.1	0.1	Liver, kidney, gastrointestinal effects
Endrin	0.002	0.002	Liver, kidney, heart effects
Glyphosate	0.7	0.7	Liver, kidney effects
Hexachlorocyclopentadiene	0.05	0.05	Kidney, stomach effects
Picloram	0.5	0.5	Kidney, liver effects
Nickel	0.1	0.1	Liver effects
Oxamyl (Vydate)	0.1	0.2	Kidney effects
Simazine	0.004	0.004	Body weight and blood effects, possible carcinogen
Thallium	0.0005	0.002	Kidney, liver, brain, intestine effects
(1,2,4-)Trichlorobenzene	0.07	0.07	Liver, kidney effects

* Indicates contaminants with interim (pre-SDWAA) standards that have been or will be revised.
⁺ Less than 5% positive or greather than detections limit of 1 count/100ml
TT Treatment technique requirement
⁺⁺ Action level = mg/L
*** Regulation currently not in effect
Source: Reference 1

Other potential noncarcinogenic health benefits due to the regulation of chronic exposures to chemical contaminants are not readily quantified or valued. In general, the health benefits associated with drinking water standards for systemics are not expected to be as significant as the lead and copper rule benefits. However, their relative efficacy can be evaluated, at least in part, by applying the same type of cost-effectiveness assessment to these systemics as was described above for carcinogens.

For systemic contaminants, changes in exposures are not directly linked to quantified expected reductions in adverse health effects (i.e. there is usually no estimate of reduced cases of illness). Instead, risk assessments typically relate exposure levels (doses) to a benchmark, threshold-like value called the oral reference dose (oral RfD), which is the chronic exposure level below which no adverse affects are anticipated in individuals, allowing for several uncertainty factors. The ratio of the expected exposure levels to the oral RfD is called the Hazard Quotient (HQ); an $HQ > 1.0$ implies that the dose is above the no effects (i.e. safe) threshold-like value. Likewise, an HQ value < 1.0 indicates chronic exposures are below the concentration at which no adverse health effects are anticipated.

To estimate the cost-effectiveness of reducing drinking water-related exposures to systemics, a Health Effectiveness Index (HEI) can be developed to weigh changes in the HQ due to alternative regulatory options. The HEI is intended to indicate a level of public health achieved by a standard (with HEI increasing to reflect gains in public health protection). Thus, the HEI can be defined generally as

$$\text{HEI} = g(N, HQ_b, HQ_m), \qquad\qquad 1.$$

where N = the number of individuals for whom exposures are reduced (e.g. the number of individuals residing in communities whose water supplies have baseline concentrations of the contaminant exceeding the MCL), HQ_b = Hazard Quotient at baseline, pre-regulatory levels of contaminant concentrations (i.e. expected individual exposure levels from drinking water intake in systems above the MCL under consideration, divided by the oral RfD), HQ_m = Hazard Quotient at the MCL (individual exposure levels, under standard consumption assumptions, at drinking water concentrations equal to the MCL, divided by the oral RfD), and where $g' > 0$ with respect to N and HQ_b, and $g' < 0$ with respect to HQ_m.

Thus, HEI is a function of the number of individuals for whom exposures will be reduced by a standard, and it increases with the number of people for whom exposures will be reduced because of a regulation. HEI values are also an increasing function of HQ at baseline, so the greater the initial risk, the greater the HEI (all else constant). The HEI is a decreasing function of the HQ_m because as more stringent MCLs are set (MCLs of declining numerical value), HQ_m decreases, and the HEI measure of public health increases.

To operationalize the HEI within the conceptual framework established above, the following specification is used here

$$\text{HEI} = N * f(HQ_b/HQ_m), \qquad\qquad 2.$$

with

$$(HQ_b/HQ_m) = \min [HQ_b^3, HQ_b] / [(HQ_m^2/2) + 0.5]. \qquad\qquad 3.$$

This functional form is depicted in Figure 2 and has several advantages. With respect to HQ_b, where baseline exposure levels are below the oral RfD, anticipated public health benefits to be gained from further reducing exposures are limited. Thus, where HQ_b is <1, its cubed value is used. This replicates a threshold-like dose response function in that f'>0 and f''>0 (i.e. the HEI will rise in value at an increasing rate as HQ_b moves from 0.0 and approaches 1.0). In essence, this formulation places greater weight on regulatory changes that reduce the HQ from a baseline value exceeding 1, and decreasing weight as baseline HQ drops further below 1. In effect, this provides more weight where exposures are being reduced from a point above the no effects dose than where the baseline exposure is already below the no effects threshold.

With respect to HQ_m, the formulation depicted in Eq. 3 allows HEI to increase as MCLs become more stringent, but also limits the extent to which the HEI increases as MCLs approach zero. As MCLs become more stringent and HQ_m drops, the HEI will increase, but at a decreasing rate.

The average cost-effectiveness of existing MCLs for systemics can then be calculated by dividing regulatory costs by reductions achieved in the HEI for a contaminant. Results for regulated systemics with positive occurrence estimates are demonstrated in Table 5 and displayed in Figure 3. The results are comparable to those derived for carcinogens: cost-effectiveness varies considerably (*a*) according to the contaminant selected (although the HEI does not attempt to reflect differences in terms of the potential severity of the health effect endpoint for which the oral RfD is established), and (*b*) across systems serving different-sized populations (e.g. residents of smaller-sized water systems pay considerably more per unit of risk reduction than do individuals served by larger water suppliers).

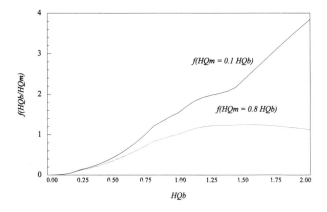

Figure 2   Health Effectiveness Index formulation reflecting threshold-like values for HQ_b <1.

Table 5   Average cost per health effectiveness index (millions of 1992 dollars per HEI)

| Contaminant | HQb | HQm | System size (population served) | | | | | Avg. cost per HEI |
			25–100	101–500	501–3,300	3,301–10,000	>10,000	
Mercury	0.9	0.1	$190	$107	$56	$29	$53	$52
Antimony	2.5	0.3	$547	$290	$80	$60	$39	$74
Cadmium	0.6	0.2	$388	$208	$100	$64	$97	$108
Nitrate	0.4	0.1	$816	$481	$304	$193	$217	$282
Nickel	0.2	0.1	$9712	$4305	a	a	a	$5679

[a]No occurrence above MCL anticipated

Microbials

The risks posed by microbials (bacteria, viruses, and parasites) in community water systems has re-emerged as a primary public health concern in recent years. In contrast, the SDWA and SDWAA clearly emphasized controlling chemical contaminants, in part because of the perception that outbreaks of waterborne infectious disease (WBID) were no longer likely to be a major public health issue, and also because of the heightened public and scientific concern over carcinogenic risks potentially posed by chlorine disinfection, hazardous wastes, pesticide products, and other synthetic (and natural) compounds introduced into the environment.

The large-scale outbreak of cryptosporidiosis (a parasitic disease) in Milwaukee in 1993 restored microbials and associated WBIDs to the spotlight.

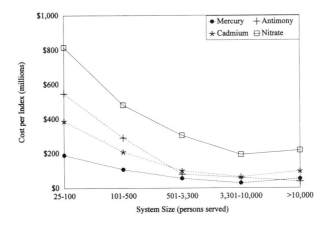

Figure 3:   Average cost per Health Effectiveness Index

Table 6 Summary estimates of the incidence of and mortality from waterborne infectious disease[a]

	Estimated incidence (high–low)[b]		Estimated incidence	Estimated mortality
Moderate-to-severe infections				
Salmonella	22,000 –	170,000	59,000	59
Shigella	30,000 –	49,000	35,000	70
E. coli	not available		150,000	300
Campylobacter	not available		320,000	320
Total	520,000 –	690,000	560,000	750
Mild-to-moderate infections				
Giardia	40,000 –	690,000	260,000	1
Cryptosporidium	64,000 –	1,500,000	420,000	130
Viruses	300,000 –	25,000,000	6,500,000	330
Total	400,000 –	27,000,000	7,100,000	460

[a] From Reference 6
[b] This range uses the point estimates of illness related to E. coli and Campylobacter to calculate both the high and low values.

The Milwaukee incident, which occurred in a chlorinated, filtered system that met all applicable federal standards, contributed to an estimated 104 fatalities, 4000 hospitalizations, and 403,000 illnesses (3, 4). This and other outbreaks revealed the failure of the federal regulatory program in ensuring that public water supplies be completely free of microbial-related risks to health.

With the re-emergence of microbials as an issue of concern, the incidence of WBID in the U.S. has come under close scrutiny. A recent review by Morris & Levin (6) suggests that over half a million cases of "moderate-to-severe" WIDB occur in the United States annually, with an additional 7 million "mild-to-moderate" cases. They derive an associated expected mortality rate from WBID of 1200 cases per year. A more detailed summary of the Morris & Levin findings is presented in Table 6.

Although achieving a risk-free network of public water supplies is not a practical reality, the accumulating evidence of actual and potential microbial-related risks to public health has raised the question of how to define (and achieve) a reasonable degree of safety from the risks posed by microbials in drinking water. This issue has become the focus of attention for US EPA and water suppliers.

The current federal regulatory program for microbial-related risks consists mainly of the Total Coliform Rule (TCR) and the Surface Water Treatment Rule (SWTR). The TCR establishes monitoring and sanitary survey requirements for surface and groundwater systems. Treatment requirements for pathogen removal and disinfection (CT) are established in the SWTR for systems using surface waters or groundwaters directly influenced by surface waters.

US EPA estimates a reduction of over 80,000 cases of waterborne disease annually due to the Surface Water Treatment Rule, with consequent benefits valued at $280 million to $615 million per year based on its estimates of cost per case of disease (15, 19). This benefit-cost analysis of the SWTR indicates the potential for negative net benefits on the basis of just the expected value of avoided health effects (i.e. costs were expected to exceed benefits unless a margin of safety was included in the analyses).

Control of microbial contaminants in drinking water has traditionally been treated conservatively by public health officials because of concern over outbreaks of waterborne disease. The notion of adding a margin of safety for microbials in some manner replicates the conservatism embodied into risk assessments (and hence standard setting) for chemical contaminants. Nonetheless, the Milwaukee episode and a previous cryptosporidium incident in Georgia demonstrated that meeting the TCR and SWTR standards was not sufficient to preclude the possibility of sizable outbreaks of microbial-related disease.

Several other federal rule-making activities are now under way to address microbial risks. Foremost among these is the intensive effort in "negotiated rulemaking" by US EPA and other interested parties to address the challenge of balancing disinfection (D) requirements with concerns over disinfection byproducts (DBP). This D/DBP issue raises the complex problem of assessing and regulating tradeoffs between WBID and elevated cancer risks.

In light of this public health challenge and the need for more information to develop a sound drinking water policy, a massive effort to collect data on source water quality parameters and water system treatment operations and performance is anticipated through the Information Collection Rule (ICR). The Agency will likely use the ICR data in developing an Enhanced Surface Water Treatment Rule. US EPA is also considering disinfection requirements for groundwater systems. Concurrently, US EPA has asked for relief from court-imposed schedules for promulgating additional standards, as mandated by the SDWAA, so that it can prioritize its resources on microbials and their associated public health issues.

CONCLUSIONS

The public health and regulatory aspects of drinking water in the United States have come full circle over the course of the 20th century. In the early 1900s, gastrointestinal infections were the third leading cause of death in the USA. The widespread implementation of filtration and chlorination early in the century (in conjunction with improved antibiotic therapy) significantly reduced the incidence of WBID (6).

In the 1960s, the federal government modestly expanded its role in drinking water quality, with the Public Health Service issuing voluntary guidelines for a limited number of contaminants. By the early 1970s, emerging evidence of elevated cancer risks posed by drinking water contributed to the passage of the SDWA of 1974, which created a federal regulatory role for the newly formed Environmental Protection Agency.

The limited progress made in issuing standards under the SDWA led to the very prescriptive Amendments to the SDWA Act in 1986. The mandatory regulation of a long list of chemical contaminants under the SDWAA reflected the perceived need to establish a strong federal regulatory presence to address carcinogenic and other chronic exposure health risks. However, although the aggressive and rigid regulatory requirements imposed by the SDWAA have yielded appreciable public health benefits, they have failed to do so in a cost-effective manner.

In the mid 1990s, the regulatory pendulum has swung back. Evidence from the regulatory record and WBID outbreaks has demonstrated a need for rational public health and drinking water priorities regarding what to regulate, how to regulate, and whom to regulate. Public health focus is again on microbials in drinking water and related waterborne risks, although chemical contaminants remain a concern. The high cost of complying with drinking water standards, particularly as related to contaminants for which the regulations provide minimal and/or non cost-effective public health protection, has shifted current SDWA reauthorization efforts into the spotlight of broader public policy debates on regulatory burdens, unfunded mandates, the role of the federal government in regulating state and local issues, the equitable distribution of envi- ronmental risks and compliance costs, and the use of risk assessment and benefit-cost techniques in developing environmental, health, and safety regulations.

It remains to be seen how, or when, the SDWA will be reauthorized. However, relative to the program driven by the 1986 SDWAA, the regulatory aspects of drinking water and public health at the end of this century will entail greater relative emphasis on microbials, a higher degree of risk-based priori-tization, and additional attention to how cost-effectively the rules can, with limited resources, obtain the most significant gains in protecting and enhancing public health.

ACKNOWLEDGMENTS

The author gratefully acknowledges the significant contributions made by Eloise Trabka Castillo, Julie Sommer, Jeni Biodrowski, and other Hagler Bailly staff who assisted in this and related previous efforts, and by Dr. Joseph A. Drago of Kennedy/Jenks Consultants.

Portions of the analysis were derived from a project supported by the Water Industry Technical Action Fund (WITAF). The author gratefully acknowledges the insights and contributions made by the Safe Drinking Water Act Technical Advisory Workgroup and other participants on the Project Advisory Committee.

Finally, this paper reflects the opinions and efforts of the author. It does not necessarily reflect the opinions or policies of Hagler Bailly Consulting, EPA, AWWA, or any individuals or organizations noted above. Any errors or omissions are the responsibility of the author.

Literature Cited

1. Auerbach J. 1994. Costs and benefits of current SDWA regulations. *J. Am. Water Works Assoc.* 86:69–78
2. Clark RM. 1978. The Safe Drinking Water Act: its implications for planning. In *Municipal Water Systems*, ed. Holtz, Sebastian, p. 136. Bloomington: Indiana Univ. Press
3. Davis J. 1993. *A massive outbreak of Cryptosporidium infection associated with a filtered public water supply.* Presented at Annu. Meet. Am. Water Works Assoc., Miami, FL
4. MacKenzie WR, Hoxie NJ, Proctor ME, Gradus MS, Blair KA, et al. 1994. A massive outbreak in Milwaukee of *Cryptosporidium* infection transmitted through the public water supply. *N. Engl. J. Med.* 331:161–67
5. McDermott JH. 1973. Federal drinking water standards past, present, future. *J. Environ. Eng. Div.* 99:469–72
6. Morris RD, Levin R. 1995. Estimating the incidence of waterborne infectious disease related to drinking water in the United States. *Proc. IAHS/ISS Int. Symp. Manag. Health Risks from Drink. Water Contam.: Approach. Appl.* Rome, Italy, 1994, ed. E. Reichard, G Zapponi, pp. 75–88. Publ. 233. Wallingford, UK: IAHS Press
7. Natl. Acad. Sci. 1977. *Drinking Water and Health*, pp. 2–5. Washington, DC: Natl. Acad. Press
8. Natl. Acad. Sci. 1977. *Drinking Water and Health*, Appendix A, p. 905 (provides summary of HR No. 93–523, SR No. 93–231, and PL 93–523). Washington, DC: Natl. Acad. Press
9. Page T, Harris RH, Epstein SS. 1976. Drinking water and cancer mortality in Louisiana. *Science* 193:55–57
10. Raucher RS, Drago JA, Castillo ET, Dixon A, Breffle W, Waldman D. 1996. *Estimating the Cost of Compliance with Drinking Water Standards: A User's Guide for Developing or Auditing Estimates of Water Supply Regulatory Compliance Costs. Final Report., 1996.* Am. Water Works Assoc. Res. Found., Denver
11. RCG/Hagler Bailly. 1993. *An Evaluation of The Federal Drinking Water Regulatory Program Under The Safe Drinking Water Act as Amended in 1986.* Am. Water Works Assoc. Safe Drink. Water Act Tech. Advis. Workgroup
12. Reichard E, Cranor C, Raucher RS, Zapponi G. 1990. *Groundwater Contamination Risk Assessment: A Guide to Understanding and Managing Uncertainties.* IAHS Publ. No. 196
13. Rogers PG. 1978. Opening address to the Conference on Safe Drinking Water, conducted by Resources for the Future. In *Safe Drinking Water: Current and Future Problems*, ed. C Russell, p. 5. Washington, DC: Resources for the Future
14. US EPA. 1986. Guidelines for Carcinogenic Risk Assessment. *Fed. Regist.* 51:33992–4003
15. US EPA. 1993. *Technical and Economic Capacity of States and Public Water Systems to Implement Drinking Water Regulations. Report to Congress.* Prepared by US EPA, Off. Water, Washington, DC. EPA 810-R–93–001
16. Violette DM, Chestnut LG. 1983. Valuing reduction in risks: a review of the

empirical estimates. In *Environmental Benefits Analysis Series*, Washington, DC: US EPA. EPA–230–05–83–003

17. Violette DM, Chestnut LG. 1986. *Valuing risks: new information on the willingness to pay for changes in fatal risks.* Rep. US EPA, Washington, DC. Contract 68–01–7047

18. Vitruvius MP. 1960. *The Ten Books on Architecture*, Book 8, Chap. 6. Transl. MH Morgan, New York: Dover. As cited in Options for Coping with the Safe Drinking Water, *Safe Drinking Water: Current and Future Problems*, ed. C Russell, p. 412. Washington, DC: Resources for the Future

19. Wade Miller Assoc. 1987. *Regulatory Impact Analysis: Benefits and Costs of Proposed Surface Water Treatment Rule and Total Coliform Rule. Draft Rep.*. Prepared for US EPA Off. Drink. Water

20. Wade Miller Assoc., Abt Assoc. 1991. *Final Regulatory Impact Analysis of Proposed National Primary Drinking Water Regulations for Lead and Copper*. Prepared for US EPA, Off. Drink. Water. EPA Contract 68-CO–0069

Annu. Rev. Public Health. 1996. 17:203–19

BENEFIT-COST ANALYSIS IN PUBLIC HEALTH

Lester B. Lave[1] and Satish V. Joshi[2]

[1]Graduate School of Industrial Administration and Heinz School of Public Policy,
[2]PhD Student, Heinz School of Public Policy, Carnegie Mellon University,
Pittsburgh, Pennsylvania 15213

KEY WORDS: benefit-cost analysis, cost-benefit analysis, cost-effectiveness, evaluation,
              monetizing

ABSTRACT

This chapter gives an overview of benefit-cost analysis (BCA) and similar evaluation tools, such as cost-effectiveness analysis and technology-based standards, in the context of public health. We describe these evaluation tools, how they are used, their shortcomings, and how they should be interpreted. As with other powerful tools, they are subject to misuse and misinterpretation, even by professionals doing the analysis.

INTRODUCTION

The rising costs of health care and a general desire to lower government expenditures have led to a close scrutiny of public health programs. For more than 20 years, public health officials have had to justify many programs by an analysis of their social benefits and costs. Although benefit-cost analysis (BCA) may often require extensive data collection and analysis, public health professionals should welcome the use of this tool. It is helpful in making public health programs more efficient and effective while providing evidence to convince decision makers that these programs are worthy of support. However, BCA is not a panacea. Public health professionals have much to gain from knowing what the tool is and is not, and how the results should be interpreted.

One of the first official acts of President Reagan was to promulgate Executive Order 12291 requiring agencies to conduct a BCA of all major rules (those imposing costs on the economy of at least $100 million). Requiring this analysis was not peculiar to President Reagan. Rather, some form of White House review of the benefits and costs of regulation had been required since President Nixon. President Clinton modified the executive order slightly, but

203

the essential parts remain in force. Just before the 1994 elections, Congress came close to enacting legislation requiring BCA. The Republicans made BCA a part of the "Contract with America" and the House of Representatives moved quickly after the election to pass legislation.

The 1995 House and Senate hearings on legislation to require BCA of major rules had many environmentalists and public health professionals testifying against the legislation (27). Both Carol Browner, Administrator of EPA, and Donna Shalala, Secretary of Health and Human Services, expressed vigorous disagreement with the notion of requiring BCA. They seemed to regard the proposed legislation as a means of slowing or stopping new government regulation rather than as a means of improving the programs and isolating those programs that should be rejected. We agree that requiring BCA could impede regulation, particularly if existing programs must be evaluated and no new resources are available, but we praise BCA for the good it can do for public health programs. However, to reap these benefits, the community must have a good understanding of what BCA is, what it is not, and how it can be helpful in improving the quality of public health decisions.

THE BENEFITS OF BENEFIT-COST ANALYSIS

Although they do not agree on the precise interpretation of BCA, practitioners agree that their tool is useful for posing the right questions and collecting and analyzing the relevant data. They disagree on whether the tool should dictate decisions, but agree that where decisions involve the health of many individuals or millions of dollars, the BCA framework can inform decision makers. However, as shown below, BCA can be expensive and time-consuming. The depth of analysis, and even the decision as to whether to do an analysis, must depend on the value of the information to be gleaned and the importance of the decision. The tool must be used with discretion and flexibility.

BCA should be thought of as a framework to improve the quality of decisions. For example, myriad screening programs have been suggested for breast, prostate, colon, skin, and other cancers; stringent regulations exist for abating air and water pollution, occupational exposure to toxicants; and control of drinking water quality and pesticide residues in food. Each of these programs is potentially expensive but each also offers large potential health benefits. Should society require that every screening and environmental quality program be funded? Should all programs shown to be efficacious be funded? Should society offer first the programs that are most cost-effective, i.e. those giving the greatest health improvement per dollar expended? Should programs be offered only if their social benefits exceed their social costs?

A tool to help policy makers decide among programs is likely to be most helpful if it examines the following issues:

1. Problem definition and statement of objectives: What is the problem we are trying to solve? Often people have different perceptions of the problem and thus come to very different conclusions about the desirability of proposed interventions. For example, is the problem excessive deaths from breast cancer? Is it excessive incidence? Or is it a lack of concern for women's health problems? These three definitions would give rise to very different interventions, from better screening and treatment to prevention programs to broader attention to women's health problems.

2. Identification of all reasonable means to accomplish the stated objectives: What is the full panoply of interventions? For example, the goal of fewer breast cancer deaths could be accomplished by improved treatment, by improved screening, or by primary prevention. Resources would be spent in quite different ways in each of these interventions. Tools are needed to compare the efficacy and costs of each program.

3. Analysis of the benefits and costs of each alternative: The benefits and costs must be quantified and, if reasonably possible, be translated into dollars. Where the translation is controversial, the analysis must be careful to summarize the effects in terms of a multidimensional array. If the goal is fewer breast cancer deaths, a variety of interventions could improve treatment at increasing costs, with an extreme case being establishing tertiary medical care centers in every community to treat breast cancers. How many deaths would be prevented by each type of intervention to improve treatment? What is the estimated cost of each intervention? What are the life expectancy and the quality of life of women who have been treated? What is the quality of life during treatment? Analogous questions should be asked for early detection programs: How many deaths would be prevented? What is the increase in life expectancy? What is the quality of life for each group —particularly women who are incorrectly diagnosed as having breast cancer or as not having breast cancer? How should the inconvenience and discomfort of screening be weighed against the increased life-expectancy of the small proportion who are helped? There might be significant psychological and medical costs associated with a false positive, requiring a woman to undergo further tests and undergo the anxiety of thinking that she may have breast cancer. Primary prevention has the virtue of requiring fewer women to undergo treatment. However, prevention might require a change in diet or other habits that could be costly to the individual, and might lower the quality of life.

4. Use of all relevant data: The analysis should emphasize a systematic, analytic approach that uses all relevant data and helps to structure a research agenda for gathering the crucial missing data. For example, at what age should

breast cancer screening start? How often should women be screened? How should information on family and personal history of breast cancer be used?

5. Perspective and values used in the analysis: We suggest using a social perspective, but this is not uniquely defined. An analyst who is 25, black, and was raised in Harlem probably has a different perception of the social perspective than an analyst who is 65, white, and was raised in a small town in Washington. To be most helpful, the analysis should consider a range of important perspectives and values, corresponding to the range of most groups in society.

6. The time pattern of benefits and costs: Programs generally involve expenditures and benefits that extend over many years. A dollar spent now is more costly than one spent a decade from now, if only because the dollar could be put into the bank to grow in value. Similarly, benefits a decade from now are worth less than benefits today. For example, suppose that one program would prevent 100 breast cancer deaths each year starting now; a second program has the same costs and prevents 101 deaths each year, but there is a ten-year lag before any deaths are prevented. Which program is preferred?

7. Analysis of uncertainties: Each of the previous steps is filled with uncertainties, from quantification to discounting. The analysis should examine the uncertainties explicitly to discover which are most important for the conclusions. For example, what is the detection rate and increase in life expectancy associated with screening women aged 40–49 for breast cancer? We present below the range of outcomes from various studies of mammography. A sensitivity analysis is needed to account for the likely range of outcomes.

8. Interpretation of the results: Neither the facts nor the analysis "speak for themselves"; the analyst must interpret these for the reader.

These eight steps define an approach to gathering information and performing an analysis to inform social decisions (adapted from Reference 17). They can be thought of as providing a framework for asking questions, collecting data, and deciding which questions are most important. It is hard to quarrel with these steps for evaluating large-scale public health programs, such as removing toxic substances from drinking water or screening for breast cancer: The price is large and the health implications are potentially large. Good decision making requires a careful analysis using all steps.

For major public health decisions, such as setting drinking water standards or urging people to get more exercise, the resources required for the analysis are small compared to the social costs and benefits of selecting the best program. An elaborate analysis is not appropriate to decide the operating hours for a public health clinic. While that decision is important, an elaborate analysis would be far more expensive than the value of the information gained.

Even when the decision does not justify an elaborate analysis, these steps provide a good template for thinking through the problem. What is the problem and what are the goals? What are the benefits and costs of alternative actions? What do available data show about these benefits and costs?

Strictly speaking, these steps constitute a BCA only if all the effects are quantified and then monetized. The benefits and costs that occur over a period of time must be brought to the present so that they are fully commensurate with current benefits and costs. These steps are necessary since a BCA requires calculating the present dollar value of benefits, the present dollar value of costs, and the net benefit of each program.

The Reagan Executive Order requires an agency to choose the alternative with the greatest net benefit, unless this is precluded by law. This requirement meant that failure to quantify or to monetize a benefit or cost implied that the benefit or cost was ignored. For example, if the psychological costs of a false positive on the breast cancer screen were not quantified and evaluated in dollar terms, they were ignored in the subsequent decision making. As shown below, there is no realistic hope of quantifying and monetizing all important benefits and costs. Unquantified or unmonetrized benefits and costs that are omitted from the analysis will bias decision makers. If the quantification or monetization is biased or done badly, decision makers will be misled.

A different problem is the distribution of benefits and costs: Who pays and who is benefitted? For public health programs, most of the costs are borne by individuals other than those who reap the benefits. The implied income redistribution can be an important attribute of a program. There is no realistic attempt to account for these distributional issues in the analysis.

Thus, a BCA emphasizes systematic analysis and use of data. No one should claim that BCA will find a social optimum. "Once benefit-cost analysis is understood as a process meant to yield information rather than to make decisions, practitioners of benefit-cost analysis need not take sides in controversies over the nature of justice" (21).

ALTERNATIVE FRAMEWORKS AND CRITERIA

BCA is one of several decision frameworks that Congress has written into legislation. Others include: (a) no risk, (b) risk-risk, (c) technology-based standards, (d) risk-benefit analysis, and (e) cost-effectiveness analysis (11). (a) No risk framework is exemplified by the Delaney Clause that forbids the Food and Drug Administration from permitting carcinogens to be added to food, no matter how small the risk or how large the benefit. When Congress adopts the no risk framework, it is assuming that benefits are trivially small and the consequences of permitting the action are horrendous. (*b*) Risk-risk analysis is used by the FDA to regulate drugs and medical devices. Drugs and X rays have some risk of harming the patient; thus the FDA trades off the possible risk of the intervention against the possible risk of no intervention. The FDA does not account for the cost of treatment and other factors and does not compare one type of treatment to another, e.g. pharmaceuticals vs surgery for coronary artery disease. (*c*) Technology-based standards are frequently used for regulation of industrial emissions to air or water; agencies are instructed to choose a control technology with no explicit consideration of costs and health or other benefits. (*d*) Risk-benefit analysis attempts to weigh the risks of a technology or intervention against the benefits of that technology or intervention. Costs and other issues are not considered. (*e*) Cost-effectiveness analysis attempts to achieve a specified goal, e.g. lowering the infant mortality rate by 20%, at the least cost. (*f*) Benefit-cost analysis attempts to identify, quantify, monetize, and then compare all of the social benefits with all of the social costs.

These frameworks, (*a*)–(*f*), are arrayed in rough order with respect to the breadth of considerations, tradeoffs considered, and thus efficiency. The frameworks are also in rough order in terms of the amount of data and analysis required. For example, cost-effectiveness analysis requires that the various costs be combined into a total cost but does not require analysis of the benefits; the framework does not require that benefits and costs be compared (25a). Despite these limitations, cost-effectiveness will result in the socially efficient outcome if the goal chosen happens to be the efficient one, the one that would be selected by a benefit-cost analysis.

Each framework makes implicit assumptions about ethics. For example, the "no risk" framework assumes that protecting human health is the only goal; no tradeoffs are relevant concerning such other attributes as health vs private or public consumption. The no risk framework is simplistic in not recognizing more complicated implications, such as the risk-risk tradeoffs of the second framework. The risk-risk framework continues to focus only on health. Technology-based standards rest upon a naive assumption that the technology drives the solution and that other considerations, including health and consumption, are either not important or are handled in an obvious fashion. Risk-benefit analysis examines the health risks and general benefits of a technology. It assumes that other types of risk are not relevant. Finally, cost-effectiveness is based on the premise that efficiency is the most important attribute, that choosing the desired goal is simple or not possible analytically. Although Congress could be forthright in declaring its goals, more often it expresses its values more subtly by choosing one of these decision frameworks.

DIFFICULTIES IN BENEFIT-COST ANALYSIS

A host of difficulties impede BCA. The most important difficulty is quantifying the effects of an intervention. How much additional life expectancy, on average, will result from screening women aged 40 to 49 years for breast cancer? Screening detects breast tumors earlier than they would be detected without screening. The increase in the survival rate comparing those screened with those not screened is due, in part, to detecting the disease earlier than if the woman were symptomatic. Meanwhile, some abnormalities will be detected and treated that may not have progressed to breast cancer in the absence of treatment. Women with these abnormalities bias upward the survival rate attributed to screening. In addition, these women suffer psychological trauma, a decrease in the quality of life, and may even have their lives shortened as an adverse effect of the mistaken treatment of these abnormalities.

Whether the analyst is trying to estimate the effect of breast cancer screening, suspended particles in the air, trihalomethanes in drinking water, pesticide residues in food, or occupational exposures to toxic substances, quantifying all the health effects of an intervention is difficult. We emphasize that the difficulty is inherent, not a problem caused by appealing to BCA. Sensible decisions cannot be made without good estimates of the health benefits of the intervention. Criticism of BCA tends to focus on the monetization of these effects, rather than on the magnitude of effects. This criticism is misguided insofar as the real problem is the quantification of the benefits of intervention.

Monetizing the benefits of health improvements does add controversy to the analysis. What is the dollar value of adding a year of life expectancy to the population of 50–59 year old women? Some studies look at decisions that people currently make, such as taking risky jobs or purchasing less safe products, such as cars without air bags or cars that are smaller and lighter (28). Few people are skeptical of using market prices for the supplies used in a public health clinic. There is less comfort in using market prices in other areas, such as the risk premium in the pay of underground coal miners who may have little alternative employment.

The way in which economists value most goods and services not traded in the market is via surveys that ask individuals how much they would be willing to pay to get something they desire or how much they would have to be paid to give it up (contingent valuation). This technique has been used for valuing an additional asthma attack, other kinds of morbidity, and the rate of time preference in saving lives (5, 26). People are asked how much they would be willing to pay to lower their chance of being killed this year in a highway crash by one chance in 100,000. In many cases, the answers can be compared to actual purchasing decisions that people make, such as buying cars with air bags or antilock brakes or buying larger, safer cars (28).

In some cases, monetization can be avoided by concluding that the health benefits of the intervention are small or nonexistent. No further analysis is needed. When the intervention does produce substantial benefits, they will need to be monetized in a BCA. This monetization cannot be done with mathematical precision. However, in many cases, the uncertainty about the valuation estimate is smaller than the uncertainty in quantifying the health benefits. For example, there is considerable uncertainty about how much women would be willing to pay to lower their chance of dying of breast cancer by one chance in 1000 per year. However, there is still greater uncertainty concerning the reduction in relative risk as a result of an annual screening program in 40–49 year-old women.

Since quantification and valuation are fraught with uncertainty, the question is whether the estimates help or mislead government officials. Miller has no patience with this question: "If we have given government officials the power to impose costs on the activities of private citizens or otherwise control them, we cannot say they cannot be trusted to weigh benefits and costs in determining what they do. If regulatory statutes allow discretion, the enforcing agency would be irresponsible—and in my view unfair—not to weight the benefits and costs of its policies" (16).

BCA is filled with uncertainties concerning the health benefits of the intervention, their monetization, the costs of the intervention, and other aspects of the analysis. To be helpful to decision makers, the analyst should be careful to present the data and assumptions clearly. The analyst should undertake a sensitivity analysis and state clearly which of the results are most sensitive to the uncertainties in the data and monetization.

IMPLEMENTATION DIFFICULTIES

Whatever the theoretical difficulties, they are dwarfed by the difficulties of implementing BCA. For example, the tool has been criticized as biased and as serving the incumbent politicians. However, "any technique employed in the political process may be distorted to suit parochial ends and particular interest groups. Cost-benefit analysis can be an advocacy weapon, and it can be used by knaves. But it does not create knaves, and to some extent it may even police their behavior. The critical question is whether it is more or less subject to manipulation than alternative decision processes. Our claim is that its ultimate grounding in analytic disciplines affords some protection" (13).

In practice, BCA is an unimaginative, bookkeeper's activity. The tool seems to encourage a narrow analysis. All too often economists miss the primary benefits (or costs) in doing the analysis. The conceptual difficulties are the grist for academic theorists. Reality is more bleak. In a few cases catching national attention, BCAs are careful and complete (16a). Even these analyses are subject to the limitations described above. More generally, BCA is done by apprentice analysts without the time or resources for careful analysis (8). Still, a conceptually correct BCA that is done quickly can be helpful, even in a limited way. Conversely, analyses that are not conceptually correct can mislead. For example, a novice analyst might count the jobs created by an air pollution control program as a social benefit; in fact they are a social cost. The benefit consists of clear air; program expenditures needed to achieve clear air are a cost, not a benefit.

In practice, what decision makers learn from BCA comes from the executive summary. But no one- or two-page summary can indicate the range of uncertainties and other qualifications that a decision maker must know to use the analysis intelligently. Furthermore, reading the report might detect fundamental conceptual flaws in the analysis, something the summary is unlikely to indicate.

CASE STUDIES

To complement the theoretical discussion above of the strengths and weaknesses of BCA, we illustrate the tool by applying it to three case studies.

A: Regulating Coke Oven Emissions

Coke making is the first step in steel making. It involves heating coal to a high temperature in an airtight chamber. The impurities are volatilized, leaving almost pure carbon. The volatilized coke oven gas (COG) is a complex mixture of over 10,000 different chemicals in the form of gases, vapors, and particles. Modern coke ovens collect the COG produced in coke making and further process it or use it as a fuel. However, some of the COG is released to the environment during charging, discharging, and cooling operations, and due to leakages through imperfect seals around doors and pipes (fugitive emissions). Among the diseases associated with COG are lung and urinary tract cancers, skin tumors, bronchitis, and emphysema. There is strong scientific evidence, based on epidemiological surveys, animal studies, and chemical analyses, that coke oven emissions are carcinogenic at exposure levels experienced by coke oven workers. Since these emissions pose health hazards for both the workers and the populace living around coke ovens, they have been regulated by OSHA and the EPA.

BCA can be very useful in evaluating these regulations. However, estimating the benefits of regulating industrial emissions such as COG requires data on current emissions rates, prospective control technologies and the extent to which they reduce emissions, the ambient concentrations associated with different emission rates, populations exposed and the exposure rates, the dose-response rates for the relevant diseases and populations, and the timing and intensity of various health effects. Estimating costs requires information on costs and disruptions, including productivity changes, of each relevant control technology.

Here we outline the procedures used by EPA in developing coke oven regulations to highlight some of the subjective decisions and assumptions often necessary in carrying out a practical BCA, which may not be apparent from the executive summaries and how systematic biases in these can misinform and mislead (see References 12, 23 for more detailed analyses).

To estimate the uncontrolled emission rates, the EPA study assumed that coke ovens operate at full capacity 90% of the time. Three control options were considered that were estimated to cost $7 million, $19 million and $81 million per year of operations, and reduce annual coke oven emissions to 450 Mg, 420 Mg, and 100 Mg, respectively, from base emissions of 720 Mg. EPA chose to use analytic diffusion models instead of actual site measurements to estimate ambient concentrations due to these emissions. Generic air dispersion models were used to estimate the ambient air concentrations in an area within a radius of 50 km from each source. EPA also developed some site-specific dispersion models based on local meteorological conditions but did not use them in their final analyses. To estimate lifetime exposure to COG, EPA assumed that individuals are exposed 24 h per day, 365 days per year for 70 years to these ambient concentrations.

Similarly, EPA used a series of conservative procedures to arrive at the estimates of cancer risk from these exposures. NIOSH and the steel industry conducted an elaborate ongoing epidemiological study that discovered and quantified the excess cancer deaths for coke oven workers (14, 15, 22). One major limitation of these epidemiological studies was that they collected no data on individual exposure levels or cigarette smoking habits. EPA risk analysis assumed that coke oven workers had smoking habits similar to other steel workers and that exposure levels were the same as those observed in coke plants in the 1960s, both of which are likely to overstate risks. The next step was to estimate the cancer risks to the population that is exposed to much lower doses than were the coke oven workers for whom data were available. The EPA study chose to extrapolate using the linear functional form, which gave the greatest estimated risk level. However, the quadratic functional form fitted the data best and gave much lower estimates for disease incidence. EPA followed its standard procedure of using the linear dose-response relationship and the upper bound of the 95% confidence interval, instead of the maximum likelihood estimates on the parameters to calculate unit risks of exposure. The number of cancer deaths averted was calculated based on the population living within the 50-km radius. Under these assumptions, control option 1 was estimated to save 2.6 lives per year at a cost of $2.7 million/life saved; option 2, an additional 0.3 lives at $41million/life saved; and option 3, 3.1 lives at $26 million/premature death averted. Using maximum likelihood estimates for the linear dose-response relationship or the quadratic dose-response relationship would have lowered the estimated number of deaths by at least factors of 10 and 19; thus the cost per premature death averted would be $27–51 million for option 1, $410–800 million for option 2, and $260–500 million for option 3 (12).

The process of cascading conservative estimates at each stage led to risk estimates that are orders of magnitude greater than estimates based on more realistic or "best" estimates. The result is regulation calling for much greater control—and greater expense. Lave & Leonard (12) argue that true cancer risk to people living around coke ovens may be almost zero and the most likely cost per life saved is in the order of $270–$4100 million. Reuter & Steger (23) studied geographical patterns of cancer incidence around coke ovens in Allegheny county and found no evidence of increased cancer risk due to closeness to coke ovens.

B: Mammography Screening for Women under Age 50 Years

The effectiveness of mammography screening in reducing breast cancer mortality in women older than 50 years is well established. In contrast, mammography screening for women under age 50 years has been the subject of a continuing debate among medical professionals. Twelve medical groups, including the American Cancer Society (ACS), American Medical Association (AMA), National Cancer Institute (NCI), and American College of Radiology, recommend mammography at 1–2 year intervals for women in the age group 40–49 years, whereas the US Preventive Services Task Force, the Canadian Task Force on Periodic Health Examination, the International Union Against Cancer (UICC), and the American College of Gynecology and Obstetrics declined to recommend mammography for women with average risk in this age group (3).

The issue is important. Estimates of new cases of breast cancer found each year in this age group vary from 18,300 (7) to 29,000 (6). There are about 17 million women in this age group. Assuming 25% coverage and a cost of $100/screen, the annual cost of screening at one-year intervals would be about $425 million.

The difference in recommendations concerning screening may be due to differences in goals. Possible goals of early detection, preventing premature deaths, improving the well-being of women, appear to be similar, but actually differ significantly. The American Cancer Society appears to focus on the first goal: "American Cancer society feels that the value of screening transcends cost .... As long as mammography represents the only method by which breast cancers can be diagnosed in a subclinical stage, adequate screening opportunities must be provided to women as a whole" (6). The implicit assumption is that early detection will improve survival rates and well-being. Kerlikowske et al focus on the second goal when they state: "The goal of screening mammography is to reduce mortality from breast cancer" (10). For this goal, improving treatment after detection is an alternative to screening for early detection. Costs are not important in either goal. ACS explicitly rejects consideration of costs, whereas Kerlikowske et al do not comment on costs. The third goal focuses on improving well-being, which suggests an examination of primary prevention through changes in lifestyle, such as diet, instead of focusing only on early detection (secondary prevention). Indeed, changing lifestyle might be more cost-effective than screening.

Estimating the benefits of mammography screening requires quantifying the following linkages: the relationship between prevalence and incidence of breast cancer by age group and by other risk factors such as genetics, personal habits, and medical history; the relationship between timing of screening procedures and proportion of cancers detected by various combinations of procedures; additional risks due to screening procedures; lead time gained through screening and the effectiveness of available therapy in terms of reductions in morbidity and mortality as a function of time of detection. The outcomes of the screening program include reduction in premature deaths due to early detection; gains/losses in quality of life due to changes in morbidity levels; the extra years of life gained; premature deaths due to screening radiations; and unnecessary biopsies in the case of false positive screenings. Quantifying the (financial and other) costs of screening requires consideration of the costs of false positives and additional cancers due to screening radiation.

Breast cancer is a relatively well studied problem. However, evidence on the most important health outcome, i.e. effectiveness of routine mammography screening in reducing mortality in this age group, is inconclusive. Table 1 summarizes the estimated relative risks of mortality for the screened with respect to unscreened populations, obtained in major studies of breast cancer.

Kerlikowske et al (10) find that the overall summary relative risk of cancer deaths in the screened and unscreened populations arrived at by the meta-analyses of all the nine studies was 0.93 (95% CI, 0.76 to 1.13), and for randomized controlled trials was 0.92 (95% CI, 0.75 to 1.13). They also find that the studies that had 10-12 years of follow-up had a lower summary RR than those that had only 7-9 years follow-up (0.83 and 1.02, respectively). Smart et al (24) conduct meta-analysis of a subset of the above trial results and estimate the relative risk to be 0.84 (95% CI, 0.69 to 1.02).

Screening appears to increase the risk of cancer death in the short run. In general, the RR declines with increased number of years of follow-up.

Table 1 Relative Risks (RR), odds ratios and 95% confidence intervals (CI) of screening mammography in women aged 40-49 years: results from major studies.[a,b]

Study[a]	RR and CI	Years follow-up
1. Edinburgh	0.98 (0.45–2.10)	7
	0.78 (0.46–1.51)	10
2. Malmo	1.29 (0.74–2.25)	8
	0.51 (0.22–1.17)	12
3. Kopparberg	0.76 (0.32–1.77)	8
	0.75 (0.41–1.36)	12
4. Ostergotland	1.03 (0.50–2.10)	8
	1.28 (0.76–2.33)	12
5. Canadian I	1.36 (0.84–2.21)	7
6. HIP	0.81 (0.53–1.24)	9
	0.77 (0.50–1.16)	10
7. Stockholm	1.04 (0.53–2.05)	8
8. Gothenberg	0.73 (0.27–1.97)	7
9. Nijmegen	1.23 (0.31–4.81)	8

[a]Source: Reference 10, Table 2
[b]All except Nijmegen are randomized control trials, while Nijmegen is a case-control study.

However, the changes in mortality risks are not statistically significant, even when results from many studies are combined to gain more statistical power. Kerlikowske et al (10) hypothesize that the key to increases in mortality in the short run, but better performance with longer follow-up, may be the timing of menopause. They suggest that screening begin at menopause, or at age 50 if menopause has not occurred. However, if the cancers occurring before age 50 are more aggressive, annual screening may not be frequent enough to detect the tumor early enough for effective intervention. If so, more frequent screening would be required. The higher frequency of screening must balance the risks of additional screening against the benefits of early detection (see below).

A detailed BCA would also require relative risk estimates at various time intervals of follow-up. Eddy et al (7) combine results from four short-term studies (BCDDP, Swedish, Nijmegen, and Florence) and one longer-term study (HIP in New York), using "confidence profile" method, and estimate that annual mammography for women aged 40–49 years would decrease mortality by 6% at five years, 14% at 10 years, 19% at 15 years, 22% at 20 years, and 26% at 30 years, and add an average of 3.5 years to the life of a woman destined to get cancer. However, they warn that there is considerable uncertainty about these estimates. They estimate that the savings in initial and terminal treatment costs due to early detection are very small (about 1%)

compared to the total costs of a screening program. They do not attempt to value the quality of the life in the additional years of life gained.

Screening is not risk free. Exposure to screening radiation may increase risk of cancer. Eddy et al (7) estimate the lifetime risk of cancer due to ten screening radiations at 1/25,000, and the natural risk of cancer in the age group 40–49 years at 128/10,000. As seen from Table 1, the reduction in mortality due to screening can vary from 2% to 20% of this risk, i.e. about 6/25,000 to 102/25,000. In other words, the risk induced by screening radiations can alone offset between 1.6% to 16% of the benefits of screening. Confirmatory testing of false positive screens may impose further avoidable risks, and there will be roughly 100 false positives for every cancer case detected (at 1% FP rate) or between 50 and 226 FPs per cancer death avoided (7). In addition to risks due to biopsies and costs of testing, there are nontrivial psychological costs of false positives.

In conclusion, in breast cancer screening in younger women, the main tradeoff is between the likely number and quality-of-life years saved, and the costs and risks of the screening program. The current evidence is too weak to draw firm conclusions. There is a good case to be made for putting more resources into primary prevention compared to screening.

C: Promotion of Exercise as a Preventive Health Measure

Of the three examples, defining the goals is most important for promoting exercise. The goals might be: (a) the reduction of mortality and morbidity, (b) reductions in health care expenses, (c) Improvement of well-being, (d) improvement of appearance, or (e) reducing obesity and eliminating sedentary lifestyles. The choice of goals is likely to shape the type of intervention that is desired. If we assume that the goal is to improve longevity by reducing CHD deaths, we neglect reductions in morbidity, improvements in fitness and improved lifestyles; a BCA should account for all the outcomes.

The linkage between physical activity and longevity is as follows: Physical activity→physical fitness→higher quality life→low hypertensive-metabolic-arteriosclerotic disease (HMAD) risk→longer life (18, 19). However, these linkages are confounded by interrelationships between different types of physical activity (leisure time, occupational, and other chores), levels/intensities of activities, different types of fitness, (morphological, muscular, motor, cardio-respiratory, and metabolic), heredity, lifestyle (sleep, stress, smoking), personal attributes (age, sex, motivation), nutrition, physical environment (weather), social environment (marriage, children, pets, other social networks), and different physiological mechanisms through which increased fitness affects health outcomes in terms of mortality, morbidity, and wellness. Additional complications arise due to the dynamic nature of exercise programs and progression of CHD, and health risks due to exercise itself (adapted from Reference 2).

The problem of accurate and consistent measurement of these factors is not a trivial one. Hence it is almost impossible to design studies that control for all the factors and also establish causality.

So far, most research pertaining to the relationship between physical activity and CHD has been epidemiological; many studies are only suggestive because of small numbers of subjects or failure to control for important factors. In all studies, uncontrolled factors mean that the observed association may not be causal. The studies, especially the earlier ones, suffer from problems of self-selection, crude measures of exercise and CHD, dependence on self-reports, and inadequate control of confounding and covariate factors. Very few of the studies are RCTs (1, 18–20). The estimated summary relative risk of CHD associated with inactivity varies among studies, but generally ranges from 1.5 to 2.4 with a median of about 1.9 (20). Though it is well accepted that exercise improves fitness defined as capacity for work, little is known about how exercise and improved fitness protect against heart disease. Researchers have hypothesized that exercise affects CHD by preventing development of athero-sclerosis or the accumulation of fatty deposits on blood vessels; or through secondary prevention by affecting blood pressure, HDL levels, blood coagulation, collateral blood flows to the heart, etc. However, the evidence is weak (4, 25).

As with any preventive activity, there are risks associated with exercise. They include increased risk of CHD events during and after exercise, and risk of muscular and skeletal injuries. These risks vary by age, sex, and exercise intensity. Other risks typically not considered include increased road and other accidents, dog bites, increased effect of urban pollution, heightened risks in conventional diseases if one exercises during illness, osteoporosis, cumulative damage to heart muscles due to exercise during infections, etc. Few data exist to quantify these risks. Also, CHD incidences attributable to exercise are likely to be underreported due to delayed effects, confusion with normal aches and pains of exercise, and deliberate concealing when they occur in commercial facilities.

The financial costs of exercise would include direct costs of equipment, facilities, counseling, initial medical evaluation, and medical care for injuries. Indirect costs include the value of time spent exercising and time lost to injury.

Inability to quantify the medical benefits and costs means that there are very few full-fledged BCAs of exercise programs. We could find one study that attempted a CEA of exercise as a health promotion activity. Hatziandreu et al (9) made several assumptions in their CEA to overcome data limitations. For example, they used the age-specific incidence rates of CHD from the Framingham study to calculate separate rates for exercisers and non-exercisers, by assuming that 10% of all men exercise, and that exercise reduces the rate of CHD by 50%. Similarly, they assume that people who are neutral toward exercise value the time spent in exercise at the prevailing wage rate, those who dislike it at twice the wage rate, and those who like exercise as costless. They consider only THE medical costs and lost wages due to increased risk of injury as the value of risks associated with exercise. They estimate the direct and indirect cost per CHD death avoided at $250,000.

In conclusion, in all these cases the main difficulty is in quantifying the health effects with adequate accuracy and establishing a prima facie case for the intervention. The issues of valuation, distributional justice, ethics, and achievement of social optimum, which have been the focus of much of the academic and political debate, are of secondary importance in many practical BCA in public health.

CONCLUSION

Benefit-cost analysis can be an extremely useful tool for public health professionals. It is a systematic, scientific approach to evaluation of programs; it uses analysis rather than emotion to inform difficult decisions. BCA focuses on the need to justify programs before recommending them to the public. It can serve to convince political leaders and the public of the social benefits of public health programs.

Despite the real advantages of BCA, one must take care that it is used properly and the results are not over-interpreted. For example, the Reagan Executive Order directing agencies to choose the alternative with the greatest net benefits makes no sense either in theory or practice. Public health professionals and political decision makers must be aware of the limitations of the tool and know how to interpret the analysis.

Literature Cited

1. Berlin AJ, Colditz GA. 1990. A meta-analysis of physical activity in the prevention of coronary heart disease. *Am. J. Epidemiol.* 132:612–28
2. Bouchard C. 1994. Physical activity, fitness, and health: overview of consensus symposium. In *Toward Active Living; Proc. Int. Conf. Physical Activity, Fitness, and Health*, ed. AH Quinney, L Gauvin, TAE Wall, pp. 7–14. Champaign, IL: Hum. Kinet. Publ.
3. Canadian Coord. Off. Health Technol. Assess. 1992. *An Overview of Major Breast Screening Studies and Their Findings.* Ottawa, Ont.
4. Consensus Statement. 1994. In *Physical Activity, Fitness, and Health. Int. Proc. Consensus Statement*, ed. C Bouchard, RJ Shephard, T Stephens, pp. 9–76. Champaign, IL: Hum. Kinet. Publ.
5. Cropper M, Aydede SK, Portney P. 1992. Rates of time preference for saving lives. *Am. Econ. Rev. Pap. Proc.* 82 (May):469–72
6. Dodd GD. 1993. American Cancer Society Guidelines from the Past to the Present. *Cancer* 72:1429–32 (Suppl.)
7. Eddy DM, Hasselblad V, McGivney W, Hendee W. 1988. The value of mam-

mography screening in women under age 50 years. *JAMA* 259:1512–19

8. Grubb WN, Whittington D, Humphries M. 1984. The ambiguities of benefit-cost analysis: an evaluation of regulatory impact analyses under Executive Order 12291. In *Environmental Policy Under Reagan's Executive Order*, ed. K Smith, pp. 121–64. Chapel Hill, NC: Univ. N. Carolina Press

9. Hatziandreu EI, Koplan JP, Weinstein MC, Caspersen CJ, Warner KE. 1988. A cost effectiveness analysis of exercise as a health promotion activity. *Am. J. Public Health* 78:1417–21

10. Kerlikowske K, Grady D, Rubin SM, Sandrock C, Ernster VL. 1995. Efficacy of screening mammography: a meta-analysis. *JAMA* 273:149–54

11. Lave LB. 1981. *The Strategy of Social Regulation.* Washington, DC: Brookings Inst.

12. Lave LB, Leonard BA. 1988. Regulating coke oven emissions. In *The Risk Assessment of Environmental and Human Health Hazards: A Text Book of Case Studies,* ed. DJ Paustenbach, pp. 1064–81. New York: Wiley

13. Leonard HB, Zeckhauser RJ. 1986. Cost benefit analysis applied to risks: its philosophy and legitimacy. In *Values at Risk,* ed. D Maclean, pp. 31–48. Totowa, NJ: Rowman Allanheld

14. Lloyd JW. 1971. Long-term mortality study of steel workers. V. Respiratory cancer in coke oven workers. *J. Occup. Med.* 13:53–68

15. Mazumdar S, Redmond CK, Sollecito W, Sussman N. 1975. An epidemiological study of exposure to coal tar pitch volatiles among coke oven workers. *J. Air Pollut. Control Assoc.* 25: 382–89

16. Miller JC III. 1989. *The Economist as Reformer: Revamping the FTC. 1981–85.* Washington DC: Am. Enterp. Inst. Public Policy Res.

16a. Niskanen WA, Harberger AC, Haveman RH, Turvey R, Zeckhauser R, eds. 1972. *Benefit-Cost and Policy Analysis.* Chicago: Aldine

17. Off. Technol. Assess. 1982. *Evaluation of Medical Technology.* Washington, DC: GPO

18. Paffenbarger RS Jr, Hyde RT, Wing AL, Min-Lee I, Kampert JB. 1994. An active and fit way-of-life influencing health and longevity. In *Toward Active Living; Proced. Int. Conf.*

Physical Activity, Fitness, and Health, ed. AH Quinney, L Gauvin, TAE Wall, pp. 61–68. Champaign, IL: Hum. Kinet. Publ.

19. Paffenbarger RS Jr, Hyde RT, Wing AL, Min-Lee I, Kampert JB. 1994. Some interrelations of physical activity, physiological fitness, health and longevity. In *Physical Activity, Fitness, and Health. Int. Proc. Consensus Statement,* ed. C Bouchard, RJ Shephard, T Stephens, pp. 119–33. Champaign, IL: Hum. Kinet. Publ.

20. Powell KE, Thomson PD, Caspersen CJ, Kendrik JS. 1987. Physical activity and the incidence of coronary heart disease. *Annu. Rev. Public Health* 8:253–87

21. Railton P. 1990. Benefit cost analysis as a source of information about welfare. In *Decision Making: Report of a Conference,* ed. RB Hammond, R Coppock, pp. 55–82. Washington, DC: Natl. Acad. Press

22. Redmond CK, Cicco A, Lloyd JW, Rush HW. 1972. Long-term mortality study of steel workers. VI. Mortality from malignant neoplasms among coke oven workers. *J. Occup. Med.* 14:621–29

23. Rueter FH, Steger WA. 1990. Air toxics and public health, exaggerating risk and misdirecting policy. *Regulation* 3: 51–60

24. Smart CR, Hendrick RE, Rutledge JH, Smith RA, 1995. Benefit of mammography screening in women ages 40–49 years. *Cancer* 75:1619–25

25. Solomon HA. 1984. *The Exercise Myth.* New York: Harcourt Brace Jovanovich

25a. Tengs TO, Adams ME, Pliskin JS, Safran DG, Siegel JE, et al. 1995. Five-hundred life-saving interventions and their cost-effectiveness. *Risk Anal.* 15: 369–90

26. Tolley G, Kenkel D, Fabian R. 1994. State-of-the-art health values. In *Valuing Health for Policy,* ed. G Tolley, D Kenkel, R Fabian, pp. 323–44, Chicago, IL: Univ. Chicago Press

27. US Congress. House Subcomm. Commer., Trade, Hazard. Mater. and the Subcomm. Health Environ., Comm. Commer. 1995. *Joint Hearings on Risk Assess. and Cost/Benefit Analysis for New Regulations,* Feb. 1, 2. US GPO, Ser. No. 104-3, Washington, DC

28. Viscusi KW. 1993. The value of risks to life and health. *J. Econ. Lit.* 31:1912–46

Annu. Rev. Public Health. 1996. 17:221–45

HEALTH HAZARDS TO HUMANS ASSOCIATED WITH DOMESTIC PETS[1]

Marshall Plaut, Eugene M. Zimmerman, and Robert A. Goldstein

Division of Allergy, Immunology and Transplantation, National Institute of Allergy and Infectious Diseases, National Institutes of Health, Bethesda, Maryland 20892

KEY WORDS: asthma, hypersensitivity diseases, bites by animals, infectious diseases, immunocompromised patients

---

ABSTRACT

Allergy to pets, particularly when manifested as asthma, is an important health hazard. The health impact of severe clinical disease associated with allergy to pets can be minimized by avoidance of pets. Many individuals with milder disease keep their pets and obtain medications for relief of their allergy symptoms. Bird fancier's disease can result in profound deterioration of pulmonary function, and requires avoidance of bird exposure. Animal bites are the commonest health hazard of domestic pets and result in tissue damage and infection risk. Bites are treated by cleaning the wound, and appropriate use of antibiotics and tetanus prophylaxis. Diverse infectious diseases are transmitted to humans by their pets; these diseases are particularly dangerous to immunocompromised individuals. The infectious diseases can be partly prevented by avoiding ill animals and by washing of hands following exposure to pets or pet-derived secretions. They can be treated by appropriate antibiotics and/or specific immune globulins and/or vaccines.

INTRODUCTION

This review discusses the potential health hazards to humans from their pets. These hazards are divided into three categories of diseases: (*a*) immunologic responsiveness to pets, resulting in allergic disease, asthma, and/or hypersensitivity pneumonitis; (*b*) bites and or scratches from pets, which cause tissue damage and may induce infections, and (*c*) infectious diseases associated with pets. Table 1 gives an overview of the major diseases reviewed in this chapter, and the pets responsible.

---

[1]The US Government has the right to retain a nonexclusive, royalty-free license in and to any copyright covering this paper.

Table 1 Diseases associated with domestic pets

Disease	Pet
IMMUNOLOGICAL DISEASE	
Allergic diseases	Cat (commonest), dog; rarely, hamster, rabbit, rodent, bird
Asthma	Same as allergic diseases
Hypersensitivity pneumonitis	Birds (pigeon, budgerigar, canary, chicken)
INJURY	
Bite, scratch (laceration, puncture, contusion, infection risk)	Dog (commonest), cat; others including rodent, bird
INFECTIOUS DISEASES	
Campylobacteriosis *(Campylobacter jejuni Campylobacter coli)*	Dog, cat, horse, hamster
Capnocytophaga canimorsus (DF-2)	Dog, cat (rare)
Leptospirosis	Dog, rat, cat (rare)
Lyme disease *(Borrelia burgdorferi)*	Mice, dog
Meliodosis *(Pseudomonas pseudomallei)*	Fish (exotic)
Mycobacteria marinum	Fish
Pasteurella multocida	Cat, dog, rabbit, rodent (bite)
Plague *(Yersinia pestis)*	Cat, dog, rabbit
Rat-bite fever *(Streptobacillus moniliformis* and (in Asia) *Streptobacillus minus)*	Rodent, cat (rare)
Salmonellosis (not S. *typhi)*	Chicken, dog, cat, rabbit, rodent, ferret, turtle, iguana, other reptiles
Tetanus	Dog, cat (bites)
Tularemia *(Francisca tularensis)*	Rabbit, rodent; rarely bird, dog (bite), cat (bite)
Yersiniosis *(Yersinia enterocolitica* and *Yersinia pseudotuberculosis)*	Rodent, cat, dog, rabbit
Fungal diseases	
Cryptococcosis	Pet birds, especially pigeons
Histoplasmosis	Birds (especially starlings)
Ringworm *(Microsporum, Trichophyton)*	Cat, dog, rabbit, rodent, ferret, horse
Sporotrichosis *(Sporothrix schenckii)*	Cat, dog, rodent
Parasitic diseases	
Cestiodiasis *(Hymenodepsis nana)*	Hamster and other rodents
Cryptosporidiosis	Cat, dog, ferret, rodent, reptile (rare)
Cutaneous larva migrans *(Ancylostoma braziliensis, Ancylostoma caninum)*	Dog, cat
Echinococcosis *(Echinococcus granulosis)*	Dog (rare)
Ectoparasites [*Cheyletiella* infestation and sarcoptic mange (scabies) *(Sarcoptes scabiei)*]	Cat, dog, rabbit
Giardiasis	Dog, cat, rodent, ferret, bird
Toxoplasmosis *(Toxoplasma gondii)*	Cat; rarely dog
Visceral larva migrans *(Toxocara canis, Toxocara cati)*	Dog, cat, ferret
Chlamydial and rickettsial diseases	
Cat scratch disease *(Bartonellosis) (Bartonella henselae)*	Cat, rarely dog
Chlamydiosis (Psittacosis)	Psittacine (parrots) and domestic birds
Rocky Mountain spotted fever *(Rickettsia rickettsii)*	Dog, rabbit
Viral diseases	
Rabies	Dog, cat, ferret
Lymphocytic choriomeningitis	Hamster and other rodents

The review focuses on pet-related diseases in the United States. Parasitic and other infectious diseases transmitted by pets are much more frequent in some countries than in the United States, but these are not described unless they occur in the United States. This review emphasizes allergic diseases and, in particular, the most important clinical manifestation of allergy to pets, asthma and rhinitis. Advances in understanding the pathophysiology of allergic diseases and asthma have resulted in a new view: Pet (especially cat) exposure is more important in asthma than previously appreciated (59, 63). The magnitude of exposure to cat and other allergens is an important determinant of asthma severity and perhaps of irreversible reduction in pulmonary function.

ALLERGY TO PETS

Definition

Allergic diseases are characterized by the production of IgE antibodies directed against proteins or glycoproteins that serve as antigens. Those proteins and glycoproteins that induce an IgE antibody response are a subset of antigens, called allergens. Once IgE antibody molecules are present, allergen cross-links the IgE antibody and induces mediator release from mast cells and basophils. As described below, these mediators are responsible for increases in blood vessel permeability, smooth muscle tone, mucus production, and inflammatory cell accumulation that are the manifestations of allergic diseases. Atopic patients, with a genetic predisposition to allergic diseases, express one or more of the three major allergic diseases: allergic rhinitis, asthma, and atopic dermatitis.

Among the most common manifestations of allergy to pets are allergic rhinitis, allergic conjunctivitis, and asthma. Other allergic diseases less commonly induced by pet allergens include atopic dermatitis (eczema) and urticaria. The immune mechanisms involved in atopic dermatitis are poorly understood. Allergic rhinitis, asthma, conjunctivitis, and urticaria are mediated, at least in part, by IgE antibodies (62).

Allergic rhinitis is characterized by an inflammatory infiltrate in the nasal mucosa, and is associated with symptoms of sneezing and nasal congestion. The disease may be complicated by sinusitis. Allergic conjunctivitis is characterized by an inflammatory conjunctival infiltrate, associated with pain, itching, and redness of the conjunctiva. Asthma is defined (23a) as "a lung disease with the following characteristics: 1. Airway obstruction (or airway narrowing) that is reversible (but not completely so in some patients) either spontaneously or with treatment; 2. Airway inflammation; 3. Airway hyperresponsiveness to a variety of stimuli."

Diagnosis

The diagnosis of allergy to pets consists of medical history, physical examination, and laboratory tests establishing that (*a*) the patient makes IgE antibody to allergens derived from the pet; and (*b*) the patient is exposed to the pet (i.e. allergen is found in deposited house dust and/or in the air of the home or other environment) (58). If a pet lives in the home, the allergen will certainly be there. Pet-derived allergen may be found in homes even if the pet is not there (see below). Other diagnostic procedures include nasal and/or bronchial challenge with allergens; and/or exposure to the pet in a room containing a controlled ventilation system, a more "natural" setting than challenge with soluble allergens. Medical history reveals the symptoms of allergic diseases, which lead to diagnoses of rhinitis and/or asthma and/or atopic dermatitis, conjunctivitis, and urticaria.

Most pet-allergic individuals are "atopic," in that they have a familial tendency to produce IgE antibodies to a large number of the aeroallergens to which they are exposed. Thus, in addition to symptoms from pet exposure, they react to many other allergens. They usually have symptoms of allergic rhinitis corresponding to seasons when certain plants pollinate. It may be difficult to distinguish between allergic disease induced by pets vs other allergens.

Relationship of Exposure to Symptoms

Pet exposure may induce acute and/or chronic symptoms. Acute symptoms can most readily be linked to the pet. For example, if symptoms develop within minutes of entering an environment with a pet, then the pet is a possible or likely cause of the symptoms. Chronic symptoms are difficult to relate to specific environmental exposures. The most useful diagnostic test is a reduction in symptoms related to prolonged removal from pet exposure (73). Because it is virtually impossible to remove residual cat or dog allergen rapidly from a home even after removing the pet, it is useful for the patient to move, temporarily, to a pet-free environment.

Laboratory Tests

Laboratory tests are important for establishing that individuals are "sensitized" to pet allergens, i.e. they produce IgE antibodies to the allergens, which can be determined by skin testing or by testing the blood.

Pathophysiology

The relationship between pet exposure and clinical symptoms requires two separable events: sensitization (induction of an IgE antibody response) and symptoms (seen following aeroallergen exposure by a sensitized individual).

The capacity of individuals to make an IgE antibody response to airborne allergens (aeroallergens) depends upon the genetic background of that individual. Atopic individuals do make IgE antibodies to allergens, whereas most individuals are nonatopic and do not make IgE antibodies to these allergens (62). The capacity to make an IgE response also depends upon the extent of allergen exposure; allergen concentrations above a minimal threshold substantially increase the likelihood of stimulating IgE antibody production in atopics. Thus, atopic individuals produce IgE antibodies to a wide variety of aeroallergens. As a high proportion of atopic individuals are frequently exposed to cats and dogs, which both express allergens, not surprisingly, a high proportion of atopic patients are allergic to these pets. Prolonged exposure and exposure to high concentrations of allergen are both risk factors for the production of IgE antibodies to allergens from pets (24). Approximately 20% of the population of the USA is atopic, and approximately 1/7 of these atopic individuals (i.e. 3% of the population) is allergic to cat allergens, while a smaller fraction is allergic to dog allergens (26, 32).

While most individuals with allergy to pets are atopic, some individuals are not atopic and may have IgE antibody predominantly against pet allergens. For example, one group of elderly patients with asthma have been described who are not atopic but are allergic to cats (45, 54).

Induction of Disease

In sensitized individuals, repeated allergen exposure stimulates a variety of allergic symptoms including allergic rhinitis and asthma (and perhaps atopic dermatitis). However, only some allergic patients have clinical manifestation of asthma. The reasons why the pathology involves distinct target organs (i.e. nose or lung) are not known.

The most severe clinical allergic disease (other than acute anaphylaxis) is asthma, which is present in about 5% of individuals in the United States (10) and is associated with high economic costs, high morbidity, and occasional mortality. Allergy to pets is important because IgE antibody to pet allergens, like other indoor allergens, is a significant risk factor for asthma. Indeed, exposure to cat or dog allergen can (rarely) induce fatal and near-fatal asthma (13). In contrast, IgE antibody to outdoor allergens like ragweed pollen or grass pollen is a risk factor for allergic rhinitis but, in most patients, is not a risk factor for asthma (59, 63, 71).

Relationship of Indoor Allergens to Asthma

The induction of asthma by pet allergens (and other indoor allergens) may reflect some combination of the following seven factors: high concentrations of airborne allergens in a closed environment; long-term exposure to high concentrations of allergens; other as yet unidentified factors in the environment, like pollutants; the nature and size of the particle that carries the allergen;

biochemical properties of the allergen (e.g. many allergens have protease activity); genetic factors; and age when exposed to allergen.

Allergens Associated with Pets

A series of allergens derived from pets have been identified (60). For example, the major cat allergen is found in the saliva and on the fur. Cat allergens are widely distributed, presumably because they adhere to many surfaces (e.g. furniture, carpeting, clothing) (22, 27, 50, 86). This property means that (a) individuals who contact pets in their own home may bring substantial amounts of pet allergen into environments that they visit; and (b) once the allergen is in a new environment, it persists unless extraordinary cleaning measures are undertaken (49, 51). Thus schools with no cats have substantial levels of cat allergen in dust (49, 52), as do homes without cats (although generally at lower concentrations).

The particle distribution of cat allergen has been determined. In an undisturbed room, 25% of cat allergen is on small particles (<2.5 μ) and thus will be airborne and readily deposited on the respiratory tract of individuals in a room containing allergen (46). In contrast, the major allergen of house dust mite is on large particles and is not airborne in an undisturbed room.

The Natural History of Cat Allergy

Asthma is a clinical diagnosis, and the definition of asthma (see above) includes the phrase: "Airway obstruction (or airway narrowing) that is reversible (but not completely so in some patients)." Asthma is associated with long-term irreversible, but relatively slow, worsening of pulmonary function.

There is no information about the long-term natural history of asthma due to pet allergens, but one study of laboratory animal allergy indicates that asthma induced by laboratory animals is not progressive, in that bronchial reactivity remained constant over a 12-month period of allergen exposure (53). Based on our present knowledge of the natural history of asthma, asthma induced by pet allergens is likely associated with a (slow) deterioration of pulmonary function, given continued and long-term exposure.

Age of Exposure

Exposure to allergen in infancy appears to be a risk factor for the development of allergy and asthma. Dust mite exposure at age <2 predisposed to both IgE antibody to house dust mite and asthma at age 10; other data have confirmed and extended the original study. Pet exposure at ages 0–5 years correlates with wheezing at ages 8–13 (72).

Treatment

Treatment of allergy to pets consists of at least four approaches (27, 84): removal of pet; extensive cleaning, removal of carpets, air filtration, and denaturation; symptomatic treatment with standard medication ("pharmaco-therapy"); and immunotherapy

REMOVAL OF PET: EXTENSIVE CLEANING TO REMOVE ALLERGEN   The major reasons to remove the pet are (*a*) the importance of pet allergen exposure on both the induction and the severity of asthma; and (*b*) the possible importance of pet allergen exposure on long-term irreversible deterioration of pulmonary function tests. Removal of the pet is considered to be effective in diminishing the severity of asthma and allergic diseases induced by the pet, yet pets are not always removed. Indeed, many individuals whose livelihood depends on pets (e.g. veterinarians) attempt to continue to work with pets after making some attempts to reduce exposure. The risks and the benefits of pet ownership need to be balanced.

Management of asthma now focuses on using antiinflammatory glucocorti-coids and of allergen avoidance. The rationale of pet allergen avoidance is based in part on research studies of asthma in a "cat room," a room with controlled ventilation in which cats live, and into which cat-allergic patients are brought for varying periods of time, as an in vivo challenge model (81). Antiinflammatory medications (glucocorticoids) do block cat-induced rhinitis and asthma symptoms, but only partially (85). The magnitude of symptoms induced in a cat room may be quite high, and these symptoms are not entirely relieved by antiinflammatory medications. The results also suggest that heavy allergen exposure induces airway inflammation (53, 81, 85), possibly by stimu-lating production of high concentrations of proinflammatory cytokines. Thus, reduction in allergen exposure is necessary to control airway inflammation, perhaps by reducing cytokine production.

Allergen avoidance may be important for modifying the long-term natural history of asthma (59, 60, 84). If early intervention to avoid pet allergens prevents deterioration in pulmonary function, then pet allergen avoidance is critical for maintenance of lung function. These types of results suggest that allergen avoidance is extremely important for at least some patients with allergy to pets.

In contrast, pet allergen avoidance may be of limited clinical efficacy be-cause (*a*) in many individuals, pet allergens are either not the most important allergen or are not the only important allergen; and (*b*) the physical and chemical properties of pet allergens make it extremely difficult to remove these allergens from the environment.

Thus, allergy to pets occurs typically in atopic individuals who are allergic to multiple allergens. In cold, dry and/or mountain environments, IgE antibody to cats is the predominant risk factor for asthma (50, 52, 76). However, other allergens are also important even in these environments. In temperate climates, house dust mite, not pet, is considered the major indoor (and asthma-inducing) allergen, and in some inner-city environments, cockroach allergens may be most important (59–61). Pet allergen avoidance may have limited clinical efficacy in patients in whom pet allergens are not the most important ones.

After removal of the pet, removal of pet-derived allergens requires aggressive cleaning, and removing of carpets and upholstery (51, 60). With the most effective cleaning strategies, it may take six months after removal of cats before cat allergen concentrations are reduced. Although frequent washing of cats, in conjunction with other measures such as removing furniture and improving air filtration, has been reported to be effective in reducing airborne cat allergen concentrations (6), other data suggest that washing of cats does not significantly reduce levels of cat allergens (41). Even when the home environment is cleaned, exposure may recur because allergen is encountered at many environments elsewhere.

Some data suggest that the development of allergic diseases and asthma may be prevented by avoiding allergens in infancy (38). However, the protocols used up to now suggest that the magnitude and duration of this prevention effect appears to be limited.

SYMPTOM RELIEF   Symptom relief of rhinitis involves the use of antihistamines, decongestants, nasal cromolyn, and intranasal glucocorticoids. Symptom relief of asthma involves the use of beta-adrenergic agents (usually inhalers), cromolyn, and glucocorticoids. These agents are useful even for moderate and severe asthma, but they are not effective unless they are used in combination with environmental controls to reduce allergen exposure. Avoidance of house dust mite allergen is effective in reducing symptoms of asthma (59–61). Although similar studies have not been performed with pet allergens, it is likely that allergen avoidance would be effective clinically.

IMMUNOTHERAPY   Altering the immune response by repeated injections of allergens has been used as specific treatment in allergic patients who continue to be exposed to the allergens. None of the newer approaches to immunotherapy has yet been shown to be superior to standard immunotherapy.

One consistent effect of immunotherapy is to increase substantially the specific IgG antibody response. It is considered to be contraindicated in certain diseases where IgG antibody, and not just IgE antibody, induces some of the pathophysiological changes (e.g. pigeon breeder's disease—see below).

Although immunotherapy reduces symptoms (e.g. upon exposure in a cat room) and allergen responsiveness in cat allergy (37, 55, 82), it is not clear that it is as effective as cat allergen avoidance. There are data suggesting that an important clinical effect of immunotherapy is to reduce the intensity of late-phase reactions (62), perhaps by some (poorly understood) antiinflammatory effect. As noted above, antiinflammatory glucocorticoids are only partially effective when patients are heavily exposed to cats. We hypothesize that immunotherapy with cats will be only partially effective if patients are heavily exposed to cats.

Allergens Derived from Pets Other Than Cats

Allergy to any pet is possible. Contact with virtually any pet can induce IgE antibody production to some allergens and can induce allergic rhinitis or asthma. Since cats and dogs have the run of the indoor environment, these pets are associated with the highest and second highest frequency of IgE antibody production, and asthma. For other pets that are often kept in cages, high concentrations of allergens are limited to the environment around the cages. Allergens are shed on animal fur and bird feathers and on droppings in the cages. Of course, exposure to the environment of the cages, depending on the amount of time exposed, and activities such as cleaning the cages increase the likelihood of sensitization.

Rats, mice, rabbits, guinea pigs, and hamsters also induce allergy in susceptible individuals (both laboratory animal workers and people who own these animals as pets) (74). Birds also induce sensitivity (e.g. pigeon, budgerigar, canary, chicken, etc) (48, 83). Exposure to multiple birds increases the likelihood of an immune response. Pigeon breeders disease is associated with an IgE response (associated with rhinitis and asthma) and/or other immune responses (associated with inflammatory alveolitis), as discussed below (28, 29).

IMMUNOTHERAPY FOR ALLERGENS DERIVED FROM PETS OTHER THAN CATS There is limited information on this subject. It is reported that immunotherapy with dog allergens is not effective clinically (37). There is insufficient information on the basic mechanisms of immunotherapy to explain this clinical ineffectiveness.

BIRD FANCIER'S DISEASE

Immune reactions to bird antigens in some patients are remarkably similar to reactions to cat and dog allergens: immediate hypersensitivity reactions, including asthma, upon exposure to birds (29, 48, 83). Rhinitis and asthma are presumably mediated by IgE antibodies (just as rhinitis and asthma to cats and dogs). The precise antigens of birds have not yet been identified in bird droppings, feathers, and/or serum proteins (77).

In addition to immediate hypersensitivity reactions, bird exposure may induce a different type of inflammatory reaction in the lung, called hypersensitivity pneumonitis or extrinsic allergic alveolitis (28, 29). (Bird exposure can induce immediate reactions, alveolitis, or both.) Alveolitis is presumed to be induced by the immune response to antigens carried on small particulates that reach the lung alveoli. The reaction is reproduced by antigen inhalation and is dose dependent. Most patients are exposed chronically to large numbers of birds kept in cages in a closed environment. In the United States, pigeon breeders disease is the most frequent example of this alveolitis. Symptoms are related to the intensity of exposure (hours per day of exposure × the number of pigeons). Almost all symptomatic breeders, and 50% or more of asymptomatic breeders, produce IgG antibodies to pigeon proteins (against pigeon IgA, pigeon IgG, and pigeon mucin), although the identity of the pathogenic protein is unclear (79). Many patients with hypersensitivity pneumonitis have laboratory evidence of nonspecific activation of the immune response, such as increased total IgG levels. In addition to specific IgG antibodies, patients also have cell-mediated immune responses to bird antigens. IgE antibodies are thought to be irrelevant to hypersensitivity pneumonitis since hypersensitivity pneumonitis induced by other antigens, such as farmer's lung disease, is not associated with IgE antibodies. It is not known whether asthma and alveolitis are induced by the same, or different, bird-derived antigens.

Inhalation challenge to pigeon-dropping extracts or pigeon serum induces immediate and late symptoms and changes in pulmonary function. Immediate reactions include bronchospasm in some patients; the late reaction is quite different in patients with alveolitis from that in asthmatic patients, in that it consists of fever, alveolitis, and pulmonary function changes consistent with restrictive lung disease (28, 29, 65).

The birds that induce alveolitis include budgerigars, pigeons, canaries, and chickens. Breeders are typically exposed to 20 or more pigeons for several hours per day for several years before becoming symptomatic. Approximately 6–21% of pigeon breeders have symptoms of alveolitis. For example, one recent study found that, among pigeon breeders in the Canary Islands, 31% had rhinitis, 19% had asthma, 15% had symptoms resembling chronic bronchitis, and 8% had symptoms resembling alveolitis (66).

Treatment of alveolitis consists of (a) avoidance of antigen, and (b) systemic glucocorticoids. The alveolitis is reversed in many patients when exposure is avoided (28, 29, 40), but fibrotic changes (which also occur in some patients upon chronic antigen exposure) are irreversible.

BITES BY PETS

Bites represent the commonest type of hazard of pets. In the United States, there are an estimated 1–2 million dog bites and 400,000 cat bites each year. These may be profound underestimates, as only 10% of bites receive medical attention (9). Dogs are by far the commonest source of bites (63 to 93% of bites). Physicians are seen because of the severity of bite, fear of rabies or tetanus, and/or consideration of legal action. Bite wounds represent 1% of emergency room visits. These bites can cause abrasion, laceration, puncture or crush injuries, and may get infected. The potentially serious infectious complications include septic arthritis and osteomyelitis. Some dogs can generate enormous forces in their jaws, which can cause crush injuries. Deaths from pet bites, though rare, are usually due to dog bites, which can cause massive blood loss from very young children; pit bulls are the most commonly identified dog that can kill. Cats cause significant puncture injuries that can penetrate joints, but these injuries are often overlooked because cat teeth are small. Bites are generally from one's own pet (e.g. breaking up a fight between dogs) or the pet of an acquaintance; caution is needed in invading a dog's territory (33).

Treatment includes evaluation of the severity of injury and of the risk of infection, wound cleaning, and in certain circumstances, debridement (5, 25).

The major infectious organisms to be considered are mixed flora (in dogs); *Pasteurella multocida* (which causes rapid-onset infections; it is in 26% of dog wounds but is the major infectious organism in cat oral flora and is in 50% of cat wounds); *Capnocytophaga canimorsus*; and rabies and tetanus (36). Because of concern of infection, some physicians recommend that all patients with pet bites should receive prophylactic antibiotics. Tetanus prophylaxis (e.g. a booster immunization with tetanus toxoid in a previously immunized individual) is indicated. In individuals with remote (>10 years) immunization with tetanus toxoid and/or with a severe wound, both a tetanus toxoid booster and tetanus immune globulin are given.

INFECTIOUS DISEASES

Many infectious diseases are termed "zoonoses" because they are transmitted by animals, including domestic pets (11, 16, 43, 47, 58a). Humans are infected either by direct contact with pets (e.g. with the skin, nasopharyngeal or respiratory secretions, urine, or feces), or by indirect contact (with water or food that has been contaminated with infectious secretions of the pet). In addition, pet ownership is a risk factor for infections with agents that are transmitted by means other than direct or indirect contact. Two examples of the latter are the tick-transmitted diseases, Lyme disease and Rocky Mountain spotted fever. Although these diseases are usually not transmitted by pets, on occasion the ticks are carried by the pets to the vicinity of humans, and the ticks then bite humans.

Some of these infectious diseases are mild. However, there are more severe and even fatal variants of these diseases. Reduction of infectious diseases transmitted by pets can be partially achieved by avoiding contact with animals less than six months of age and animals with diarrhea. Since many pets that carry infectious agents do not appear ill, an additional preventive measure is to wash hands thoroughly after contact with pets, their secretions, or potentially contaminated food and water derived from pets.

Immune Protection from Infectious Diseases in Immunocompromised Patients

Deficient function of one or more components of the immune response of immunocompromised individuals increases susceptibility to certain infectious agents. The deficient immune component most commonly associated with increased susceptibilty to pet-transmitted infections is cell-mediated immunity. The immunocompromised patients not only are more susceptible to acquiring infections, but also are more likely to develop a severe form of the infection.

The immunocompromised patients for whom precautions on exposure to pets and pet-derived secretions are most critical are (*a*) patients being treated with immunosuppressive agents, and (*b*) patients with HIV infection. Infants and elderly individuals may also need to observe precautions. These precautions include not only avoiding young and sick animals and thorough handwashing after contact with pets and pet secretions, but also two more stringent measures: avoiding all contact with pet feces and potentially contaminated water; and avoiding all contact with reptiles or amphibians (the latter because of the risk of Salmonella infections).

Immunocompromised patients are at risk of the following pet-transmitted disease: three bacterial infections [campylobacteriosis, *Mycobacterium marinum* infections, and salmonellosis (not *S. typhi*)]; two fungal infections (cryptococcosis and histoplasmosis); three parasitic infections (cryptosporidiosis, giardiasis, and toxoplasmosis); and one rickettsial infection (cat scratch disease).

SPECIFIC INFECTIOUS DISEASES

The following is a list of important infectious diseases transmitted by pets. Each disease also lists those pets that transmit the disease. Not discussed are several diseases for which pets are known to be reservoirs for the infectious agent, but for which there is no evidence that pets transmit the agent to humans (e.g. group A streptococcal infections, where dogs and cats do harbor the bacteria).

Bacterial Diseases

CAMPYLOBACTERIOSIS (*CAMPYLOBACTER JEJUNI, CAMPYLOBACTER COLI*)   This bacterial infection has a reservoir in domestic and wild birds and animals. While the commonest mode of transmission is via ingestion of contaminated food or water, some cases are transmitted from contact with pets (4, 58a).

Infected pets (dogs, cats, horses, and hamsters) shed bacteria in their feces, and this shedding is age dependent (notably in the first year of life) and is increased if the pet has diarrhea. About 2 million cases occur per year in the United States, but only a small minority are due to pet exposure. Epidemiologic analysis shows that contact with animals is not a risk factor for illness, but exposure to pets with diarrhea is a risk factor, accounting for 6.3% of cases (67). Rare cases result from exposure to apparently healthy young pets.

The clinical illness is associated with a self-limited gastroenteritis, but occasionally septicemia and death (an estimate of 120–360 deaths/year in the United States) occur from these bacteria.

CAPNOCYTOPHAGA CANIMORSUS (DF-2)   This organism, found in the oral cavity of dogs and, rarely, of cats is a potential cause of infections following pet bites (36, 58a). In immunosuppressed patients, *Capnocytophaga canimorsus* (dysgonic fermenter (DF-2)) infection, from dog flora, is a cause of sepsis even in the absence of local signs of infection.

LEPTOSPIROSIS   This disease is transmitted by urine of sick or carrier animals. Human infection occurs when urine contaminates food or water (11, 16). Mucus membrane contact is an alternate mode of transmission. Rodents are the most common source. Vaccination of pets protects against clinical disease but does not prevent infection following exposure.

LYME DISEASE *(BORRELIA BURGDORFERI)*   Household pets are relatively rare sources of this infection. However, pet ownership in rural areas is a risk factor for this disease (70), and dogs acquiring vector ticks may become ill. The ticks carried by the pets may infect the human owners (75).

MELIODOSIS *(PSEUDOMONAS PSEUDOMALLEI)*   This is a rare human disease in the United States, but it is more common in Southeast Asia where the organism is endemic. Aquarium tank water with exotic imported fish may be contaminated (16). Bleach disinfection of tanks is recommended to control this disease.

MYCOBACTERIA MARINUM   These are rare infections in public swimming areas. Infection occurs when areas of minor skin trauma are exposed to water contaminated with these organisms. The disease is characterized by cutaneous granulomas. HIV-infected individuals are especially susceptible and can acquire this infection from contaminated aquariums (34).

PASTEURELLA MULTOCIDA   These infections occur from cat and dog bites and scratches (16, 36, 58a). This organism, found in the oral flora of most cats and many dogs, induces a cellulitis with very rapid onset (within 24–48 h). Signs and symptoms include regional lymphadenopathy, chills, and fever. Septic arthritis, osteomyelitis, and tenosynovitis also occur. Treatment is with penicillin or ampicillin, with wound drainage needed at times.

PLAGUE *(YERSINIA PESTIS)* This disease is typically transmitted by rats and other rodents (19, 58a). In endemic areas (i.e. California, Arizona, and New Mexico), cats are infected by eating rodents or by being bitten by rat fleas (17). Thus, oropharyngeal secretions in cats (and occasionally in other pets) are a source of aerosol exposure (31).

RAT-BITE FEVER *(STREPTOBACILLUS MONILIFORMIS* AND (IN ASIA) *STREPTOBACIL-LUS MINUS)* This disease is usually transmitted by bites from rat and, rarely, cat (16, 36, 43).

SALMONELLOSIS (NOT *S. TYPHI)* Species of Salmonella, other than *Salmonella typhi*, have an animal reservoir, and serotyping often can identify the likely reservoir. The most common cause of *Salmonella* infections is transmission from undercooked food including poultry, meat, eggs, and unpasteurized milk. Transmission from pets (chicken, dog, cat, rabbit, rodent, ferret, turtle, iguana, and other reptiles) accounts for 15–20% of total cases of *Salmonella* (18). The disease can be transmitted by direct or indirect contact (e.g. with water that pets swim in or drink). About 60–80% of pet-associated cases are in children aged 1–9 years, and none of the pet-associated cases occur in individuals over aged 50 years.

Patients at high risk for pet-transmitted salmonellosis include not only infants and young children, but also patients with HIV infection. Patients with malignancy and with hemoglobinopathies such as sickle cell disease are also at increased risk of salmonellosis, presumably including pet-transmitted salmonellosis.

Many species, such as amphibians and reptiles, have high fecal carriage rates without signs of illness. The fecal carriage rates for reptiles is more than 90% (58a). Treating reptiles with antibiotics has not been successful but rather has increased the antibiotic resistance of the Salmonella. The organism is transmitted transovarially so that eggs are infected; in addition, some species such as iguanas eat feces.

In the 1970s, the number of households having small pet turtles rose to 4%, with large, parallel, increases in human salmonellosis of turtle-associated serotypes (18). A requirement that turtles be certified *Salmonella*-free was ineffective in halting cases of turtle-associated serotypes of *Salmonella*. Thus, in 1975, the FDA banned all interstate shipments of pet turtles in the United States, resulting in a 14% reduction in cases of *Salmonella* (an 18% decrease in the population ages 1–9 years). More recently, lizards, notably iguanas, have become more popular as pets, with over 795,000 green iguanas imported into the United States in 1993; 7.3 million pet reptiles are now present in 3% of homes. Substantial increases in human *Salmonella* infections of reptile serotypes have occurred concomitantly (14, 23).

Salmonella typically causes an uncomplicated gastroenteritis that does not require antibiotic therapy (58a). Antimicrobial agents are indicated for patients with underlying diseases listed above, infants, and patients with severe colitis, and for those with invasive *Salmonella* disease. Effective antibiotics include ampicillin, amoxicillin, trimethoprim-sulfamethoxazole, etc, for gastroenteritis; and chloramphenicol or one of the above agents for invasive salmonellosis. A vaccine for typhoid fever is not effective against the pet-derived serotypes of *Salmonella*.

TETANUS Dog and cat oropharynx contain these organisms, so puncture wounds represent a risk factor for this infection (16, 36, 43, 58a). As discussed in the section on pet bites, tetanus toxoid alone, or with tetanus immune globulin, is useful for preventing such infections.

TULAREMIA (*FRANCISCA TULARENSIS*) The major vectors for this organism in the United States are rabbits, ticks, and rodents; rarely birds, dogs, or cats. Pets may harbor the organism in their oral secretions, so the infection is transmitted by bites, or occasionally by contact with oral secretions (e.g. licking) (44, 47, 58a).

YERSINIOSIS (*YERSINIA ENTEROCOLITICA* AND *YERSINIA PSEUDOTUBERCULOSIS*) These diseases are usually transmitted by contaminated food (meat, milk) or water, but they can be transmitted by infected pets such as rodents, cats, dogs, rabbits (43, 58a).

Fungal Diseases

CRYPTOCOCCOSIS This fungal disease is transmitted by inhalation of organisms from bird droppings, especially pigeon droppings. It causes a systemic disease including meningoencephalitis and pneumonia and requires prolonged, combined antifungal systemic therapy (e.g. six weeks for meningitis). The treatment is potentially toxic. For patients at risk, avoidance of areas contaminated with pigeon droppings is advisable. Elderly patients are at somewhat increased risk, and 5 to 10% of patients with AIDS are infected with the organism (15, 34). In patients with advanced HIV infection, prophylaxis with fluconazole is useful in reducing the infection rate.

HISTOPLASMOSIS This fungal infection is transmitted in histoplasma-endemic areas (eastern and central United States) by inhalation of soil or dust in barnyards, bat droppings, and bird droppings, especially from starlings. For high-risk individuals, it is advisable to avoid high-risk activities such as cleaning chicken coops, disturbing soil under bird-roosting sites, and exploring caves (15, 47).

RINGWORM (*MICROSPORUM, TRICHOPHYTON*)   These cutaneous fungal agents are transmitted by direct contact with infected animals (cats, dogs, rabbits, rodents, ferrets, and horses) (11, 16, 43, 57).

SPOROTRICHOSIS (*SPOROTHRIX SCHENCKII*)   This organism is widely distributed in the soil. It infects pets (cats, dogs, rodents) following wound infection (e.g. cat-fight wounds) and is excreted in the feces. It can be transmitted by direct contact with pet wounds (58a, 64).

Parasitic Diseases

CESTIODIASIS (*HYMENODEPSIS NANA*)   This tapeworm is transmitted from ingesting eggs after handling rodent species or contaminated food or water. Infection occurs mainly in children (16).

CRYPTOSPORIDIOSIS   This occurs usually via transmission in contaminated water, and by human to human (fecal-oral) transmission. Contamination from feces of pets [e.g. cats, dogs, ferrets, rodents, reptiles (rare)] is a risk factor, although a less common cause of transmission (58a). Children and patients with HIV infections are most susceptible (15, 34). The organism is resistant to chlorine and thus requires effective water filtration systems.

CUTANEOUS LARVA MIGRANS (*ANCYLOSTOMA BRAZILIENSIS, ANCYLOSTOMA CANINUM*)   While most cases of hookworm infections are transmitted from human to human in rural, tropical, and subtropical areas, on rare occasions human disease, presenting as eosinophilic enteritis, has been transmitted by the feline and canine hookworm, *Ancylostoma braziliensis* (in the Gulf coast and New World tropics), and more recently by the canine hookworm, *Ancylostoma caninum* (68). These latter cases have been identified in Queensland, Australia, mostly in dog owners (21). The precise mode of transmission is believed to be through walking barefoot in soil contaminated by dog feces. In some surveys, more than 20% of dogs not only in Australia but also in the United States have hookworms, and sporadic cases have been seen in the United States; the disease may therefore be more widespread than so far thought (20, 43).

ECHINOCOCCOSIS (*ECHINOCOCCUS GRANULOSIS*)   This particular species of *Echinococcus* is acquired by dogs (43). It is a rare disease in the United States, but is seen occasionally in endemic areas in Arizona, California, New Mexico, and Utah. Exposure to dog feces–contaminated food or water can result in development of cysts in humans.

ECTOPARASITES [*CHEYLETIELLA* INFESTATION AND SARCOPTIC MANGE (SCABIES) (*SARCOPTES SCABIEI*)]   *Cheyletiella* infestation is transmitted by direct contact from animals (cats, dogs, and rabbits). Scabies is most commonly transmitted by direct human-to-human contact. Direct contact with pets carrying this organism can transmit the disease (43, 57).

GIARDIASIS   Although humans are the principal reservoir of *Giardia* infections, pets (dogs, cats, rodents, ferrets, and birds) can be infected and can contaminate water with infectious cysts (58a). Humans are infected by direct contact with feces and with contaminated water. The organism is widely disseminated (depending on location and age, positive cultures are obtained from 1–20% of the population of the United States). Patients with cellular immune deficiency (notably patients with HIV infection), with humoral immunodeficiency, and with cystic fibrosis are at increased risk of infection.

TOXOPLASMOSIS (*TOXOPLASMA GONDII*)   This protozoa is very common; the cat is the major vehicle for transmission, rarely dogs (47, 58a). Serologic tests indicate that 30% of cats, and humans, have been exposed. Cat-to-cat transmission is by the fecal-oral route. Oocytes are excreted in the feces of cats, but become infectious only after sporulating, which requires 1–3 days. Humans are exposed by the fecal-oral route, for example after changing cat litter–boxes. In addition, the organism is found in many animals; raw or undercooked meat is therefore another source of infectious material.

The incubation period is approximately seven days. Immunocompetent individuals have subclinical disease, or a mild flulike illness. However, in primary exposure of women during gestation, toxoplasmosis acquired 6–8 weeks before gestation can also be transmitted to the fetus, although this is rare. Infection of women during the first two trimesters of pregnancy results in infection of 50% or more fetuses, with severe clinical disease in 10% or more of fetuses. This congenital disease can present with meningoencephalitis (which may lead to mental retardation and blindness), as well as hepatosplenomegaly, jaundice, and thrombocytopenia (43, 47).

Immunocompromised patients, notably those with HIV infections, are at increased risk for acquiring severe form of disease (systemic toxoplasmosis and/or encephalitis), and/or reactivation of an endogenous tissue cysts leading to disseminated disease and/or encephalitis (15, 34).

Pet-transmitted infection, in pregnant women and in HIV-infected individuals, is reduced by extensive handwashing after contact with cat feces or residue of cat feces in sandboxes or in soil. More effective measures include avoidance of contact with cat feces. Thus cat litter should be changed daily (i.e. before the oocysts sporulate) by a nonsusceptible individual. Cats should be kept from hunting and ideally be confined indoors and fed only canned or dried commercial food or well-cooked meats. Fresh fruit and vegetables should be well washed.

Toxoplasma infections are treated with pyrimethamine and sulfonamides. Immunocompromised patients are at risk of recurrence. Such individuals should have lifetime suppressive therapy, with pyrimethamine plus sulfadiazine and leucovorin.

VISCERAL LARVA MIGRANS (*TOXOCARA CANIS, TOXOCARA CATI*) The primary cause of visceral larva migrans and ocular larva migrans is the dog roundworm, *Toxocara canis*. A second but considerably less frequent cause is the cat roundworm, *Toxocara cati*. The seroprevalence of infection in children in the United States is between 2 and 10%, with higher rates among minorities (African-Americans, Hispanics) and persons of lower socioeconomic status. This disease is the most frequent of animal-transmitted human infection (12, 35, 47, 58a). Although some cases of toxocariasis are caused by eating contaminated food (lightly cooked liver or other meat), most are transmitted from puppies. Eggs of *T. canis* are recovered from yards of homes and parks where untreated puppies roam. Nearly all puppies are infected at birth by transplacental larval transmission. Worm eggs are released in the feces of 5- to 6-week-old puppies and contaminate soil. Toddlers with pica are at highest risk of infection. Direct contact does not cause the disease because the eggs are not immediately infectious.

Once infected, most children are asymptomatic. Some develop ocular larva migrans (more common in older children), which is typically unilateral and can result in an intense chorioretinitis leading to blindness. Visceral larva migrans (commonest in children aged 1–4) is associated with eosinophilia, liver granulomas, and occasionally, complications including intractable asthma and encephalitis.

Treatment of ocular larva migrans is with antiinflammatory glucocorticoids. The role of antihelmintic drugs is unclear. Treatment of visceral larva migrans is symptomatic, with glucocorticoids effective in reducing the eosinophilic infiltrations in the myocardium and/or central nervous system. The value of antihelminthic agents in killing larva is not known, and the drugs have toxic side effects.

Control measures include controlling pets in the household—disposing of visible cat and dog feces (including closing sandboxes, since cats often defecate there), eliminating causes of pica, and treating puppies and kittens with antihelminthics at 2, 4, 6, and 8 weeks of age. Thus, an appropriately treated pet is unlikely to transmit the disease to its owner.

Chlamydial and Rickettsial Diseases

CAT SCRATCH DISEASE (BARTONELLOSIS) (*BARTONELLA HENSELAE*)   The etiology of cat scratch disease was discovered only recently and was called *Rochalimaea henselae*, and now *Bartonella henselae*. Other members of this genus of Rickettsia include *Bartonella quintana, Bartonella elizabethae*, and *Bartonella bacilliformis*. These are causes of diseases ranging from bacillary angiomatosis and bacillary peliosis hepatitis, to cat scratch disease, and trench fever. Immunocompromised individuals, including HIV-positive individuals, are susceptible to severe forms of *Bartonella* infection (15). However, only *Bartonella henselae* has been linked to cats (42, 80). This bacteria is a cause of bacillary angiomatosis and bacillary peliosis hepatitis (which occurs most frequently in HIV-infected individuals) and cat scratch disease (which occurs most commonly in healthy individuals). There are estimates of up to 9.3 cases per 100,000 (about 22,000 cases) per year in the United States of cat scratch disease (39).

The symptoms of cat scratch disease include regional lymphadenopathy, occasionally associated with fever and with skin papules. Complications include encephalitis, hepatitis, and chronic systemic disease; these complications are rare except in immunosuppressed patients. Bacillary angiomatosis is occasionally fatal. The disease is presumed to be transmitted by cat fleas, and it is epidemiologically linked to owning a kitten younger than 12 months and to being scratched, and (less frequently) to being licked in the face by a cat (87). Both ill cats and apparently healthy cats may harbor *Bartonella*. Dogs may rarely transmit the disease, but the epidemiologic link to cats is very strong. The incubation period is approximately three weeks.

Treatment of humans consists of doxycycline or erythromycin; however, this treatment is generally not necessary for healthy individuals, and may not be fully effective in immunocompromised individuals.

CHLAMYDIOSIS (*PSITTACOSIS*)   Psittacosis is a chlamydial disease caused by *Chlamydia psittaci*, which is transmitted by infected birds (11, 13a, 47, 58a, 69). Any species of bird, including members of the parrot family, can be a source of this organism. Imported, exotic birds (some imported illegally), including members of the parrot family, pigeons, and turkeys are common sources (13a). Most patients have had contact with a pet bird. The organism is found in 5–8% of birds, and certain environments (e.g. crowding of birds during shipping) may markedly increase the prevalence of infection in the birds. The birds may be symptomatic or asymptomatic, but continue to shed the organism intermittently for many months. Up to 10% of infected birds may become chronic carriers. The organism is most commonly transmitted by the airborne route, but all excreted material of the birds, and feathers and dust derived from the birds, are contaminated.

Incubation periods following exposure are approximately 7–14 days. Both sporadic and epidemic forms of the illness have been reported. The illness may vary from a acute febrile, flu-like illness with a severe headache, to an atypical pneumonia with a nonproductive cough, but extensive changes detectable by X ray.

Prevention involves treating infected birds with a tetracycline antibiotic for 45 consecutive days. Legally imported birds are quarantined and treated with chlortetracycline for 30 days, but this time interval is too short, and some infected birds continue to shed. Birds should be kept isolated from wild birds and from newly arrived birds (e.g. in a pet store). Cages, droppings, and other materials must be disinfected.

Untreated patients have a mortality of 20%. Treatment with tetracycline or doxycycline for 10–21 days is effective, and reduces the mortality rate to 1% (47).

ROCKY MOUNTAIN SPOTTED FEVER (*RICKETTSIA RICKETTSII*)   This disease is widespread in the south Atlantic, southeastern, and south-central United States in particular, especially in spring and summer. It is transmitted by tick bites. Although the exact role of dogs in transmitting this disease is unknown, it is presumed that dogs carry ticks to the vicinity of humans. Humans exposed to ticks are at increased risk of infection (11, 47, 58a)

Viral Diseases

RABIES   Rabies is a viral disease that infects principally animals. Its primary reservoir consists of wild animals, including bats, raccoons, skunks, foxes, and mongooses; raccoons have become a significant source in parts of the United States (7, 30, 58a); and cats and horses are also potential reservoirs. Dogs are a major reservoir in many countries other than the United States, including Mexico. Dogs may become infected by bites or saliva of infected animals. In the United States, rabies has been well controlled by vaccinating dogs (and cats); in nonendemic areas, 0.1% or less of dogs and cats are rabid. In endemic areas of the United States, 0.1 to 2% of dogs are positive for rabies. In contrast, in developing countries and in parts of Mexico, up to 80% of tested dogs are positive and 90% of human rabies is transmitted by dogs. The infection is usually transmitted by biting, but the virus is present in saliva and is transmissible by licking. Most dogs and cats become ill within five days. Diagnoses can be made by demonstrating viral antigen in the brain.

The incubation period in humans is variable but averages two months.

Symptoms include central nervous system manifestations, commonly including dysphagia and convulsions, with a fatality rate approaching 100% (47, 58a).

Although there is considerable fear of rabies transmission from dogs, since untreated rabies is uniformly fatal, the disease is quite rare in the United States (except along the Mexican border); only 200 cases are reported annually despite a population of 50 million dogs. Treatment is typically delayed while the dog or cat from a low-risk area (i.e. there are very few positive tests, and the animals are typically vaccinated also) is confined for observation for ten days.

Treatment consists of three phases, each of which must be done properly: (a) clean the wound extensively with soap and water (which alone substantially reduces risk); and, if a decision is made to treat, (b) administer rabies immune globulin both into the wound and in the gluteal area and (c) with a separate syringe, administer one of two approved rabies vaccines (human diploid-cell rabies vaccine and rabies vaccine absorbed), on days 3, 7, 14, and 28, intramuscularly in the deltoid area. Treatment is begun as soon as possible after exposure, but empirical data indicate that the average delay after exposure is five days, yet treatment is fully effective. A genetically engineered oral rabies vaccine is currently being tested in humans.

LYMPHOCYTIC CHORIOMENINGITIS   This is a chronic infection occurring in hamsters and other rodents. Humans are infected by inhalation or ingestion of dust or food contaminated with virus from urine, feces, blood, or nasopharygeal secretions of rodents. Pet hamsters have been implicated as the source of some human infections (16). Surveys indicate that 5% of individuals in large cities in the United States have serologic evidence of infection. Most infections of adults cause mild disease, although some patients develop meningitis. Lymphocytic choriomeningitis virus infection of pregnant women results in transmission of the infection to the fetus. Fetal infection may be complicated by hydrocephalus and chorioretinitis.

Literature Cited

1. Deleted in proof
2. Deleted in proof
3. Deleted in proof
4. Altekruse SF, Hunt JM, Tollefson LK, Madden JM. 1994. Food and animal sources of human *Campylobacter jejuni* infection. *J. Am. Vet. Med. Assoc.* 204: 57–61
5. Anderson CR. 1992. Animal bites: guidelines to current management. *Anim. Bites* 92:134–49
6. Avner D, Woodfolk JA, Platts-Mills

TAE. 1995. Washing cats: quantitation of Fel dl allergen removed by water immersion. *J. Allergy Clin. Immunol.* 95:262 (Abstr.)

7. Baevsky RH, Bartfield JM. 1993. Human rabies: a review. *Am. J. Emer. Med.* 11:279–86

8. Deleted in proof

9. Beck AM. 1991. The epidemiology and prevention of animal bites. *Semin. Vet. Med. Surg. (Small Anim.)* 6:186–91

10. Benson V, Marano MA. 1994. *Current Estimates from the National Health Interview Survey,* 1993. Natl. Cent. Health Stat. Vital Health Stat. 10 (190)

11. Beran GW. 1993. Zoonoses in practice. *Vet. Clin. N. Am. Small Anim. Pract.* 23:1085–1107

12. Buijs J, Boorsboom G, van Germund JJ, Hazebroek A, van Dongen PAM, et al. 1994. Toxocara seroprevalence in 5-year-old elementary schoolchildren: relation with allergic asthma. *Am. J. Epidemiol.* 140:839–47

13. Call RS, Ward G, Jackson S, Platts-Mills TAE. 1994. Investigating severe and fatal asthma. *J. Allergy Clin. Immunol.* 94:1065–72

13a. Cent. Dis. Control Prevent. 1992. Human psittacosis linked to a bird distributor in Mississippi-Massachusetts and Tennessee, 1992. *Morbid. Mortal. Wkly. Rep.* 41:794–97

14. Cent. Dis. Control Prevent. 1995. Reptile-associated salmonellosis—selected states, 1994–1995. *Morbid. Mortal. Wkly. Rep.* 44:347–50

15. Cent. Dis. Control Prevent. 1995. USPHS/IDSA guidelines for the prevention of opportunistic infections in persons infected with human immunodeficiency virus: a summary. *Morbid. Mortal. Wkly. Rep.* 44:1–34

16. Chomel BB. 1992. Zoonoses of house pets other than dogs, cats and birds. *Pediatr. Infect. Dis. J.* 11:479–87

17. Chomel BB, Jay MT, Smith CR, Kass PH, Ryan CP, Barrett LR. 1994. Serological surveillance of plague in dogs and cats, California, 1979–1991. *Comp. Immunol. Microbiol. Infect. Dis.* 17:111–23

18. Cohen ML, Potter M, Pollard R, Feldman RA. 1980. Turtle-associated salmonellosis in the United States. Effect of public health action, 1970 to 1976. *JAMA* 243:1247–49

19. Craven RB, Maupin GO, Beard ML, Quan TJ, Barnes AM. 1993. Reported cases of human plague infections in the United States, 1970–1991. *J. Med. Entomol.* 30:758–61

20. Croese J, Loukas A, Opdebeeck J, Fairley S, Prociv P. 1994. Human enteric infection with canine hookworms. *Ann. Intern. Med.* 120:369–74

21. Croese J, Loukas A, Opdebeeck J, Prociv P. 1994. Occult enteric infection by *Ancylostoma caninum*: a previously unrecognized zoonosis. *Gastroenterology* 106:3–12

22. Custovic A, Taggart SCO, Woodcock A. 1994. House dust mite and cat allergen in different indoor environments. *Clin. Exp. Allergy* 24:1164–68

23. Dalton C. 1995. Iguana-associated salmonellosis in children. *Pediatr. Infect. Dis. J.* 14:319–20

23a. Dep. Health Hum. Serv. 1991. *Guidelines for the diagnosis and management of asthma.* Natl. Asthma Educ.Program Expert Panel Rep. DHHS Publ. No. (PHS) 91–3042

24. Desjardins A, Benoit C, Ghezzo H, L'Archeveque J, Leblanc C, et al. 1993. Exposure to domestic animals and risk of immunologic sensitization in subjects with asthma. *J. Allergy Clin. Immunol.* 91:979–86

25. Dire DJ. 1992. Emergency management of dog and cat bite wounds. *Emer. Med. Clin. N. Am.* 10:719–36

26. Duff AL, Platts-Mills TAE. 1992. Allergens and asthma. *Pediatr. Clin. N. Am.* 39:1277–91

27. Eggleston PA, Wood RA. 1992. Management of allergies to animals. *Allergy Proc.* 6:289–92

28. Fink JN. 1992. Hypersensitivity pneumonitis. *Clin. Chest Med.* 13:303–9

29. Fink JN. 1993. Hypersensitivity pneumonitis. In *Allergy, Principles and Practice,* ed. E Middleton Jr, CE Reed, EF Ellis, NF Adkinson Jr, JW Yunginger, WW Busse, pp. 1415–31. St. Louis: Mosby. 4th ed.

30. Fishbein DB, Robinson LE. 1993. Rabies. *N. Engl. J. Med.* 329:1632–38

31. Gasper PW, Barnes AM, Quan TJ, Benziger JP, Carter LG, et al. 1993. Plague (*Yersinia pestis*) in cats: description of experimentally induced disease. *J. Med. Entomol.* 30:20–26

32. Gergen PJ, Turkeltaub PC. 1992. The association of individual allergen reactivity with respiratory disease in a national sample: data from the second National Health and Nutrition Examination Survey, 1976080 (NHANES II). *J. Allergy Clin. Immunol.* 90:579–88

33. Gershman KA, Sacks JJ, Wright JC. 1994. Which dogs bite? A case-control study of risk factors. *Pediatrics* 93:913–17

34. Glaser CA, Angulo FJ, Rooney JA. 1994. Animal-associated opportunistic

infections among persons infected with the human immunodeficiency virus. *Clin. Infect. Dis.* 18:14–24

35. Glickman LT, Magnaval JF. 1993. Zoonotic roundworm infections. *Infect. Dis. Clin. N. Am.* 7:717–32
36. Goldstein EJC. 1992. Bite wounds and infection. *Clin. Infect. Dis.* 14:633–40
37. Haugaard L, Dahl R. 1992. Immunotherapy in patients allergic to cat and dog dander. I. Clinical results. *Allergy* 47:249–54
38. Hide DW, Matthews S, Matthews L, Stevens M, Ridout S, et al. 1994. Effect of allergen avoidance in infancy on allergic manifestations at age two years. *J. Allergy Clin. Immunol.* 93:842–46
39. Jackson LA, Perkins BA, Wenger JD. 1993. Cat scratch disease in the United States: an analysis of three national databases. *Am. J. Public Health* 83:1707–11
40. Johnson MA, Nemeth A, Condez A, Clarke SW, Poulter LW. 1989. Cell-mediated immunity in pigeon breeders lung: the effect of removal from antigen exposure. *Eur. Respir. J.* 2:444–50
41. Klucka CV, Ownby DR, Green J, Zoratti E. 1995. Cat shedding of Fel d 1 is not reduced by washings, Allerpet-C spray, or acepromazine. *J. Allergy Clin. Immunol.* 95:1164–71
42. Koehler JE, Glaser CA, Tappero JW. 1994. *Rochalimaea henselae* infection. A new zoonosis with the domestic cat as reservoir. *JAMA* 271:531–35
43. Lappin MR. 1993. Feline zoonotic diseases. *Vet. Clin. N. Am. Small Anim. Pract.* 23:57–78
44. Liles WC, Burger RJ. 1993. Tularemia from domestic cats. *West. J. Med.* 158:619–22
45. Long A, Sparrow D, Weiss ST, O'Connor G, Ardman BS, Jones N, et al. 1995. Sensitization to cat allergen is associated with asthma in older men and predicts airway hyperresponsiveness. *J. Allergy Clin. Immunol. 1995;* 95:185 (Abstr.)
46. Luczynska CM, Li Y, Chapman MD, Platts-Mills TAE. 1990. Airborne concentrations and particle size distribution of allergen derived from domestic cats (*Felis domesticus*). *Am. Rev. Respir. Dis.* 141:361–67
47. Mandell GL, Bennett JE, Dolin R, eds. 19XX. *Mandell, Douglas and Bennett's Principles and Practice of Infectious Diseases.* New York: Churchill Livingstone. 4th ed.

48. Marks MB. 1984. Respiratory tract allergy to household pet birds. *Ann. Allergy* 52:56–57
49. Munir AKM, Einarsson R, Dreborg SKG. 1995. Mite (Der-p-I, Der-f-I), cat (Fel-d-I) and dog (Can-f-I) allergens in dust from Swedish day-care centers. *Clin. Exp. Allergy* 25:119–26
50. Munir AKM, Bjorksten B, Einarsson R, Schou C, Ekstrand-Tobin A, et al. 1994. Cat (Fel-d-I), dog (Can-f-I), and cockroach allergens in homes of asthmatic children from three climatic zones in Sweden. *Allergy* 49:508–16
51. Munir AKM, Einarsson R, Dreborg SKG. 1994. Indirect contact with pets can confound the effect of cleaning procedures for reduction of animal allergen levels in house dust. *Pediatr. Allergy Immunol.* 5:32–39
52. Munir AKM, Einarsson R, Schou C, Dreborg SKG. 1993. Allergens in school dust. I. The amount of the major cat (Fel d I) and dog (Can F I) allergens in dust from Swedish schools is high enough to probably cause perennial symptoms in most children with asthma who are sensitized to cat and dog. *J. Allergy Clin. Immunol.* 91:1067–74
53. Newill CA, Eggleston PA, Prenger VL, Fish JE, Diamond EL, et al. 1995. Prospective study of occupational asthma to laboratory animal allergens: stability of airway responsiveness to methacholine challenge for one year. *J. Allergy Clin. Immunol.* 95:707–15
54. Ohman JL Jr, Sparrow D, MacDonald MR. 1993. New onset wheezing in an older male population: evidence of allergen sensitization in a longitudinal study. Results of the normative aging study. *J. Allergy Clin. Immunol.* 91:752–57
55. Ohman JL, Findlay SR, Leiterman KM. 1984. Immunotherapy in cat-induced asthma. Double-blind trial with evaluation of in vivo and in vitro responses. *J. Allergy Clin. Immunol.* 74:230–39
56. Deleted in proof
57. Parish LC, Schwartzman RM. 1993. Zoonoses of dermatologic interest. *Semin. Dermatol.* 12:57–64
58. Patterson R. 1987. Diagnosis of animal allergy. *N. Engl. Reg. Allergy Proc.* 8:167–68
58a. Peter G, ed. 1994. *Red Book: Report of the Committee of Infectious Diseases.* Elk Grove, IL: Am. Acad. Pediatr. 23rd ed.
59. Platts-Mills TAE. 1993. Allergen-specific treatment for Asthma: III. *Am. Rev. Respir. Dis.* 148:553–55

60. Platts-Mills TAE, Chapman MD, Squillace SP, Sporik RB, Call RS, Heymann PW. 1993. The role of allergens. In *Asthma: Physiology, Immunopharmacology and Treatment, 4th. Int. Symp.*, pp. 27–39. New York: Academic

61. Platts-Mills TAE, Sporik RB, Wheatley LM, Heymann PW. 1995. Is there a dose-response relationship between exposure to indoor allergens and symptoms of asthma? *J. Allergy Clin. Immunol.* 96:435–40

62. Plaut M, Zimmerman EM. 1993. Allergy and mechanisms of hypersensitivity. In *Fundamental Immunology*, ed. WE Paul, pp. 1399–425. New York, Raven. 3rd ed.

63. Pollart SM, Chapman MD, Fiocco GP, Rose G, Platts-Mills TAE. 1989. Epidemiology of acute asthma: IgE antibodies to common inhalant allergens as a risk factor for emergency room visits. *J. Allergy Clin. Immunol.* 83:875–82

64. Reed KD, Moore FM, Geiger GE, Stemper ME. 1993. Zoonotic transmission of sporotrichosis: case report and review. *Clin. Infect. Dis.* 16:384–87

65. Reynolds SP, Jones KP, Edwards JH, Davies BH. 1993. Inhalation challenge in pigeon breeder's disease: BAL fluid changes after 6 hours. *Eur. Respir. J.* 6:467–76

66. Rodriguez de Castro F, Carrillo T, Castillo R, Blanco C, Diaz F, et al. 1993. Relationships between characteristics of exposure to pigeon antigen. *Chest* 103:1059–63

67. Saeed AM, Harris NV, DiGiacomo RF. 1993. The role of exposure to animals in the etiology of *Camplyobacter jejuni/coli* enteritis. *Am. J. Epidemiol.* 137:108–14

68. Schad GA. 1994. Hookworms: pets to humans. *Ann. Intern. Med.* 120:434–35

69. Schlossberg D, Delgado J, Moore M, Wishner A, Mohn J. 1993. An epidemic of avian and human psittacosis. *Arch. Intern. Med.* 153:2594–96

70. Schwartz BS, Goldstein MD, Childs JE. 1994. Longitudinal study of *Borrelia burgdorferi* infection in New Jersey outdoor workers, 1988–1991. *Am. J. Epidemiol.* 139:504–12

71. Sears MR, Hervison GP, Holdaway MD, Hewitt CJ, Flannery EM, Silva PA. 1989. The relative risks of sensitivity to grass pollen, house dust mite, and cat dander in the development of childhood asthma. *Clin. Exp. Allergy* 19:419–24

72. Shaw R, Woodman K, Crane J, Moyes C, Kennedy J, Pearce N. 1994. Risk factors for asthma symptoms in Kawerau children. *NZ Med. J.* 107:387–91

73. Siraganian RP. 1987. Allergy to animals: principles of clinical management. *N. Engl. Reg. Allergy Proc.* 8:181–83

74. Slavin RG. 1987. Clinical aspects of allergies to animals: overview and definition. *N. Engl. Reg. Allergy Proc.* 8:163–66

75. Smith RP Jr, Rand PW, Lacombe EH, Telford SR III, Rich SM, et al. 1993. Norway rats as reservoir hosts for Lyme disease spirochetes on Monhegan Island, Maine. *J. Infect. Dis.* 168:687–91

76. Sporik R, Ingram JM, Price W, Sussman JH, Honsinger RW, Platts-Mills TA. 1995. Association of asthma with serum IgE and skin test reactivity to allergens among children living at high altitude. Tickling the dragon's breath. *Am. J. Respir. Crit. Care Med.* 151:1388–92

77. Tauer-Reich I, Fruhmann G, Czuppon AB, Baur X. 1994. Allergens causing bird fancier's asthma. *Allergy* 49:448–53

78. Deleted in proof

79. Todd A, Coan R, Allen A. 1993. Pigeon breeders' lung; IgG subclasses to pigeon intestinal mucin and IgA antigens. *Clin. Exp. Immunol.* 92:494–99

80. Tompkins LS. 1994. Rochalimaea infections: are they zoonoses? *JAMA* 271:553–54

81. Van Metre TE Jr, Marsh DG, Adkinson NF Jr, Fish JE, Kagey-Sobotka A, et al. 1986. Dose of cat (*Felis domesticus*) allergen 1 (Fel d I) that induces asthma. *J. Allergy Clin. Immunol.* 78:62–75

82. Van Metre TE Jr, Marsh DG, Adkinson NF Jr, Kagey-Sobotka A, Khattignavong A, et al. 1988. Immunotherapy for cat asthma. *J. Allergy Clin. Immunol.* 82:1055–68

83. Van Toorenenbergen AW, Van Wijk RG, Van Dooremalen G, Dieges PH. 1985. Immunoglobulin E antibodies against budgerigar and canary feathers. *Int. Arch. Allergy Appl. Immunol.* 77:433–37

84. Warner JA, Marchant JL, Warner JO. 1993. Allergen avoidance in the homes of atopic asthmatic children: the effect of Allersearch DMS. *Clin. Exp. Allergy* 23:279–86

85. Wood RA, Eggleston PA. 1995. The Effects of intranasal steroids on nasal and pulmonary responses to cat expo-

sure. *Am. J. Respir. Crit. Care Med.*
151:315–20

86. Wood RA, Mudd KE, Eggleston PA.
1992. The distribution of cat and dust
mite allergens on wall surfaces. *J. Allergy Clin. Immunol.* 89:126–30

87. Zangwill KM, Hamilton DH, Perkins
BA, Regnery RL, Plikaytis BD, Hadler
JL, et al. 1993. Cat scratch disease in
Connecticut. Epidemiology, risk factors,
and evaluation of a new diagnostic test.
N. Engl. J. Med. 329:8–13

Annu. Rev. Public Health. 1996. 17:247–57

HEALTH ENHANCEMENT AND COMPANION ANIMAL OWNERSHIP

Alan M. Beck[1] and N. Marshall Meyers[2]

[1]School of Veterinary Medicine, Purdue University West Lafayette, Indiana
47907-1243 and [2]Pet Industry Joint Advisory Council, 1220 19th Street, N.W.,
Washington, D.C. 20036

KEY WORDS: animals interaction, pets, epidemiology

ABSTRACT

The relationship between people and companion animals, on the one hand,
explains the bites and zoonotic diseases that occur among those with companion
animals and, on the other hand, appears to enhance the psychological and physiological well-being of many people. Presently, no less than 56% of households
in the United States have animals, typical of developed countries around the
world. It is well documented that people denied human contact do not thrive
well. All indications are that companion animals play the role of a family
member, often a member with the most desired attributes. Animals play special
roles for children, aiding the teaching of nurturing behavior and appreciation of
nonverbal communication. Ordinary interactions with animals can reduce blood
pressure and alter survival after a heart attack. For some, pets increase the
opportunities to meet people, while for others pets permit them to be alone
without being lonely.

Introduction

In 1994, no less that 56% of U.S. households (53 million) have companion
animals and more than half of these owners have more than one animal (1).
In addition to animals that live in the home, 2% of the households own an
average of 2.54 horses for a horse population of 4.9 million, down, in 1991,
from 6.6 million horses four years earlier (2).

In Australia, approximately 60% of the 6.2 million households have one or
more pets; 53% of the households have either a dog or a cat (44). Examples
of dog, cat, and/or bird ownership in European households include Belgium
(71%), France (63%), Netherlands (60%), Britain (55%), Italy (61%), Germany
(West) (37%), Ireland (70%), and for all 17 European countries surveyed (52%)

247

Table 1   U.S. Animal ownership and population estimates, 1991

Species	Households with at least one animal (percent)	Estimated population of species (millions)
Dogs	38.2	55.0
Cats	32.3	63.8
Caged birds	7.7	31.0
Small animals	5.0	12.2*
Reptiles	3.0	7.3*
Freshwater fish	10.0	82.7*
Marine fish	0.6	4.6*
Total	56.0	256.6

*Unpublished industry data and U.S. Fish and Wildlife Service import data indicate substantially greater populations. For example, current Iguana imports approximate 800,000 animals annually; domestic ferret population estimated at 5 million animals; reptiles are the fastest growing area with more than 4 million reptiles imported annually. Source: References 2, 36, 50.

(52). All existing cultures keep pets, although the favorite species vary. The sheer numbers of pet animals is only one facet of the "pet phenomenon"; one also has to appreciate who are the benefactors of the "pet experience" (11). As clearly demonstrated by the data, companion pet ownership is neither rare nor random; it is an integral part of society (see Table 1).

Changing social attitudes toward companion pets, along with changing lifestyles, influence decisions regarding ownership. Major demographic trends, notably smaller households, aging populations, coupled with increasingly hectic lifestyles and reduced leisure time, are altering pet population demographics. While more U.S. households own dogs than any other pet, the number of households with a dog or cat is declining (50). Conversely, ownership of birds, small animals, reptiles, and freshwater fish is increasing (1).

In the United States, the people who associate with pets tend to be younger than the general population; dogs, cats, and small mammals are far more common in families that have children. For instance, while young and middle-aged people without children compose 5.2% and 10.9%, respectively, of all U.S. households, only 4.3% and 8.1% of these households, respectively, have any pet, which is less than expected. However, young and middle-aged parents with children at home compose 12.6% and 12.9% of all households, and of these 14.6% and 17.5%, respectively, have a pet—more than expected (2). It is believed the same general pattern exists among European countries (44).

Children with pets in their homes enjoy more leisure activities and work not related with school than their counterparts. Pets are a common and relatively important feature of children's social network (41). Children also learn important values and attitudes from animals. By preschool, children can appreciate the differences between dogs, cats, puppies, and kittens. They begin to understand the role of the adult animals as caregivers for baby animals. Boys as they mature usually increase their knowledge of and caring for animals, while there is typically a decline in their interest and care for human infants (42). Boys, in particular, may be helped to understand the importance of nurturing by watching pet behaviors and by interacting with their pets. Pets are nonjudgmental in their love and facilitate a child's learning about responsibility. There is even evidence that the mere presence of animals positively alters children's attitudes about themselves and increases their ability to relate to others (39, 45). Animals as varied as dogs, birds, and spiders facilitate social interaction and are catalysts for social and verbal interaction. Live animals are focal points of interest; toy animals do not hold a child's interest in the same degree (47).

Animals are perceived to be especially valued as companions for older adults (15, 24, 48, 53, 58, 59). Animals may replace children who have grown and moved away or perhaps those who were never born. They may afford opportunities for an increase of human-to-human social interaction and, finally, they may permit older adults to live alone without being lonely.

Various studies have found that the household pet is perceived to be a member of the family, sharing many of the attributes of a favored family member. It is typical to talk to the animal as if it were a person. Carrying its photograph and sharing a bedroom are also within the norm (8). While nearly half of adults confide in their pet, more than 70% of adolescents do so (10, 30, 31).

At the very least, interaction with animals positively influences transient physiological states, resulting in improved morale. The impact may be mediated directly, involving physiological functions like blood pressure, or by influencing the person's psychological well-being (e.g. improving morale and lessening risky behaviors) or psychosocial interactions with others. Besides immediate changes in blood pressure and feelings of well-being, there appear to be long-term effects of animal interaction, most notably influencing the attitudes and behaviors of young children. "The basis for the positive effect of health and well-being resulting from the interactions with a pet has come to be known as the companion-animal bond or the human-companion animal bond" (51). Preserving the bond between people and their animals, like encouraging good nutrition and exercise, appears to be in the best interests of those concerned with public health.

Epidemiological Findings

There is a long history of using animals as sentinels for humans at risk. "Birds and mice may be used to detect carbon monoxide, because they are much more sensitive to the poisonous action of the gas than are men" (14).

Epidemiological studies of pet animals with spontaneously occurring disease could serve as sentinels and supplement human epidemiological research (6). Compared with humans, animal diseases have a shorter latency after exposure and occur with less confounding factors, such as occupational or self-selected exposures like workplace pollutants or smoking tobacco. In contrast to laboratory experiments, spontaneous tumors in pets reflect natural exposures to a wide variety of environmental carcinogens; pets could therefore be sentinels for the humans that share the home (25, 46).

Companion animals may receive detailed physical evaluations comparable to those of their owners. The veterinary community stands ready to be part of the human health research team, but for the most part is rarely asked to participate. Companion animals are an unrecognized alternative to study many of the health problems facing people today (6).

While there is no clearly identified *single* explanation for the positive effect pets have on their owners, there is growing epidemiologic evidence that people who feel an attachment for nature (57) or for companion animals have lessened risks of disease and disease processes compared with people without such experiences (8). It is well documented that people denied good human contact and interaction do not thrive well (40). One way people can be protected from the ravages of loneliness is through animal companionship.

A 1980 report first documented the value of pet ownership. A study of people hospitalized after a heart attack found that ownership of any animal correlated with improved survival: 94% of those who owned pets were alive after the first year compared with 72% of those who did not own any animal. A discriminate analysis demonstrated that pet ownership accounted for 2–3% of the variance (22). Although 2–3% may seem small, the impact is significant and cost effective considering the frequency of heart disease.

A more recent study of the benefits of interactions with animals found that pet owners had reductions in some common risk factors for cardiovascular disease, lower systolic blood pressures, plasma cholesterol, and triglyceride values (3). Socioeconomic profiles of the two groups were very similar and although pet owners engaged in more exercise, they also ate more meat and "take-out" foods.

Physiological Effects

Differences were observed in the way pet owners talk to their animals by species (28, 30); these are influenced by the handling needs of the animals and social stereotypes, but people find comfort in talking to their animals (32, 33). Unlike talking to other humans, people experience a decrease of blood pressure talking to pets, indicating that they are more relaxed than with people (5, 23, 33). Even in the presence of unfamiliar dogs, people experience a temporary decrease in blood pressure (23). Blood pressure also decreases for people with normal pressures and those with hypertension when watching fish in a standard aquarium; systolic and diastolic levels for hypertensive subjects often fall within normal ranges. The decreased physiological arousal indicated by the reduction of blood pressure is associated with stereotypical changes in facial expression and vocal pattern; the face becomes more relaxed with a decrease in muscle tension, especially around the eyes (29), and subjects talking to their companion dogs, cats, and birds talk more slowly and with a more relaxed mode (30), which, in itself, tends to reduce blood pressure.

Psychological/Social Effects

It has been hypothesized that pet ownership improves survival because it influences psychosocial risk factors that lessen the risk of coronary heart disease (49).

The general tendency to overestimate the importance of personal factors relative to environmental considerations in making judgments about a person or situation is well recognized and has been named "the fundamental attribution error" (53a, 53b, 60). A good example is that people perceive others observed in the company of animals more positively and with more favorable attributes than observed without animals present. This "fundamental attribution error" occurs when people are observed live or in photographs (39). Our experimental observations of normal and handicapped subjects in public situations, and anecdotal accounts of the behavior of politicians, suggest that the presence of pet animals improves the social attractiveness of human subjects.

There may also be less dramatic effects from pet ownership than increasing survival rates or reducing anxiety. Serpell (54) reported that dog owners experienced fewer minor health problems and increased the number and durations of their recreational walks. The effects persisted over the ten-month study period and there was no clear explanation for the results.

Many naturally occurring events are enhanced by animal companionship. People walking with their dog experience more social contact and longer conversations than when walking alone (45). Even rabbits and turtles can encourage approaches by other people and stimulate conversations between children and unfamiliar adults in a community park setting (27). Wilson (58) reported that companion animals alleviate anxiety and relax college students of all ages and races.

Probably the most conclusive study of the stress-managing value of animal interaction used subjects who were scheduled for molar extractions at a School of Dental Medicine. People who contemplated an aquarium underwent dental surgery very much like those who were hypnotized prior to the procedure (34). Although measuring the anxiolytic effect of a pet on a human companion is not a simple task, there appears to be a real effect (12).

Companion animals could have a positive impact on societal health. Katcher & Wilkins (35) used carefully designed educational programs structured around animal contact with children who had attention-deficit hyperactive disorders (ADHD) and defiant disorders (CD). The children in the animal contact groups had better attendance and improved measurements in a variety of knowledge and skills objectives. The children whose educational experiences included animal contact exhibited significantly less antisocial and violent behavior.

Abusing animals and abusing other humans are related behaviors (4, 19). Prisoners with crimes involving aggression to others are statistically more likely to have a history of multiple acts of cruelty to animals than noncriminals or those whose crimes did not involve violence (37). Nearly a century ago, Sigmund Freud (21) suggested that clinicians attend to "children who are distinguished by evincing especial cruelty to animals and playmates," but it was not until 1987 that cruelty to animals was added to the list of diagnostic criteria for *Conduct Disorders in the Diagnostic and Statistical Manual of Mental Disorder,* 3rd revised (DSM-III-R).

If being cruel to animals is associated with being cruel to people, it is reasonable to hypothesize the opposite effect, i.e. that good animal contact reduces anti-social behavior. There is a need to assess the widespread but largely untested belief that we should teach children to be kind to animals. For example, children exposed to humane education programs displayed enhanced empathy for humans compared with children who were not exposed to such programs (4).

One long-recognized but often ignored value of animal contact is that many people find joy and even humor in interacting with animals. Animals often permit people to laugh at themselves or at their surroundings; note the role animals play in cartoon humor. The writer Norman Cousins described the role of laughter in diminishing pain, even reducing the inflammatory process that afflicted him (17). McCulloch observed that animals owned by his psychiatric outpatients played a clear and identified role in their lives; the animals helped all the patients to laugh and maintain a sense of humor (43). Laughter, or at least encouragement to find humor, is a recognized medical intervention, and animals are a frequent source of that humor.

Animals As Therapy

In the last few years, popular and scientific discussion of pet therapy or, more appropriately, Animal Facilitated Therapy (AFT) has flourished. Much of the early literature documents nothing more than fortuitous interactions with animals that happen to be present in a therapeutic setting (8). There were no scientific goals or expected effects other than what normally occurs when people and animals interact (9). The animals were to provide a diversion from routines in institutional settings or companionship to those living alone.

In one study, nearly 1000 noninstitutionalized older adult Medicare patients were evaluated prospectively. Those subjects who owned pets appeared to experience less distress and to require fewer visits to their physicians than nonowners. While animal ownership generally had value, the most remarkable benefits to health were for dog owners (55). Most people noted that the pets provided them with companionship and a sense of security and the opportunity for fun/play and relaxation. Animals allowed people to experience bonding. Siegel (56) suggested that pets have a stress-reducing effect. As a result, support has grown for protecting the right of pet ownership for senior citizens living in the community and for encouraging animal contact for patients in long-term nursing home settings.

Animals can also play a role in improving the well-being of people of all ages who are stigmatized or whose special needs make them less able to function in normal settings. Kidd & Kidd (38) interviewed 105 homeless people and noted the importance of pets for companionship, friendship, and love for this population, although the provision of food and veterinary care for the animals was a problem. Wheelchair-users were more likely to experience positive social interactions when with a dog (26, 18). Psychiatric inpatients were more comfortable talking and participating in group therapy sessions in the presence of birds than in the same room with no animals present (13). Animals are becoming a frequent adjunctive in many therapeutic settings, for all ages and for a wide variety of circumstances (8).

Conclusion

Animals have been part of human households since humans started living in villages, some 12,000 years ago. Interaction with companion animals may well be one of our more successful strategies for survival. All cultures have maintained a commitment to carrying for and protecting animals kept solely for companionship. Today, animals continue to play a major role in the lives of many people. Nevertheless, the medical history of our relationship with animals documents mostly the detrimental effects of animal contact, addressing allergies, infectious diseases, zoonoses, parasitism, and traumatic injury from bites and kicks. To be sure, animal contact carries risk, but the frequency of most zoonotic diseases can be lessened, even eliminated, with animal management practices that would serve both humans and the animals themselves. Veterinary care to manage bacterial, viral, and parasitic infections, mechanical restraints like leashes and cages, selective breeding, responsible legislation, and owner education have made animal ownership a safe and rewarding experience for many.

The reports by Friedmann et al (22) and Anderson et al (3) have not promoted interest in funding studies on the links between human-animal interactions and cardiovascular health. The reports have had a limited impact on subsequent cardiovascular research since few researchers have added questions about pet ownership and attachment to animals. One independent ancillary study to the Coronary Arrhythmia Suppression Trial (CAST) (16), a National Institutes of Health (NIH) clinical trial, is finding that pet ownership, lower anxiety, and social support are all associated with an increased likelihood of one-year survival after a myocardial infarction (23a).

Research on human-animal interactions is needed for reasonably large study populations. Most grants to study human-animal interactions are for less than $10,000, whereas large epidemiological studies are much more expensive. Such an amount would be sufficient to support the addition of a few questions on human-animal interactions to larger epidemiological surveys, but only if those controlling the large study are supportive; they are usually not.

The lack of funding is not exclusive to the study of human-animal interactions. People who pray and participate more actively in their religions have better health at all ages. People associated with conservative religious affiliations have poorer health than those with more liberal affiliations (20). While society generally believes that being religious is valuable to health, there have been few studies (12). There is stronger evidence for the benefit of animal contact than there is for the benefit of being religious, yet we still have trouble accepting animals as more than the "therapeutic clown" of society (8).

At the final presentation of the 1987 NIH Technology Assessment Workshop, *Health Benefits of Pets,* Beck & Glickman (7) proposed that "All future studies of human health should consider the presence or absence of a pet in the home and, perhaps, the nature of this relationship with the pet, as a significant variable. No future study of human health should be considered comprehensive if the animals with which they share their lives are not included."

In sum, there is substantial evidence to support the positive benefits of animal companionship for various segments of the population, especially children, the elderly, socially isolated, and the handicapped. Research needs to be directed to establish both the scope of these benefits and ways to channel them more effectively to improve the public health of the community.

Literature Cited

1. American Pet Products Manufacturers Association (APPMA). 1994. *1994 National Pet Owners Survey*. Scarsdale, NY; NFO Research, Inc.
2. American Veterinary Medical Association (AVMA). 1993. *US Pet Ownership and Demographic Sourcebook*. Schaumburg, IL: Cent. Inform. Manage.
3. Anderson WP, Reid CM, Jennings GL. 1992. Pet ownership and risk factors for cardiovascular disease. *Med. J. Aust.* 157:298–301
4. Ascione, FR. 1992. Enhancing children's attitudes about the humane treatment of animals: generalization to human-directed empathy. *Anthrozoös* 5:176–91
5. Baun MM, Bergstrom, N, Langston NF, Thoma L. 1984. Physiological effects of petting dogs: influences of attachment. In *The Pet Connection*, ed. RK Anderson, BL Hart, LA Hart, 18:162–70. Minneapolis: Univ. Minnesota Press. 451 pp.
6. Beck AM. 1995. Animals and Society. In *The World Congress on Alternatives and Animal Use in Life Sciences: Education, Research, Testing*, ed. A Goldberg, LFM Van Zutphen, H:59–64, New York: Mary Ann Liebert
7. Beck AM, Glickman LT. 1987. Future research on pet facilitated therapy: a plea for comprehension before intervention. *Health Benefits of Pets*, NIH Technol. Assess. Workshop, Sept. 10–11
8. Beck AM, Katcher AH. 1983. *Between Pets and People: The Importance of Animal Companionship*. New York: Putman. 317 pp.
9. Beck AM, Katcher AH. 1984. A new look at pet-facilitated therapy. *J. Am. Vet. Med. Assoc.* 184:414–21
10. Beck AM, Katcher AH. 1989. Bird-human interacton. *J. Assoc. Avian Vet.* 3:152–53
11. Beck AM, Meyers NM. 1987. The pet owner experience. *N. Engl. Reg. Allergy Proc.* 8:29–31
12. Beck AM, Rowan AN. 1994. The health benefits of human-animal interactions. *Anthrozoös* 7:85–89
13. Beck AM, Serarydarian L, Hunter GF. 1986. Use of animals in the rehabilitation of psychiatric inpatients. *Psychol. Rep.* 58:63–66
14. Burrell GA, Seibert FM. 1916. *Gases Found in Coal Mines, Miner's Circular*

14. Bur. Mines, Washington, DC: Dep. Interior
15. Bustad LK. 1980. *Animals, Aging, and the Aged*. Minneapolis: Univ. Minnesota Press. 227 pp.
16. CAST. 1989. The Coronary Arrhythmia Suppression Trial Investigators. Preliminary report: effect of encainide and flexainide on mortality in a randomized trail of arrhythmia suppression after myocardial infarction. *N. Engl. J. Med.* 321:406–12
17. Cousins N. 1979. *Anatomy of an Illness as Perceived by the Patient: Reflections on Healing and Regeneration*. New York: Norton. 215 pp.
18. Eddy J, Hart LA, Bolts RP. 1988. The effects of service dogs on social acknowledgements of people in wheelchairs. *J. Psychol.* 122:39–45
19. Felthous AR, Kellert SR. 1986. Violence against animals and people: Is aggression against living creatures generalized? *Bull. Am. Acad. Psychiatr. Law* 14:55–69
20. Ferraro KF. Albrecht-Jensen CM. 1991. Does religion influence adult health? *J. Sci. Study Relig.* 30:193–202
20a. Fogle B, ed. 1981. *Interrelations Between People and Pets*. Springfield, IL: Charles C Thomas. 352 pp.
21. Freud S. 1905. Three contributions to the theory of sex. In *The Basic Writings of Sigmund Freud*, ed. AA Brill, 1938, pp. 594. New York: Random House
22. Friedmann E, Katcher AH, Lynch JJ, Thomas SS. 1980. Animal companions and one-year survival of patients after discharge from a coronary care unit. *Public Health Rep.* 95:307–12
23. Friedmann E, Katcher AH, Thomas SA, Lynch JJ Messent PR. 1983. Social interaction and blood pressure: influence of animal companions. *J. Nerv. Mental Dis.* 171:461–65
23a. Friedmann E, Thomas SA. 1995. Pet ownership, social support and one year survival after acute myocardial infarction in the cardiac suppression trial (CAST). *Am. J. Cardiol.* In press
24. Garrity TF, Stallones L, Marx MB, Johnson TP. 1989. Pet ownership and attachment as supportive factors in the health of the elderly. *Anthrozoös* 3:35–44
25. Glickman LT, Domanski LM. 1986. An alternative to laboratory animal experi-

mentation for human health risk assessment: epidemiological studies of pet animals. *ATLA* 13:267–85

26. Hart LA, Hart BL. 1987. Socializing effects of service dogs for people with disabilities. *Anthrozoös* 1:41–44

27. Hunt SJ, Hart LA, Gomulkiewicz R. 1992. The role of small animals in social interactions between strangers. *J. Soc. Psychol.* 132:245–56

28. Katcher AH. 1981. Interactions between people and their pets: form and function. See Ref. 20a, 3:41–67

28a. Katcher AH, Beck AM, eds. 1983. *New Perspectives on Our Lives with Companion Animals.* Philadelphia: Univ. Pennsylvania Press. 588 pp.

29. Katcher AH, Beck AM. 1983. Safety and intimacy: physiological and behavioral responses to interaction with companion animals. *The Human-Pet Relationship: Proc. Int. Symp. Occas. 80th Birthday Nobel Prize Winner Prof. DDr. Konrad Lorenz,* pp. 122–28. Vienna: IEMT

30. Katcher AH, Beck AM. 1986. Dialogue with animals. *Trans. Stud. Coll. Phys. Phila.* 8:105–12

31. Katcher AH, Beck AM. 1987. Health and caring for living things. *Anthrozoös* 1:175–83

32. Katcher AH, Beck AM. 1989. Human-animal communication. In *International Encyclopedia of Communica- tions,* ed. E Barnow, 2:295–96. London: Oxford Univ. Press

33. Katcher AH, Friedmann E, Beck AM, Lynch JJ. 1983. Looking, talking and blood pressure: the physiological consequences of interaction with the living environment. See Ref. 28a, 31:351–59

34. Katcher AH, Segal H, Beck AM. 1984. Comparison of contemplation and hypnosis for the reduction of anxiety and discomfort during dental surgery. *Am. J. Clin. Hypnosis* 27:14–21

35. Katcher A, Wilkins G. 1993. Dialogue with animals: its nature and culture. In *The Biophilia Hypothesis,* ed. SR Kellert, EO Wilson, 5:173–97. Washington, DC: Island Press. 484 pp.

36. Kaytee Products. 1994. *Bird Study.* Chilton, WI

37. Kellert S, Felthouse A. 1983. Noncriminals and criminals in Kansas and Connecticut. See Ref. 29, pp. 72–81.

38. Kidd AH, Kidd RM. 1994. Benefits and liabilities of pets for the homeless. *Psychol. Rep.* 74:715–22

39. Lockwood R. 1983. The influence of animals on social perception. See Ref. 28a, 8:64–71

40. Lynch JJ. 1977. *The Broken Heart: The Medical Consequences of Loneliness.* New York: Basic Books. 271 pp.

41. Melson GF. 1988. Availability of and involvement with pets by children: determinants and correlates. *Anthrozoös* 2:45–52

42. Melson, GF, Fogel A. 1989. Children's ideas about animal young and their care: a reassessment of gender differences in the development of nurturance. *Anthrozoös* 2:265–73

43. McCulloch MJ. 1981. The pet as prosthesis defining criteria for the adjunctive use of companion animals in the treatment of medically ill, depressed outpatients. See Ref. 20a, 6:101–23

44. McHarg M, Baldock C, Headey B, Robinson A. 1995. *National People and Pets Survey.* Urban Animal Management Coalition. Aust.

45. Messent PR. 1983. Social facilitation of contact with other people by pet dogs. See Ref. 28a, 5:37–46

46. National Research Council (NRC). 1991. *Animals As Sentinels of Environmental Health Hazards,* chair. LT Glickman. Washington, DC: Natl. Acad. Press

47. Neielsen JA, Delude LA. 1989. Behavior of young children in the presence of different kinds of animals. *Anthrozoös* 3:119–29

48. Ory MG, Goldberg EL. 1983. Pet possession and life satisfaction in elderly women. See Ref. 28a, 26:303–17

49. Patronek GJ, Glickman LT. 1993. Pet ownership protects the risks and consequences of coronary heart disease. *Med. Hypotheses* 40:245–49

50. Pet Food Institute. 1995. *US Pet Trends.* Washington, DC

51. Pritchard WR, ed. 1988. *Future Directions for Veterinary Medicine.* Durham, NC: Pew Natl. Vet. Educ. Progr.

52. Reader's Digest Association, Inc. 1991. *A Consumer Survey of 17 European Countries.* London: Reader's Digest Eurodata

53. Robb SS, Stegman CE. 1983. Companion animals and elderly people: a challenge for evaluation of social support. *Gerontologist* 23:277–82

53a. Ross L. 1977. The intuitive psychologist and his shortcomings: distortions in the attribution process. In *Advances in Experimental Social Psychology,* ed. L Berkowitz, pp. 173–220. New York: Academic

53b. Ross L, Nisbett RE. 1991. *The Person and the Situation.* Philadelphia: Temple Univ. Press

54. Serpell J. 1991. Beneficial effects of pet

ownership on some aspects of human health and behavior. *J. Roy. Soc. Med.* 84:717–20

55. Siegel JM. 1990. Stressful life events and use of physician services among the elderly: the moderating role of pet ownership. *J. Pers. Soc. Psychol.* 58:1081–86

56. Siegel JM. 1993. Companion animals: in sickness and in health. *J. Soc. Issues* 49:157–67

57. Ulrich RS. 1993. Biophilia, biophobia, and natural landscapes. See Ref. 35, 3:73–137.

58. Wilson CC, Netting FE. 1983. Companion animals and the elderly: a state-of-the-art summary. *J. Am. Vet. Med. Assoc.* 183:1425–29

59. Zasloff RL, Kidd AH. 1993. Loneliness and pet ownership among single women. *Psychol. Rep.* 75:747–52

60. Zebrowitz X. 1990. *Social Perception.* Pacific Grove, CA: Brooks/Cole. 231 pp.

Annu. Rev. Public Health. 1996. 17:259–73

CRACK COCAINE ABUSE: An Epidemic with Many Public Health Consequences[1]

James W. Cornish and Charles P. O'Brien

Department of Psychiatry, University of Pennsylvania, Philadelphia, Pennsylvania
19104; and Department of Veterans Affairs Medical Center, Philadelphia,
Pennsylvania 19104

KEY WORDS: substance abuse/dependence, toxicity, epidemiology, HIV, pregnancy

ABSTRACT

In the mid-1980s a new, smokable form of cocaine, called crack, was introduced
in the United States. Soon thereafter, it became apparent that crack cocaine abuse
was a serious and important public health concern. Over the past several years,
crack cocaine use has increasingly been associated with a myriad of immediate
and long-term adverse effects. Duing this same period, crack cocaine use has
progressively moved away from experimentation and recreational use to chronic
and compulsive drug use.

The aim of this chapter is to present several topics concerning compulsive
crack cocaine use that have particularly important consequences for public
health. Crack cocaine use associated with pregnancy and with sexually transmitted diseases is highlighted.

WHAT IS CRACK?

Despite the widespread use of crack cocaine, there is quite a bit of confusion
among the lay public regarding its definition. Therefore, it is important for
health care providers to educate the public that crack is cocaine that is in a
smokable form.

Until the late 1970s, the usual form of cocaine available on the street was
cocaine hydrochloride. This salt form of cocaine is usually sniffed (snorted)

---

[1]The US Government has the right to retain a nonexclusive, royalty-free license in and to any
copyright covering this paper.

nasally or mixed with water and injected intravenously. Occasionally, cocaine hydrochloride is combined with heroin and the mixture (called a "speedball") is injected. The hydrochloride salt can not be smoked because it is quickly destroyed at high temperatures. Cocaine is smokable in its freebase alkaloid form which is easily extracted from the hydrochloride salt (30). Freebase cocaine is generally prepared by one of two techniques. In one method the hydrochloride salt is first mixed with buffered ammonia, then the alkaloidal cocaine is extracted from the solution using ether, and finally the ether is evaporated to yield cocaine crystals. When heated the crystals liberate a vaporized cocaine that can be inhaled. Upon heating, the crystals make a popping sound and it is this characteristic sound that is the origin of the term "crack". This form of cocaine is very pure and is generally called "free base" on the street. The other method of producing free base cocaine is to combine cocaine hydrochloride with sodium bicarbonate (baking soda) and heat the solution until a solid forms. The resultant pieces of the solid, also called "rock", when heated release vaporized cocaine (30). Since the mid-1980s this has been the preferred method of production for smokable cocaine because it is simpler and safer than the ether extraction method. Today most of the available crack cocaine in the United States has been produced in this manner.

HISTORY

It is ironic yet important to know that our country had suffered through a previous cocaine epidemic. From the 1880s to the early 1900s, there was an epidemic of cocaine use in the United States and also in Europe. Some of the purported therapeutic uses for cocaine began to appear in the early 1880s. In his 1884 paper entitled *On Cocaine,* Sigmund Freud recommended that cocaine be used as a local anesthetic, an aphrodisiac and as a pharmacotherapy for depression, alcoholism and morphine addiction (18). Unfortunately, some of the patients who had substituted cocaine for either alcohol or morphine, subsequently became addicted to cocaine. By 1887 Freud had changed his opinion on the merits of cocaine and wrote an article in which he said that cocaine was much more dangerous for public health than morphine (5). During this time there was widespread use of cocaine and it was touted as a treatment for almost every imaginable illness. Cocaine could be found in a variety of goods ranging from patent medicines and tonics to soft drinks, In 1886 John Styth Pemberton, a druggist, formulated the syrup base for Coca-Cola. He blended a whole-leaf extract of coca with an extract from the African kola nut which is also a stimulant. Coca-Cola was initially manufactured and marketed as medicine. Later it was touted as a temperance drink despite the fact that cocaine was still a key ingredient. The manufacturer believed that their product should not only be strongly associated with cocaine by the product name but also by the product package. Thus, the unique shape of the Coca-Cola bottle was originally intended to resemble the shape of a coca bean. In reality, the bottle shape resembles a cocoa bean because the production artists mistakenly used a cocoa bean, instead of a coca bean, as the model for the bottle design. In 1903, soon after the dangers of cocaine were publicized, the manufacturer of Coca-Cola removed cocaine from its formulation (23, 40). Congress passed The Harrison Narcotic Act of 1914 as a method of controlling the manufacture, sale, distribution and prescription of narcotics. Interestingly, cocaine, a stimulant, was included in the list of narcotics covered by these federal narcotic regulations. Consequently, cocaine was only available through a doctor's prescription. The public perception that cocaine was a dangerous drug was reinforced by these restrictions. Cocaine use decreased and remained low through the 1960s. In the early 1970s, cocaine abuse re-emerged, particularly among middle-class Americans. As Gold noted (23) all that had been learned about the dangers of cocaine from the previous epidemic had been forgotten.

EPIDEMIOLOGY

Cocaine abuse in the United States has maintained epidemic status since the early 1980s. Estimates from a recent National Household Survey on Drug Abuse (50), based on a sample of 22,181 individuals, indicate that in 1994 there were 1.4 million current cocaine users in the United States. The estimated number of crack abusers was 500,000. This represents a marked reduction in cocaine usage compared to peak use, 5.8 million persons, in 1985, and is also a significant decrease from the 1.9 million users in 1991. Almost all of the reduction in use is accounted for by occasional cocaine users, people who used in the past year but less frequent than monthly (Figure 1). Despite the dramatic change in pattern of cocaine consumption, the number of frequent cocaine abusers, defined as those who use cocaine on a weekly basis during the past year, has remained constant since 1985 at about 640,000 persons. Most of the current cocaine users were in the age bracket 18 to 34. Men used cocaine twice as frequently as women. With regard to ethnicity, blacks and Hispanics had higher rates of cocaine use, 1.3% and 1.1%, respectively, compared to whites who used at a rate of 0.5%. In terms of absolute number of current cocaine abusers, whites accounted for 62%, blacks 22%, and Hispanics 16%.

Cocaine abuse and dependence appear even more serious considering that chronic cocaine users are developing a significant number of medical and psychosocial problems. According to data from the Drug Abuse Warning Network (51), cocaine-related hospital emergencies continue to increase, especially for individuals 35 years of age and older (11).

Unlike the United States, European countries have not experienced dramatic increases in cocaine abuse. Ingold et al (29) describe an overall low level of

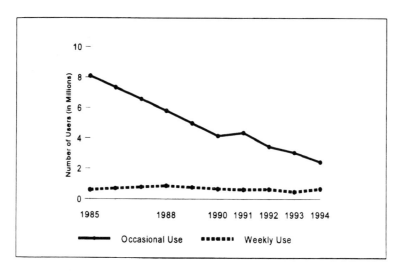

Figure 1   Cocaine use in past year, 1985–1994

crack cocaine use in France; however, in the last few years there has been a progressive increase in the number of crack abusers. In 1991 there were 51 known crack abusers in all of France but by 1993 there were 226 abusers in Paris alone. These authors believe that France and other European countries may be on the eve a crack cocaine epidemic. Recently, there has been research directed at understanding the meaning of the reported differences in prevalence rates of cocaine use for the race/ethnic demographic characteristic. In the last two National Household Surveys on Drug Abuse (NHSDA), the prevalence rates for lifetime use of crack cocaine for African Americans were more than twice those for white Americans. In a recently reported study (39), investigators conducted a reanalysis of the original data for the 1988 NHSDA to examine the extent to which cocaine smoking is associated with race/ethnic factors. The hypothesis was that the reported racial/ethnic group differences might be an artifact of environmental risk factors. In the reanalysis the survey respondents were grouped into neighborhood clusters. In this manner, shared characteristics such as drug availability and social conditions could be held constant. The results showed that the odds of cocaine use did not differ by race and ethnicity. In other words, environmental influences increase the risk of cocaine use regardless of race and ethnicity.

COCAINE AND ADDICTION

Cocaine abuse refers to a pattern of drug use that produces recurrent and significant adverse consequences related to repeated use of the drug. Cocaine addiction, which is also referred to as dependence, involves compulsive drug use that causes interference with normal activities and may include tolerance and physical dependence. Crack cocaine smoking and intravenous cocaine are associated with a rapid progression from cocaine use to cocaine abuse and addiction. Over the past two decades, health care providers and researchers have increasingly used criteria of the *Diagnostic and Statistical Manual of Mental Disorders* of the American Psychiatric Association (1) to characterize individuals with substance use disorders. The reader is referred to this manual for a full discussion of these specific diagnostic criteria.

Drugs that reliably produce pleasure (euphoria) are more likely to be taken repeatedly. Reinforcement refers to the quality of drugs to produce effects that make the user wish to take them again. The more strongly reinforcing a drug is, the greater the likelihood that the drug will be abused. Studies in animal models have associated reinforcement with the ability to increase extracellular levels of the neurotransmitter dopamine in critical brain areas, particularly the nucleus accumbens. Cocaine, amphetamine, ethanol, opioids and nicotine all reliably increase extracellular dopamine levels in the nucleus accumbens region. In contrast, drugs that block dopamine receptors generally produce unpleasant feelings. Neither laboratory animals nor humans will spontaneously take such drugs. The abuse liability of a drug is enhanced if it has a rapid onset of action. Effects that occur soon after administration are more likely to initiate the chain of events that lead to loss of control over drug taking. The time that it takes the drug to reach critical receptor sites in the brain and the concentrations achieved can be influenced by the form of the drug, route of administration and rate of absorption, metabolism and entry into the brain.

The history of cocaine illustrates the changes in abuse liability of the same compound, depending on the form and the route of administration. Coca leaves can be chewed and the alkaloidal cocaine is slowly absorbed through the oral mucosa. This method produces low cocaine blood levels and correspondingly low levels in the brain. The mild stimulant effects produced by the chewing of coca leaves have a gradual onset, and this practice has produced little, if any, abuse or dependence despite thousands of years of use by natives of the Andes mountains. Natives in several of the cocaine-producing countries in South America use coca paste which is the product of a crude extraction of the coca plant. This paste, which is locally called basulca, is smoked. Basulca frequently contains leftover hydrocarbons and chemicals which when smoked exposes the user to the additional dangers of inhaling these contaminants.

Beginning in the late nineteenth century, scientists isolated cocaine hydrochloride from coca leaves and the extraction of pure cocaine became possible. Cocaine could be taken in higher doses by oral ingestion or by absorption through the nasal mucosa, producing higher cocaine levels in the blood and a more rapid onset of stimulation. Subsequently, it was found that a solution of cocaine hydrochloride could be administered via the intravenous route giving the ultimate in rapidity of blood levels and speed of onset of stimulatory effects. With each "advance" in cocaine administration, there was an associated increment in blood level and speed of onset of the drug. Consequently, the drug became more likely to produce addiction. In the 1980s, the availability of cocaine to the American public was increased further with the invention of crack cocaine. Crack, which is sold at a very low price on the street ($1 to $3 per dose), is alkaloidal cocaine (free base) that can be readily vaporized by heating. Simply inhaling the vapors produces blood levels comparable to intravenous cocaine. The pulmonary route is highly effective because the lungs provide a large surface area for absorption into the pulmonary circulation. The cocaine-containing blood then enters the left side of the heart and reaches the cerebral circulation without dilution by the systemic circulation. The pulmonary route rapidly delivers the drug to the brain and is also the preferred route for users of nicotine and cannabis. Inhalation of crack cocaine is thus more likely to produce addiction than chewing, drinking or sniffing cocaine.

The behavioral effects of a cocaine "high" are manifested by an extreme euphoria, increased sense of self-confidence, hyperalertness, hyperactivity, restlessness, decreased appetite, decreased need for sleep and impaired judgment (30). Users frequently report that when cocaine is available it is difficult to avoid using it and that it is almost impossible to resist completely ingesting all of the cocaine that is available. The effects of cocaine are so powerful that the abuser often neglects personal care and health, sleep, employment and even child care (23). The cocaine high lasts only for about 10-20 minutes, and is quickly followed by anxiety, depression and an immense craving to re-experience the high. These symptoms are relieved by taking more cocaine.

Only a minority of cocaine-dependent persons who discontinue use manifest cocaine withdrawal symptoms. When present, cocaine withdrawal occurs within hours to days after the last dose and is manifested by dysphoria, depression with suicidal ideation, fatigue, hypersomnia, and increased appetite. These symptoms usually do not require specific treatment, other than rest, and they usually subside within 3 to 4 days.

TOXICITY

Cocaine abuse has been associated with a variety of systemic complications involving all the major organ systems. Cardiovascular, neurologic, psychiatric, pulmonary, gastrointestinal, musculoskeletal and dermatologic manifestations have been reported. Several reviews of cocaine toxicity are available (23, 37, 38, 53).

Cardiovascular

The most frequently occurring toxic complications involve the cardiovascular system and are manifested by arrhythmias, coronary vasospasm, myocardial ischemia, myocardial infarction, and cardiomyopathy. Cocaine is a powerful vasoconstrictor whose effects are dose dependent. The toxic effects of cocaine are the result of direct stimulation of the cardiovascular system and the prolonged catecholamine stimulation following reuptake blockade (16).

Several studies have reported an increased incidence of strokes in persons who smoke crack cocaine (12, 32). In most cases strokes occurred in young adults who had few, if any other, risk factors for stroke. Cerebral hemorrhages and ischemic infarcts are seen with about equal frequency.

The pressor effects of cocaine can cause a sudden increase in arterial pressure that may cause a cerebral vessel to rupture. In addition, cocaine may cause constriction of cerebral vessels and lead to ischemic brain infarction. In persons who have risk factors for stroke, such as hypertension, renal failure and diabetes mellitus, the additional risk of smoking crack cocaine may be particularly harmful.

Neurological

Seizures are the most frequent neurological complication associated with cocaine use. The seizures occur because cocaine, through its local anesthetic action, lowers the seizure threshold. The seizures usually occur within minutes after cocaine use, are generalized tonic-clonic type, and have a short duration (30, 44, 52)

Several studies have found evidence of the neurotoxic effects of cocaine (28, 46, 54). Cerebral atrophy, between 20% and 40%, has been described for a chronic cocaine abusers (46). Strickland et al (54) studied cerebral perfusion and neuropsychological function in a group of 8 chronic cocaine abusers who had been abstinent for at least 6 months. All the subjects showed abnormal brain perfusion and neuropsychological deficits. Hypoperfusion, which varied in location and severity, was observed in all 8 subjects during single-photon emission computed tomography (SPECT) studies. Deficits in attention, concentration, and new learning were seen in all subjects.

Pulmonary

Difficulty breathing is a frequent complaint of crack cocaine smokers and often leads the abuser to seek medical attention. There are a variety of reported pulmonary problems associated with the inhalation of crack cocaine. Pulmonary pathology and crack cocaine use has been reviewed elsewhere (37). This review emphasized that cocaine abuse may cause several diverse, pulmonary disorders such as pulmonary hemorrhage, pulmonary edema, asthma, and barotrauma manifested as pneumothorax, pneumomediastium and pneumop-ericardium.

COMBINATIION OF COCAINE WITH ALCOHOL

Between 60% and 90% of cocaine abusers also abuse alcohol (24, 49). Co-caethylene, an ethyl ester of benzoylecgonine, is formed in the liver when cocaine and alcohol are consumed together. High blood levels of cocaethylene following cocaine and alcohol use have been found in persons admitted to the emergency room and in persons who died as a result of cocaine overdose (25). This metabolite has behavioral effects similar to those of cocaine. It is as potent as cocaine in animal self-administration studies and thus it has significant abuse potential (31). Cocaethylene is more toxic than cocaine and its half-life is twice as long as that of cocaine (15, 26). Compared to using cocaine alone, a person who consumes both alcohol and cocaine may experience more intense pleas-urable sensations, but he may also develop the combined toxicities of cocaine and cocaethylene (26).

SEXUALLY TRANSMITTED DISEASES

Several investigators have described an increased incidence of sexually trans-mitted diseases (STD), including human immunodeficiency virus (HIV) infec-tion, in crack cocaine abusers as a consequence of these abusers participating in high risk sexual behaviors (4, 9, 19, 43). Two recently reported studies, each involving a large patient cohort, provide additional clinical evidence that links crack cocaine abuse to infections with STD. Edlin et al (14) investigated the relationship between crack cocaine addiction and HIV infection in crack co-caine abusers in three cities. The study consisted of interviewing and testing for HIV all participants. Subjects for this study were adults, 18 to 29 years of age, who either smoked crack cocaine regularly or who had never smoked crack cocaine, and who were recruited from inner-city areas in New York, Miami and San Francisco. The reported findings were for 1967 participants who had never injected drugs. Of these, 1137 were regular (at least 3 days a week during the prior 30 days) crack cocaine users and the remaining 830 had never smoked crack. Half the subjects in each group were males. African Americans represented 87% of crack smokers and 81% of nonsmokers. The crack users had been smoking crack for a median of 5 years, used crack regularly (at least 3 days a week) a median of three years, and had used crack a median of 28 of the prior 30 days.

The authors stated that the study has three limitations: (*a*) study participants were recruited from the streets and thus, there is probably an overrepresentation of people who live or spend a lot of time in public places; (*b*) participants were either regular crack cocaine users or nonusers, therefore no information was collected regarding infrequent and former crack cocaine smokers; and (c) information regarding drug use and sexual behaviors were from the participants' self-reports. Overall these limitations did not seriously weaken the importance of the findings from this study.

Several important findings were cited: prevalence of HIV infection among crack smokers (15.7%) was 2.4 times that of the nonsmokers (5.2%); the highest prevalence of HIV infection was among the women crack smokers in New York (29.6%) and Miami (23%). The lowest prevalence was among nonsmoking women; in women there was a stronger association between crack smoking and HIV infection than among men; four sexual practices were the strongest risk factors for HIV infection and accounted for the higher prevalence of HIV infection among the crack cocaine smokers. The four high-risk sexual practices are: (a) sexual work (meaning sex in exchange for money or drugs) at any time; (b) recent unprotected sexual work, (c) anal sex between men; and (d) homosexual anal intercourse with 50 or more male partners. Women who used crack were more likely than men who used crack to report high risk sexual practices.

The authors conclude that crack cocaine smoking is associated with high-risk sexual practices, which in turn results in the transmission of HIV. Eighty percent of the crack smokers reported having had a sexually transmitted disease.

The females who abused crack were also more likely to report ever having had a sexually transmitted disease, in particular genital ulcer disease. DeHovitz et al (13) studied a group of 372 sexually active inner-city women in Brooklyn, New York in order to determined the prevalence of untreated sexually transmitted diseases. Women 18 to 50 years old who had at least one male sex partner in the prior year were eligible for the study. Women with a history of intravenous drug use or a positive HIV antibody test were excluded.

Each participant had an extensive evaluation that included questionnaires to collect demographic data and historical information regarding alcohol consumption, drug use and sexual practices, medical history, physical examination, pelvic examination, routine laboratory blood studies, and a urine toxicological analysis. STD's were assessed using medical history, culture, serologic analyses.

Three-hundred and seventy-two women were studied, of whom 92% were black and 49% were US-born. Thirty-five percent of all the women had at least one STD. The rate of STD among US-born women was 50% compared to a rate of 22% among foreign-born women. A total of nine women (2.4%), seven US-born and two foreign-born, had a positive HIV antibody test. All seven US-born reported recent crack cocaine use and three reported having six or more sexual partners during the prior year. The researchers found large differences between crack cocaine use, sexual behavior, and place of birth, and consequently they examined the US-born and foreign-born groups separately. Among the US-born women, 61% of the cocaine users had an STD compared to 34% of nonusers. Recent crack cocaine use was the strongest predictor of syphilis infection.

The authors summarized the study findings as showing three important relationships: (a) that undiagnosed and untreated STD was significantly associated with a history of crack cocaine use; (b) and to a lesser extent to a history of multiple sex partners; and (c) that there was a very strong association in women between crack cocaine use and syphilis and HIV.

PREGNANCY

It is reported that in urban areas as many as 18% of all newborns infants are delivered to women who in the prenatal period test positive for cocaine (17). It is difficult to gather accurate self-report data from pregnant women who use cocaine because they fear that they may lose custody of their newborn because of their drug use. This is also a principal reason that they delay or avoid seeking prenatal care. One report found that 25% of prenatal mothers currently abusing cocaine denied drug use (17).

Over the past decade there have been several reports of the negative effects on the infant of prenatal cocaine exposure (7, 8, 42). The detrimental effects included depressed growth manifested as low birth weight, a variety of neurological abnormalities, and behavioral disturbances. Richardson et al (48) found that many of the reported studies on the effects of prenatal cocaine exposure have significant methodological problems such as failure to control for the prenatal use of other drugs, or the failure to control for other important variables such as prenatal care and environmental conditions. In one recent study, when these types of confounding variables were controlled, the analysis revealed no difference between infants of women who abused cocaine and those who did not use cocaine (48).

Lutiger et al (41) performed a meta-analysis of studies on the effects of prenatal cocaine use on fetal development. They found that of all the reported detrimental effects, only low birth weight could be specially attributed to the mother's prenatal use of cocaine. Although a significant number of pregnant women use cocaine, it is not clear what effects this intrauteral cocaine exposure has on the fetus, infant, and child.

TREATMENT

Detoxification is simply accomplished by abstinence. Cocaine withdrawal symptoms are not life-threatening and rarely require treatment.

Psychosocial Therapies

RELAPSE PREVENTION   The therapeutic goal of relapse prevention is to achieve and maintain abstinence from drugs and alcohol. Psychosocial treatments are the modal form of therapy for cocaine dependence. Most of the treatment programs last about 30 days and have been patterned after alcohol treatments (2). Treatment is usually provided through a variety of modalities, and urinary drug screens are an integral part of the program. Group and individual therapies are combined in varying amounts, with family/couples therapy and self-help groups (20).

Treatment results from research studies on cocaine dependence indicate that long-term care is needed because brief treatments are ineffective (33). A typical protocol may require a short in-patient stay or an intensive outpatient program; then treatment is tapered and continued for one to two years.

Recent reports for outcome studies involving intensive psychosocial treatments for cocaine dependence show good rates of abstinence: Alterman et al (2) 60% for 7 months; Carroll et al (6) 30% for a year; Higgins et al (27) report that for patients who received behavioral treatment with an added incentive program, 55% achieved 10 weeks of continuous abstinence and 30% achieve 20 weeks. Although these kinds of programs appear effective, they are not practical as standard treatments for huge numbers of patients because they are very expensive, long-term and require specialized staff. On the other hand, they are less expensive than long-term inpatient care.

Medication

Many patients are unable or unwilling to undergo therapy without the support of medication. Unfortunately, there is no medication clearly identified as an effective pharmacotherapy for cocaine-dependent persons.

Our current understanding of the neurochemical changes that result from chronic stimulant use has been the basis for the selection of potential pharmacotherapies for cocaine dependence. The nucleus accumbens is an important part of the brain reward pathways. Cocaine administration, in rats, results in increased levels of dopamine in the region of the nucleus accumbens. Cocaine and other abused substances that increase nucleus accumbens dopamine also decrease the threshold for brain-stimulation reward (34).

Medications for the treatment of cocaine dependence must be considered separately from medications used to treat complications involved in cocaine abuse such as depression and psychotic reactions. Although a withdrawal syndrome for cocaine dependence has been proposed (21), this withdrawal generally consists simply of tiredness, somnolence, lack of energy, craving for cocaine and periods of depression. It usually resolves spontaneously over several days but there is evidence from brain imaging studies that receptor changes and even brain metabolic effects from chronic cocaine may persist for weeks or months after the last dose of cocaine. Several types of medications have been used in an effort to correct the biochemical changes that are thought to play a role in relapse to compulsive cocaine use. Antidepressant medications have been used, based on the theory that they, like cocaine, block reuptake of biogenic amines and therefore, may correct some of the deficit produced by the abrupt withdrawal of cocaine (11). The antidepressant medication most studied has been desipramine. It has also yielded the best results in specific populations. Several double-blind studies with desipramine (22) indicate that it has a modest effect, at best, in inducing abstinence from cocaine. Two recently reported studies of Arndt et al (3) and Kosten et al (35) both involved methadone maintenance patients who were abusing cocaine, mainly intravenously, and they did not find desipramine to be an effective pharmacotherapy. Possibly cocaine abusing methadone patients who primarily use cocaine by the intravenous route may be more difficult to treat and less likely to respond to desipramine. Research is needed, particularly in nonintravenous abusers, in order to determine which population of cocaine abusers benefits most from desipramine pharmacotherapy.

Another approach has been based on animal studies that indicate that cocaine can produce kindling of seizure activity. Kindling is an electrical phenomenon that refers to the increase in seizure activity when a standard sub-threshold stimulus is applied repeatedly to certain brain structures, especially the amygdaloid nucleus. Small doses of cocaine applied to the amygdala have also been shown to produce kindling and thus, the drug carbamazepine which blocks the production kindling (47), might have a role in the treatment of cocaine dependence. Thus far, double-blind studies have not shown any benefit from carbamazepine in preventing relapse to cocaine use (10, 36, 45).

SUMMARY

This review has briefly described the history of cocaine use over the past century in the United States. Although crack cocaine is a relatively recent development, it has already been shown to be highly addicting and associated with numerous medical problems. Treatment of compulsive users is difficult, but behavioral treatments have achieved success with about half of the cocaine addicts requesting treatment. There is a great deal of interest in finding a medication that will improve the treatment of cocaine addiction, but so far no medication has been consistently successful in controlled clinical trails.

Literature Cited

1. American Psychiatric Association. 1994. *Diagnostic and Statistical Manual of Mental Disorders.* Washington, DC: Am. Psychiatric Assoc.
2. Alterman AI, McLellan AT, O'Brien CP, August DS, Snider EC, et al. 1994. Effectiveness and costs of inpatient versus day hospital cocaine rehabilitation. *J. Nerv. Ment. Dis.* 182:157–63
3. Arndt IO, Dorozynsky L, Woody GE, McLellan AT, O'Brien CP. 1992. Desipramine treatment of cocaine dependence in methandone-maintained patients. *Arch. Gen. Psychiatr.* 49:888–93
4. Booth RE, Watters JK, Chitwood DD. 1993. HIV risk-related sex behaviors among injection drug users. *Am. J. Public Health* 83:1144–48
5. Brain PF, Coward GA. 1989. A review of the history, actions, and legitimate uses of cocaine. *J. Subst. Abuse* 1:431–51
6. Carroll KM, Power ME, Bryant K, Rounsaville BJ. 1993. One-year follow-up status of treatment-seeking cocaine abusers. Psychopathology and dependence severity as predictors of outcome [see comments]. *J. Nerv. Ment. Dis.* 181:71–79
7. Chasnoff IJ, Burns WJ, Schnoll SH, Burn KA. 1985. Cocaine use in pregnancy. *N. Engl. J. Med* 313:666–69
8. Chasnoff IJ, Griffith DR, MacGregor S, Dirkes K, Burns KA. 1989. Temporal patterns of cocaine use in pregnancy: perinatal outcome. *JAMA* 261:1741–44
9. Chiasson MA, Stoneburner RL, Hildebrandt DS, Ewing WE, Telzak EE, Jaffee HW. 1991. Heterosexual transmission of HIV-1 associated with the use of smokable freebase cocaine (crack). *AIDS* 5:1121–26
10. Cornish JW, Maany I, Fudala PJ, Neal S, Poole SA, et al. 1995. Carbmazepine treatment for cocaine dependence. *Drug Alcohol Depend.* 38:221–27
11. Cornish JW, McNicholas LF, O'Brien CP. 1995. Treatment of substance-related disorders. In *The American Psychiatric Press Textbook of Psychopharmacology,* ed. AF Schatzberg, CB Nemeroff, pp. 707–24. Washington, DC: Am. Psychiatric Press
12. Daras M, Tuchman AJ, Koppel BS, Samkoff LM, Weitzner I, Marc J. 1994. Neurovascular complications of cocaine. *Acta Neurol. Scand.* 90:124–29
13. DeHovitz JA, Kelly P, Feldman J, Sierra MF, Clarke L, et al. 1994. Sexually transmitted diseases, sexual behavior, and cocaine use in inner-city women. *Am. J. Epidemiol.* 140:1125–34
14. Edlin BR, Irwin KL, Faruque S, McCoy CB, Word C. 1994. Intersecting epidemics—crack cocaine use and HIV infection among inner-city young adults. Multicenter Crack Cocaine and HIV Infection Study Team. *N. Engl. J. Med.* 331:1422–27
15. Foltin RW, Fischman MW. 1989. Ethanol and cocaine interactions in humans: cardiovascular consequences. *Pharmacol. Biochem. Behav.* 31:877–83
16. Foltin RW, Fischman MW. 1991. Smoked and intravenous cocaine in humans: acute tolerance, cardiovascular and subjective effects. *J. Pharmacol. Exp. Ther.* 257:247–61
17. Frank D, Zuckerman B, Reece H, Amaro H, Hingson R, et al. 1988. Cocaine use during pregnancy: prevalence and correlates. *Pediatrics* 82:888–95
18. Freud S. 1974. Uber Coca (On cocaine). In *Cocaine Papers,* ed. R Byck, pp. 49–73. New York: Stonehill Publ.
19. Fullilove MT, Golden E, Fullilove RED, Lennon R, Porterfield D, et al. 1993. Crack cocaine use and high-risk behaviors among sexually active black adolescents. *J. Adolesc. Health* 14:295–300
20. Gawin FH, Khalsa ME, Ellinwood E. 1994. Stimulants. In *The American Psychiatric Press Textbook of Substance Abuse Treatment,* ed. M Galanter, HD Kleber, pp. 111–39. Washington, DC: Am. Psychiatric Press
21. Gawin FH, Kleber HD. 1986. Abstinence symptomatology and psychiatric diagnosis in cocaine abusers. *Arch. Gen. Psychiatr.* 43:107–13
22. Gawin FH, Kleber HD, Byck R, Rounsaville BJ, Kosten TR, et al. 1989. Desipramine facilitation of initial cocaine abstinence. *Arch. Gen. Psychiatr.* 46:117–21
23. Gold MS. 1992. Cocaine (and crack): clinical aspects. In *Substance Abuse: A Comprehensive Textbook,* ed. JH Lowinson, P Ruiz, RB Millman, JGAE Langrod, pp. 205–21. Baltimore: Williams & Wilkins
24. Grant BF, Harford TC. 1990. Current and simultaneous use of alcohol with cocaine: results of a national survey. *Drug Alcohol Depend.* 25:97–104
25. Hearn WL, Flynn DD, Hime GW, Rose S, Cofino JC, et al. 1991. A unique cocaine metabolite displays high affinity for the dopamine transporter. *J. Neurochem.* 56:698–701

26. Hearn WL, Rose S, Wagner J, Ciarleglio A, Mash DC. 1991. Cocaethylene is more potent than cocaine in mediating lethality. *Pharmacol. Biochem. Behav.* 39:531–33

27. Higgins ST, Budney AJ, Bickel WK, Foerg FE, Donham R, Badger GJ. 1994. Incentives improve outcome in outpatient behavioral treatment of cocaine dependence. *Arch. Gen. Psychiatr.* 51:568–76

28. Holman BL, Carvalho PA, Mendelson J, Teoh SK, Nardin R, et al. 1991. Brain perfusion is abnormal in cocaine-dependent polydrug users: a study using technetium-99m-HMPAO and SPECT. *J. Nuclear Med.* 32:1206–10

29. Ingold FR, Toussirt M. 1994. [The consumption of "crack" in Paris in 1993. Epidemiological and ethnographic data]. *Ann. Med. Psychol.* 152:400–6

30. Jaffe JH. 1990. Drug addiction and drug abuse. In *The Pharmacological Basis of Therapeutics*, ed. AG Gilman, TW Rall, AS Nies, P Taylor, pp. 522–45. New York: Pergamon

31. Jatlow P, Elsworth JD, Bradberry CW, Winger G, Taylor JR, et al. 1991. Cocaethylene: a neuropharmacologically active metabolite associated with concurrent cocaine-ethanol ingestion. *Life Sci.* 48:1787–94

32. Kaku DA, Lowenstein DH. 1990. Emergence of recreational drug abuse as a major factor for stroke in young adults. *Ann. Intern. Med.* 113:821–27

33. Kang SY, Kleiman PH, Woody GE, Millman RB, Todd TC, et al. 1991. Outcomes for cocaine abusers after once-a-week psychosocial therapy. *Am. J. Psychiatr.* 148:630–35

34. Kornetsky C, Porrino LJ. 1992. Brain mechanisms of drug-induced reinforcement. In *Addictive States*, ed. CP O'Brien, JH Jaffe. pp. 59–77 New York: Raven

35. Kosten TR, Morgan CM, Falcione J, Schottenfeld RS. 1992. Pharmacotherapy for cocaine-abusing methadone-maintained patients using amantadine or desipramine. *Arch. Gen. Psychiatr.* 49:894–98

36. Kranzler HR, Bauer LO, Hersh D, Klinghoffer V. 1995. Carbamazepine treatment of cocaine dependence: a placebo-controlled trial. *Drug Alcohol Depend.* 38:203–11

37. Laposata EA, Mayo GL. 1993. A review of pulmonary pathology and mechanisms associated with inhalation of freebase cocaine ("crack"). *Am. J. Forensic Med. Pathol.* 14:1–9

38. Lee HO, Eisenberg MJ, Drew D, Schiller NB. 1995. Intraventricular thrombus after cocaine-induced myocardial infarction. *Am. Heart J.* 129:403–5

39. Lillie-Blanton M, Anthony JC, Schuster CR. 1993. Probing the meaning of racial/ethnic group comparisons in crack cocaine smoking [see comments]. *JAMA* 269:993–97

40. Louis JC, Yazijian HZ. 1980. *The Cola Wars*, pp. 13–38. New York: Everest House Publ.

41. Lutiger B, Graham K, Einarson TR, Koren G. 1991. Relationship between gestational cocaine use and pregnancy outcome: a meta-analysis. *Teratology* 44:405–14

42. MacGregor SN, Keith LG, Chasnoff IJ, Rosner MA, Chisum GM, et al. 1987. Cocaine use during pregnancy: adverse perinatal outcome. *Am. J. Obstet. Gynecol.* 157:686–90

43. Marx R, Aral SO, Rolfs RT, Sterk CE, Kahn JG. 1991. Crack, sex and STD. *Sex. Transm. Dis.* 18:92–101

44. Miller BL, Chiang F, McGill L, Sadow T, Goldberg MA, Mena I. 1992. Cerebrovascular complications from cocaine: possible long-term sequelae. *NIDA Res. Monogr.* 123:129–46

45. Montoya ID, Levin FR, Fudala PJ, Gorelick DA. 1995. Double-blind comparison of carbamazepine and placebo for treatment of cocaine dependence. *Drug Alcohol Depend.* 38:213–19

46. Pascual-Leone A, Dhuna A, Anderson DC. 1991. Cerebral atrophy in habitual cocaine abusers: a planimetric CT study. *Neurology* 41:34–38

47. Post R. 1988. Time course of clinical effects of carbamazepine: implications for mechanisms of action. *J. Clin Psychiatr.* 49 (Suppl. 1):35–46

48. Richardson GA, Day NL. 1994. Detrimental effects of prenatal cocaine exposure: illusion or reality? *J. Am. Acad Child Adolesc. Psychiatr.* 33:28–34

49. Rounsaville BJ, Anton SF, Carroll K, Budde D, Pursoff BA, Gawin F. 1991. Psychiatric diagnoses of treatment-seeking cocaine abusers. *Arch. Gen. Psychiatr.* 48:43–51

50. SAMHSA. 1995. *Preliminary Estimates From The 1994 National Household Survey on Drug Abuse.* Washington, DC: US GPO

51. SAMHSA. 1993. *Preliminary Estimates From the Drug Abuse Warning Network—Third Quarter 1992 Estimates of Drug-Related Emergency Room Episodes.* Washington, DC: US GPO

52. Schrank KS. 1992. Cocaine-related emergency department presentations. *NIDA Res. Monogr.* 123:110–28

53. Smart RG. 1991. Crack cocaine use: a review of prevalence and adverse effects. *Am. J. Drug Alcohol Abuse* 17:13–26

54. Strickland TL, Millanueva-Meyer J, Miller BL, Cummings J, Mehringer CM, et al. 1993. Cerebral perfusion and neuropsychological consequences of chronic cocaine use. *J. Neuropsychiatr. Clin. Neurosci.* 5:419–27

Annu. Rev. Public Health. 1996. 17:275–98

PERVASIVE MEDIA VIOLENCE

C. Schooler and J. A. Flora

Stanford Center for Research in Disease Prevention, Stanford University School of
Medicine, 1000 Welch Road, Palo Alto, California 94304-1885

KEY WORDS: mass media violence, youth media habits, media effects

ABSTRACT

In this review, we focus our discussion on studies examining effects on children
and young adults. We believe that the current epidemic of youth violence in the
United States justifies a focus on this vulnerable segment of society. We consider
media effects on individual children's behaviors, such as imitating aggressive
acts. In addition, we examine how the media influence young people's perceptions of norms regarding interpersonal relationships. Next, we assess mass media
effects on societal beliefs, or what children and adolescents think the "real world"
is like. We suggest these media influences are cumulative and mutually reinforcing, and discuss the implications of repeated exposure to prominent and prevalent
violent media messages. Finally, we catalog multiple intervention possibilities
ranging from education to regulation. From a public health perspective, therefore,
we evaluate the effects that pervasive media messages depicting violence have
on young people and present multiple strategies to promote more healthful
outcomes.

The effects of mass media violence have been the subject of scientific inquiry
and public concern since the 1920s when motion pictures became a major
source of mass entertainment (23, 67). The growth of television in the 1950s
provoked concerns about potential harms for young people, and researchers
examined the relationship between watching violence and aggressive behavior
(173). The causal connection between media violence and aggression has been
the subject of over 1000 studies, including a Surgeon General's special report
in 1972 (13) and a National Institute of Mental Health report ten years later
(151). The many reviews of this large empirical literature generally distinguish
various research methodologies such as laboratory experiments, cross-sectional surveys, field experiments, and longitudinal analyses. Moreover, reviews
typically differentiate behavioral, attitudinal, and cognitive effects. Such reviews, however, neglect a public health framework: analysis of multiple levels
of effects (e.g. individual, interpersonal, societal) and comprehensive examination of intervention possibilities.

275

0163-7525/96/0510-0275$08.00

In this review, we focus our discussion on studies examining effects on children and young adults. We believe that the current epidemic of youth violence in the United States justifies a focus on this vulnerable segment of society. We consider media effects on individual children's behaviors, such as imitating aggressive acts. In addition, we examine how the media influence young people's perceptions of norms regarding interpersonal relationships. Next, we assess mass media effects on societal beliefs, or what children and adolescents think the "real world" is like (88). We suggest these media influences are cumulative and mutually reinforcing (99), and discuss the implications of repeated exposure to prominent and prevalent violent media messages.

To provide a context for our discussion of mass media effects on violence, we begin this chapter by presenting relevant background information. This includes a brief discussion of the epidemiology of youth violence. To frame our discussion of media effects, we discuss the many different types and genres of media to which young people are exposed. Following this material, we review evidence regarding effects of mass media violence on youth at the individual, interpersonal, and societal levels. Finally, we catalog multiple intervention possibilities ranging from education to regulation. From a public health perspective, therefore, we evaluate the effects that pervasive media messages depicting violence have on young people and present multiple strategies to promote more healthful outcomes.

YOUTH VIOLENCE IN AMERICA

The United States has the highest rate of violence of any industrialized nation. From 1968 through 1991, the number of firearm-related deaths increased by 60% (74). For several years, firearm injuries have been the leading cause of death among African-American and white teenage males (38, 116). A study of inner-city African American and Latino youth revealed that over half had lost relatives or close friends to homicide (165). Moreover, a survey of 3735 public high school students found that over 10% of males reported being beaten or mugged, attacked or stabbed with a knife, or being shot or shot at; and over 10% of females reported being sexually abused/assaulted. In addition, this study indicates that 33% of boys and 27% of girls reported they had recently witnessed someone else shot at or shot. Exposure to violence is strongly associated with psychological trauma, including serious developmental and emotional sequelae such as depression and suicidal ideation (79, 95, 164, 165, 186). Moreover, exposure to violence is associated with adolescents' use of violence (66, 208).

YOUTH AND MASS MEDIA

Exposure to media

It is estimated that the average American child watches approximately 23 hours of TV per week; the average teenager watches nearly 22 hours per week (167). Young people spend more time watching television than doing any other leisure time activity except sleeping and spend more time watching TV by the time they complete high school (15,000–18,000 hours) than in the classroom (12,000) hours (196). As youngsters proceed through school, they turn increasingly to adult programs; by the sixth grade, about 80% of children's preferences consist of adult programs (68, 179). The average American child will view more than 200,000 acts of violence (111), including at least 18,000 murders on television (87) by the time he or she reaches 18.

Viewing of television peaks in early adolescence, then gradually declines in response to increasing interest in competing media and the demands of school and adolescent social life (53, 130, 139). As television viewing declines, the use of music media—radio, CDs and tapes, music videos—increases to four to six hours per day by middle adolescence (29, 30, 44). Approximately 70% of American households now receive cable TV so most teenagers have access to music television and spend up to two hours per day watching it (45, 197). In addition, as teenagers get older, movie attendance increases, with over 50% of teenagers reporting at least monthly attendance (73). Furthermore, approximately 77% of American homes have videocassette recorders (VCRs) (167). It is estimated that teenagers spend from 13 to 30 hours per week watching movies and playing video games (93, 115, 205).

The use of print media also grows throughout the teenage years. Newspaper reading begins at around 11 or 12 and gradually increases until 60 to 80% of late adolescents report at least some daily newspaper reading (24, 47). Similarly, magazine and book reading slowly climbs until over a third of high school juniors and seniors read magazines and over 20% say they read nonschool books (24, 47). Comic book reading, however, declines steadily from ages 10 to 18 (24, 47).

When time devoted to all of these media is combined, even allowing for instances when reading and listening, or even reading and television viewing occur simultaneously, the average adolescent spends roughly eight hours daily with some form of mass media (73). Although most research focuses on television, all types of media play important roles in the lives of youngsters. For example, teenagers spend more time with radio than with television. Moreover, many films, videos, and print materials are produced primarily for youth.

Processing of Media Messages

Children process mass media differently than older youth. For television, young children do not have sufficiently developed cognitive skills to comprehend fully what they are seeing and hearing, to attend to more than a few aspects of the situation, to remember such aspects, or to make appropriate inferences about them (49, 50, 182). For example, young children are less able to understand the fine points of plot, characterization, and motivation (31). Very young children cannot distinguish between commercials and regular programs (6, 122). Moreover, young children make no connection between a murder at the beginning of a half-hour show and the man led away in handcuffs at the end (33) and often do not understand death to be a permanent condition (180). Whatever the eventual outcome, TV supplies numerous instances in which aggressive and antisocial behavior is immediately rewarded.

Actions and ideas learned by children may result in behavioral consequences when they are older (195). With violence and aggression, this is quite likely the case (70, 107). The years between 2 and 8 are thought to be crucial in determining attitudes about violence (196).

Repeated Exposure

A survey of 2750 14- to 16-years olds revealed that adolescents who listened to more radio and watched more music videos, cartoons, and soap operas were more likely to engage in risky behaviors (drinking alcohol, having sex, smoking cigarettes) (115). This study corroborates other research demonstrating that risk-taking teens are more likely to read sports and music magazines, and to listen to punk or heavy metal rock music (45, 115). This implies that the prevalence of violent content in a wide array of mass media is an important consideration for assessing effects. Youth are repeatedly exposed to depictions of violence in all forms of mass media. This iteration may serve to firmly establish information and ideas about the utility and acceptability of violence into young minds. Moreover, findings that at-risk teens are more likely to consume more violent media implies that the reinforcement of violence through multiple media channels over time may lead to cumulative, deleterious effects.

CONTENT AND EFFECTS OF MASS MEDIA

Television

Television is perhaps the most ubiquitous form of mass media in young people's lives, portraying a world that is significantly more violent than reality. Compared to real crime, TV crime is 12 times more likely to be violent, and

100 times more likely to involve murder (119). Moreover, there are approximately five violent acts per hour in primetime television, and almost three times as many in children's Saturday morning programming (87). The level of violence is higher for cartoons and toy commercials than in any other genre of programming, and these scenes usually depict children or animated characters playing with guns (38a). In addition, 48% of television news stories about children are related to crime (55).

Many genres of television programming influence violence-related outcomes. For example, Atkin (5) demonstrated that a violent incident presented as a television news story had a greater impact on children's aggressiveness than the same scene portrayed as part of a movie. Exposure to real-life violence reported on television news may have just as powerful an effect on young emotions as graphically violent crime shows (213) and can elicit symptoms of traumatic stress such as fear, depression, and loss of sleep in young viewers (26, 192). In addition, coverage of live sports action and sports news on television highlights violent action (32, 51, 214), and exposure to this content has been linked to higher levels of aggression in young athletes (171, 188).

Movies

High levels of violence are present in many types of motion pictures such as horror, action/crime, and science fiction (203). The popularity of fright (or "slasher") movies among adolescents has led to a plethora of such films that depict extreme forms of violence, usually with erotic overtones. Moreover, the emergence and growth of cable television, home video, and pay-per-view television have increased the availability to children of adult-themed feature films, many of which contain graphic depictions of violence.

Videos and Video Games

Use of VCRs enables young people to watch movies and movie scenes that would not be broadcast on television. Adolescents commonly rent and watch videos in groups, and the combination of pressure and bravado inherent in the adolescent peer group context helps explain why much adolescent video viewing involves R-rated and even X-rated films (73).

Consistent with trends in other media, violence is a prominent theme in most popular video games (76, 77, 163)[a]. The primary audience for video games is boys between 8 and 14 years-of-age (90), the majority of whom report that they prefer video games with fantasy violence and human violence (90). In fact, the majority of video games feature violent content, promoting destruction

---

[a]Many popular video games are available for use on computers; we use the term video games as a generic label.

of objects or individuals (25). Many video games reward players for using violence (90). The story-directing, interactive, repetitive nature of game-playing may amplify the deleterious effects of playing video games (78), and research indicates that playing or observing violent video games is linked to increased aggressiveness and antisocial behavior among adolescents and children (3, 42, 98, 178).

Music Media

Young people spend a lot of time listening to music on the radio, on music television, and on CDs and cassettes. A survey of middle and high-school students revealed that nearly one fifth had favorite rock songs that describe homicide, suicide, and satanism (206). These fans were more likely to be male and to know all the lyrics to the songs. Content analyses reveal that violence and crime are depicted in over half the music videos shown on cable and network television (11, 28, 176), and that they depict almost twice the amount of violence as primetime programming (approximately ten violent acts per hour) (35). Hard-rock music and violent music videos have been shown to promote callous, negative, and antagonistic attitudes toward women (154, 191). Violent music videos have also been demonstrated to desensitize young viewers to violence (97, 166) and to promote aggressiveness in viewers (101). Music videos, moreover, are self-reinforcing: if viewers hear a song after having seen the video version, they immediately "flash-back" to the visual imagery of the video (96).

Newspapers, Magazines, Books, and Comics

Although network and local news programs are the media of choice for many youth, a survey of 850 10- to 16-year-olds revealed that 44% reported reading a newspaper the day before they were questioned (42a). Moreover, 60% of those surveyed said stories related to youth usually involve drugs, violence, or crime—sometimes with children as perpetrators, sometimes as victims. Content analysis reveals that 40% of all newspaper stories about children are related to crime (55). A lot of popular fiction (horror, adventure, science fiction, detective, and western) contains high levels of violence (203). Sales of adult comics and violent, sexually suggestive comics for children are rising (177). Belsen (15) found that exposure to violence in comic books and films was positively associated with both aggressive behavior and criminal acts.

MASS MEDIA AND VIOLENCE

Individual Behavior

A substantial number of experimental studies demonstrate that media violence can teach specific acts or social scripts of violence (105). In the 1960s, Bandura and colleagues demonstrated that children could learn and subsequently enact novel aggressive responses by watching filmed depictions (7, 8). Aggressive effects have also been demonstrated among children who view violent cartoons (129, 193). In addition, many studies have explored the impact of media violence on real-life aggression under realistic conditions and have determined that exposure to depictions of violence is related to aggressiveness (94, 102, 136–138).

A meta-analysis of studies examining media effects on young people's spontaneous aggression in unstructured social interaction reveals that exposure to media violence significantly enhances viewers' aggressive behavior (212). This study identified small-to-moderate media effects on children's and adolescents' aggression in interactions with strangers, classmates, and friends. Other research indicates that the amount of variance in aggression explained by television violence is 9–10% (70). In addition, exposure to media violence has been shown to be related to aggressive behavior and crime, even after controlling for the effects of socioeconomic class, education, and race (103). Observing this effect size for relatively brief exposures to media violence suggests that across multiple exposures and multiple social interactions, the impact of mass media on violence may be substantial.

In fact, research indicates there is a cumulative effect of TV viewing over an extended period of time (183, 184). A compelling demonstration of the long-term effects is provided by research by Huesmann and colleagues. The researchers first showed that viewing TV violence in the third grade was significantly related to aggressive behavior 10 years later (aggressive behavior in the third grade was not predictive of violent TV consumption at age 19) (118). When the researchers restudied the original population 11 years later, they found that among 30-year-old adults, exposure to TV violence at age 8 was associated with antisocial behavior 22 years later (109). Further evidence that aggressive habits can be learned from television early in life is provided by a unique naturalistic study by Williams (210). Researchers compared a town that had no television (Notel) in Canada with nearby communities that received either one station (Unitel) or multiple stations (Multitel). These three communities were practically identical except for the presence of television, and data could be collected on children in Notel before and after TV was introduced. Initially lower in aggressiveness than students in Unitel or Multitel, children in Notel caught up to their peers within two years of the introduction of television into their community.

Research also demonstrates that media can affect actual crime rates. A series of studies by Phillips and colleagues links acts of violence on television and similar acts in real life (155–161). This research has been both replicated and criticized by other investigators (114, 140, 190). In one of the most compelling examinations of television's impact on crime, Centerwall (40) compared homicide rates over a 30-year period (1945–1975) among white populations in the United States, Canada, and South Africa. During the period of observation, both the United States and Canada experienced a dramatic growth in television set ownership, particularly in the mid-1950s. In South Africa, there was no television. The homicide rate in the United States and Canada doubled 10 to 15 years after the introduction of television; homicide rates in South Africa remained more stable. There were no differences between the three nations in terms of changes in age distribution, urbanization, economic conditions, alcohol consumption, capital punishment, civil unrest, or availability of firearms that could account for differences in homicide rates, which suggests that TV was the causal agent. In addition, homicide rates among whites rose 10 to 15 years after television was introduced to South Africa in 1973 (39, 41). Centerwall argues that the 10- to 15-year lag between the introduction of TV and changes in the homicide rate indicates "that the behavioral effects of TV are primarily exerted upon children" (40, p. 15).

Interpersonal Norms

Mass media depictions of violence can shape young people's attitudes regarding the favorability of behaving aggressively, and about the acceptability and prevalence of violence (94). A survey of 838 children (ages 9–12) revealed that frequent viewers of TV violence expressed a greater willingness to resort to violence to resolve conflict situations than infrequent viewers (58). In addition, children who believe their favorite television characters would respond to interpersonal conflict violently are more likely to believe that this is the right thing to do (142). Exposure to media violence also increases audience members' perceptions that violence is quite frequent and normatively accepted (105). Children can learn aggressive attitudes from certain programs and come to believe that violence is a commonplace, useful, and appropriate solution to complex problems (54, 200). Furthermore, depictions of violence in the media can legitimize the use of violence in real life by undermining social sanctions against behaving violently towards others that normally work to inhibit such behavior (16, 17).

Compelling evidence that media messages promote interpersonal aggression comes from research demonstrating that young men's propensities to behave aggressively toward women are influenced by exposure to violent sexually explicit mass media (59, 61, 132, 133). For example, watching feature-length films that portray women enjoying sexual and nonsexual aggression[b] is related

---

[b]None of the films were X-rated, and edited versions of them have been shown on TV. Many R-rated films contain far more graphic violence than X-rated pornography, and much of it is directed toward women (213a).

to young men reporting higher acceptance of violence against women (131). Exposure to R-rated "slasher" films, in which women are often the victims of extremely brutal acts juxtaposing violence and eroticism, desensitizes men to violence against women (124, 125). In general, research demonstrates that violence that is perceived to be justified, especially against women when there is often an erotic undertone, is a powerful facilitator of violence (127).

Exposure to graphic portrayals of violence can also reduce young people's emotional responsiveness to violence and increase acceptance of this behavior in real life (34, 105). Children who watch a lot of television (25 or more hours per week) are much less responsive to TV violence in terms of physiological arousal than light viewers (46). Moreover, experiments have shown that even a brief exposure to violent programming affects how 8-year-olds respond to a real fight between two other children in a playroom: Children who watch violent material are less likely to seek the help of an adult to stop a "real" fight (64, 65, 201).

Societal Beliefs

Extensive portrayal of violence in the media shapes young people's ideas about what the "real world" is like (84). Most adolescents believe that television represents reality (207), and children who watch large amounts of television think the world is a "mean and scary" place (181). Violent media content also affects adults. Gerbner and colleagues (87) describe the "mean world syndrome" whereby heavy viewing of television is associated with beliefs that the world is a violent and threatening place, overpopulated with criminals. Apparently, viewers draw inferences from antisocial television content that they generalize to the real world (83–86, 89).

Mass media, therefore, shape what people think about and which issues they consider to be most important (48). This is known as the agenda setting function of the media (135). For example, most people believe that crime has increased in the country, as well as in their own communities, despite the fact that the nation's overall crime rate is quite stable (171a). People's perceptions of increased crime and victimization have been linked to increasing media attention to these topics (92, 198, 199). The three network evening newscasts continue to increase their coverage of crime and violence (162), and newspaper coverage of murder was three times as high in 1993 as in 1992, while the murder rate remained virtually unchanged (209). Not surprisingly, crime is gaining momentum at an incredible pace as a political issue (110), replacing the economy in public opinion polls as the single most important problem facing the country (144).

An important characteristic of media violence is that it fails to provide an explanation of the sociopolitical context and consequences of violence (105).

Thus the social and economic roots of violence are seldom illuminated or explored, leaving the impression that violence is predominantly an interpersonal issue. This means that audience members do not receive adequate information upon which to base political choices regarding crime issues. Research demonstrates that what is presented in the media influences the policy preferences of the American public (14, 91, 112, 123, 148). In fact, several studies reveal an association between mass media consumption and support for punitive measures toward individual criminals (10, 134). Moreover, adolescents who are heavy viewers of crime shows measure lower on knowledge of criminal justice processes and favor incarceration-based crime policies (36), which likely has implications for the types of policies they will support as adults.

Implications of Pervasive Media Violence

Research reveals four important dimensions that affect the likelihood of media violence influencing young people's behavior: (a) violence that is rewarded or has no negative consequences (7, 9, 21, 117, 170); (b) violence that is justified (21, 18, 81, 141); (c) violence that is pertinent or relevant to the viewer (1, 19, 20, 72, 169); and (d) violence that emotionally involves the viewer (19, 60–62, 69, 80, 187, 215, 216). It is essential to remember, moreover, that children and adolescents in this country are exposed to hours and hours of many kinds of mass media, and much of this content is violent, which doubtless enhances the probability that an audience member will remember the violence and consider it a worthwhile behavioral option (22).

Josephson (113) demonstrated that visual cues can reawaken or activate aggressive ideas from earlier exposure to violent media content. The ubiquity of violence in young people's media environments, therefore, may reinforce or exacerbate deleterious effects. For example, a child may watch a Batman movie that contains many violent scenes. Each time that child reads a Batman comic, watches a Batman television show, sees a Batman glass at a fast-food restaurant, plays with a Batmobile toy car, or wears a Batman T-shirt, he may remember the violent content of the movie, which can influence his thoughts, attitudes, or behaviors.

Lippmann's (128) "pictures in our heads" metaphor, Schramm's (172) stalagmite analogy, and Becker's (12) mosaic model of communication all suggest that the effects of mass media usually come not from a single message or source of messages, but from regular exposure to certain images, ideas, or attitudes over a long period of time. In other words, repeated exposure to violent content helps to more firmly entrench information and attitudes about violence in a young audience member's mind. The pervasiveness of media violence, and the iterative nature of consumption behavior, serve to inculcate the idea that violence is a widely accepted and generally successful way to solve interpersonal problems.

RESEARCH GAPS

Measures of Violence

Violence usually refers to serious or extreme behavior that is intended to cause physical harm to the self or another person. Violent behavior should be distinguished from aggressive behavior, which is often less extreme and does not necessarily lead to physical harm. Moreover, aggression is more normatively accepted in US society. From a practical perspective, however, studies have rarely differentiated aggressive behavior from violent behavior (38b). The most frequently measured outcomes in media effects research are surrogate measures of aggression: "aggressive" responses in laboratory experiments such as hitting toys, pushing "shock" buttons, or responses to questions about hypothetical situations (75). Attitudes about aggression are also commonly used to assess impact of media violence. Measures of actual aggressive acts are quite rare, and most of the studies that examine real-life behavior measure relatively mild forms of aggression. The preponderance of these substitute measures is due to ethical concerns about possibly inducing antisocial or dangerous behavior during the research process, and the desire to have standardized, quantitative effects measures (194). The difficulty of observing serious aggression or violence because of time delay and the relative rarity of such acts doubtless also contribute to the prevalence of surrogate measures. The use of such measures, however, raises questions about the relevance of this research for the issue of real-life violence.

Measures of Exposure

In experimental studies, exposure is manipulated by the researcher. Experimental stimuli often differ dramatically from naturally occurring media content (e.g. selected parts of films or television programs, materials created expressly to be clear and unambiguous). The viewing context may also differ because experimental subjects likely are more attentive than ordinary audience members, who may be doing other activities while using mass media or using several media simultaneously. Surveys and field experiments are hampered by their reliance on recall, viewing diaries, and other measures that are likely subject to reporting biases and error. These studies typically concentrate on number of hours spent with various types of content, and do not consider such variables as attention or comprehension.

Cumulative Effects

As discussed above, most of the studies examining media effects on violence are controlled experiments. Although these are useful for establishing causality, design constraints mean that they often measure effects immediately after exposure. Some studies examining effects over time rely on retrospective measures of media exposure, which may suffer from poor reliability due to errors in recall. Several longitudinal studies have used cohorts, although these typically fail to assess the cumulative effects of exposure to violent content in a wide array of media. Surveys of youth indicate that most watch television, listen to music, view movies, read print media, and many play video games. There is a dearth of studies examining the effects of repeated exposure to violent content in multiple media over many years. The research literature, therefore, fails to capture the public health implications of the pervasiveness of media violence.

POSSIBILITIES FOR INTERVENTION

Pervasive messages regarding the frequency, acceptability, and utility of violence permeate most young people's lives. Rapidly changing technology such as interactive multimedia, fiber-optic "information highways," computer bulletin boards, and home satellite services provide an increasingly wide array of mediated depictions of more and more graphically sophisticated violence. Violence is largely a function of social learning and environmental contingencies, and multiple factors are involved in the facilitation and occurrence of antisocial behavior (105). Although media portrayals of violence may not be the sole or primary factor promoting violence, they do appear to be important influences on this behavior. In fact, a considerable body of research points to a consistent and causal relationship between viewing TV violence and aggressive behavior in children and adolescents (1a, 13, 52, 53, 122, 138, 151, 174, 179). Moreover, studies reveal a significant relationship between violent media exposure and serious aggressive behavior resulting in contacts with the criminal justice system (39, 41, 136, 168). Intervention possibilities include education regarding the effects of media experiences, the mediation of media experiences both at home and in the community, and programs and policies to restrict the accessibility of certain media programming (174, 189).

Education

MEDIA LITERACY   Because television indiscriminately exposes children to adult actions and relationships before they have the cognitive development to cope with them, several programs have been introduced to teach children critical viewing skills. Researchers have identified five critical media-evaluation skills for young people: explicit and spontaneous reasoning, readiness to compare media content to outside information sources, readiness to refer to industry knowledge in reasoning about media content, tendency to find media depictions more fabricated or inaccurate, and less positive evaluation of media content (4, 63). Researchers hoping to inoculate children against television's detrimental influences have sought to improve young viewers' television literacy, that is, their critical appraisal and understanding of television content. Although school-based curricula have demonstrated effects on children's knowledge and attitudes, it is not clear if these educational programs affect aggressive behavior (106, 108, 175, 184). Similarly, educational interventions appear to mitigate the adverse attitudinal effects of media portrayals of violence against women, but influence on actual behavior is not clear (126).

MEDIA CAMPAIGNS   Various public information campaigns have been launched to combat youth violence. One campaign that has been evaluated is "Take a Bite Out of Crime," which was initiated in the 1970s under the sponsorship of the National Crime Prevention Coalition and the US Bureau of Justice. Media materials feature an animated trench-coated dog, McGruff, who calls on Americans to help "take a bite out of crime." Evaluation data reveal widespread penetration of radio and television public service announcements, as well as increases in knowledge and participation in violence prevention activities (145–147). Other anti-violence campaigns include The California Wellness Foundation's Violence Prevention Initiative, geared toward reducing youth access to guns, and programs sponsored by the Centers for Disease Control and the Children's Defense Fund. Television networks and cable companies such as Fox, HBO, TNT, MTV, and the National Cable Television Association are also participating in anti-violent media campaigns.

PARENTAL MEDIATION   The family plays an important role in developing attitudes and behavior patterns that either facilitate or hinder aggression. Research indicates that strong parental disapproval of using aggressive behavior to resolve conflicts attenuates the deleterious effects of exposure to media violence (104, 137, 138, 185). Educational programs teaching parents to supervise and monitor their children's viewing, however, have not met with great success (184). Television, apparently, is a convenient baby-sitter for many parents who may have little motivation to control and limit their children's television time. Working with parents of children who have been determined to be predelinquent or delinquent, however, has been more effective in helping parents reduce the antisocial behavior of preadolescent children (149, 150).

Regulatory and Policy Change

COOPERATIVE CONSULTATION   This process involves cooperation between media and public health professionals to change media content to discourage violent content and encourage the inclusion of prosocial behavior. Breed &

DeFoe (27), for example, worked with interested professionals in the television industry to analyze scripts, rewrite material, and supply specific suggestions about the treatment of alcohol. The Center for Population Options has long appealed directly to program creators to influence media content (143). Likewise, public health professionals from the Harvard School of Public Health worked with the creators of entertainment programming in integrating messages about the selection of a designated driver in many 1989, 1990, and 1991 television shows (82).

MEDIA ADVOCACY   The "strategic use of mass media for advancing social or public policy initiatives" (153) is known as media advocacy. This process involves stimulating media coverage in order to reframe public debate to increase public support for more effective policy level approaches to public health problems (204). To achieve these goals, public health professionals utilize public relations techniques to enhance and influence media coverage of health topics. An example of media advocacy to reduce violence is the work of Wintemute and colleagues (211). Wintemute found that over a six-year period, 88 children in California were unintentionally shot and killed by other children or themselves. Handguns were involved in 58% of these incidents. At a news conference, Wintemute mounted real guns paired with their toy replicas on plywood and challenged reporters to identify the real guns, a difficult task even on close visual examination. The resulting coverage was extensive and succeeded in bringing national attention to the issue of injury and death from firearms. Moreover, Toys "R" Us, the nation's largest toy retailer, pulled replica guns from their shelves.

SELF-REGULATORY CODES AND RATINGS   Movies are rated by the Classification and Ratings Administration, a division of the Motion Picture Association of America, a film industry trade group. Criticisms of this self-regulatory system concern the issue that sexual content and profanity are weighed more heavily than violence and that the system is based on assumptions about what is offensive to parents instead of what is scientifically established as harmful to children.

Pressure continues to mount for regulation that would require ratings for broadcast and cable programming according to its violent content and parental-discretion warnings before violent television shows. The networks are already using such parental warnings voluntarily, but sitcoms and cartoons are exempt from warning labels. Research reveals that viewer discretion advisories result in 14% less viewing of network primetime movies by children aged 2–11 (100). These results provide statistical support from ratings data for the conclusion that parents do act upon information contained in program advisories to discourage the viewing of violent programming among children.

Responding to public concern about youth access to adult-themed movies via video rental stores, the Video Software Dealers Association, the home video trade organization, has developed a "Pledge to Parents." Individual stores that adopt this voluntary Pledge agree to withhold from children films rated NC-17, and refuse to sell or rent R-rated films without some form of parental consent. In practice, parental consent arrangements vary by retailer, although it is unclear how many retailers have adopted the Pledge and how consistently the policy is enforced.

Following public outcry over some particularly graphic, violent video games, the video game producer Sega independently established a three-part rating system with games either recommended for all audiences, for "mature" audiences (over age 13), or for adults only. Subsequently, Sega and the other major game producer Nintendo, through the Interactive Digital Software Rating Board, have developed proposed standards for a four-part rating system.

Since 1985, record companies have been voluntarily adding parental advisory labels to record albums, tapes, or compact discs that they judge to be violent, sexually explicit, or potentially offensive. An experimental study indicates that adolescents like labeled music less, but the impact is limited; teens apparently react primarily to the music per se, rather than to the lyrics (43). These findings do not, however, support the contention that labeling would make certain recordings more appealing to adolescents.

The Comics Code Authority prohibits cartoonists from depicting graphic and other antisocial behavior. Many publishers, however, do not seek a seal from the Comics Code Authority. In addition, many comics carrying the code's seal contain sexual or violent acts that, if they were films, would probably earn them a PG-13 or R rating.

GOVERNMENT POLICIES   The Children's Television Act of 1990 provides for the regulation of children's television and an endowment for the production of quality programming. The Act seeks to maximize prosocial content by providing for the Federal Communications Commission (FCC) to mandate that every commercial television station serve the "educational and informational needs of children." The goal of the Act is to increase the quantity and quality of educational and prosocial programming for children and adolescents.

The 1990 Television Violence Act provides a mechanism for the networks to collaborate and develop voluntary guidelines to discipline the degree of violent material aired during times when children are most likely to be viewing television. The industry has compiled guidelines sensitive to the scheduling of programs. It remains to be seen how effective these guidelines will be as there is no oversight mechanism. In addition, the FCC has tried to establish a "safe harbor period" prohibiting the broadcast of indecent material from 06:00 to

24:00, but this has been contested in the courts, with broadcasters questioning the FCC's definition of indecent material.

The v-chip is a device allowing viewers to automatically block out violent programs. Proposed legislation would require broadcasters and cable television operators to set up a system for rating the level of violence in a television program. Television stations would then have to transmit a special signal for programs deemed to be violent, which the new chip would detect. Parents could use this system to restrict their children's exposure to violent television content.

CONCLUSION

Many Americans believe that Hollywood, the networks, and other media professionals are doing more than simply entertaining the American public and giving it what it wants. Although there is little empirical evidence addressing whether people indeed prefer violent programming, a series of studies by Diener and colleagues demonstrate that level of violence is not reliably related to how much a program is liked (56, 57). Public opinion data suggest, in fact, that people do not like the degree of violence portrayed in mass media. A 1995 survey revealed that over two thirds of American adults are concerned about violence in the media, believing it numbs people to violence, inspires young people to behave violently, and tells people that violence is fun and acceptable (37).

Aggression and violence, however, are multi-determined behaviors stemming from inequities in access to social and economic resources, inequities in the adequacy of medical and educational services, persistent racism and social oppression, and ready access to handguns and firearms. Depictions of violence in the mass media serve to validate and perhaps exacerbate this culture. Decreasing violent content in mass media and the exposure of children and adolescents to such violence, and encouraging parents to monitor and critically discuss media violence are important elements of a multifaceted public health violence prevention effort. Interventions must emphasize both the undesirability of aggressive behavior and the lack of reality of many media characterizations, as well as provide young people with alternative problem-solving behaviors (70). Moreover, such interventions must be instituted early in children's development, both because of the persistence of aggressive behavior once it is learned (71, 109) and because of the massive amount of time spent with media by children even as young as two years of age (53).

Our review of relevant literature indicates, however, that intervention practice far exceeds the empirical base demonstrating positive effects. Moreover, there is no framework for comprehensive public health action concerning media violence effects. Media effects studies have typically investigated narrow questions and failed to examine the multiplicity of violent messages that pervade young people's media environments. This suggests that media effects research should examine the developmental, cognitive, and social processes for media effects, as well as move away from a concentration on the individual level of analysis to consider effects at interpersonal, social network or organizational, and societal levels. In addition, there is a dearth of studies empirically evaluating intervention effects on youth behavior, particularly policy strategies.

Successful youth violence prevention programs need information regarding how to attenuate the deleterious effects of exposure to violent media content, and also how to best encourage policy action to reduce young people's exposure to pervasive messages touting the benefits of violence. We argue that research and interventions should focus on the wide array of violent cues and messages bombarding young people from mass media, consumer items such as toy guns and action figures, and policies encouraging punitive, incarceration-based approaches to crime reduction. The prevalence and severity of the youth violence problem in the United States call for comprehensive and integrated prevention efforts focusing on many facets of young people's lives including the mass media they consume, as well as the communities in which they live, the schools they attend, and the family members and friends who share their lives.

Literature Cited

1. *ABC*. 1975. Children's reaction to violent material on television

1a. Am. Acad. Pediatrics. 1984. *Task Force on Children and Television*. Elk Grove Village, IL: Am. Acad. Pediatr.

2. *Am. Psychol. Assoc.* 1988. Div. 37, Newsl., p. 1

3. Anderson C, Ford C. 1986. Affect of the game player: Short-term effects of highly and mildly aggressive video games. *Pers. Soc. Psychol. Bull.* 12: 390–402

4. Anderson J. 1980. The theoretical lineage of critical viewing curricula. *J. Commun.* 30:64–70

5. Atkin C. 1983. Effects of realistic TV violence vs. fictional violence on aggression. *Journal. Q.* 60:615–21

6. Atkin C. 1982. Television advertising and socialization to consumer roles. In *Television and Behavior: Ten Years of Scientific Progress and Implications for the Eighties,* ed. D Pearl, L Bouthilet, J Lazar, pp. 191–200. Rockville, MD: Natl. Inst. Ment. Health

7. Bandura A. 1965. Influence on models' reinforcement contingencies on the acquisition of imitative responses. *J. Pers. Soc. Psychol.* 1:589–95

8. Bandura A, Ross D, Ross S. 1963. Imitation of film-mediated aggressive peer and adult models. *J. Abnorm. Soc. Psychol.* 66:3–11

9. Bandura A, Ross D, Ross S. 1963. Vicarious reinforcement and imitative learning. *J. Abnorm. Soc. Psychol.* 67: 601–7

10. Barrile L. 1980. *Television and attitudes about crime*. PhD Diss. Boston College, Sociology

11. Baxter R, DeRiemer C, Landini A, Leslie L, Singletary M. 1985. A content analysis of music videos. *J. Broadcast. Electron. Media* 29:333–40

12. Becker S. 1978. Visual stimuli and the construction of meaning. In *Visual Learning, Thinking and Communication*, ed. B Randhawa, W Coffman, p. 44. New York: Academic

13. Behavior USGSACoTaS. 1972. *Television and Growing Up: The Impact of Televised Violence: Rep. Surg. Gen., US Public Health Serv.* Washington, DC: US GPO

14. Belenko S. 1993. *Crack and the Evolution of Anti-Drug Policy.* Westport, CT: Greenwood

15. Belson W. 1978. *Television Violence and the Adolescent Boy.* Hampshire, England: Saxon House

16. Berkowitz L. 1974. Some determinants of impulsive aggression: The role of mediated associations with reinforcements for aggression. *Psychol. Rev.* 81:165–76

17. Berkowitz L. 1962. Violence in the mass media. In *Aggression: A Social Psychological Analysis*, ed. L Berkowitz, pp. 229–55. New York: McGraw-Hill

18. Berkowitz L, Alioto J. 1973. The meaning of an observed event as a determinant of aggressive consequences. *J. Pers. Psychol.* 28:206–27

19. Berkowitz L, Geen R. 1966. Film violence and the cue properties of available targets. *J. Pers. Psychol.* 3:525–30

20. Berkowitz L, Geen R. 1967. Stimulus qualities of the target of aggression: A further study. *J. Pers. Soc. Psychol.* 3:364–68

21. Berkowitz L, Rawlings E. 1963. Effects of film violence on inhibitions against subsequent aggression. *J. Abnorm. Soc. Psychol.* 66:405–12

22. Berkowitz L, Rogers K. 1986. A priming effect analysis of media influences. In *Perspectives on Media Effects*, ed. J Bryant, D Zillmann, pp. 57–81. Hillsdale, NJ: Erlbaum

23. Blumer H, Hauser P. 1933. *Movies, Delinquency and Crime.* New York: Macmillan

24. Bogart L. 1978. *Children, Mother, and Newspapers.* New York: Newsp. Advert. Bur.

25. Braun C, Giroux J. 1989. Arcade video games: Proxemic, cognitive and content analyses. *J. Leis. Res.* 21:92–105

26. Braun S. 1994. "TV stations moving away from gory crime coverage." *San Jose Mercury News*, Nov. 6, p. 12A

27. Breed W, De Foe J. 1982. Effective media change: The role of cooperative consultation on alcohol topics. *J. Commun.* 32:88–99

28. Brown J, Campbell K. 1986. Race and gender in music videos: the same beat but a different drummer. *J. Commun.* 36:94–106

29. Brown J, Campbell K, Fischer L. 1986. American adolescents and music videos: Why do they watch? *Gazette* 37:19–32

30. Brown J, Childers K, Bauman K, Koch G. 1990. The influence of new media and family structure on young adolescents' TV and radio use. *Commun. Res.* 17:65–82

31. Bryant J, Anderson D. 1983. *Children's Understanding of Television.* New York: Academic

32. Bryant J, Zillman D. 1983. Sports violence and the media. In *Sports Violence*, ed. J Goldstein, pp. XX–xx. New York: Springer-Verlag

33. Cannon C. 1993. Honey, I warped the kids. *Mother Jones,* 18:16–21

34. Cantor J, Sparks G, Hoffner C. 1988. Calming childrens' television fears: Mr. Rogers vs. The Incredible Hulk. *J. Broadcast. Electron. Media* 32:271–88

35. Caplan R. 1985. Violent program content in music video. *Journal. Q.* 62:144–47

36. Carlson J. 1985. *Prime Time Law Enforcement.* New York: Praeger

37. Carney J, Duffy M, Cole P, Hornblower M, Moody J. 1995. *Time* 145:24–28

38. CDCP. 1994. Deaths resulting from firearm- and motor-vehicle-related injuries—United States. *Morbid. Mortal. Wkly. Rep.* 43:37–42

38a. Cent. Media Public Affairs. 1992. *A Day of Television Violence*, ed. SR Lichter, D Amundson

38b. Cent. Study Prev. Violence. 1994. *What Works in Reducing Adolescent Violence: An Empirical Review of the Field.* Boulder, CO: Cent. Study Prev. Violence

39. Centerwall B. 1992. Children, television and violence. In *Children and Violence*, ed. D Schwartz, pp. 87–97. Columbus, OH: Ross Labs.

40. Centerwall B. 1989. Exposure to television as a cause of violence. *Public Commun. Behav.* 2:1–58

41. Centerwall B. 1992. Television and violence: The scale of the problem and where to go from here. *JAMA* 267:3059–63

42. Chambers J, Ascione F. 1987. The effects of video game playing on children's donating and helping. *J. Genet. Psychol.* 148:499–505

42a. Children Now. 1994. *Tuned In or Tuned*

Out?: America's Children Speak Out on the News Media

43. Christenson P. 1992. The effect of parental advisory labels on adolescent music preferences. *J. Commun.* 42:106–13
44. Christenson P, Lindlof T. 1985. Children's use of audio media. *Commun. Res.* 12:327–43
45. Christenson P, Roberts D. 1990. *Popular Music in Early Adolescence.* Washington, DC: Carnegies Couc. Adolesc. Dev.
46. Cline V, Croft R, Courrier S. 1973. Desensitization of children to television violence. *J. Pers. Soc. Psychol.* 27:260–365
47. Cobb C. 1986. Patterns of newspaper readership among teenagers. *Commun. Res.* 13:299–326
48. Cohen B. 1963. *The Press and Foreign Policy.* Princeton, NJ: Princeton Univ. Press
49. Collins W. 1978. Temporal integration and children's understanding of social information on television. *Am. J. Orthopsychiatry* 48:198–204
50. Collins W, Wellman H, Keniston A, Westby S. 1978. Age related aspects of comprehension of televised social content. *Child Dev.* 49:389–94
51. Comisky P, Bryant J, Zillman D. 1977. Commentary as a substitute for action. *J. Commun.* 27:150–52
52. Comstock G. 1983. Media influences on aggression. In *Prevention and Control of Aggression,* ed. A Goldstein, pp. 241–72. New York: Pergamon
53. Comstock G, Chaffee S, Katzman N, McCombs M, Roberts D, et al. 1978. *Television and Human Behavior.* New York: Columbia Univ. Press
53a. Comstock G, Rubinstein E, eds. 1972. *Television and Social Behavior: Television and Adolescent Aggressiveness,* Vol. 3. Washington, DC: US GPO
54. Comstock G, Strasburger V. 1990. Deceptive appearances: television violence and aggressive behavior. *J. Adolesc. Health Care* 11:31–44
55. Curtis D. 1994. "Youths call media too negative: 60% say they dislike emphasis on child-related violence, drugs." *San Francisco Chronicle,* March 1, p. A7
56. Diener E, DeFour D. 1978. Does television violence enhance programme publicity? *J. Res. Soc. Psychol.* 36:333–41
57. Diener E, Woody L. 1981. TV violence and viewer liking. *Commun. Res.* 8:281–306
58. Dominick J, Greenberg B. 1972. Attitudes toward violence: The interaction of television, exposure, family attitudes, and social class. See Ref. 53a, pp. 314–35
59. Donnerstein E. 1980. Pornography and violence against women: Experimental studies. *Ann. NY Acad. Sci.* 347:277–88
60. Donnerstein E, Barrett G. 1978. The effects of erotic stimuli on male aggression against women. *J. Pers. Soc. Psychol.* 36:180–88
61. Donnerstein E, Berkowitz L. 1981. Victim reactions in aggressive erotic films as a factor in violence against women. *J. Pers. Soc. Psychol.* 41:710–24
62. Donnerstein E, Hallam J. 1978. The facilitating effects of erotica on aggression against women. *J. Pers. Soc. Psychol.* 36:1270–77
63. Dorr A, Graves S, Phelps E. 1980. Developing a curriculum for teenagers. *J. Commun.* 30:71–83
64. Drabman R, Thomas M. 1974. Does media violence increase children's tolerance of real-life aggression? *Dev. Psychol.* 10:418–21
65. Drabman R, Thomas M. 1974. Exposure to filmed violence and children's tolerance of real life aggresion. *Pers. Soc. Psychol. Bull.* 1:198–99
66. Durant R, Cadenhead C, Pendergrast R, Slavens G, Linder C. 1994. Factors associated with the use of violence among urban Black adolescents. *Am. J. Public Health* 84:612–17
67. Dysinger WS, Ruckmick CA. 1933. *The Emotional Responses of Children to the Motion Picture Situation.* New York: Macmillan
68. Eastman H, Liss M. 1980. TV preferences of children from four parts of the U.S. *Journal. Q.* 57:488–90
69. Ekman P, Liebert R, Friesen W, al et. 1972. Facial expressions of emotion while watching televised violence as predictors of subsequent aggression. See Ref. 53a, pp. 22–58
70. Eron L. 1986. Interventions to mitigate the psychological effects of media violence on aggressive behavior. *J. Soc. Issues* 42:155–69
71. Eron L, Huesmann L. 1984. The relation of prosocial behavior to the development of aggression and psychopathology. *Aggress. Behav.* 10:201–12
72. Feshbach S. 1972. Reality and fantasy in filmed violence. See Ref. 53a, pp. 318–45
73. Fine G, Mortimer J, Roberts D. 1990. Leisure, work, and the mass media. In *At the Threshold: The Developing Adolescent,* ed. S Feldman, GR Elliott, pp. 225–52. Cambridge, MA/London: Harvard Univ. Press

74. Fingerhut L, Jones C, Makuc D. 1994. Firearm and motor vehicle injury mortality: Variations by state, race and ethnicity: United States, 1990–91. In *Advance Data From Vital and Health Statistics,* pp. 1–12. Hyattsville, MD: DHHSS, Natl. Cent. Health Stat.

75. Freedman J. 1984. Effect of television violence on aggressiveness. *Psychol. Bull.* 96:227–46

76. Funk J. 1993. Reevaluating the impact of video games. *Clin. Pediatr.* 32:86–90

77. Funk J. 1993. Video games. *Adolesc. Med: State Art Rev.* 4:589–98

78. Funk J, Buchman D. 1995. Video game controversies. *Pediatr. Ann.* 24:91–94

79. Garbarino J, Dubrow N, Kostelny K, Prado C. 1992. *Children in Danger: Coping with the Consequences of Community Violence.* San Francisco: Jossey-Bass

80. Geen RG. 1968. Effects of frustration, attack, and prior training in aggressiveness upon aggressive behavior. *J. Pers. Soc. Psychol.* 9:316–21

81. Geen RG, Stoner D. 1972. Context effects in observed violence. *J. Pers. Soc. Psychol.* 25:145–50

82. Gelman M. 1989. Drunk driving TV campaign a success. *Variety* 4

83. Gerbner G. 1972. Violence in television drama: Trends and symbolic functions. In *Television and Social Behavious: Media Content and Control,* ed. G Comstock, E Rubinstein, 1:28–187. Washington, DC: US GPO

84. Gerbner G, Gross L. 1976. Living with television: The violence profile. *J. Commun.* 26:173–99

85. Gerbner G, Gross L, Eleey MF, Jackson-Beeck M, Jeffries-Fox S, Signorelli N. 1977. Television profile No. 8: The highlights. *J. Commun.* 27:171–80

86. Gerbner G, Gross L, Jackson-Beeck M, Jeffries-Fox S, Signorelli N. 1978. Cultural indicators: Violence profile No. 9. *J. Commun.* 28:176–207

87. Gerbner G, Gross L, Morgan M, et al. 1980. The "mainstreaming" of America: Violence profile No. 11. *J. Commun.* 30:10–29

88. Gerbner G, Gross L, Morgan M, Signorelli N. 1986. The dynamics of the cultivation process. In *Perspectives on Media Effects,* ed. J Bryant, D Zillman, pp. 17–48. Hillsdale, NJ: Erlbaum

89. Gerbner G, Gross L, Signorelli N, Morgan M, Jackson-Beeck M. 1979. The demonstration of power: Violence profile No. 10. *J. Commun.* 29:177–96

90. Ginsburg M. 1994. "Violence backlash on video: Rating games meant for kids called overdue." *San Francisco Examiner,* May 22, p. B1

91. Gonzenbach W. 1992. A time-series analysis of the drug issue, 1985–1990: The press, the president, and public opinion. *Int. J. Public Opin. Res.* 4:126–47

92. Gordon M, Heath L. 1981. The news business, crime and fear. In *Reaction to Crime,* ed. D Lewis. Beverly Hills, CA: Sage

93. Greenberg B. 1982. Television and role socialization: An overview. In *Television and Behavior: Ten Years of Scientific Progress and Implications for the Eighties,* ed. L Pearl, L Bouthilet, J Lazar, pp. 179–90. Rockville, MD: US Dep. Health Hum. Serv.

94. Greenberg G. 1975. British children and televised violence. *Public Opin. Q.* 38:531–47

95. Greene M. 1993. Chronic exposure to violence and poverty: Interventions that work for youth. *Crime Delinq.* 39:106–24

96. Greenfield P, Beagles-Roos J. 1988. Television vs. radio: The cognitive impact on different soci-economic and ethnic groups. *J. Commun.* 38:71–92

97. Greeson L, Williams R. 1986. Social implications of music videos for youth: An analysis of the content and effects of MTV. *Youth Soc.* 18:177–89

98. Griffiths M. 1991. Amusement machine playing in childhood and adolescence. *J. Adolesc.* 14:53–73

99. Gunter B. 1994. The question of media violence. In *Media Effects,* ed. J Bryant, D Zillman, pp. 163–211. Hillsdale, NJ: Earlbaum

100. Hamilton J. 1994 *Marketing Violence: The Impact of Labeling Violent Television Content.* Durham, NC: Dewitt Wallace Cent. Commun. J., Duke Univ.

101. Hansen C, Hansen R. 1990. The influence of sex and violence on the appeal of rock music. *Commun. Res.* 17:212–34

102. Hartnagel T, Teevan J, McIntyre J. 1975. Television violence and violent behavior. *Soc. Forces* 54:341–51

103. Heath L, Bresolin L, Rinaldi R. 1989. Effects of media violence on children. *Arch. Gen. Psychiatry* 46:376–79

104. Hicks D. 1968. Effects of co-observer's sanctions and adult presence on imitative aggression. *Child Dev.* 38:308–9

105. Hoberman H. 1990. Study group report on the impact of television violence on adolescents. *J. Adolesc. Health Care* 11:45–49

106. Huesmann L. 1986. Psychological processes promoting the relation between exposure to media violence and agres-

sive behavior by the viewer. *J. Soc. Issues* 42:125–39

107. Huesmann L. 1982. Television violence and aggressive behavior. In *Television and Behavior: Ten Years of Scientific Progress and Implications for the Eighties,* ed. D Pearl, L Bouthilet, J Lazer, pp. 126–37. New York: Academic

108. Huesmann L, Eron L, Klein R, Brice P, Fischer P, et al. 1983. Mitigating the imitation of aggressive behaviors by changing children's attitudes about media violence. *J. Pers. Soc. Psychol.* 44:899–910

109. Huesmann L, Eron L, Lefkowitz M, Walder L. 1984. Stability of aggression over time and generations. *Dev. Psychol.* 20:1120–34

110. Hull T. 1994. "Californians: Get tough on crime." *San Francisco Chronicle,* Jan. 16, pp. A1, A10

111. Huston AC, Donnerstein E, Fairfield H, Feshbach ND, Katz PA, et al. 1992. *Big World, Small Screen: The Role of Television in American Society.* Lincoln, NE: Univ. Nebr. Press

112. Jordan D. 1993. Newspaper effects on policy preferences. *Public Opin. Q.* 57:191–204

113. Josephson W. 1981. *Television violence and childrens' aggression: disinhibition, elicitation, or catharsis?* Presented at Meet. Can. Psychol. Assoc.

114. Kessler R, Stipp H. 1984. The impact of fictional television suicide stories on U.S. fatalities: A replication. *Am. J. Sociol.* 90:151–67

115. Klein JD, Brown JD, Childers KW, Oliveri J, Porter C, Dykers C. 1993. Adolescents' risky behavior and mass media use. *Pediatrics* 92:24–31

116. Koop C, Lundberg G. 1992. Violence in America: A public health emergency: Time to bite the bullet back. *JAMA* 267:3075–76

117. Lefcourt H, Barnes K, Parke R, Schwartz F. 1966. Anticipated social censure and aggression-conflict as mediators of response to aggression induction. *J. Soc. Psychol.* 70:251–63

118. Lefkowitz M, Eron L, Walder L, Huesmann L. 1972. Television violence and child aggression: A follow-up study. See Ref. 53a, pp. 35–135

119. Media Inst. 1983. *Prime Time Crime*

120. Deleted in proof

121. Deleted in proof

122. Liebert R, Sprafkin J, eds. 1988. *The Early Window - Effects of Television on Children and Youth.* New York: Pergamon

123. Linsky M. 1986. *Impact: How the Press Affects Federal Policy Making.* New York: Norton

124. Linz D, Donnerstein E, Penrod S. 1984. The effects of long term exposure to violence against women. *J. Commun.* 34:130–47

125. Linz D, Donnerstein E, Penrod S. 1988. Effects of long-term exposure to violent and sexually degrading depictions of women. *J. Pers. Soc. Psychol.* 55:758–68

126. Linz D, Fuson I, Donnerstein E. 1990. *Mitigating the Negative Effects of Sexually Violent Mass Communications Through Preexposure Briefings.* Beverly Hills, CA: Sage

127. Linz D, Malamuth N. 1993. *Pornography.* Newbury Park, CA: Sage

128. Lippmann W. 1921. In *Public Opinion,* pp. 3–32. New York: Macmillan

129. Lovaas O. 1961. Effect of exposure to symbolic aggression on aggrssive behavior. *Child Dev.* 32:37–44

130. Lyle J, Hoffmann H. 1972. Childrens' use of television and other media. In *Television and Social Behavior: Reports and Papers: Television in Day-to-Day Life: Patterns of Use,* ed. E Rubenstein, G Comstock, J Murray, 4:129–256. Washington, DC: US GPO

131. Malamuth N, Briere J. 1986. Sexual violence in the media: Indirect effects on aggression against women. *J. Soc. Issues* 42:75–92

132. Malamuth N, Check J. 1980. Penile tumescence and perpetual responses to rape as a function of victim's perceived reactions. *J. Appl. Soc. Psychol.* 10:528–47

133. Malamuth N, Donnerstein E. 1982. The effects of aggressive pornographic mass media stimuli. In *Advances on Experimental Social Psychology,* ed. L Berkowitz, pp. 103–36. New York: Academic

134. Marks A. 1987. *Television Exposure, Fear of Crime and Concern About Serious Illness.* PhD Diss. Northwestern Univ., Evanston, IL

135. McCombs M, Shaw D. 1972. The agenda-setting function of mass media. *Public Opin. Q.* 36:176–87

136. McIntyre J, Teevan J, Hartnagel T. 1972. Television violence and deviant behavior. *Television and Social Behavior,* ed G Comstock, E Rubinstein, 3:383–435

137. McLeod J, Atkin C, Chaffee S. 1972. Adolescents, parents and television use: Self-report and other measures from the Wisconsin samples. See Ref. 53a, pp. 239–335

138. McLeod J, Atkin C, Chaffee S. 1972.

Adolescents, parents and television use: adolescent self-report measures from Maryland and Wisconsin samples. See Ref. 53a, pp. 173–238

139. Medrish E. 1979. Constant television: A background to daily life. *J. Commun.* 29:171–79

140. Messner S. 1986. Television violence and violent crime: An aggregate analysis. *Soc. Probl.* 33:218–35

141. Meyer T. 1972. Children's perceptions of favorite television characters as behavioral models. *Educ. Broadcast. Rev.* 7:25–33

142. Meyer T. 1973. Childrens' perceptions of favorite television characters as behavioral models. *Educ. Broadcast. Rev.* 7:25–33

143. Montgomery K. 1989. *Target: Prime Time.* New York: Oxford Univ. Press

144. Morin R. 1994. "Media have stoked anxiety on crime." *San Francisco Chronicle,* Jan. 25, p. A8

145. O'Keefe G. 1986. The "McGruff" national media campaign: its public impact and future implications. In *Community Crime Prevention: Does it Work?,* ed. D Rosenbaum, pp. xxx–xx. Beverly Hills, CA: Sage

146. O'Keefe G. 1985. "Taking a bite out of crime": The impact of a public information campaign. *Commun. Res.* 12:147–78

147. O'Keefe G. 1993. *The Social Impact of the National Citizens' Crime Prevention Campaign.* Washington, DC: Bur. Justice

148. Page B, Shapiro R, Dempsey G. 1987. What moves public opinion. *Am. Polit. Sci. Rev.* 81:23–43

149. Patterson G. 1979. A performance theory for coercive family interactions. In *Social Interaction: Methods, Analyses and Illustrations,* ed. R Cairns, pp. 119–62. Hillsdale, NJ: Erbaum

150. Patterson G, Chamberlain P, Reid J. 1982. A comparative evaluation of parent training procedures. *Behav. Ther.* 13:638–50

151. Pearl D, Bouthilet L, Lazar J. 1982. *Television and Behavior: Ten Years of Scientific Progress and Implications for the Eighties.* Washington, DC: US GPO

152. Deleted in proof

153. Pertschuck M. 1988. In *Smoking Control: Media Advocacy Guidelines.* Washington, DC: Advocacy Inst. Natl. Cancer Inst., Natl. Inst. Health

154. Peterson D, Pfost K. 1989. Influence of rock videos on attitudes of violence against women. *Psychol. Rep.* 64:319–22

155. Phillips D. 1980. Airplane accidents,

murder and the mass media: Towards a theory of imitation and suggestion. *Soc. Forces* 58:1001–23

156. Phillips D. 1980. The deterrent effect of capital punishment: New evidence on an old controversy. *Am. J. Sociol.* 86:139–47

157. Phillips D. 1982. The impact of fictional television stories on U.S. adult fatalities: New evidence on the effect of mass media on violence. *Am. J. Sociol.* 87:1340–59

158. Phillips D. 1983. The impact of mass media violence on U.S. homicides. *Am. Sociol. Rev.* 48:560–68

159. Phillips D. 1974. The influence of suggestion on suicide: Substantive and theoretical implications of the Warner Effect. *Am. Sociol. Rev.* 39:340–54

160. Phillips D. 1981. Strong and weak research designs for detecting the impact of capital punishment on homicide. *Rutgers Law Rev.* 33:790–98

161. Phillips D. 1979. Suicide, motor fatalities, and the mass media: Evidence toward a theory of suggestion. *Am. J. Sociol.* 84:1150–73

162. Post W. 1994. "Afraid of crime? Don't watch TV." *San Jose Mercury News,* March 3, p. 1A

163. Provenzo E. 1991. *Video Kids: Making Sense of Nintendo.* Cambridge, MA: Harvard Univ. Press

164. Pynoos R, Eth S. 1985. Children traumatized by witnessing acts of personal violence. In *Post-Traumatic Stress Disorder in Children,* ed. S Eth, R Pynoos, pp. xxx–xx. Washington, DC: Am. Psychiatr. Press

165. Rathus J, Wetzler S, Asnis G. 1995. Posttraumatic Stress Disorder and exposure to violence in adolescents. *JAMA* 273:1734

166. Rehman S, Reilly S. 1985. Music videos: A new dimension of televised violence. *Penn. Speech Commun. Ann.* 41:61–64

167. Research NM. 1993. *1992–1993 Report on Television.* New York: Nielsen Media Res.

168. Robinson J, Bachman J. 1972. Television viewing habits and aggression. In *Television and Social Behaviour:* Vol. 3. *Television and Adolescent Aggressiveness,* ed. G Comstock, E Rubinstein. Washington, DC: US GPO

169. Rosekrans M. 1967. Imitation in children as a function of perceived similarities to a social model of vicarious reinforcemen. *J. Pers. Soc. Psychol.* 7:305–17

170. Rosekrans M, Hartup W. 1967. Imitative influences of consistent and inconsistent

response consequences to a model on aggressive behavior in children. *J. Pers. Soc. Psychol.* 7:429–34

171. Russell G. 1979. Hero selection by Canadian hockey players: Skill or aggression? *Can. J. Appl. Sport Sci.* 4:309–13

171a. *San Francisco Chronicle.* 1993. "Anxiety over crime is growing, poll finds," Dec. 17, p. A4

172. Schramm W. 1954. Procedures and effects of mass communication. In *Mass Media and Education II: 53rd Yearbook of the National Society for the Study of Education,* ed. N Henry, pp. 113–38. Chicago: Univ. Chicago Press

173. Schramm W, Lyle J, Parker E. 1961. *Television in the Lives of Our Children.* Stanford, CA: Stanford Univ. Press

174. Shelov S, Nar-On M, Beard L, Hojan M, Holroyd HJ, et al. 1995. Media violence. *Pediatrics* 95:949–51

175. Sheppard A, Sheehy N, Young B. 1989. *Violence on Television: An Intervention: A Report to the Independent Broadcasting Industry.* Leeds: Univ. Leeds

176. Sherman B, Dominick J. 1986. Violence and sex in music videos: TV and rock'n'roll. *J. Commun.* 36:79–93

177. Shetterly W. 1991. In *Utne Reader,* May/June, pp. 32–34

178. Silvern S, Williamson P. 1987. The effects of video game play on young childrens' aggression, fantasy, and prosocial behavior. *J. Appl. Dev. Psychol.* 8:453–62

179. Singer D. 1985. Does violent television produce aggressive children? *Pediatr. Ann.* 14:804–10

180. Singer D, Benton W. 1989. Caution: Television may be hazardous to a child's mental health. *Dev. Behav. Pediatr.* 10: 259–61

181. Singer D, Singer J. 1984. What's all the fuss about. *Television Child.* Spring:30–41

182. Singer D, Zuckerman D, Singer J. 1980. Teaching elementary and school children television viewing skills: an evaluation. *J. Commun.* 30:84–93

183. Singer J, Singer DG, Rapaczynski W. 1984. Family patterns and television viewing as predictors of children's beliefs and aggression. *J. Commun.* 34:73–89

184. Singer J, Singer D. 1981. *Television, Imagination, and Aggression: A Study of Preschoolers.* Hillsdale, NJ: Erlbaum

185. Singer J, Singer D, Desmond R, Hirsch B, Nicol A. 1988. Family mediation and childrens' cognition, aggression, and comprehension of television: A longitudinal study. *J. Appl. Dev. Psychol.* 9:329–47

186. Singer M, Anglin T, Song L, Lunghofer L. 1995. Adolescents' exposure to violence and associated symptoms of psychological trauma. *JAMA* 273:477–82

187. Slife B, Rychiak J. 1982. Role of affective assessment in modeling behavior. *J. Pers. Soc. Psychol.* 43:861–68

188. Smith M. 1974. Significant others' influence on the assaultive behavior of young hockey players. *Int. Rev. Sport Sociol.* 3–5:45–56

189. Deleted in proof

190. Stack S. 1987. Celebrities and suicide: A taxonomy and analysis, 1948–1983. *Am. Sociol. Rev.* 52:401–12

191. St. Lawrence J, Joyner D. 1991. The effects of sexually violent rock music on males' acceptance of violence against women. *Psychol. Women Q.* 15:49–63

192. Stein S, Kraemer H, Spiegel D. 1995. *The impact of media coverage of a violent crime on children in 3 states.* Presented at Ann. Meet. Am. Psychiatr. Assoc.

193. Steuer F, Applefield J, Smith R. 1971. Televised aggression and the interpersonal aggression of preschool children. *J. Exp. Child Psychol.* 11:442–47

194. Stipp H, Milavsky J. 1988. U.S. television programming's effects on aggressive behavior of children and adolescents. *Curr. Psychol: Res. Rev.* 7:76–92

195. Strasburger V. 1993. Adolescents and the media: Five crucial issues. *Adolesc. Med: State Art Rev.* 273:479–93

196. Strasburger V. 1995. *Adolescents and the Media: Medical and Psychological Impact.* Thousand Oaks, CA: Sage

197. Sun S-W, Lull J. 1986. The adolescent audience for music videos and why they watch. *J. Commun.* 36:115–25

198. Surette R. 1990. Criminal justice policy and the media. In *The Media and Criminal Justice Policy: Recent Research and Social Effects,* ed. R Surette, pp. 3–17. Springfield, IL: Charles C. Thomas

199. Swank D, Jacob H, Moran J. 1982. Newspaper attentiveness to crime. In *Governmental Responses to Crime,* ed. H Jacob, R Lineberry, pp. 77–117. Washington, DC: Natl. Inst. Justice

200. Thomas M, Drabman R. 1978. Effects of television violence on expectations of others' aggression. *Pers. Soc. Psychol. Bull.* 4:73–76

201. Thomas M, Horton R, Lippincott E, Drabman R. 1977. Desensitization to portrayals of real-life aggression as a function of exposure to television violence. *J. Pers. Soc. Psychol.* 35:450–58

202. Deleted in proof

203. Walker J. How viewing of MTV relates

to exposure to other media violence. *Journal. Q.* 64:756–62

204. Wallack L. 1990. Improving health promotion: Media advocacy and social marketing approaches. In *Mass Communication and Public Health,* ed. C Atkin, L Wallack, pp. 41–51. Newbury Park, CA: Sage

205. Wartella E, Heintz K, Aidman A, Mazzarella S. 1990. Television and beyond: Childrens' video media in one community. *Commun. Res.* 17:45–64

206. Wass H, Raup J, Cervillo K, Martel L, Mingione L, Sperring A. 1989. Adolescents' interest in and view of destructive themes in rock music. *Omega* 19:177–86

207. Wass H, Raup J, Sisler H. 1989. Adolescents and death on television: A follow-up study. *Death Stud.* 13:161–73

208. Widom C. 1989. Does violence beget violence?: A critical review of the literature. *Psychol. Bull.* 106:3–28

209. Williams S. 1994. "It's a crime, the way news scares us." *San Jose Mercury News,* April 21, p. 5E

210. Williams T. 1986. *The Impact of Television: A Natural Experiment in Three Communities.* New York: Academic

211. Wintemute G, Teret S, Kraus J, Wright M, Bradford G. 1987. When children shoot children: 88 unintended deaths in California. *JAMA* 257:3107–9

212. Wood W, Wong F, Chachere J. 1991. Effects of media violence on viewers' aggression in unconstrained social interaction. *Am. Psychol. Assoc.* 109:371–83

213. Workman B. 1994. "TV news linked to children's stress: Stanford researchers report on effects of Klaas kidnap coverage." *San Francisco Chronicle,* April 27, p. A2

213a. Yang N, Linz D. 1990. Movie ratings and the content of adult videos: the sex violence ratio. *J. Commun.* 40:28–42

214. Young K, Smith M. 1988. Mass media treatment of violence in sports and its effects. *Curr. Psychol: Res. Rev.* 7:298–311

215. Zillman D. 1971. Excitation transfer in communication-mediated aggressive behavior. *J. Exp. Soc. Psychol.* 7:419–34

216. Zillman D, Johnson R, Hanrahan J. 1973. Pacifying Effect of a happy ending of communications involving agresion. *Psychol. Rep.* 32:967–70

Annu. Rev. Public Health. 1996. 17:299–309

HEALTHY CITIES: Toward Worldwide Health Promotion

Beverly Collora Flynn

Indiana University School of Nursing, WHO Collaborating Center in Healthy Cities, 1111 Middle Drive, Indianapolis, Indiana 46202-5107

KEY WORDS: health promotion, primary health care, policy, public health, urbanization

---

ABSTRACT

Healthy Cities is a community problem-solving process for health promotion that began in Canada and Europe in the mid-1980s. Although Healthy Cities have expanded worldwide, there is limited scientific literature that documents the effects of these efforts. This review describes the dynamic status of Healthy Cities globally and summarizes what is known about these efforts. It is difficult to draw generalizations or clear differences between Healthy Cities and other efforts with similar objectives in the United States. There appears to be less variation among Healthy Cities in Europe, most likely because of the extensive technical support provided by the WHO European Regional Office to the Healthy Cities Project. Case descriptions present the diversity and types of activities of Healthy Cities. It is concluded that community participation and broad involvement from different sectors of the community are promising approaches to addressing urban problems.

INTRODUCTION

The purpose of this review is describe Healthy Cities globally and to evaluate critically what is known about these activities and their effects. I conducted computer on-line searches of Healthy Cities and Healthy Communities and reviewed bibliography research for Healthy Cities (42, 46) and a vast array of Healthy Cities materials on file at the WHO Collaborating Center in Healthy Cities at Indiana University School of Nursing. Only literature available in English was included in this chapter. Because of the youth of the Healthy Cities movement and the variety of the organizational forms and processes working under this banner, limited scientific literature exists to assess the effects of these efforts.

299

WHAT IS HEALTHY CITIES?

The most widely used definition of Healthy Cities is, "a Healthy City is one that is continually creating and improving those physical and social environments and strengthening those community resources which enable people to mutually support each other in performing all the functions of life and achieving their maximum potential" (26). This definition is process oriented and consistent with the *Ottawa Charter for Health Promotion* (41). The Healthy Cities process involves the following steps: establishing a broad-based structure for Healthy Cities, encouraging community participation, assessing community needs, establishing priorities and strategic plans, soliciting political support, taking local action, and evaluating progress (14, 38, 45, 55).

Healthy Cities began in Canada (now called Healthy Communities) in 1984 (24, 34), and the WHO European Healthy Cities Project was initiated by Ilona Kickbusch in 1986 (32, 51). These Healthy Cities projects were built on the concepts of primary health care and health promotion, which included challenging communities to develop projects that reduce inequalities in health status and access to services, and to develop healthy public policies at the local level through a multisectoral approach and increased community participation in health decision making (2, 32, 41, 50, 51, 54). The role of local government is central to the Healthy Cities concept and one that distinguishes Healthy Cities from other community-level health promotion programs (25). Also, the Healthy Cities concept involves focusing on the whole community, with its strengths and problems, rather than being established under the rubric of categorical problems such as tobacco, hypertension, cancer, or child abuse. Healthy Cities is not confined to one or more health problems, but "is intended to build health into the decision-making processes of local governments, community organizations and businesses, to develop a broad range of strategies to address the broad social, environmental and economic determinants of health" and to change the ..."community culture by incorporating health" (25). The Healthy Cities concept suggests a restructuring of the health decision-making process, shifting power to the local level.

HEALTHY CITIES: WHAT WE KNOW

Nationally

Healthy Cities in the United States is also called Healthy Communities and is one of several health promotion models found to support communities in improving their health (17). Within Healthy Cities and Communities there are multiple approaches that are often not well defined. Healthy Cities projects are initiated independently, based on a range of philosophical orientations and with different sponsoring organizations and funding.

As of mid-1995, there were more than 200 self-proclaimed Healthy Cities and Communities in the United States. Individual Healthy Cities have been initiated throughout the country at the city and state levels. Some examples of cities include Atlantic City, Boston, Pittsburgh, and Philadelphia. Healthy Cities began in the United States with two statewide initiatives, Healthy Cities Indiana and the California Healthy Cities Project. Healthy Cities Indiana was begun in 1988 by Indiana University School of Nursing in partnership with six cities and with funding from the W. K. Kellogg Foundation (19). The dissemination of this model is called CITYNET Healthy Cities. California initiated a Healthy Cities Project about the same time and continues to receive prevention block grant money for their activities (52). Maine and New Mexico have Indian communities involved in their networks. The Colorado Healthy Communities Initiative was organized through the National Civic League (NCL) with a grant from the Colorado Trust. South Carolina and Massachusetts also have announced the formation of Healthy Communities (4; T Wolff, unpublished letter).

Several years ago, the United States Public Health Service (USPHS) funded the NCL for a Healthy Communities Initiative and continues to disseminate information about Healthy Cities and Communities in the United States. CITYNET Healthy Cities and the WHO Collaborating Center in Healthy Cities at Indiana University School of Nursing provide materials, consultation, leadership training, and technical support to communities interested in Healthy Cities and conduct research in the field. The National Association of County and City Health Officials (NACCHO) and CDC conducted a survey of about 2000 local health departments in 1994 and documented the planning tools they used (35). It was found that 32% used APEX/PH, 12% used PATCH, and 6% used Healthy Cities.

Based on meeting with Healthy Cities and Communities coordinators of the California, Colorado, and New Mexico projects and information from CITYNET Healthy Cities, the organizations with the most experience in Healthy Cities in the United States, common action areas emerged. They are the environment (recycling, land use and protection, air and water quality); community safety (youth gangs and domestic violence); immunizations; tobacco; and youth (teenage pregnancy, recreation for youth, job training, family life skills, immigrants, and school-based services). Initiatives in these areas differ across cities in stage of development, Healthy Cities method used, and level of activity. It is difficult to draw generalizations or clear differences between the Healthy Cities/Healthy Communities efforts and others with similar objectives. For example, the American Hospital Association Research and Educational Trust is involved with other organizations, including the Voluntary Hospitals of America, in developing community care networks with a grant from the W. K. Kellogg Foundation (53). The Healthcare Forum, an organization of primarily hospital leaders, initiated a Healthier Communities Fellows Program in 1993 and presents annual Healthier Communities Awards (28, 29). And the Institute for Healthcare Improvement has initiated a community-wide health improvement learning collaborative in ten communities throughout the country, using continuous quality improvement principles (5).

Globally

There are over 1000 Healthy Cities established throughout the world, including every WHO region. However, the majority are in Europe (see Table 1). Since the WHO European Regional Office has provided extensive technical support and has developed and disseminated many documents on methods and processes to implement Healthy Cities, there appears to be less variation in the approaches employed by European Healthy Cities than by their counterparts in the United States. Healthy Cities in Europe are designated by WHO as Healthy Cities by their continued commitment to specified actions, such as participating in an international network, to exchanging information, and working systematically to make their cities healthier (11). In addition to the 35 WHO European Project Cities, there are 23 national networks of Healthy Cities throughout Europe that have facilitated the development of approximately 650

Table 1 Globalization of Healthy Cities: the regional situation

African Region (N = 30)[a]	American Region (N = 300)[a]	Mid-Eastern Region (N = 30)[a]	European Region (N = 650)[a]	S.E. Asian Region (N = 10)[a]	W. Pacific Region (N = 30)[a]
Congo	Bolivia	Algeria	23 Countries	Bangladesh	Australia
Ghana	Brazil	Cyprus		Nepal	China
Ivory Coast	Canada	Egypt	35 WHO Project Cities	Thailand	Japan
Niger	Chile	Iran			Malaysia
	Colombia	Kuwait			New Zealand
Senegal	Costa Rica	Oman			Vietnam
South Africa	Cuba	Pakistan			
		Tunisia			
Tanzania	Mexico				
	United States				
	Venezuela				

[a] Approximate numbers
Sources: References 13, 22

Healthy Cities. The national networks provide training, research, organization, planning of activities, and networking across cities. Goumans (23) analyzed networks in the WHO Healthy Cities project. She concluded that there was no uniformity across national networks, but the strength of networks was that they had the potential to sustain Healthy Cities over time. In addition to national networking, there are two networks based on language, a French-speaking network that includes Healthy Cities in Africa, Canada, and France, and Spanish-speaking network between Healthy Cities in Spain and Latin America (13).

The WHO Healthy Cities Project also has initiated Multi-City Action Plans (MCAP), in which a number of participating Healthy Cities collaborate closely in addressing common health problems. MCAP goals are to take action in primary health care and health promotion as well as produce knowledge useful to other cities (43). Problems being addressed by the MCAPs include accidents, alcohol, environment and health among Baltic cities, diabetes, disabled and elderly people, drugs, nutrition, sports and active living, tobacco-free cities, unemployment, urban primary health care, and women's health. It is interesting to note that these are common problems being addressed by Healthy Cities in other parts of the world (3, 7, 8, 34, 44).

In 1997, the WHO participation in the existing European Healthy Cities Project will end (13). To assist with this transition an organization of European National Healthy Cities Networks, EURONET, was created by national network coordinators to establish self-sustainable mechanisms to promote Healthy Cities throughout Europe (59; WHO Regional office for Europe unpublished meeting report; WHO Regional Office for Europe, unpublished communication on EURONET). EURONET works jointly with WHO in developing and strengthening national Healthy Cities networks and in establishing mechanisms for information exchange and support between networks and their member cities. For example, during 1994–1998, the Association is working to identify minimum criteria of accreditation for network cities; support and establish systems for communication, information exchange, research and training; support the involvement of national networks and member cities with the WHO Healthy Cities Project, MCAP, twinning arrangements, and special projects; and to develop action on peace and human rights in the context of the new public health. The WHO Regional Office for Europe is also interested in building on the efforts of the Healthy Cities Project in Europe by developing Healthy Cities in Eastern Europe and the Balkan countries (WHO Regional Office for Europe, unpublished communication on EURONET).

HEALTHY CITIES PROJECTS AND ACTIVITIES

Most of the information on how Healthy City projects assess needs and operate has been gleaned from the European experience (10, 12, 13, 23, 51, 57). Across these cities common problems identified included aging, migrants and refugees, cardiovascular disease and cancer, economic decline, inadequate housing, and traffic.

Major activities were community assessment, communication and information exchange, and training of various categories of workers to promote health. Development of city health plans and technical and financial assistance were provided to community groups to start action throughout the city or in neighborhoods.

Promotion of healthy public policy has been noted as central to the Healthy Cities approach (16, 31, 33, 48, 51). The European Healthy Cities projects have been broadly involved in policy issues such as promoting equity, altering lifestyles, improving political environment for a health agenda, and reorienting health services toward prevention and health promotion (13). Cities follow four common approaches to policy change: They adopt position statements and advocate for city council resolutions; they facilitate adoption of policies on particular health issues, population groups, geographic areas, or services; support the formulation and adoption of comprehensive city health plans; and finally, they advocate for assessments of the impact of city policies on health and the use of assessments by decision makers.

An analysis of the location of 32 Healthy Cities project offices within the city structure and project linkages with other city organizations found that the the majority of projects were located within city administration departments (57). Projects were found to act through both formal and informal relationships with a wide range of organizations including other city departments, district and regional health organizations, and universities and academic institutes.

No consensus exists on the best indicators of Healthy Cities despite considerable effort to construct a valid set (6, 12, 27, 37–40, 44, 45, 48, 49, 56, 58; Thurnhurst, unpublished paper). However, the WHO European Healthy Cities Project requires reporting on a common set of selected MCAP indicators that are categorized as health, health services, environment, and socioeconomic indicators (9). A number of problems with the variety of Healthy Cities indicators used include uncertain relevance of these indicators to health promotion; use of static methods in attempting to measure dynamic community processes; and questionable validity of applying indicators to compare cities that have different physical, social, political, and cultural contexts and different local needs and priorities (27, 37; WHO Regional Office for Europe, unpublished Workshop on Indicators Report).

Characteristics of successful Healthy Cities have been reported based on experiences in Europe, Quebec, Canada, and Indiana (20, 21, 51). These characteristics include effective leadership; a multisectoral Healthy City committee or steering group that directs the project; strong economy; community participation; information used in citywide planning; obtaining needed technical support; being viewed as a credible resource for health in the community; effective networking; smaller city size or neighborhoods in large cities. However, since these characteristics are community and process variables, conclusions about the effects of these variables on achievement of project goals (outcomes) cannot be made.

Case Descriptions

To provide a more concrete picture of the diversity and types of activities of Healthy Cities, five projects are briefly described in differing levels of detail below.

Healthy City Toronto (Canada)

Healthy City Toronto is noted as the birthplace of Healthy Cities (34). Healthy City Toronto began in 1984, and as early as 1985 was building alliances with key people in city departments. The public planning process was initiated by the city's Board of Health in 1986 and included vision workshops, a comprehensive environmental scan, development and distribution of issue papers, and public forums that resulted in *Healthy Toronto 2000*. This report contained specific recommendations for action that were accepted by the Board of Health and unanimously approved by the City Council. In 1989, the City Council formally launched the Healthy City Toronto project and established a Healthy City office. This office has focused on connecting the economy, environment, and equity in solving urban problems. Citizen participation and partnerships have lead to numerous projects including the following: Healthy Neighborhoods and Communities that promote citizen participation in health; Sustainable Development that builds partnerships on environmental issues such as clean air; and Homeless Persons Self-Help and Community Economic Development that create opportunities for economic ventures and housing by involving marginalized communities. The Healthy City project office studies urban problems and develops coordinated practical solutions through partnerships and sharing of resources.

Tokyo Healthy City (Japan)

Tokyo Healthy City (population approximately 12 million people) provides an example of a megacity's approach to building healthy public policy (36). The Action Plan for Tokyo Healthy City entitled, "Towards Healthy City Tokyo—Our Action Plan for Health Promotion" was adopted in 1993 by the Tokyo Citizens' Council for Health Promotion and endorsed by municipal governments. This plan defined priority areas for action, roles of citizens and the public and private sectors, and proposed strategies for action. The strategies were for development of comprehensive housing policy; recycling-oriented urban planning; innovations to the urban traffic policy; and infrastructure development. The Action Plan also encouraged research in health promotion. For example, Image-Diagnosis, which is a geographic information system or a form of computer mapping, was used to delineate health and environmental conditions of the city and was reported to be used to predict the impact of changes in health determinants on the public's health. Although it was reported that teamwork of citizens, administrators, and academics developed multisectoral programs and policies based on scientific knowledge of health and environment, it is difficult to assess the extent to which broad participation existed in a city of this size.

Bialystock Healthy City (Poland)

Bialystock, Poland, has undergone rapid change during the transition from a centrally planned economy to a democracy with a free-market economy (30). A history of heavy industrial development resulted in environmental degradation. The Bialystock Healthy City has been active in health and environmental issues and has sought public environmental education methods that involved active community participation. The city participated in the international Clean Up the World Campaign in September 1994, which offered the opportunity to use the experiences of others to promote citizen environmental action at low cost. An organizing committee was formed and plans were made for litter cleanups and a festival for participants. The city government approved the project, and the media and other forms of publicity announced the events and solicited citizen participation. The organizing committee planned the logistics of action and solicited in-kind support of businesses who provided garbage bags, gloves, and transportation for participants and removal of litter. An analysis of this Healthy City event indicated that approximately 14,000 citizens or 5% of the city's population participated over a five-day period and removed approximately 1000 cubic meters of garbage and litter. As a result of the campaign, a recycling program was initiated in the city of Bialystock. It was concluded that several factors contributed to the project's success; these include the level of public interest and willingness to respond, a catalyzing event, early initiation of the project, emphasis on adequate publicity, in-kind support from local businesses, and sufficient attention to logistics.

Copenhagen Healthy City (Denmark)

Copenhagen Healthy City developed The Copenhagen Healthy City Plan that was endorsed by the Copenhagen City Council in 1994 (15). The plan provided a framework for a number of preventive and health-promoting initiatives in the city. High priority was given to developing personal skills around lifestyle issues that were health damaging, including alcohol, tobacco smoking, nutrition, physical exercise, accidents, and unwanted pregnancies. The plan also focused on four key settings for health promotion: local communities, schools, workplaces, and health services. Its formation led to an increased allocation of resources for health to the city plan.

Jeffersonville Healthy City (Indiana, USA)

Jeffersonville Healthy City in Indiana (now called Healthy Communities of Clark County) was initiated in 1988 and soon gained recognition as a resource to the community. In 1991, Congressman Lee Hamilton requested that the Indiana Primary Health Care Association address the need for indigent care within Southern Indiana (18). This request was channeled to the Jeffersonville Healthy City Committee, which formed an Indigent Health Care Coalition. Although the local hospital provided approximately one million dollars per year to Clark County residents for indigent care services, neither the hospital nor any nearby resources were set up for primary care services for the indigent. Planning began for the development of a primary health care clinic for this population, which opened its doors in 1992. Except for a part-time coordinator, all health professionals providing services in the clinic were volunteers. An expanded partnership between the clinic and Indiana University School of Nursing led to funding from the Indiana State Department of Health for nurse-managed primary health care services at the clinic (1, 47).

IMPRESSIONS AND CONCLUSIONS

Much remains unexplained about Healthy Cities. The process of Healthy Cities is often not well documented, nor are the community factors that influence the process and outcomes. For example, the extent to which the local government was involved in initial development of the project is not always clear. Also unclear is the general extent of community participation in Healthy Cities and Communities projects. Conclusions about the relationships between the context of Healthy Cities or community factors, the Healthy Cities process, and outcomes cannot be made.

Despite uncertainty as to the effects of Healthy Cities, principles of community participation in local decisions that affect health have broad appeal in many parts of the world. The broad involvement of different segments of the community remains a promising approach to dealing with urban problems.

ACKNOWLEDGMENTS

The author wishes to thank Drs. Jean Goeppinger, Dixie Ray, and Phyllis Stern for their review of this manuscript and helpful suggestions given in its revision, and Amy Steinke and Debbie Corson for their conscientious assistance in compiling the manuscript.

Literature Cited

1. Adams C, Flynn BC. 1995. Indigent health care reform in a healthy city. *Am. J. Public Health.* In press
2. Ashton J. 1992. The origins of healthy cities. See Ref. 3, pp. 1–12
3. Ashton J, ed. 1992. *Healthy Cities.* Milton Keynes/Philadelphia: Open Univ. Press. 235 pp.
4. Blueprint. 1995. *Columbia: Healthy Communities Initiative.* SC Dep. Health Environ. Control Plan. Policy Dev. 2. 6 pp.
5. Boisvert L. 1993. Building community collaborations beyond the hospital walls. *Qual. Connect.* 2:1, 6
6. Cappon D. 1989. *Indicators for a healthy city.* Presented at Int. Conf. Res. Healthy Cities, The Hague
7. Case Studies and Sub-Plenary Present. 1995. *International Healthy and Ecological Cities Congress, Madrid,* Vol. 1. 250 pp.
8. Case Study Poster Presentations. 1995. *International Healthy and Ecological Cities Congress, Madrid,* Vol. 2. 198 pp.
9. Collin J. 1992. *Healthy City—Guide Note for the Healthy-Cities Indicators MCAP Indicators.* Copenhagen/Nancy: WHO Reg. Off. Eur. 124 pp.
10. Curtice L. 1993. Strategies and values research and the WHO healthy cities project in Europe. See Ref. 12, pp. 34–54
11. Curtice L, Minay R, eds. 1994. *Action for Health in Cities.* Copenhagen: WHO Reg. Off. Eur. 113 pp.
12. Davies JK, Kelly MP, eds. 1993. *Healthy Cities Research and Practice.* London/New York: Routledge. 188 pp.
13. Draper R, Curtice L, Hooper J, Goumans M. 1993. *WHO Healthy Cities Project: Review of the First Five Years (1987–1992).* Copenhagen: WHO Reg. Off. Eur. 137 pp.
14. Duhl L. 1986. The healthy city: Its functions and its future. *Health Promot.* 1:55–60

15. Egsgaard J. 1995. Copenhagen city health plan. See Ref. 7, pp. 128–32
16. Evers A, Farrant W, Trojan A, eds. 1990. *Healthy Public Policy at the Local Level.* Frankfurt am Main: Campus Verlag/Boulder, CO: Westview. 242 pp.
17. Flynn BC. 1993. Healthy cities within the American context. See Ref. 12, pp. 112–26
18. Flynn BC. 1995. Health care reform in Jeffersonville healthy city, Indiana, USA. See Ref. 8, pp. 37–42
19. Flynn BC, Rider MS. 1991. Healthy cities Indiana: mainstreaming community health in the United States. *Am. J. Public Health* 81:510–11
20. Flynn BC, Rider MS, Ray DW. 1991. Healthy cities: the Indiana model of community development in public health. *Health Educ. Q.* 18:331–47
21. Fortin JP, Groleau G, O'Neill M, Lemreux V. 1991. *The Evaluation Tool for the Quebec Healthy City (Town) Projects.* Quebec, Can: Cent. Res., Laval Univ. (From French)
22. Goldstein G. 1995. WHO Healthy cities—towards an interregional programme framework. See Ref. 7, pp. 1–9
23. Goumans M. 1992. What about healthy networks? An analysis of national healthy cities networks in Europe. *Health Promot. Int.* 7:273–81
24. Hancock T. 1987. Healthy cities: the Canadian project. *Health Promot.* 26:2–4, 27
25. Hancock T. 1993. The evolution, impact and significance of the healthy cities/healthy communities movement. *J. Public Health Policy* 14:5–18
26. Hancock T, Duhl L. 1988. *Promoting Health in the Urban Context.* WHO Healthy Cities Pap. No. 1. Copenhagen: FADL. 54 pp.
27. Hayes MV, Willms SM. 1990. Healthy community indicators: The perils of the research and the paucity of the find. *Health Promot. Int.* 5:161–66
28. Healthcare Forum. 1994. *Creating Healthier Communities Fellowship for*

Healthcare Leaders. San Francisco: Heathcare Forum. Program announc.

29. Healthcare Forum. 1994. *Healthier Communities Award.* San Francisco: Healthcare Forum. Program announc.

30. Kent MM. 1995. Clean up Bialystock 1994—successful implementation of large- scale citizen environmental action in central Europe. See Ref. 8, pp. 1–6

31. Kickbusch I. 1989. *Good planets are hard to find.* WHO Healthy Cities Pap. No. 5. Copenhagen: FADL. 31 pp.

32. Kickbusch I. 1989. Healthy cities: a working project and a growing movement. *Health Promot.* 4:77–82

33. Milio N. 1990. Healthy cities: the new public health and supportive research. *Health Promot. Int.* 5:291–97

34. Mitchell D, ed. 1994. *Using Stories to Guide Action.* Toronto: Ontario Prev. Clearinghouse

35. NACCHO, Cent. Dis. Control. 1995. *1992–1993 National Profile of Local Health Departments.* Washington, DC: NACCHO. 116 pp.

36. Nakamura K. 1995. A megacity's approach: Tokyo healthy city. See Ref. 7, pp. 117–22

37. Noack H, McQueen D. 1988. Towards health promotion indicators. *Health Promot.* 3:73–78

38. Norris T. 1993. *The Healthy Communities Handbook.* Denver, CO: Natl. Civic League. 155 pp.

39. Oers JAM van, Reelick NF. 1992. Quantitative indicators for a healthy city. *Int. J. Epidemiol. Commun. Health* 46:293–96

40. O'Neill M. 1993. Building bridges between knowledge and action: the Canadian process of healthy communities indicators. See Ref. 12, pp. 127–47

41. *Ottawa Charter for Health Promotion.* 1986. Copenhagen: WHO Reg. Off. Eur. 2 pp.

42. Polman L, Goumans M, de Leeuw E. 1993. *Bibliography Research for Healthy Cities.* RHC Monogr Ser. 1. Maastricht. 167 pp.

43. Price C, ed. 1994. *Briefings on Multi-City Action Plans. WHO Healthy Cities Project Phase II 1993–1997.* Copenhagen: WHO Reg. Off. Eur. 32 pp.

44. Rees A, ed. 1992. *Healthy Cities: Reshaping the Urban Environment.* *Proc. Natl. Conf. Healthy Cities Aust., 2nd. Bondi Junction.* 312 pp.

45. Rider MS, Flynn BC, Yuska TP, Ray DW, Rains J. 1994. *The CityNet Manual: How Communities Can (And Do!) Create Healthy Cities.* Indianapolis: Inst. Action Res. Commun. Health/Indiana Univ.

46. Sanders M, de Leeuw E, Polman L. 1995. *Bibliography Research for Healthy Cities Suppl. 1995.* RHC Monogr. Ser. 8. Maastricht. 57 pp.

47. Saywell RW, Lassiter WL, Flynn BC. 1995. A cost analysis of a nurse-managed, voluntary community health center. *J. Nurs. Admin.* 25:17–27

48. Takano T, Ishidate K, Nagasaki M, eds. 1992. *Formulation and Development of a Research Base for Healthy Cities. Proc. Int. Symp. Formulation Dev. Res. Base Healthy Cities, Oct. 17–20, Tokyo.* Tokyo: Kyoiku Syoseki. 215 pp.

49. *The Quality of Life in Pasadena: An Index for the 90's and Beyond.* 1992. Pasadena, CA: Public Health Dep. 36 pp.

50. Tsouros AD. 1989. Equity and the healthy cities project. *Health Promot.* 4:73–75

51. Tsouros AD. 1990. *World Health Organization Healthy Cities Project: A Project Becomes a Movement.* Copenhagen: FADL. 80 pp.

52. Twiss JM. 1991. The healthy city: An idea whose time is right. *West. City* 67:6–9

53. Voluntary Hospitals of America. 1994. Community health improvement. *Bulletin,* p. 1

54. WHO. 1978. *Primary Health Care.* Geneva: WHO/UNICEF. 78 pp.

55. WHO. 1992. *Twenty Steps for Developing a Healthy Cities Project.* Copenhagen: Reg. Off. Eur. 61 pp.

56. WHO. 1992. *The Multi-City Action Plan on Baltic Cities and Indicators.* Copenhagen: Reg. Off. Eur.

57. WHO. 1994. *Healthy City Project Organigrams.* Copenhagen: Reg. Off. Eur. 77 pp.

58. WHO. 1995. *City Health Profiles: How to Report on Health in Your City.* Copenhagen: WHO Reg. Off. Eur. 50 pp.

59. WHO. 1995. *Healthy Cities Net News.* No. 1. (Jan.) Copenhagen: WHO Reg. Off. Eur.

Annu. Rev. Public Health. 1996. 17:311–36

MENTAL HEALTH PROBLEMS OF HOMELESS WOMEN AND DIFFERENCES ACROSS SUBGROUPS

Marjorie J. Robertson

Alcohol Research Group, Western Consortium for Public Health, 2000 Hearst Avenue, Berkeley, California 94709; e-mail: marjorie@cygnus.ucsf.edu

Marilyn A. Winkleby

Stanford Center for Research in Disease Prevention, Stanford University School of Medicine, Stanford, California 94305

KEY WORDS: mental disorders, parent, Diagnostic Interview Schedule, distress

ABSTRACT

Homeless women are a large and diverse group, constituting one fifth of the US homeless adult population. Although most homeless women do not have major mental illness, homeless women exhibit disproportionately high rates of major mental disorders and other mental problems. Rates of mental disorders are highest among whites and women without children, and important variations by subgroups of homeless women reinforce the need for disaggregated analysis. Many homeless women with serious mental illness are not receiving needed care, apparently due in part to the lack of perception of a mental health problem and the lack of services designed to meet the special needs of homeless women.

INTRODUCTION

The growing literature on homelessness comes from a wide array of disciplines including anthropology, epidemiology, medicine, psychology, social welfare, and sociology (50). Although women constitute about 20% of homeless adults in the United States, women's concerns are underrepresented in the survey literature on homeless people (4, 35, 36). Most studies include samples in which the vast majority is male, and they often report findings for men and women combined, obscuring important findings about women. Even among

311

0163-7525/96/0510-0311$08.00

studies that are stratified by gender, there is little discussion of implications specifically for women or for subgroups of women.

Where gender comparisons are available, studies usually report higher rates of mental health problems among homeless women than men (22, 49), a finding that warrants an in-depth analysis of findings for women. Furthermore, the literature suggests important differences in mental health problems among subgroups of women (57). Consequently, this review has two goals: to document the prevalence and types of mental health problems among homeless women, and to consider how mental health problems are distributed among different groups of homeless women.

THE PREVALENCE OF MENTAL HEALTH PROBLEMS AMONG HOMELESS WOMEN

Overview of the Literature Reviewed

This review is based on reports of original research that met the following criteria: (*a*) use of nonclinical, noninstitutional samples of homeless women in the United States; (*b*) adequate description of the study methodology; (*c*) use of at least one indicator of mental health status for adult women; and (*d*) publication or release since 1975. Thirty-one reports met these selection criteria (5–7, 13–15, 17, 21, 23, 27–29, 31, 32, 37, 44, 47, 51, 52, 55, 56, 59, 61, 62, 65–68, 70, 72–74).

The primary sources of material were bibliographic data bases including PsychInfo and Medline and reference lists from recent published literature reviews and the National Resource Center on Homelessness and Mental Illness (22, 49). The focus of the literature was the prevalence and distribution of mental health problems among homeless women. Other important aspects of mental health status, such as resilience, coping strategies, subsistence adaptation, and availability of social supports, were not included.

All identified studies used cross-sectional designs, and most were descriptive and depended exclusively on self-report. None of the samples is representative of the population of homeless women nationally. Studies varied in definitions of homelessness; indicators of mental health problems; sample selection, sizes and sites; and geographic locations. Because of the variety of mental health indicators reported, findings for homeless women were divided into three categories for discussion: history of psychiatric hospitalization, current distress or demoralization, and psychiatric diagnoses.

PSYCHIATRIC HOSPITALIZATION   Researchers suggest that despite its popularity, psychiatric hospitalization is a highly imperfect and questionable proxy for psychiatric morbidity. For example, as reported by Breakey and colleagues, many homeless respondents in Baltimore who reported previous hospitalization did not have major mental disorders (false positives), while many who reported no previous hospitalization met diagnostic criteria for major mental illness (false negatives) (49). Furthermore, rates of hospitalization may be inflated because they include persons who enter psychiatric facilities for treatment of alcohol or drug problems (45, 60) or for a place to stay (2). Nevertheless, despite its limitations, previous psychiatric hospitalization was the most frequently reported mental health indicator for homeless women among the studies reviewed. Psychiatric hospitalization was reported in 26 studies, and findings from these studies are presented in Table 1. The rates of hospitalization among homeless women ranged from 8 to 35%, which is high compared to less than 3% among women in the general population. Nevertheless, Smith and colleagues (59) reported that when stratified by specific psychiatric disorders, rates of hospitalization for homeless women were similar to those for women in the general population. The question of sampling effects arises in the Baltimore study reporting the highest prevalence (7) and may be due in part to including jailed women who had higher rates of mental disorders than women in shelters (8, 71).

Rates of hospitalization for subgroups of women based on parenting status are also presented in Table 1. Among subgroups of women, rates of psychiatric hospitalization were consistently lower among women with children in their care. This finding is clearest within studies that stratify by parenting status (13, 27, 30, 49, 51, 55, 70, 72); homeless women with children in their care reported lower rates of psychiatric hospitalization (2 to 14%) compared to homeless women without children (10 to 27%). In turn, homeless women with children demonstrated a higher prevalence of previous hospitalization (8 to 14%) than did comparison groups of poor but housed women with children (<1 to 6%) (Table 1) (5, 68, 73). In another example of effects of sampling, the highest rate of hospitalization for women with children is reported in a Richmond, Virginia study (23%) that included a domestic violence shelter among its sampling sites. Shinn & Weitzman found that although the prevalence of mental hospitalization was low among homeless women with children, for those who had a mental health problem, hospitalization was a significant predictor of homelessness (57).

The importance of subgroup analysis among homeless populations is reinforced by the consistent difference among women and other groups. Figure 1 presents findings from three studies in which rates for men, women with children, and women without children are contrasted.

CURRENT DISTRESS OR DEMORALIZATION   It is understandable that homeless women experience high rates of emotional distress and demoralization (22), and symptom scales have often been used to evaluate distress among homeless

Table 1 Lifetime prevalence of psychiatric hospitalization among homeless women (U.S. studies: 1980–1995)

| Authors | Sample | | Number of women | Psychiatric hospitalization among women | | | Comments |
	Location	Sites		Overall (%)	With children (%)	Without children (%)	
Bassuk & Rosenberg, 1988 (5)	Boston, MA	Shelters	49	8[c]	8[c]	—	Compared to 4% of poor housed mothers
Bassuk et al, 1986 (6)	Massachusetts	Shelters	80	8[?]	8[c]	—	
Breakey et al, 1989 (7)	Baltimore, MD	Shelters, jail[a]	229[a]	33	—	—	Hospitalized in past 12 months; compared to 23% of men in sample
Burt & Cohen, 1989 (13)	20 large cities nationally	Shelters, meal programs	512[a]	19	8	27	Compared to 17% of men in sample
Crystal & Goldstein, 1984 (14)	New York City, NY	Shelters	1602	28	—	—	
Crystal & Goldstein, 1984 (15)	New York City, NY	Shelters	152	27	—	—	
Gelberg et al, 1988 (23)	Los Angeles County, CA	Shelters, food programs agencies, streets, other	143	22[b]	—	—	
Johnson & Krueger, 1989 (27)	St. Louis, MO	Shelters	240	9[c]	6	25	Hospitalized in previous five years
Khanna et al, 1992 (28)	Richmond, VA	Shelters	100	23	23	—	Study sites included one domestic violence shelter
Koegel et al, 1995 (31)	Los Angeles County, CA	Shelters, meal programs, streets	379[a]	9[c]	2[c]	10[c]	Compared to 8%[c] of men in sample

Table 1 (*continued*)

Authors	Location	Sites	Number of women	Psychiatric hospitalization among women Over-all (%)	With children (%)	Without children (%)	Comments
Morse, 1985 (37)	St. Louis, MO	Shelters	122	25[b]	—	—	
Padgett & Streuning, 1992 (44)	New York City, NY	Public shelters	311	19	—	19	Compared to 9% of men in sample
Ritchey et al, 1991 (47)	Birmingham, AL	Shelters, meal programs, streets	28[a]	29	—	—	Women ages 18–44 only
Robertson et al, 1993 (51)	Alameda County, CA	Shelters, meal programs, drop-in centers	179[a]	16	11	21	Compared to 11% of men in sample
Robertson et al, 1985 (52)	Los Angeles County, CA	Shelters, meal programs, streets	55	27	—	—	Compared to 3% of householders in Los Angeles ECA study
Roll & Toro, 1995 (55)	Buffalo, NY	Agency intake site	97[d]	8[c]	7[d]	11[d]	Compared to 12% of men in sample
Roth et al, 1992 (56)	19 counties in Ohio		186	30	—	—	
Smith et al, 1993 (59)	St. Louis, MO	Shelters and day centers[a]	300	26	—	—	
Solarz, 1985 (61)	Detroit, MI	Shelter	46[c]	35	—	—	
Solarz & Mowbray, 1985 (62)	Detroit, MI	Shelters	21	35	—	—	

Table 1 *(continued)*

Authors	Sample			Psychiatric hospitalization among women				Comments
	Location	Sites	Number of women	Over-all (%)	With children (%)	Without children (%)		
Toro, 1993 (65)	Buffalo, NY	Shelters, meal programs, agencies, streets	110	17[b]	—	—		
Toro, 1993 (65)	Detroit, MI	Shelters, meal programs, agencies, streets	81	23[b]	—	—		
Wagner et al, 1994 (66)	11 rural counties in Ohio	Shelters, agencies	76	7	7	—		
Weitzman et al, 1992 (68)	New York City, NY	Public shelter intake site	677	4	4	—		Compared to 0.8% of poor housed women with children
Winkleby, 1992, 1994 (70, 72)	Santa Clara County, CA	Shelters	269	—	6	22		Compared to 18% of single men in sample
Wood et al, 1990 (73)	Los Angeles, CA	Shelters	192	14	14	—		Compared to 6% for comparison group of housed mothers

[a] Probability sample
[b] Unpublished data provided by first author
[c] Extrapolated from data provided in article
[d] Unpublished data provided by second author

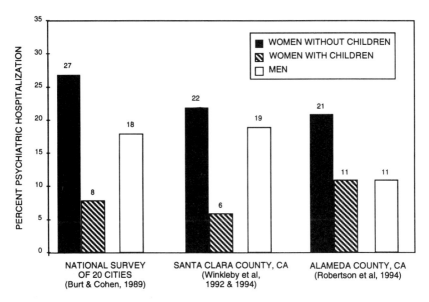

Figure 1   Lifetime prevalences of psychiatric hospitalizations by demographic subgroups for three US surveys.

women. Measures of current symptoms may not be specific enough to be useful at times since they may reflect not only ongoing psychiatric conditions but also reactions to trauma, stressful environments, strategies of adaptation, or behaviors perpetuated by an institutional environment (33, 34, 64).

Nevertheless, findings for symptom scales were reported in ten studies and are summarized in Table 2. Findings suggest that homeless women have higher levels of distress or depressed mood than the general population. The most frequently used indicator was emotional distress or depressed mood assessed with the Center for Epidemiologic Studies Depression Scale (CES-D) in four studies. One study used a form modified for use with homeless respondents, and one used six items from the 20-point scale. Three studies reported that the majority of women in their samples exceeded the CES-D threshold (16), with rates of distress from two to four times higher than the general population. One study reported that mean scores were higher than a community sample, but lower than an inpatient sample (17). The study of 20 large cities nationally reported that distress was higher for women with children (59%) compared to women without children (46%) (13). Findings on the Brief Symptom Inventory (BSI) indicated homeless women scored in the 90th percentile.

PSYCHIATRIC DIAGNOSES   Rates of specific psychiatric disorders among homeless women were reported in eight studies that varied widely in geogra-

Table 2 Mental health symptoms among homeless women (U.S. studies 1980–1995)

Authors	Location	Sample Sites	Number of women	Symptom scale[b]	Findings
Bassuk et al, 1986 (6)	Massachusetts	Shelters[a]	80	BPRS	Among women with children, the majority were described with moderate to extremely severe symptoms of anxiety (72%), depression (67%), and tension (58%)
Burt & Cohen, 1989 (13)	20 large cities nationally	Shelters, meal programs[d]	512	CES-D (modified)	Used 6 of 20 CES-D items; rate of distress higher for women with children (59%) than for women without (46%)
D'Ercole & Streuning, 1990 (17)	New York City, NY	Shelter	141	CES-D (revised)	Mean score of 19.4, higher than a community sample (9.1) but lower than acutely depressed inpatients (38.3). Depressive symptoms were related to victimization
Fischer & Breakey, 1987 (17)	Baltimore, MD	Shelters, jail[d]	78	GHQ	Women higher than men (61 vs 49%)
Klein et al, 1993 (29)	Flint, MI	Shelters	112	CES-D	Sample of women with children; 80% exceeded the cutoff indicating probable depression/distress, a rate four times higher than the general population
Padgett & Streuning, 1992 (44)	New York City, NY	Shelters	311	CES-D	45% exceeded cutoff indicating probable depression/distress compared to <20% in general population
Roth et al, 1992 (56)	Ohio	Shelters	186	PSS	One third were assessed with psychiatric symptomatology (35%) or behavioral disturbance (36%)
Solarz & Mowbray, 1985 (62)	Detroit, MI	Shelters	21	BSI	Women scored in 90th percentile and men in 95th percentile
Wagner et al, 1994 (66)	11 rural counties in Ohio	Shelters, agencies	76	SCL-90-R	3% exceeded cutoff scores suggesting need for further evaluation

Table 2 *(Continued)*

| Authors | Sample | | | | |
	Location	Sites	Number of women	Symptom scale	Findings
Warren et al, 1992 (67)		Shelters, meal programs, agencies, other	126	SCL-90-R	Three quarters (74%) exceeded cutoff suggesting need for further evaluation; no differences by race

Source: [a] Census
[b] BPRS, brief Psychiatric Rating Schedule: CES-D, Center for Epidemiological Studies Depression Scale; PSS, Psychiatric Status Schedule; SCL-90-R
[c] Estimated from data provided in report
[d] Random or probability sample

phy, source and composition of the sample, and diagnostic method. Psychiatric interviews were used in three studies, and the Diagnostic Interview Schedule (DIS, versions III and III-R), a standardized instrument that provides a structured diagnostic interview for use by trained nonclinicians (53), was used in five studies. Studies documented a wide range of psychopathology. Despite differences in diagnostic procedures, diagnostic criteria in all eight studies were based on the Diagnostic and Statistical Manual of the American Psychiatric Association (DSM-III or DSM-III-R) (1).

The prevalence of disorders among homeless women varied considerably across studies. Rates of major mental illnesses and substance use disorders are summarized in Table 3. Also included are rates for women in the general population for comparison, based on household samples of the Epidemiologic Catchment Area Study (53). Although rates of major mental disorders fail to converge, rates were consistently higher for homeless women than for women in the general population. For example, the lifetime rates of schizophrenia in homeless women ranged from 2.5 to 17.1%, compared to 1.7% for women in the general population. Rates of major depression ranged from 15.8 to 32% compared to 10.2% for women in the general population. Bipolar disorders ranged from 3.3 to 12% compared to less than 1% in the general population. Substance use disorders were also higher among homeless women; alcohol disorders ranged from 16.8 to 42.5% and drug disorders ranged from 16.7 to 51.2%. These prevalences were much higher compared to 4.8% for women in the general population.

Key Studies

Four recent studies reviewed below illustrate the diversity and mental health status of homeless women. These studies are presented in chronological order and report significant findings.

SANTA CLARA COUNTY SURVEYS   The Santa Clara County surveys of homeless adults in Northern California had two main objectives: to distinguish personal characteristics and other risk factors that preceded homelessness from those that were a consequence of homelessness (72); and to examine how homeless adults with children differed from homeless adults who were alone (70). Over 1500 homeless women and men in the county were surveyed in late 1989 and early 1990. This county, with a population of 1.5 million people, has a large population of homeless people, one third of whom are estimated to be women with children. Women (n=100) and men (n=41) with children were sampled from the two largest county family shelters; women (n=169) and men (n=1268) without children were sampled from the three main county adult shelters. Data were collected through the use of a 58-item questionnaire administered by

Table 3 Lifetime prevalence of psychiatric disorders among homeless women and women in the general population (U.S. studies: 1980–1995)

Authors	Location	Sample — Sites	Number of women	Any major mental disorder (%)	Schizophrenia (%)	Major affective disorders (%) — Any	Major depression	Bipolar	Substance use disorders (%) — Any	Alcohol	Drug
Bassuk & Rosenberg, 1988 (5)[a]	Boston, MA[b]	Shelters	49	—	6.3[c]	2.0[c]	—	—	8.2[c]	—	—
Bassuk et al, 1986 (6)[a]	Massachusetts[d]	Shelters	80	—	2.5[c]	10.0	—	—	9.0	—	—
Breakey et al, 1989 (7)[a]	Baltimore, MD[d]	Shelters and jail	78	48.7	17.1	33.7	15.8	7.9	38.2	31.6	16.7
Koegel et al, 1995 (31)[f]	Los Angeles County, CA[d]	Shelters, meal programs, drop-in centers, streets	379	—	5.0	—	26.0	7.0	—	—	—
Robertson et al, 1993 (51)[f]	Alameda County, CA[d]	Shelters, meal programs, drop-in centers	179	33.6	3.4	33.0	32.0	12.0	62.5	40.3	51.2
Smith et al, 1993 (59)	St. Louis, MO[d]	Shelters and day centers	300	—	3.7	—	24.7	3.3	30.8	16.8	23.1
Toro, 1993 (65)[e]	Buffalo, NY[f]	Shelters, meal programs, agencies, streets	110	30.0[e]	3.6[e]	29.1[e]	20.9[g]	6.5[e]	40.9[e]	25.5[e]	30.0[e]
Toro, 1993 (65)[e]	Detroit, MI[f]	Shelters, meal programs, agencies, streets	81	32.1[e]	8.6[e]	25.9[e]	16.0[e]	3.7[e]	62.5[e]	42.5[e]	43.8[e]
Robins & Regier, 1991[h]	ECA sites[d,i]	Households		—	1.7	10.2[g]	7.0	<1.0	—	4.8	4.8

[a] Diagnostic assessment through psychiatric examination, DSM-III criteria
[b] Census
[c] Extrapolated from data provided
[d] Probability sample
[e] Unpublished data provided by author
[f] Diagnostic assessment through Diagnostic Interview Schedule, DSM-III-R criteria
[g] Includes dysthymia
[h] Diagnostic assessment through Diagnostic Interview Schedule, DSM-III criteria
[i] Epidemiologic Catchment Area Study

registered nurses and health interviewers. Although this survey did not emphasize mental health outcomes, it provides estimates of prevalences of psychiatric hospitalizations and substance use problems before homelessness as well as a perspective on the heterogeneity of the homeless population. Furthermore, it is one of the few studies that sampled a geographic area with diverse ethnic groups. Results for women that pertain to sociodemographic characteristics and factors potentially related to mental health outcomes are summarized below.

Homeless women with children were significantly different from homeless women living alone. Compared to women living alone, women with children were significantly younger (mean age 29.3 vs 34.1 years), less educated (10.9 vs 11.6 mean years of education), less likely to have ever experienced full-time employment (74 vs 86%), and more likely to have been supported by public assistance before first becoming homeless (55 vs 29%). In addition, women with children became homeless at younger ages and had been homeless for less time.

Further differences were found for mental health measures. The question regarding lifetime psychiatric hospitalization, adapted from the NIMH Epidemiologic Catchment Area Study questionnaire (54), asked whether respondents had been admitted overnight to a hospital or treatment program for family or personal problems, emotional problems, or problems with drugs or alcohol. An additional question asked whether psychiatric hospitalization had occurred before first becoming homeless. Women with children were significantly less likely than women without children to report a lifetime history of hospitalization (6 vs 22%, respectively) and to report psychiatric hospitalization before first becoming homeless (2 vs 16%, respectively). Similar differences were evident for substance use. Before their first episode of homelessness, women with children were less likely than women without children to report excessive alcohol intake (3 vs 14%) or illegal drug use (8 vs 16%).

Adverse childhood experiences were common among women from both groups including placement in foster care (15% for women with children and 17% for women living alone); physical abuse (23 vs 28%, respectively); and sexual abuse (22 vs 33%). Seventeen percent of women with children had repeated a grade in school, and 31% had run away from home before the age of 18. (These data were unavailable for women living alone).

The women in this study were ethnically diverse, with African Americans, Hispanics, and whites each comprising about one third of the sample. There were few age or educational differences by ethnicity within the two samples of women. Regardless of ethnicity, women with children were younger and less educated than women living alone, and they were less likely to enter homelessness with histories of psychiatric hospitalizations, excessive alcohol intake, or illegal drug use. The most striking ethnic differences were that

Hispanic women with and without children were the least educated of all women; white women without children reported the highest prevalence of excessive alcohol intake; and African-American women without children reported the highest prevalence of illegal drug use.

Women with children completed a supplemental questionnaire that provided further information about family characteristics. While few of these women delivered their first child before the age of 16, over half gave birth before the age of 20. Families were small in many cases (46% had only one or two children) and most often composed of children under the age of ten. Among women with children who reported that one or more of their children were living apart from them (29%), the majority reported that their children were being cared for by grandparents or other relatives. Most women had experienced unstable housing situations before their loss of shelter; women moved an average of 2.6 times in the 12 months prior to their current episode of homelessness. Despite this instability, almost all women with children (97%) had lived with their children in the month preceding their loss of shelter.

While these findings are from cross-sectional surveys that depended on retrospective reports, and where information on mental health status was limited, they support the hypothesis that homeless women with children have fewer risk factors related to psychiatric problems or substance than women without children. Findings further suggest that homeless young women with children, who lack adequate education and stable participation in the work force, may be particularly vulnerable to the economic and social trends that have led to the recent increases in homelessness.

THE ST. LOUIS STUDY   The most detailed research to date on mental health issues and homeless women comes from a study in St. Louis, Missouri. The St. Louis study was designed to identify important subgroups among the homeless population by gender, ethnicity, and parenting status (40, 42). A randomly selected sample of 900 men and 300 women was recruited from St. Louis shelters, day centers, rehabilitation centers, and the streets (although no women were found on the streets) in 1989 and 1990. Subjects were assessed with the Diagnostic Interview Schedule that permitted diagnoses based on the Diagnostic and Statistical Manual of Mental Disorders, Third Edition-Revised (DSM-III-R) (1). Many of the women reported major mental disorders, and almost one third reported substance use disorders. (See Table 3 for rates for specific disorders.) Almost half of the women with lifetime Axis I disorders (44%) also had lifetime substance use disorders.

The authors reported that lifetime and current (six-month) rates of major mental disorders and substance use disorders were higher in homeless women compared to other low-income women, which in turn were higher than other women in St. Louis (comparisons based on ECA data for non-homeless women in St. Louis) (59). For example, lifetime major depression was twice as prevalent among homeless women (24.7%) as among their low-income counterparts (11.8%), which in turn was higher than other women in St. Louis (8.8%). Also, although rates were more similar to low-income women, homeless women had slightly higher rates of schizophrenia (3.7 vs 3.2% for low-income women and 1% for other women) and bipolar disorder (3.3 vs 2.2% for low-income women and 0.8% for other women). Homeless women reported higher rates of substance use disorders including alcohol (16.8 vs 10.3% for low-income women and 5.8% for other women) and drugs (30.8 vs 14.3% for low-income women). Again, rates were lowest for other women (5.8% for alcohol and 4.1% for drugs). Homeless women also reported strikingly high rates of posttraumatic stress disorder (PTSD) (33.8 vs 3.2% for low-income women and 1.3% for other women) (39).

Disaggregation of data unmasked important ethnic variations. To evaluate differences among homeless women by ethnicity (42), the sample of women was divided into two main ethnic subgroups, nonwhite (88%) (most of whom were African Americans) and white (12%). Nonwhite women were significantly younger (28.4 vs 32.9 years) and less likely to have ever married (38 vs 65%) compared to white women in the sample. Nonwhite women were also more likely to be mothers and to have their minor children in their physical custody (83.5 vs 45.5% of whites). Socioeconomic characteristics were similar for the two groups of women, including similar education levels (43% of nonwhites completed high school vs 38% of whites), annual incomes (60% had $4000 or more vs 43% of whites), and rates of employment (10% in both groups). However, significantly more nonwhites identified welfare as their primary income source during the previous year (47 vs 14% of whites). Nonwhites reported significantly less childhood physical and sexual abuse and fewer maternal psychiatric problems than white women (17 vs 64% of whites).

For both groups of women, family conflict, household dissolution, and eviction were the most frequently reported causes of first homelessness. The main places where women in both groups had stayed in the previous year were either their own homes or with friends or family members. However, nonwhite women reported significantly fewer episodes of homelessness and less years of homelessness overall than white women (65% homeless one year or less vs 36% of whites).

Rates of lifetime psychiatric disorders varied dramatically by ethnicity. Nonwhite women had significantly lower rates of all major mental disorders than white women, including schizophrenia (2 vs 14% for whites), bipolar affective disorder (2 vs 17%), and major depression (22 vs 44%). Nonwhites also had significantly lower rates of panic disorder, generalized anxiety disorder, and PTSD. In contrast, however, there were no significant differences in alcohol or other drug disorders. Among women with apparent need for help with mental health problems (i.e. with Axis I diagnoses), nonwhite women were only half as likely to receive inpatient care (37 vs 67% of whites) or outpatient psychiatric treatment (41 vs 84.6%). Furthermore, more nonwhites had recently desired but not obtained psychiatric treatment, suggesting dramatic differences in access to treatment by ethnicity.

The authors caution that within ethnic groups there is considerable heterogeneity, and people within a given subgroup may have a variety of problems and reasons for their homelessness. Nevertheless, they conclude that difficulties underlying homelessness for white women seemed "internal" (i.e. more likely due to psychopathology) than for nonwhite women whose difficulties may be more "external" (i.e. related to socioeconomic problems) (42).

To document variations by parenting status (58), women were divided into three groups based on whether a woman had minor children and whether the children were living with her. *Women with minor children in their care* were younger and more likely to be unemployed and to be disabled. They more often reported welfare support in the past year, and they reported the lowest rates of schizophrenia (1%) and alcohol disorders (12%). *Women with minor children not in their care* had significantly higher rates of schizophrenia (10%) and alcohol disorders (33%) (40, 58). *Women with no minor children* compared to other women were more likely to be white, to be homeless longer, and they had moderate rates of schizophrenia (7%) and alcohol disorders (19%) compared to other women in the sample. The authors suggested that mothers with minor children not in their care constituted a subgroup with more apparent personal and fewer social vulnerabilities to homelessness and may represent a target population for focused psychiatric interventions (58).

The authors further concluded that although major mental disorders are overrepresented among homeless women compared to women in the general population, mental health services are underutilized in this population (41). Underutilization was in part attributed to the lack of insight by women about their problems because only about ten percent of respondents with disorders perceived that their mental problems were serious (41). An alternative explanation might be that homeless women have competing priorities more concretely related to their survival.

LOS ANGELES COUNTY: THE COURSE OF HOMELESSNESS STUDY   A primary objective of the Course of Homelessness Study was to examine the extent to which homeless individuals in need of mental health and substance abuse services received treatment services, and to identify the characteristics that predict service use (31). The study also addressed how need and service use differed for homeless men and women and for subgroups of women. Data were collected in 1990 and 1991 through face-to-face interviews with a probability sample of 1563 homeless adults, including 379 women. Psychiatric status was assessed with the Diagnostic Interview Schedule, Version III-R (Dis-III-R). Respondents were sampled from shelters, meal programs, and street sites in the skid row and Westside areas of Los Angeles County, California.

Gender comparisons suggest that homeless men and women differ systematically in demographic and situational characteristics. Compared with men, women were younger, more likely to have a spouse or partner, more likely to have had children and to currently have children in their care, and less likely to be sampled from the downtown skid row area. Women also had more income and were more likely to have health insurance. Rates of psychiatric disorders were high across all groups, with no significant variation by gender or parental status. Although women reported higher rates of lifetime depression (26 vs 20% for men), they did not differ significantly from men in rates of lifetime, recent, or chronic major mental illness overall; nor in rates of psychiatric hospitalization. (See Table 3 for lifetime rates of specific disorders for women.) Nor did they differ in terms of use of mental health services.

As expected, and consistent with previous studies (13, 58, 70), women with children in their care were distinguished from other homeless women in demographic characteristics, history of homelessness, and lifestyle. Women with children were younger, included more nonwhites, and reported higher incomes and health coverage, presumably due to receipt of benefits from Aid to Families with Dependent Children (AFDC). They were less likely to be sampled from skid row, and they had been homeless for shorter periods of time. Women with children were also less likely to have chronic or recent alcohol dependence.

Surprisingly, however, women with children did not differ significantly from other women in their psychiatric profile. Among women with serious mental illness, recent treatment rates were low (26%), and treatment rates for women with children were extraordinarily low (4 vs 30% in other women in the previous 60 days). None of the women with children who had serious mental illness had received mental health treatment from service providers outside of formal treatment systems (compared to 23% of other women with serious mental illness). The lack of recent treatment contact was attributed to the women's lack of acknowledgment of mental health problems.

In sum, the study documented high rates of serious mental and substance use disorders among homeless women. However, despite apparent need for mental health treatment, only half of women with serious mental illness recognized their mental health problems, and few had received needed treatment. The authors conclude there is a significant amount of serious mental illness and chronic substance abuse among homeless women that is unrecognized and untreated, especially among homeless women with children. They recommended more aggressive outreach programs for homeless women with children, along with treatment programs that are more sensitive to the distinctive needs of homeless women with children in their care.

ALAMEDA COUNTY: THE STAR PROJECT   The Study of Alameda County Homeless Residents (STAR Project) is a study designed to document the relationship between serious mental disorders and the course of homelessness among women and men. Alameda County, California, has a diverse population of 1.3 million people. STAR Project findings were based on personal interviews with a countywide probability sample of 385 men and 179 women from shelters, meal programs, and drop-in centers in the spring of 1991 (51, 74). Baseline data were collected with a structured instrument that averaged two hours to administer. It included sections of the Diagnostic Interview Schedule, Version III-R (DIS-III-R), which were used to assess the prevalence of major mental disorders and substance use disorders.

General demographic characteristics were consistent with other recent studies of homeless adults, with a mean age of 37.6 years (33.9 years for women), an overrepresentation of ethnic minority groups (79%), and a male majority (78% male and 22% female) (see Figure 2). Most of the sample had lived in Alameda County for eight years or more as an adult.

Overall, 8.9% of adults had an average of two children with them, leading authors to estimate that 22.7% of the homeless population overall in Alameda County were members of homeless families with children. This estimate is lower than most anecdotal estimates of families among the homeless nationally, but consistent with other empirical estimates (13).

The ages of women in the sample ranged from 18 to 75 years, although the majority were age 35 or younger (56%). Also, the majority of women in this sample were African American (71%), high-school educated (70%), and had

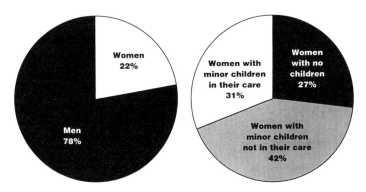

Figure 2 Composition of homeless adults and homeless women, Alameda County, California, 1991 (N=564)

been married (51%) or in a marriage-like relationship (91%). As observed elsewhere (17, 58), many homeless women in the sample had minor children living elsewhere. While about three quarters of the women (73%) had minor children, less than half of these had any children in their care. The great majority of minor children (71%) were living elsewhere, usually with the other parent, grandparents, or other family members.

Although most women reported income in the past month (87.6%), the mean income was $339, well below the federal poverty level (74). Although more than one fifth of women had employment income in the previous month (22.8%), income usually came from entitlements (51.1%), informal-sector activity (usually panhandling or selling cans and other recyclable materials) (41.8%), and gifts from family or friends (33%) (74). Although most women had been homeless previously, the majority (64.3%) had been homeless for less than a year overall. Some (15.2%) had been homeless as children. One quarter (23.3%) had been in jail at least once in the past year (51, 74).

One third of the women (33.6%) received a lifetime diagnosis of major mental illness. (See Table 3 for rates of specific lifetime disorders) (51). Among these, about half (48.8%) had been hospitalized for psychiatric treatment, most before they ever became homeless.

About one third of the women (29.5%) had "active" or current major mental disorders (i.e. they had a lifetime diagnosis *and* they experienced symptoms of the disorder in the previous 12 months). The majority of current cases (61%) had dual diagnoses: i.e. they also had current substance use disorders. Although most women with current major mental disorders perceived themselves to have a mental health problem, less than half (40.5%) received any type of mental health services in the past year, a finding suggesting that failure to recognize one's mental problems is apparently not the only barrier to treatment. Among women with current major mental disorders, perceived mental or emotional problems were predictive of recent mental health treatment. Unfortunately, women with current major mental illness were as likely to have been in jail (10.7%) as to have received inpatient mental health treatment (7.3%) in the past year.

Altogether, one sixth of the women (16.4%) reported a history of psychiatric hospitalization as adults, most (13.1%) before their first episode of homelessness.

To document differences by parenting status, women were divided into three main subgroups: *women with minor children in their care* (31%); *women with minor children who are not in their care* (42%, the largest group); and *women with no minor children* (27%) (51) (Figure 1). The authors found statistically significant differences among the three groups of women in sociodemographic background, history of homelessness, and diagnostic status. Women who had children in their care were the youngest, with a mean age of 31 years. On average, they had two children with them. Most were African Americans (73.1%). They were also the most likely to have been a primary tenant (i.e. to be named on a mortgage, lease, or rental agreement) in the past year (51.5%). They had the highest annual incomes (67% had more than $5000), and they were the most likely to report entitlement income, most of which was accounted for by AFDC benefits. Surprisingly, although all were presumably eligible for AFDC, only 62.5% of women with children in their care reported AFDC income (74). Furthermore, women with children in their care had significantly shorter histories of homelessness than the other two groups of women; less than half had been homeless before (42.7%), and very few had been homeless for one year or more (13.8%). Nearly one third of women with children in their care had current major mental disorders (30.8%) including major depression (30.8%) and schizophrenia (3.3%).

Women with minor children not in their care also had distinguishing characteristics. Their average age was 34.6 years, and they were mostly African Americans (86.1%). Almost half of these women had previously had a child removed from their custody (44%) by social service agencies. They had moderate annual incomes compared to other homeless women (41% over $5000). This group had the longest histories of homelessness; three quarters had been homeless before as adults, and more than half had been homeless for one year or longer as adults. This group of women had the lowest prevalence of major mental disorder (26.1%) accounted for entirely by major depression (26.1%).

Women with no minor children were a unique group as well. This group was the oldest, with a mean age of 36 years; had equivalent numbers of whites and African Americans (45.3% each); was the least likely to have been employed recently (5.7%); had the lowest annual incomes (29% had over $5000); and were the least likely to have been a primary tenant (9.9%). Most of this group had been homeless before (60.9%), and one third (33.1%) had been homeless for one year or longer. This group had the highest rates of major mental disorders (48.1%), including the highest rates of major depression (43.7%) and schizophrenia (8.8%).

The authors concluded that compared with the general population, the prevalence rates of lifetime and current major mental illness are disproportionately high among homeless women. Despite apparent need, few homeless women with active major mental disorders have contact with mental health treatment. In addition, most also have co-occurring substance use disorders, complicating any treatment intervention. Furthermore, diagnostic profiles vary significantly across subgroups, with major mental disorders highest among women with no minor children (48.1%) and lower among women with children in their care (30.8%) or for women with children living elsewhere (26.1%)

Findings also suggest that women without children are different from women with children: they are poorer, have more mental disorders, and have experienced recurring homelessness. In sum, women without children need to be targeted and provided a different set of services than women with children, with a greater focus on mental health services, health care, and vocational services, whereas women with children may be more likely to need parenting training, life skills, and child care.

Limitations of the Literature

The literature on homeless women presents an incomplete picture. Increasingly, researchers portray homelessness as a dynamic experience rather than a personal attribute (69). Nevertheless, most studies are epidemiological in approach, with a greater focus on characteristics or experiences of individual homeless women, and a lesser focus on the context and processes by which women become homeless (64).

The description of mental health problems among homeless women is hampered by the paucity of empirical work. Most findings on homeless women are neither comparable nor representative of the population as a whole. For example, studies of homeless adults tend to be based exclusively on sheltered samples, with little data available on women who are not in shelters. Virtually all studies are cross-sectional, likely overrepresenting the prevalence of mental health problems that are more prevalent among persons with chronic homelessness. Moreover, the lack of rigorous sampling methods often prevents generalization beyond the persons interviewed.

Research methods have become more rigorous over time. Nevertheless, research has concentrated on measuring mental health problems at the individual level, moving the focus away from larger societal problems. The persistent focus on the individual thus diverts meaningful research and dialogue from the broader questions regarding the structural causes of homelessness.

IMPLICATIONS

In sum, homelessness among women in the United States is a serious and complex problem. Homeless women are a large and diverse group, estimated to constitute about one fifth of the homeless adult population in the United States.

Most homeless women have experienced multiple episodes of homelessness, and they often have difficulty meeting basic needs, due in large part to the scarcity or inadequacy of existing services. In the short term, emergency and transitional services are needed for those who are currently homeless. However, strategies are also needed to reduce the number of women who become homeless and to reduce the time spent homeless since homelessness itself presents physical and mental health risks.

It is difficult to determine whether a homeless woman's mental
status at a given point in time is more causally associated with a
mental or emotional disorder, the exigencies of homelessness (12
stressors such as family violence or childhood trauma (3, 9, 10, 17, 29, 43,
63); their own substance abuse (48), or combinations of these or other factors.

Nevertheless, compared to women in the general population, homeless
women do exhibit relatively high rates of serious mental illness, current distress, and markers of chronic psychopathology like prior psychiatric hospitalization. While there is limited empirical evidence on which to base a specific
and reliable estimate of serious mental illness among homeless women, there
are consistent findings to suggest that homeless women have higher rates of
mental disorders than women in the general population. Despite their dispro-
portionate prevalence of psychiatric disorders, and contrary to stereotype, the
majority of homeless women do not have major mental illness (7).

Striking similarities emerge across studies, despite differences in methodology. Consistently, prevalence of major mental illness varies for different
subgroups of homeless women, which reinforces the need for disaggregated
analysis (57). Estimates are only accurate with reference to specific subgroups
of women.

Delivery of Services

Many homeless women with current serious mental illness are not receiving
needed care (7, 11). Three key studies report that a barrier to treatment among
women with current serious mental illness is the lack of perception of a mental
health problem. Other less well documented barriers include the lack of services sensitive to the special needs of homeless women (25, 46), especially
homeless women with children (31) and those with concurrent mental health
and substance use problems. As observed by Bachrach, homeless mentally ill
women comprise a diverse population with multiple and unique service needs,
although service providers often regard them in stereotyped ways.

Strategies have been developed for effective delivery of services to women
who are homeless and mentally ill. Inpatient treatment is certainly not always
indicated (22). Alternative approaches to treatment include providing community-based services (18) such as low-demand respite residences to serve "non-
compliant" and "treatment-resistant" homeless women (16); transitional residences for homeless women that require adaptations among the mental health
team and the community; and treatment programs for women with concurrent
substance abuse problems. Researchers have also suggested jails as potential
service sites for screening and treatment of mental illness (7, 20), and hospitals
as potential screening sites for ensuring that women receive adequate care and
that they do not become homeless upon release.

The Relationship between Mental Health and Homelessness

As demonstrated here, mental health problems are consistently overrepresented among homeless women compared to the general population (11, 30, 35, 38). Such findings often lead to the conclusion that mental health problems cause homelessness. Although mental health problems should not be construed as the *principal* explanation of homelessness among women, they may serve as an important contributing risk factor for some women. In the context of poverty and high housing costs (19), serious mental problems may interfere with a woman's capacity to obtain housing, employment, or services (26). Although the high rates of mental illness, substance abuse, and other problems among homeless women tend to focus our attention on the women, their homelessness also demonstrates the inadequacies of basic social systems.

Societal Factors and the Context in Which Homelessness Among Women Occurs

Stereotypes of homeless women result from seeing those who manifest the most severe mental and physical health problems and are therefore the most noticeable. Our review confirms that some homeless women have serious mental illness. However, those who are the most noticeable do not account for the largest proportion of homeless women. Homeless women without serious mental illness are less visible because their more normal appearance and behavior allow them to blend in with the larger domiciled community. They may remain unidentified as homeless and unlinked with services unless they enter the shelter system or other structured service sites. This may be especially true for certain subgroups of women such as homeless youth or undocumented Hispanic women.

Case histories concerning personal risk factors that precipitate homelessness in women include a variety of problems that are exacerbated when psychiatric problems are present: family break-ups, domestic violence, illness or death of a family member, and victimization in crimes such as robberies of rent money. While such crises are encountered by many women, they may be especially difficult to surmount for a woman with mental health problems.

Apart from their personal risk factors, virtually all homeless women have been influenced by societal forces that have occurred in the past decade (4), such as high unemployment and inflation. Such forces have likely had a special impact on women with mental health problems.

With higher levels of unemployment and declining real wages, women's need for affordable housing increased. Low-income housing, however, was substantially depleted during the 1980s due to cost restraints and the economic restructuring (49a). During this decade, for example, federal housing assistance programs for the poor were cut by over 75% and approximately 2.5 million units of low-income housing were lost to conversion, abandonment, arson, and demolition.

The economic situations of women were worsened by a number of policies implemented during the 1980s that changed social institutions in the United States. Beginning in the early 1980s, social services for poor women were cut and eligibility criteria became more stringent. Increasing numbers of women had inadequate or no health insurance coverage. Changes in the mental health care system during the 1960s and 1970s also contributed to the growing numbers of homeless women during the 1980s. A continuing lack of adequate funding for community mental health services creates competition for limited inpatient and outpatient treatment programs. This problem is compounded as women from the "baby boom" reach adulthood and increase the number of women at risk for developing serious mental disorders.

CONCLUSION

Despite limitations in study design and methods, results from recent work on homeless women present a coherent picture with implications of potential importance for the development of new policies for women who comprise about 20% of the US homeless adult population. Major mental disorders are overrepresented among homeless women. Other difficulties also confront all homeless women. In addition to their economic and housing needs, they often have special gender-related issues that include pregnancy, child care responsibilities, family violence, fragmented family support, job discrimination, and wage discrepancies.

Our review indicates that the lives of homeless women are often complicated by low utilization of mental health and other needed services. Interventions that combine targeted individual approaches with systemic approaches are especially needed for women with mental illness. Homeless women, regardless of parenting status, should be linked with social services, family support, self-help, and housing resources. Mentally ill women caring for children need additional consideration, with an emphasis on parenting skills and special services for children.

In conclusion, homelessness is a multifaceted problem related to personal, social, and economic factors. As public health policies are formulated, further epidemiologic evaluations are needed to provide a clearer understanding of the heterogeneity of homeless women and the mental health problems in this special population.

ACKNOWLEDGMENTS

This article was supported by CMHS/CSAT Cooperative Agreement # UD3 SM51800 and NIMH grant #MH51651. The authors acknowledge the contributions of Cheryl Zlotnick and Grace Lee to this article.

Literature Cited

1. American Psychiatric Association. 1987. *Diagnostic and Statistical Manual of Mental Disorders*. Washington, DC: Am. Psychiatric Assoc. DSM-III revised

2. Ball FJ, Havassey BE. 1984. A survey of the problems and needs of homeless consumers of acute psychiatric services. *Hosp. Commun. Psychiatry* 35:917–21

3. Bard M. 1994. *Organizational and Community Responses to Domestic Abuse and Homelessness* (Report). New York: Garland Publ.

4. Bassuk EL. 1993. Social and economic hardships of homeless and other poor women. *Am. J. Orthopsychiatry* 63:340–47

5. Bassuk EL, Rosenberg L. 1988. Why does family homelessness occur? A case-control study. *Am. J. Public Health* 78:783–88

6. Bassuk EL, Rubin L, Lauriat A. 1986. Characteristics of sheltered homeless families. *Am. J. Public Health* 76:1097–101

7. Breakey WR, Fischer PJ, Kramer M, Nestadt G, Romanoski AJ, et al. 1989. Health and mental health problems of homeless men and women in Baltimore. *JAMA* 262:1352–56

8. Breakey WR, Fischer PJ, Nestadt G, Romanoski A, Royall R, Ross A. 1990. Problems in reporting psychiatric disorders among homeless adults: in reply. *JAMA* 263:810–11

9. Breton M, Bunston T. 1992. Physical and sexual violence in the lives of homeless women. *Can. J. Commun. Ment. Health* 11:29–44

10. Browne A. 1993. Family violence and homelessness: The relevance of trauma histories in the lives of homeless women. *Am. J. Orthopsychiatry* 63:370–84

11. Buckner JC, Bassuk EL, Zima BT. 1993. Mental health issues affecting homeless women: implications for intervention. *Am. J. Orthopsychiatry* 63:385–99

12. Burg MA. 1994. Health problems of sheltered homeless women and their dependent children. *Health Soc. Work* 19:125–31

13. Burt MR, Cohen BE. 1989. Differences among homeless single women, women with children and single men. *Soc. Probl.* 36:508–24

14. Crystal S, Goldstein M. 1984. *Correlates of Shelter Utilization: One-Day Study*. New York, NY: Hum. Resourc. Admin. Fam. Adult Serv.

15. Crystal S, Goldstein M. 1984. *The Homeless in New York City Shelters*. New York, NY: Hum. Res. Admin. Fam. Adult Services

16. Culhane DP. 1992. Ending homelessness among women with severe mental illness: a model program from Philadelphia. *Psychosoc. Rehabil. J.* 16:63–76

17. D'Ercole A, Struening E. 1990. Victimization among homeless women: implications for service delivery. *J. Commun. Psychol.* 18:141–52

18. Dail PW, Koshes RJ. 1992. Treatment issues and treatment configurations for mentally ill homeless women. *Soc. Work Health Care* 17:27–44

19. Dolbeare CN. 1989. *Out of Reach: Why Everyday People Can't Find Affordable Housing*. Washington, DC: Low Income Hous. Inf. Serv.

20. Fischer PJ. 1992. The criminalization of homelessness. See Ref. 49a, pp. 57–64

21. Fischer PJ, Breakey WR. 1987. Profile of the Baltimore homeless with alcohol problems. *Alcohol Health Res. World* 2:36–37 61

22. Fischer PJ, Breakey WR. 1991. The epidemiology of alcohol, drug, and mental disorders among homeless persons. *Am. Psychol.* 46:1115–28

23. Gelberg L, Linn LS, Leake BD. 1988. Mental health, alcohol and drug use, and criminal history among homeless adults. *Am. J. Psychiatry* 145:191–96

24. Goodman L, Saxe L, Harvey M. 1991. Homelessness as psychological trauma. Broadening perspectives. *Am. Psychol.* 46:1219–25

25. Grella C. 1994. Contrasting a shelter and day center for homeless mentally ill women: four patterns of service use. *Commun. Ment. Health J.* 30:3–16

26. Hopper K. 1990. Deviance and dwelling space: notes on the resettlement of homeless persons with drug and alcohol

problems. *Contemp. Drug Probl.* 16:391–414

26a. Jahiel RI, ed. 1992. *Homelessness: A Prevention-Oriented Approach.* Baltimore/London: Johns Hopkins Univ. Press

27. Johnson AK, Kreuger LW. 1989. Toward a better understanding of homeless women. *Soc. Work* 34:537–40

28. Khanna M, Singh NN, Nemil M, Best A, Ellis CR. 1992. Homeless women and their families: characteristics, life circumstances, and needs. *J. Child Fam. Stud.* 1:155–65

29. Klein ME, Behnke SH, Peterson C. 1993. Depressive symptoms among sheltered homeless mothers. *Commun. Psychol.* 26:24–26

30. Koegel P, Burnam MA. 1992. Problems in the assessment of mental illness among the homeless: an empirical approach. See Ref. 49a, 77–99

31. Koegel P, Sullivan G, Burnam A, Morton SC, Wenzel S. 1995. *Utilization of Mental Health and Substance Abuse Services Among Homeless Adults.* Santa Monica, CA: RAND Corp.

32. Levine M, Toro PA, Perkins DV. 1993. Social and community interventions. *Annu. Rev. Psychol.* 44:525–58

33. Lovell AM. 1995. An analysis of psychiatric categorization in homelessness research. In *Homelessness,* ed. A Rosenblatt. Albany NY: Nelson A. Rockefeller Inst. Gov. Vol. 3. In press

34. Lovell AM, Barrows SM, Struening E. 1992. Between relevance and rigor: methodological issues in studying mental health and homelessness. See Ref. 29a, pp. 372–96

35. Merves ES. 1992. Homeless women: beyond the bad lady myth. See Ref. 49a, pp. 229–44

36. Milburn N, D'Ercole A. 1991. Homeless women: moving toward a comprehensive model. *Am. Psychol.* 46:1161–69

37. Morse G. 1985. *Homeless People in St. Louis: A Mental Health Program Evaluation, Field Study, and Follow-up Investigation.* St. Louis: Missouri Dep. Ment. Health. Vol. 1

38. Morse GA, Calsyn RJ. 1992. Mental health and other human service needs of homeless people. See Ref. 49a, pp. 3–18

39. North CS, Smith EM. 1992. Posttraumatic stress disorder among homeless men and women. *Hosp. Commun. Psychiatry* 43:1010–16

40. North CS, Smith EM. 1993a. A comparison of homeless men and women: different populations, different needs. *Commun. Ment. Health J.* 29:423–31

41. North CS, Smith EM. 1993b. A systematic study of mental health services utilization by homeless men and women. *Soc. Psychiatry Psychiatr. Epidemiol.* 28:2 77–83

42. North CS, Smith EM. 1994. Comparison of white and nonwhite homeless men and women. *Soc. Work* 39:639–47

43. North CS, Smith EM, Spitznagel EL. 1994. Violence and the homeless: an epidemiologic study of victimization and aggression. *J. Trauma. Stress* 7:95–110

44. Padgett DK, Streuning EL. 1992. Victimization and traumatic injuries among the homeless: associations with alcohol, drug, and mental problems. *Am. J. Orthopsychiatry* 62:525–34

45. Piliavin I, Sosin M, Westerfelt H. 1989. *Conditions Contributing to Long-term Homelessness: An Exploratory Study.* Univ. Madison, WI: Inst. Res. Poverty

46. Rhyns M, Rodgers HO. 1992. The unique needs and concerns of homeless women. In *Helping Homeless People: Unique Challenges and Solutions,* ed. C Solomon, P Jackson-Jobe, pp. 75–83. Alexandria VA: Am. Assoc. Couns. Dev.

47. Ritchey FJ, La Gory M, Mullis J. 1991. Gender differences in health risks and physical symptoms among the homeless. *J. Health Soc. Behav.* 32:33–48

48. Robertson MJ. 1991. Homeless women with children: the role of alcohol and other drug use. *Am. Psychol.* 46:1198–204

49. Robertson MJ. 1992. The prevalence of mental disorder among homeless people. See Ref. 26a, pp. 57–86

49a. Robertson MJ, Greenblatt M, eds. 1992. *Homelessness: A National Perspective.* New York: Plenum

50. Robertson MJ, Greenblatt M. 1992. Homelessness: a national perspective. See Ref. 49a, pp. 339–49

51. Robertson MJ, Westerfelt A, Zlotnick C. 1993. *Homeless women, children and families: identifying needs and appropriate responses.* Presented at Annu. Meet. Am. Orthopsychiatric Assoc. San Francisco, CA, May 22

52. Robertson MJ, Ropers RH, Boyer R. 1985. *The Homeless in Los Angeles County: An Empirical Assessment.* Los Angeles, CA: UCLA Sch. Public Health

53. Robins LN, Helzer JE, Przybeck TR, Regier DA. 1988. Alcohol disorders in the community: a report from the Epidemiologic Catchment Area. In *Alcoholism: Origins and Outcomes,* ed RM Rose, pp. 15–29. New York: Raven

54. Robins LN, Regier DA, eds. 1991. *Psy-*

chiatric Disorders in America: The Epidemiologic Catchment Area Study. New York: Free Press

55. Roll CN, Toro PA. 1995. *Characteristics and experiences of a homeless population: a comparison among single men, single women, and women with children.* Presented at Annu. Meet. Am. Public Health Assoc., San Diego, CA. Oct. 30–Nov. 2

56. Roth D, Toomey BG, First RJ. 1992. Gender, racial, and age variations among homeless persons. See Ref. 49a, pp. 199–212

57. Shinn M, Weitzman BC. 1995. Homeless families are different. In *Homelessness in America: A Reference Book,* ed. J Baumohl. New York: Oryx Press. In press

58. Smith EM, North CS. 1994. Not all homeless women are alike: effects of motherhood and the presence of children. *Commun. Ment. Health J.* 30:601–10

59. Smith EM, North CS, Spitznagel EL. 1993. Alcohol, drugs, and psychiatric comorbidity among homeless women: an epidemiologic study. *J. Clin. Psychiatry* 54:82–87

60. Snow DA, Baker SG, Anderson L. 1986. The myth of pervasive mental illness among the homeless. *Soc. Probl.* 33: 301–17

61. Solarz A. 1985. *Social supports among the homeless.* Presented at Annu. Meet Am. Public Health Assoc.

62. Solarz A, Mowbray C. 1985. *An examination of physical and mental health problems of the homeless.* Presented at Annu. Meet. Am. Public Health Assoc.

63. Somers A. 1992. Domestic violence survivors. See Ref. 49a, pp. 265–72

64. Susser E, Conover S, Struening EL. 1990. Mental illness in the homeless: problems of epidemiologic methods in surveys of the 1980s. *Commun. Ment. Health J.* 26:391–414

65. Toro PA. 1993. A systematic three-step methodology for representative sampling of homeless persons (August). In *Conceptual and Methodological Innovations in Research on Homelessness,* ed. PA Toro. Toronto, Canada: Am. Psychol. Assoc.

66. Wagner JD, Menke EM, Ciccone JK. 1994. The health of rural homeless women with young children. *J. Rural Health* 10:49–57

67. Warren BJ, Menke EM, Clement J, Wagner J. 1992. The mental health of African-American and Caucasian-American women who are homeless. *J. Psychosoc. Nurs.* 30:27–30

68. Weitzman BC, Knickman JR, Shinn M. 1992. Predictors of shelter use among low-income families: psychiatric history, substance abuse, and victimization. *Am. J. Public Health* 82:1547–50

69. Westerfelt H. 1990. *The ins and outs of homelessness: exit patterns and predictions.* Dissertation, Univ. Wisconsin, Madison

70. Winkleby MA, Boyce WT. 1994. Health related risk factors of homeless families and single adults. *J. Commun. Health* 19:7–23

71. Winkleby MA, Fishetti MR. 1990. Problems in reporting psychiatric disorders among homeless adults. *JAMA* 263: 810–11

72. Winkleby MA, Rockhill B, Jatulis D, Fortmann SP. 1992. The medical origins of homelessness. *Am. J. Public Health* 82:1394–98

73. Wood D, Valdez RB, Hayashi T, Shen A. 1990. Homeless and housed families in Los Angeles: a study comparing demographic, economic, and family function characteristics. *Am. J. Public Health* 80:1049–52

74. Zlotnick C, Robertson MJ. 1996. Sources of income among homeless adults with major mental disorders or substance use disorders. *Psychiatr. Serv.* 47:147–51

Annu. Rev. Public Health. 1996. 17:337–58

COMMUNITY-BASED APPROACHES FOR THE PREVENTION OF ALCOHOL, TOBACCO, AND OTHER DRUG USE

Marilyn Aguirre-Molina

Robert Wood Johnson Foundation, College Road East, Princeton, New Jersey 08543-2316

D. M. Gorman

Center of Alcohol Studies, Rutgers—The State University of New Jersey, Smithers Hall, Busch Campus, Piscataway, New Jersey 08855-0969

KEY WORDS: community-based prevention, alcohol, tobacco, other drugs

ABSTRACT

This paper summarizes what is known about community-based approaches for the prevention of ATOD problems and how the current practices in the field reflect these approaches. The first section of the chapter provides a brief summary of events early in this century when community-based approaches were central to addressing alcohol and other public health problems. The second section contains an overview of current research and empirical findings that yield consensus as to what conceptually and in practice constitutes a comprehensive, community-based prevention program for the prevention of ATOD problems. The third section reviews the literature of existing programs to assess the extent to which they include the salient elements and employ interventions determined to be fundamental to comprehensive community-based prevention programs. The final section discusses some of the challenges that confront researchers and practitioners when developing prevention initiatives and programs in high-risk environments.

INTRODUCTION

Research findings demonstrate that the risk of using alcohol, tobacco, or other drugs (ATOD) increases disproportionately with the number of risk factors

337

present in a community. For example, adolescent alcohol and other drug-related problems appear to be linked with poor family management practices, low family bonding and conflict, neighborhood deterioration, economic deprivation, and inner-city schools (21, 49). Other environmental factors have been identified as contributing to these risks. They include, for example, the easy access and availability of alcohol and tobacco in a community (70, 81, 103, 111), pricing and taxes on alcohol and tobacco (17, 103), as well as marketing and promotional activities targeted by the alcohol and tobacco industries to consumer groups such as young people, communities of color, and women (4, 34, 37, 47, 72, 88, 90). These research findings have led to an understanding of the complex etiology underlying the use of alcohol and other drugs.

This current understanding of the combined effects of environmental and social conditions on ATOD risks has resulted in an emphasis on interventions that extend beyond single-focused education programs targeting individual behavior to include comprehensive, community-based approaches. Such approaches attempt not only to influence the individual but also to incorporate the participation of the general community and its institutions to address the environmental and social factors that contribute to ATOD problems (60, 68, 79, 108, 112, 117). These approaches are characterized by systematic applications of integrated and sustained prevention strategies that are guided by public health theory and practice (8, 55, 76, 113).

Comprehensive, community-based approaches have emerged as the most viable way of reducing the risk of alcohol and other drug use (17, 21, 32, 33). As such, these prevention strategies have received substantial support from both the public and private sectors in the form of federal grants (e.g. Center for Substance Abuse Prevention-Community Partnership Program), foundation support (e.g. The Robert Wood Johnson Foundation-Fighting Back Program), and the adoption of these approaches by the voluntary sector (e.g. 4-H, the Junior League). This support is based on the observation that community-based approaches hold a great deal of promise because they endeavor to address the social context and environmental conditions that contribute to and sustain ATOD problems in a community (48, 56, 60).

EARLY COMMUNITY-BASED EFFORTS

Focus on the community as a unit of intervention is not a new phenomenon nor a unique approach to addressing problems that affect substantial numbers in a population. This focus has been at the core of public health practice in the United States since the 1800s, as the country struggled to bring under control the morbidity and mortality produced by infectious diseases and environmental conditions (58, 93, 94, 96). In like manner, community-focused action for alcohol problems has a long-standing history dating back to the 1830s and the advent of the temperance movement, when diverse constituent and citizen groups organized to address problems at the local level, where they were most directly and personally experienced (63). Although the temperance movement has been characterized by some as a failure because of the ultimate repeal of the 18th Amendment to the Constitution (which prohibited the "manufacture, sale and transportation of intoxicating liquors"), it nevertheless represents one of the most successful grass-roots, community-driven social movements in United States history. As Goldberg states, the movement's "leaders not only converted their proposals into law but achieved polity-member status" (39, p. 19).

Once again, the community is the locus of intervention as the ATOD field and grass-roots groups struggle with the public health problems posed by alcohol, tobacco, and illicit drug use. The current focus on community-based interventions for addressing ATOD problems has many parallels with early public health practice and community action. For example, then, as now, the specific mechanisms of disease were not fully understood, as is the case with the etiology of alcohol, tobacco, and other drug use today. Nevertheless, during both periods it is evident that collective action against the disease-producing agent and attention to the individual and environment (physical, social, and economic) have the greatest potential for yielding positive public health outcomes.

However, certain features distinguish current community-based action for ATOD problems from earlier efforts. For example, unlike the movements of the 1940s, 1950s, and 1960s when primary emphasis was placed on building a treatment system for alcoholics and the drug addicted, present-day community-based action for alcohol and other drug problems includes a distinct focus on prevention, the adoption of the public health model, and the use of public policy for change (92). Additionally, tobacco is prominent on the list of drugs in need of intervention. There has also been a shift away from reliance on professional change agents to the active participation of a diverse cadre of community members taking over the functions of initiating and mobilizing support for social change (10, 11). Prominent among these change agents are youth and parents, members of the faith community, local officials (elected and appointed), the business sector, and other concerned citizens.

Elsewhere, Room (92) provides an informative account of the events of the 1960s and 1970s that resulted in what he describes as the "new alcohol problems perspective" from which present-day community-based action programs for alcohol and other drugs have evolved. Additionally, Mosher & Jernigan (76), in their 1989 review of alcohol policy, provide a detailed overview and analysis of the alcohol policy movement at the core of today's public health action for the prevention of alcohol-related problems.

COMMUNITY-BASED PREVENTION

A review of the current literature reveals that community-based programs with the greatest promise for positive prevention outcomes rely heavily on the principles and models of community action for social change (11, 73) and place a high value on *community empowerment*; both concepts have their origins in the tradition of *community development* (5, 22). Programs are *comprehensive* and recognize the importance of social policy, use the tools of *public health practice*, and draw on the best available *research knowledge* to guide the interventions. Below we briefly review issues related to the comprehensiveness of programs, community empowerment, community development, and public health practice. Different types of intervention programs tend to draw upon different bodies of theory and research knowledge; for example, some draw upon studies of individual-level risk factors such as deficiencies in social skills, whereas others draw upon research pertaining to environmental factors such as drug availability. In the section discussing specific ATOD prevention interventions, we describe the underlying theory and research upon which these are based.

Comprehensive

A comprehensive community-based intervention targets multiple systems and employs multiple strategies (8). The targeting of multiple systems assures the identification of and attention to all factors within the environment that contribute to community risks (55). Equally important, targeting multiple systems enables the recruitment and participation of sectors and constituencies within a community that have an important and vital role in addressing ATOD problems. These sectors and constituencies include youth and families, the media, community organizations, and local institutions such as schools, the business sector, the faith community, government, and law enforcement.

Most prominent among the promising strategies employed at the community level are a combination of community organization (75), coalition development (13), media advocacy (118), and advocacy for public policies that influence the availability and marketing of alcohol and other drugs (25, 57, 86, 103). Embedded in an advocacy strategy for public policies is the understanding that individual behavior is shaped by the environment, which in turn is shaped by public policy. By making changes in public policy that affect the social, legal, and economic environments in which people make health decisions, there exists the opportunity for making the greatest progress.

Community Empowerment

Wallerstein & Bernstein (119, 120) provide thorough reviews of the concept of empowerment and its application in a number of community settings for varied health outcomes. They define community empowerment as ". . . a social-action process in which individuals and groups act to gain mastery over their lives in the context of changing their social and political environment" (120). The most effective community-based prevention programs are designed with the understanding that sustained change is achieved by individuals and communities that attain personal and community empowerment. This empowerment enables them to become active players (subjects) in the processes of community change vs passive recipients (objects) of prevention programs and services (73, 112, 120). It is in this domain where prevention specialists such as researchers, service providers, and health educators may encounter the greatest challenge. Many specialists approach communities as empowered experts with a ready constructed prevention model and assumptions, and thus find it difficult to hear community voices or learn ways to become part of a process that promotes social responsibility and social justice. The potential for conflict is increased when the community is ethnically, racially, or economically different from that of the specialist. Hill and colleagues (50) found that ". . . the barriers to the success of community-level prevention programs may lie more in overcoming the paternalism (by the expert) that arises as these programs actually unfold" (50, p. 86).

Community Development

Community development is the process of communities becoming invested in the identification and reinforcement of those aspects of everyday life, culture, and political activity that are conducive to health. Community development should be the ultimate goal of prevention strategies because it enables individuals and communities to increase their control over the determinants of health by securing the tools (resources, skills, authority, etc) needed to change their environment (1). These efforts are needed to change the social, political, and economic systems that contribute to neighborhood deterioration and community disorganization (see final section for details).

Public Health Model

Program interventions that are structured on the principles of the public health model take into consideration the host, agent, and environment, and focus on the interaction of this triad for the spread of alcohol and other drug-related problems. This analytic framework has moved the ATOD field away from the traditional focus on individual behavior as the primary domain of intervention to include an assessment of the drug's availability, accessibility, marketing, and the contribution of environmental structures within which these problems occur. Following Holder (53), we use the public health model to review existing community-based programs for the prevention of ATOD use and related problems.

In assessing state-of-the-art ATOD community-based prevention efforts in the United States, the following section reviews the available literature on existing community-based prevention programs. This assessment is guided by an attempt to answer the following questions: (*a*) Are the majority of the programs identified in the literature as comprehensive community-based ATOD prevention programs accurately classified, given that such programs improve their potential for success by employing multi-system/multi-strategy interventions? (*b*) Have these programs moved beyond a primary focus on individual behavior change to include environmental and public policy changes that facilitate and enhance individual behavior change? (*c*) Are the principles of community action, development, participation, and empowerment evident to the processes and interventions described? (*d*) Are these programs guided by public health theory and the best available research? The review of the literature represents a preliminary step toward answering these questions so that we might better understand the strengths and limits of the processes currently under way in the field of prevention.

COMMUNITY-BASED INTERVENTION PROGRAMS

As noted above, we use the three elements of the traditional public health model—the host, the agent, and the environment—to structure our review of community-based ATOD interventions. Of course, some programs are designed to affect more than one of the components of the public health model. For this review, a judgment has been made concerning the primary focus of the program. It should be noted that the review is restricted to programs targeted specifically at preventing drug use. Thus, it does not include programs that have a broader focus (such as preventing cardiovascular disease) and includes some types of drug use (typically cigarette smoking) among the many risk factors they target. Shea & Basch (100, 101) have reviewed these studies in detail. It also means that programs intended to reduce or stop drug use among established heavy users, such as the Community Intervention Trial for Smoking Cessation (110), are not included in the review.

Despite the attention given to community-based ATOD interventions, there are few well-designed studies reporting program effects on behavioral outcomes rather than on attitudes or knowledge. Gorman & Speer (44) conducted a detailed review of community interventions designed to prevent alcohol use and alcohol-related problems. They identified just eight studies that reported program effects on behavior and used controlled evaluation or time-series analysis to assess program impact. Most of these studies were concerned with changing the behavior of individuals rather than with influencing alcohol availability or changing the environment in which host and agent are brought together and interact. The primary focus of the present review is not methodological issues such as study design and techniques of data analysis. Such issues are discussed in detail by others (19, 54, 66, 78).

Strategies Designed to Change Host

Strategies designed to change the behavior of individuals have relied principally upon educational programs, mainly in the form of mass media interventions or community-based skills training for adolescents. Mass media programs typically target specific types of drug (i.e. alcohol or tobacco or illicit substances such as marijuana or crack cocaine). Community-based skills training programs typically target the so-called gateway substances, alcohol, tobacco, and marijuana.

MASS MEDIA INTERVENTIONS   Mass media campaigns have been widely used in the United States as part of the "war on drugs." Examples are the Just Say No campaign of the early 1980s and the succession of public service announcements (PSAs) mounted by the Partnership for a Drug-Free America since the late 1980s. As Wallack (116) observes, these campaigns are premised on the idea that ATOD use results from lack of information and focus primarily on individual behavior and personal responsibility. Advocates of this approach claim that its effectiveness can be inferred from national survey data showing a decline in drug use and in attitudes favorable to drug use since the campaigns have been in operation (87). However, there are a number of reasons why causality cannot be inferred from the association suggested by these data. For example, such an inference represents an example of the so-called ecological fallacy—meaning that changes occurring at one level of analysis (in this case, individual reports of drug use) cannot be inferred as resulting from changes occurring at another level of analysis (in this case, society-wide media campaigns) (35). Beyond such methodological issues, it has been suggested that the Partnership campaign might actually do more harm than good since it focuses attention exclusively on individual-level factors, thereby undermining potential support for initiatives that target the socioeconomic and political factors contributing to ATOD use (116).

Reviews and empirical studies from the 1980s consistently showed that broad-based mass media interventions, by themselves, had little impact on use of alcoholic beverages and cigarettes (30, 31, 77). Consequently, it was been suggested that mass media interventions be used primarily to supplement other approaches such as school-based and community-based programs. This supplementary approach has been most fully developed in the prevention of cigarette smoking among youth (30), but has also been used in community-based initiatives designed to prevent alcohol problems (14, 36, 38).

In addition to a shift toward a supplementary approach, Flay & Sobel (31) recommended more formative research into the mechanisms and processes through which media interventions work, so that messages can be more appropriately targeted at their intended audiences. Some laboratory-based research has been conducted in this area (20). Obviously, from a public health perspective, the goal of this approach is to refine media messages such that salient information reaches the largest possible number of the target high-risk audience. In one of the few evaluations of such use of mass media, Barber et al (6) assessed the effectiveness of a 30-second televised PSA designed on the principals of behavioral self-control training and targeted at heavy drinkers in North Queensland, Australia. Some subjects in the evaluation were sent a letter one week before advertisements were screened alerting them to the commencement of the campaign (it was hypothesized that forewarning the audience would enhance the effects of mass media interventions). In an evaluation involving 96 subjects, alcohol consumption was found to be significantly lower at post-test among subjects who were sent the letter and viewed the PSA compared with those who only received the letter or viewed the PSA or who got no intervention. The effects of the program were specific to alcohol use, as might be expected from such a narrowly focused clinically oriented approach. There were no effects on participants' perceptions of the dangers associated with alcohol use or attitudes toward social policies designed to control alcohol use and availability.

The key to such a targeted approach is to refine media messages such that high-quality information reaches the largest possible number of the appropriate target audience whose behavior the intervention is intended to change. This falls within what Wallack (115) refers to as the *personal-individual* approach to health promotion. In contrast, the *social-political* approach emphasizes changing the way in which a community thinks about the broader issues related to drug use and related problem, e.g. the marketing strategies of the liquor industry and laws regulating the sale of alcoholic beverages (see below).

COMMUNITY-BASED SKILLS TRAINING   Community-based skills training programs typically use curricula that are employed in school-based ATOD prevention programs. Opinion concerning the effectiveness of school-based social and resistance skills training curricula varies. Advocates claim that they are effective in preventing drug use among adolescents (9, 26, 84), whereas others maintain that their impact has been overstated (18, 35, 40, 42, 43, 67).

A number of community-based prevention programs are centered on the use of social influence curricula (e.g. 98, 109, 119). The best known of these programs is the Midwestern Prevention Project (MPP), a six-year longitudinal study targeted at youth in Kansas City and Indianapolis (59, 82, 83). The MPP consists of five components, introduced sequentially: a mass media component (comprised of television, radio, and print media events); a school-based social skills training curriculum; a parent program (oriented around six homework assignments); community organization involving training of city leaders in the planning and implementation of prevention efforts; and a health policy change component designed to initiate change in local ordinances regulating the availability of alcohol and tobacco products. Influences operating within the school (notably peer group pressure) were considered the most proximal in the sequence leading to drug use initiation, and therefore the school-based curriculum and mass media component were introduced first in the intervention sites, followed by the other three components at 6- to 12-month intervals. The school, family, and media components were concerned essentially with *demand* reduction, whereas the community organizing and policy change components were considered *supply* reduction strategies (82).

Pentz and associates (83) reported one-year follow-up data from more than 5000 students in the Kansas City site following the implementation of the school, family, and media components. Prevalence rates for cigarette, alcohol, and marijuana use were significantly lower among those who had taken part in the program than among controls. Johnson and colleagues, in a three-year follow-up study of a subsample of 1607 subjects from the Kansas City site, described two additional components: a parent organization program concerned with reviewing school prevention policy and training parents in communication skills, and initial training of community leaders in an attempt to establish a prevention task force. Significantly fewer subjects were using cigarettes and marijuana at follow-up among those who had received the program than among control subjects (25 vs 31% in the case of cigarettes, and 12 vs 20% in the case of marijuana). However, there were no differences between groups in terms of alcohol use.

One of the main weaknesses of the MPP is that allocation to study conditions was, for the most part, not random, and only limited data pertaining to initial equivalence have been reported (35). Of the 42 schools involved in the study in Kansas City, only 8 were randomly assigned to study conditions; the other 34 were allocated on administrator flexibility, with 20 rescheduling their existing activities and being assigned to the intervention group and 14 not rescheduling and being assigned to the comparison group. Also, although conceived as a comprehensive multicomponent intervention, only limited aspects of the MPP have been evaluated to date. Published accounts from the Kansas City evaluation give few details on the level of participation in the parenting program, while two other components—the mass media program and the community organization efforts—appear to have been implemented in both the intervention and control communities, which makes it impossible to assess their impact on outcome variables (59). In the Indianapolis site, participation in the parenting program was also not experimentally controlled, and the sample of self-selected participants differed in many crucial respects (e.g.

socioeconomic status, ethnicity, and reported cigarette and alcohol use) from nonparticipants (91). Those who took part in the parenting program generally engaged in the least demanding activity (namely, the homework sessions), with participation in more demanding activities (e.g. skills training and community meetings) limited to about one in five of the participants.

A methodologically more sophisticated community-based study that builds upon a school-based program was recently started in 24 public school districts located in six counties in northeastern Minnesota (85). Fourteen of the school districts have been randomly allocated to the intervention condition (Project Northland) and ten to the control condition. The intervention program employed in this project has three components: a parent program (oriented around four activity books for students to work on at home with their parents/guardians), a peer-led school-based resistance skills training program, and a community program built around task forces comprised of representatives from various community organizations. The goal of the latter is to develop strategies to reduce the access of adolescents to alcohol. These strategies fall into four broad areas: education of alcohol merchants; enforcement of existing laws on alcohol sales; development of new local ordinances regulating sales; and development of school policies concerning alcohol use. Community organizers are responsible for the formation of the task force in each community.

Strategies Designed to Change the Agent

Community-based drug prevention programs can do little to change the agent per se: They cannot reduce the production and manufacture of drugs such as alcohol, tobacco, marijuana, and cocaine. However, they can influence drug availability and access.

In recent years, field trials of illegal sales have documented the ease of availability of tobacco products to minors (16). This technique has also been employed in pretest-post-test trials to evaluate the impact of preventive measures (2, 3, 29). The outcome measure in these studies has been sales by merchants, and little is known about the effects of these efforts on use of tobacco products (2, 29). Interventions used in these studies employ one of two strategies, education of merchants and enforcement of laws. Research shows that educational approaches produce only short-term change in merchants' behavior, and that enforcement is necessary to achieve sustained reduction in availability (3, 29). However, one study (29) found that judges frequently dismissed citations against merchants for selling to minors, and observed that a successful enforcement effort could be undermined by judicial leniency. This finding suggests that interventions need to have an impact upon other institutions within a community if they are to have a sustained effect.

To date, very few studies report using field trials of merchant behavior to assess the extent of illegal sales of alcohol to minors (80, 89), and just two report employing this approach to assess the effectiveness of community prevention initiatives in reducing such sales and hence underage drinking, Project Northland (85) (see above) and Communities Mobilizing for Change on Alcohol (112) (see below).

Strategies Designed to Change the Environment

It is increasingly recognized that it is not sufficient to simply inoculate young people against the social pressures to use drugs, as is the case with many programs that target the individual without taking into consideration the enormous contribution of the social environments (51). Similarly, programs designed to limit access and availability must work through a range of institutions within a community if they are to have a sustained effect. The most comprehensive prevention programs in this area now draw upon conceptual models that emphasize the social and environmental determinants of behavior rather than individual and intrapsychic processes (e.g. 52, 112). Before discussing these broad-based initiatives, programs that target specific community agencies and organizations are discussed.

COMMUNITY ORGANIZATIONS   Sociologists argue that the social organization of communities depends to a considerable extent on the viability of its institutions (27, 121), ranging from government agencies like schools and social service departments to small private businesses such as the corner grocery store. In socially disorganized communities, institutions are typically nonexistent or function in a manner that is detrimental to local residents. Such communities are also vulnerable to the emergence of drug use, crime and delinquency, and violence (104). Conversely, communities characterized by high citizen participation in formal and informal organizations and with well-established local networks that foster meaningful social ties between individuals are more resilient to such problems and better able to respond to external pressures toward increased availability of drugs. The efforts of many community-based organizations are designed to restore local control and accountability of neighborhood institutions. Much of this effort has focused on the role of law enforcement agencies, although in recent years attempts have also been made to control the sale practices of local retail outlets for tobacco products and alcoholic beverages (see above).

Law enforcement   Community policing represents an excellent example of the attempt to rebuild communities through restructuring the role and functions of key institutions (27). In many urban minority communities, the main function of the police is to control local residents rather than to serve them. The tactics used in such areas differ markedly from those employed in white middle-class communities (17), and there is little evidence to suggest that they have much impact on the illicit drug markets (64). Community policing is intended to reduce the estrangement of the police from those they are supposed to serve, emphasizing as it does a commitment to problem-solving, two-way channels of communication between the police and citizens, responsiveness to community demands, neighborhood outreach and ministrations, and community self-help (95, 104). Drug use prevention frequently becomes the focus of community policing in urban neighborhoods since the sale and use of drugs are prominent among problems confronting residents of these areas.

Although there has been considerable rhetoric surrounding community policing, there have been relatively few systematic and methodologically sound evaluations of specific programs. Data from the few available studies show that community policing has the greatest impact upon residents' assessment of police performance, rather than on drug availability and related social disorder (69, 95, 105). As with other types of community-based programs, community policing *as implemented* often only loosely adheres to the key philosophies and principles underlying the approach (95). Police may have little enthusiasm for engaging in the activities required by community policing, and community participation is frequently hard to secure. This is especially true in socioeconomically and racially diverse neighborhoods, in which community policing can serve the needs of some members of the community (typically white, middle-class) at the expense of others (46, 95, 105).

Despite these problems and limited empirical support, community policing is likely to remain a popular drug prevention strategy given its appeal across the political spectrum: Conservatives like it because it is tough on those who sell drugs within neighborhoods and emphasizes the need for self-help, while liberals find its focus on community involvement and problem-solving attractive (41). Thus, it represents a politically expedient approach to the prevention of illicit drug use, although its capability to engage residents of those communities most affected by this problem has yet to be demonstrated (106).

Local media   As noted above, the mass media can be used to influence the way in which a community thinks about the broader issues related to ATOD use and related problems. Radio, television, and print media can provide people with the skills and information necessary to change the social and environmental factors that influence their health, rather than simply providing skills and knowledge intended to change personal behavior (115, 116). The goal of such media advocacy is to empower people such that they become active participants in the decision-making processes shaping the social and political context in which individual-level decisions about behavior are made. The behavior and health of the community, not the individual, is the central concern. Wallack and colleagues (118) discuss the principles underlying this approach to health promotion, and present a number of case studies illustrating the effective use of this strategy. The issues addressed in these case studies include the location of billboards advertising alcohol close to schools, the promotion and sale of alcohol at a large amusement park, a loophole in one state's law concerning alcohol-impaired driving, and the targeted marketing of malt liquor to African Americans.

BROAD-BASED COMMUNITY CHANGE   To date, the two most comprehensive community-based drug prevention programs have both focused on alcohol. Communities Mobilizing for Change on Alcohol (CMCA) is an 18-community trial designed to assess the effectiveness of a community mobilization strategy in reducing the availability of alcohol to those under 21 years of age and the level of alcohol use and alcohol-related health and social problems among this age group (112). The program is designed to accomplish these goals through change in community policies and practices concerning alcohol use, as opposed to simply changing "the behavior of an aggregate of individuals in the community" (112, p. 80). The project does not involve a set of pre-established program components for implementation in participating communities. Rather, the intervention entails a standardized process of community activation and mobilization, with communities free to implement whichever strategies and approaches they consider most appropriate in dealing with the problems they face. In line with this emphasis on community autonomy, the role of the research team is to help shape local policies and practices and not to try to directly control them. The research design of the CMCA is eloquent, involving both a randomized community trial and time-series analysis with multiple sources of data (e.g. school-survey, merchant survey, field trial of alcohol purchase attempts).

The Prevention Research Center (PRC) Project entails a more formal intervention than the CMCA Project, but is similar in its emphasis upon community-level processes (52). The intervention is intended to reduce the number of accidents and fatalities resulting from alcohol use, and is designed in accordance with a clearly articulated theoretical model in which the community is conceived of as a system involving the interaction of the individual and the social, economic, and physical environment. Alcohol-related accidents and fatalities are considered outputs of this system. The key factors operating within a community to produce these outputs are the level and pattern of alcohol consumption, the level of alcohol sales, the availability and marketing of alcohol, access to alcohol, community norms governing use, the enforcement of laws, community education, the level of risk-related activities (e.g. driving or using heavy machinery), and general background influences (e.g. the use of private automobiles compared to public transport).

The PRC intervention has five components: (*a*) community mobilization through the development of organizations and coalitions and increased public awareness; (*b*) training bar staff and management in responsible service practices; (*c*) community, parent, and retailer education aimed at reducing underage drinking; (*d*) increased effectiveness of DUI enforcement (both actual and as perceived by community residents); and (*e*) improved implementation of local ordinances governing youth accessibility to alcohol. The program is structured to ensure that an ongoing process of information sharing is established between the project staff and community representatives. The program has been implemented in two communities in California and one in South Carolina, each with a matched comparison community. A range of measures are being used to assess the intervention, including surveys, monitoring DUI arrest data and media accounts, and analysis of outlet densities and changes in policies.

INTERVENING IN HIGH-RISK COMMUNITIES

Despite some large-scale funding initiatives (e.g. the Center for Substance Abuse Prevention-Community Partnership Program), relatively little empirical research is available from which to assess the impact of community-based initiatives in areas most adversely affected by alcohol, tobacco, and other drugs. Although no community is immune from the adverse consequences of ATOD use, the markets for the most potent but inexpensive drugs tend to concentrate in poor, urban neighborhoods. This is true not only of illicit drug markets such as those in crack cocaine (24), but also the sale of tobacco products and alcohol (71, 102). Not surprisingly, although there has been some decline nationally in illicit drug use by adolescents since the mid-1980s (at least until the past year or two), evidence suggests that rates remain high among low-income, inner-city youth (7, 74). Consequently, many social and public health problems associated with drug use also concentrate in disadvantaged, urban communities (23, 45, 99, 114). As Kandel & Davies (62) observe, such findings suggest that drug use is becoming one further dimension of the increasing polarization evident in the United States between the economically advantaged and disadvantaged.

In communities beset by intense economic deprivation, social dislocation, and the ready availability of inexpensive drugs, the environmental factors sustaining drug use are immensely compelling, and agent-level biological and psychological risk factors (e.g. low self-esteem, poor decision-making skills) are probably of only minimal importance in explaining elevated levels of risk. Interventions that target only agent-level risk factors are likely to have minimal impact in terms of reducing ATOD use and ATOD-related problems. The need to target multiple systems, to build and develop community institutions, and to empower community members is especially acute in such settings.

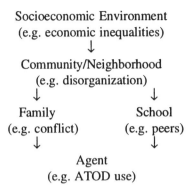

Figure 1   Hypothesized causal chain from socioeconomic factors through community and interpersonal influences to individual behavior.

Neighborhood and community social organization is crucial in mediating the impact of broader environmental influences (such as social deprivation and inequality) on ATOD use and ATOD-related problems. Neighborhood and community factors have an especially profound impact upon risk factors such as family management practices and the formation and activities of youth peer groups (28, 97). In turn, family management practices and peer group affiliations interact in influencing individual-level factors such as self-esteem, self-efficacy, and decision-making skills as well as in facilitating or discouraging children's drift into later high-risk activities such as engaging in antisocial acts (12, 61). This suggests a causal chain of the type depicted in Figure 1. Again, intervening at the lower end of this causal chain (i.e. only with the agent) is likely to prove ineffective.

Research suggests that those environmental factors that elevate the risk of drug use among the residents of impoverished urban neighborhoods (high rates of unemployment, inadequate social services, high incidence of teenage pregnancy and crime) might also mitigate against the development of community-based action. For example, Klitzner et al (65) in their study of parent-led drug prevention initiatives found that membership was comprised predominantly of white middle- and upper-class females, with "low income, minority, and high-risk youth ...largely unreached by the programs." Research in crime prevention also indicates that collective citizen action is less likely to arise in low-income, urban neighborhoods (104). However, against this, recent research shows evidence of effective community participation in prevention efforts in low-income neighborhoods beset by drug problems (69, 107). Confrontational tactics (such as marches) were most frequently used by groups in these neighborhoods, and the existing organizational capacity of the community was important in stimulating antidrug activism. One of the main challenges of future research is to find ways to engage those individuals and groups involved in prevention efforts within their communities, rather than imposing top-down prevention models and programs considered suitable by outside experts.

CONCLUSIONS

We began by presenting a brief overview of historical events showing how community-based approaches have been central to addressing issues related to alcohol use and other public health problems in the United States. We then reviewed current research indicating what conceptually and in practice constitutes a comprehensive, community-based prevention program to avert public health problems. The third section of the chapter reviewed major community-based prevention programs and initiatives in the ATOD field to assess the extent to which these include the salient elements and employ interventions determined to be fundamental to comprehensive community-based prevention programs. While it is evident from this review that there are numerous such interventions currently in progress in the field of ATOD prevention, it is also clear that the majority of these fall short of what has been described as comprehensive community-based programs. Although nearly all prevention initiatives are now conceptually driven, the focus of most of these remains to reduce demand for drugs through changing the attitudes and behavior of individuals. Programs that are truly comprehensive and attempt to change environmental-level as well as agent-level risk factors, and that empower and build community capacity for change, remain the exception. Most prevention initiatives come in the form of standardized packages and curricula devised by experts from outside the community, with minimal community participation in their design and delivery and little attention to the unique factors that contribute to ATOD problems within the target community. Not surprisingly, it has proved difficult to generate community involvement in such programs (e.g. 109). These problems are especially acute in high-risk communities—an issue addressed in the final section of this chapter.

The two most comprehensive community-based drug prevention programs described in this review both focus on alcohol (52, 112). Both draw upon the public health model in emphasizing the social and environmental determinants of alcohol use, and both attempt to foster community involvement in the design and implementation of their interventions. To date, evaluation data from these studies have yet to be reported.

Finally, it is important to note some of the factors that impede the design and implementation of comprehensive community-based ATOD prevention programs. First, such programs are difficult and complicated to set in motion and guide to completion; supervising and orchestrating the implementation of the diverse elements required of comprehensive programs is an extremely demanding enterprise (compared, for example, with delivering a tailor-made, single-focus program). Second, and related to the first issue, such activities are extremely difficult to evaluate. Expertise in methods and data analysis techniques other than those associated with traditional randomized experiments (e.g. time-series analysis) is required of the investigator. Third, when programs are truly based on the principals of community action and development, they are likely to encounter obstacles posed by the political and economic interests that are threatened by empowered communities. Fourth, to a considerable extent, the field of ATOD research is still conceptually grounded in models that attribute drug use to individual biological, psychological, and psychosocial factors such as personality traits, low self-esteem, inadequate coping skills, and peer pressure. Consequently, it is these factors that we set out to alleviate when trying to prevent drug use. Finally, an equally important deterrent to moving toward truly comprehensive community-based prevention programs is the fact that experts in the field of ATOD use (i.e. researchers, service providers, and health educators) frequently do not know how to work effectively with communities toward the empowerment and social justice that are essential for community change and the prevention of alcohol-, tobacco-, and drug-related problems. The latter requires a new way of conceiving of the community as an active partner in prevention. As case studies and accounts in the press indicate, residents of high-risk communities beset by drug problems do, of their own accord, develop and implement initiatives designed to limit the availability of alcohol, tobacco, and other drugs (97, 107, 118), and in the future prevention experts should make more effort to build upon such neighborhood-based movements.

Literature Cited

1. Aguirre-Molina M, Parra PA. 1995. Latino youth and families as active participants in planning change. In *Understanding Latino Families—Scholarship, Policy and Practice*, ed. R Zambrana, pp. 130–53. Thousand Oaks, CA: Sage
2. Altman DG, Rasenick-Douss L, Forster V, Tye JB. 1991. Sustained effects of an educational program to reduce sales of cigarettes to minors. *Am. J. Public Health* 81:891–93
3. Altman DG, School C, Basil M. 1991.

Alcohol and cigarette advertising on billboards. *Health Ed. Res.* 6:487–90
4. Altman D, Carol J, Chalkley C, Cherner J, DiFranza J, et al. 1992. Report of the Tobacco Policy Research Study Group on access to tobacco products in the United States. *Tobacco Control* 1(Suppl.): S45–S51
5. Bailey A. 1980. Community development theory and practice. *Commun. Forum* 6:1–4
6. Barber, JG, Bradshaw, R, Walsh, C.

1989. Reducing alcohol consumption through television advertising. *J. Consult. Clin. Psychol.* 57:613–18

7. Barr KEM, Farrell MP, Barnes GM, Welte JW. 1993. Race, class, and gender differences in substance abuse: evidence of middle-class/underclass polarization among black males. *Soc. Probl.* 40:314–27

8. Benard B. 1990. An overview of community-based prevention. In *Prevention Research Findings: 1988*, ed. KH Rey, CL Faegre, P Lowery, pp. 126–47. Rockville, MD: OSAP Prev. Monogr. 3

9. Botvin G. 1990. Substance abuse prevention: theory, practice and effectiveness. See Ref. 110a, pp. 461–519

10. Braithwaite RL, Lythcott N. 1989. Community empowerment as a strategy for health promotion for black and other minority populations. *JAMA* 261:282–83

11. Brown ER. 1991. Community action for health promotion: a strategy to empower individuals and communities. *Int. J. Health Serv.* 21:441–56

12. Brown BB, Mounts N, Lamborn SD, Steinberg L. 1993. Parenting practices and peer group affiliation in adolescence. *Child Dev.* 64:467–82

13. Butterfoss FD, Goodman RM, Wandersman A. 1993. Community coalitions for prevention and health promotion. *Health Ed. Res.* 8:315–30

14. Casswell S, Ransom R, Gilmore L. 1990. Evaluation of a mass-media campaign for the primary prevention of alcohol-related problems. *Health Prom. Int.* 5:9–17

15. Cent. Dis. Control. 1989. *Reducing the Health Consequences of Smoking: 25 Years of Progress. A Report to the Surgeon General.* Washington, DC: CDC

16. Cent. Dis. Control. 1993. Minors' access to tobacco—Missouri, 1992, and Texas, 1993. *Morbid. Mortal. Wkly. Rep.* 42:125–28

17. Chambliss WJ. 1994. Policing the ghetto underclass: the politics of law and law enforcement. *Soc. Probl.* 41:177–94

18. Cleary PD, Hitchcock JL, Semmer N, Flinchbaugh LJ, Pinney JM. 1988. Adolescent smoking: research and health policy. *Milbank Q.* 66:137–71

19. Collins LM, Seitz LA. 1994. *Advances in Data Analysis for Prevention Intervention Research (NIDA Res. Monogr. 142).* Rockville, MD: Natl. Inst. Drug Abuse

19a. Davis RC, Lurigio AJ, Rosenbaum DP, eds. 1993. *Drugs and the Community: Involving Community Residents in Combatting the Sale of Illegal Drugs.* Springfield, IL: Charles C Thomas

20. Donohew L, Lorch, E, Palmgreen P. 1991. Sensation seeking and targeting of televised anti-drug PSAs. In *Persuasive Communication and Drug Abuse Prevention*, ed. L Donohew, HE Sypher, WJ Bukoski, pp. 209–26. Hillsdale, NJ: Lawrence Erlbaum

21. Dryfoos JG. 1993. Preventing substance abuse: rethinking strategies. *Am. J. Public Health.* 83:793–95

22. Dubey SN. 1970. Community action programs and citizen participation: issues and confusion. *Soc. Work.* 15:76–84

23. Dunlap E. 1992. The impact of drugs on family life and kin networks in the inner-city African-American single-parent household. In *Drugs, Crime and Social Isolation: Barriers to Urban Opportunity*, ed. AV Harrell, GE Peterson, pp. 181–207. Washington, DC: Urban Inst. Press

24. Dunlap E, Johnson BD. 1992. The setting for the crack era: macro forces, micro consequences (1960–1992). *J. Psychoact. Drugs* 24:307–21

25. Edwards G, Anderson P, Babor T, Casswell S, Ferrence R, et al. 1995. *Alcohol Policy and the Public Good.* New York: Oxford Univ. Press/WHO

26. Ellickson, PL. 1995. Schools. In *Handbook on Drug Abuse Prevention: A Comprehensive Strategy to Prevent the Abuse of Alcohol and Other Drugs*, ed. RH Coombs, D Ziedonis, pp. 93–120. Boston, MA: Allyn & Bacon

27. Etzioni A. 1993. *The Spirit of Community: The Reinvention of American Society.* New York: Simon & Schuster

28. Fagan J. 1993. The political economy of drug dealing among urban gangs. See Ref. 19a, pp. 19–54

29. Feighery E, Altman DG, Shaffer G. 1991. The effects of combining education and enforcement to reduce tobacco sales to minors: a study of four northern California communities. *JAMA* 266:3168–71

30. Flay BR. 1986. Mass media linkages with school-based programs for drug abuse prevention. *J. School Health* 56:402–6

31. Flay BR, Sobel JL. 1983. The role of mass media in preventing adolescent substance abuse. In *Preventing Adolescent Drug Abuse: Intervention Strategies*, ed. TJ Glynn, CG Leukefeld, JP Ludford, pp. 5–35. Washington, DC: US GPO. NIDA Res. Monogr. 47

32. Florin P, Chavis D. 1990. Community development and substance abuse pre-

vention. In *National Training System Trainer Resource Manual*. Rockville, MD: Off. Subst. Abuse Prev.

33. Florin P, Wandersman A. 1990. An introduction to citizen participation, voluntary organizations and community development: Insights for empowerment through research. *Am. J. Comm. Psychol.* 18:41–54

34. Gerbner G. 1990. Stories that hurt: tobacco, alcohol and other drugs in the mass media. See Ref. 90, pp. 53–127

35. Gerstein DR, Green LW. 1993. *Preventing Drug Abuse: What do we Know?* Washington, DC: Natl. Acad. Press

35a. Giesbrecht N, Conley P, Denniston RW, Gliksman L, Holder HD, et al, eds. 1990. *Research, Action, and Community: Experiences in the Prevention of Alcohol and Other Drug Problems*. Washington, DC: OSAP Prev. Monogr. 4

36. Giesbrecht N, Pranovi P, Wood L. 1990. Impediments to changing local drinking practices: lessons from a prevention project. See Ref. 35a, pp. 161–82

37. Gitlin T. 1990. On drugs and mass media in America's consumer society. See Ref. 90, pp. 31–52

38. Gliksman, L, Douglas RR, Thomson M, Moffatt K, Smythe C, Caverson R. 1990. Promoting municipal alcohol policies: an evaluation of a campaign. *Contemp. Drug Probl.* 17:391–420

39. Goldberg RA. 1991. *Grassroots Resistance—Social Movements in Twentieth Century America*. Belmont, CA: Wadsworth

40. Gorman DM. 1992. Using theory and basic research to target primary prevention programs: recent developments and future prospects. *Alcohol Alcohol.* 27:583–94

41. Gorman DM. 1993. "War on drugs" continues in United States under new leadership. *Br. Med. J.* 307:369–71

42. Gorman DM. 1995. Are school-based resistance skills training programs effective in preventing alcohol misuse? *J. Alcohol Drug Ed.* 41:74–98

43. Gorman DM. 1995. Do school-based social skills training programs prevent alcohol use among young people. *Addict. Res.* In press

44. Gorman DM, Speer PW. 1995. Preventing alcohol abuse and alcohol-related problems through community interventions: a review of evaluation studies. *Psychol. Health* 10:1–38

45. Greenberg M, Schneider D. 1994. Violence in American cities: Young black males is the answer, but what was the question? *Soc. Sci. Med.* 39:179–87

46. Greene JR, McLaughlin E. 1993. Facilitating communities through police work: drug problem solving and neighborhood involvement in Philadelphia. See Ref. 19a, pp. 141–61

47. Grube JW, Wallack L. 1994. Television beer advertising and drinking knowledge, beliefs and intentions among schoolchildren. *Am. J. Public Health* 84:254–59

48. Hansen WB, Graham JW. 1991. Preventing alcohol, marijuana, and cigarette use among adolescents: peer pressure resistance training versus establishing conservative norms. *Prev. Med.* 20:414–30

49. Hawkins JD, Lishner D, Catalano R. 1992. Risk and protective factors for alcohol and other drug problems in adolescence and early adulthood: implications for substance abuse prevention. *Psychol. Bull.* 112:64–105

50. Hill H, Piper D, Moberg DP. 1995. "Us planning prevention for them": the social construct of community prevention for youth. *Int. Q. Health Ed.* 15:65–89

51. Holder HD. 1992. Undertaking a community prevention trial to reduce alcohol problems: translating theoretical models into action. See Ref. 54, pp. 227–43

52. Holder HD. 1993. Prevention of alcohol-related accidents in the community. *Addiction* 88:1003–12

53. Holder HD. 1994. Public health approaches to the reduction of alcohol problems. *Subst. Abuse* 15:123–38

54. Holder HD, Howard JM. 1992. *Community Prevention Trials for Alcohol Problems: Methodological Issues*. Westport, CT: Praeger

55. Holder HD, Wallack L. 1986. Contemporary perspectives for preventing alcohol problems: an empirically derived model. *J. Public Health Pol.* 7:324–39

56. Howard-Pitney B. 1990. Community development is alive and well in community health promotion. *Comp. Psychol.* Summer, 4–5

57. Hu T, Sung HY, Keeler T. 1995. Reducing cigarette consumption in California: tobacco taxes vs. an anti-smoking media campaign. *Am. J. Public Health* 85:1218–22

58. Institute of Medicine. 1988. *The Future of Public Health*. Washington, DC: Natl. Acad. Press

59. Johnson CA, Pentz MA, Weber MD, Dwyer JH, Baer N, et al. 1990. Relative effectiveness of comprehensive community programming for drug abuse prevention with high-risk and low-risk adolescents. *J. Consult. Clin. Psychol.* 58:447–56

60. Kaftarian SJ, Hansen WB. 1994. Improving methodologies for the evaluation of community-based substance abuse prevention programs. *J. Comp. Psychol.* 22:3–5 (OSAP Spec. Issue)

61. Kandel DB, Andrews K. 1987. Processes of adolescent socialization by parents and peers. *Int. J. Addict.* 22:319–42

62. Kandel DB, Davies M. 1991. Decline in the use of illicit drugs by high school students in New York State: a comparison with national data. *Am. J. Public Health* 81:1064–67

63. Keer KA. 1985. *Organized for Prohibition: A New History of the Anti-Saloon League.* New Haven, CT: Yale Univ. Press

64. Kleiman MAR, Smith KD. 1990. State and local drug enforcement: in search of a strategy. See Ref. 110a, pp. 69–108

65. Klitzner M, Bamberger E, Gruenewald PJ. 1990. The assessment of parent-led prevention programs: a national descriptive study *J. Drug Ed.* 20:111–25

66. Koepsell TD, Wagner EH, Cheadle AC, Patrick DL, Martin DC, et al. 1992. Selected methodological issues in evaluating community-based health promotion and disease prevention programs. *Annu. Rev. Public Health* 13:31–57

67. Kozlowski LT, Coambs RB, Ferrence RG, Adlaf EM. 1989. Preventing smoking and other drug use: Let the buyers beware and the interventions be apt. *Can. J. Public Health* 80:452–56

68. Lorion RP. 1991. Prevention research. In *DHHS Drug Abuse and Drug Abuse Research.* Trienn. Rep. Congr. Sec., 3rd, Washington, DC: DHHS, GPO

69. Lurigio AJ, Davis RC. 1992. Taking the war on drugs to the streets: the perceptual impact of four neighborhood drug programs. *Crime Delinq.* 38:522–38

70. Lynch BS, Bonnie R.J. 1994. *Growing Up Tobacco Free: Preventing Nicotine Addiction in Children and Youths.* Washington, DC: Natl. Acad. Press

71. Marriot M. 1993. For minority youths, 40 ounces of trouble. *NY Times,* April 16:A1, B3

72. Maxwell B, Jacobson M. 1989. *Marketing Disease to Hispanics.* Washington, DC: Cent. Sci. Public Interest

73. McLeroy KR, Bibeau D, Streckler A, Glanz K. 1988. An ecological perspective on health promotion programs. *Health Ed. Q.* 15:351–77

74. McNagny SE, Parker RM. 1992. High prevalence of recent cocaine use and the unreliability of patient self-report in an inner-city walk-in clinic. *JAMA* 267:1106–8

75. Minkler M. 1991. Improving health through community organization. In *Health Behavior and Health Education—Theory, Research and Practice,* ed. K Glanz, FM Lewis, BK Rimer, pp. 257–87. San Francisco, CA: Jossey-Bass

76. Mosher JF, Jernigan DH. 1989. New directions in alcohol policy. *Annu. Rev. Public Health* 10:245–79

77. Moskowitz JM. 1989. The primary prevention of alcohol problems: a critical review of the research literature. *J. Stud. Alcohol* 50:54–88

78. Murray DM, Rooney BL, Hannan PJ, Peterson AV, Ary DV, et al. 1994. Intraclass correlation among common measures of adolescent smoking: estimates, correlates, and application in smoking prevention estimates. *Am. J. Epidemiol.* 140:1038–50

79. National Cancer Institute. 1991. *Strategies to Control Tobacco Use in the United States: A Blueprint for Public Health Action in the 1990's.* Bethesda, MD: NIH. Smok. Tob. Control Monogr. 1.

80. O'Leary D, Gorman DM, Speer PM. 1994. The sale of alcoholic beverages to minors. *Public Health Rep.* 109:816–18

81. O'Malley P, Wagenaar A. 1991. The effects of minimum drinking age laws on alcohol use, related behaviors, and traffic crash involvement among American youth, 1976–1987. *J. Stud. Alcohol* 52:478–91

82. Pentz MA. 1993. Comparative effects of community-based drug abuse prevention. In *Addictive Behaviors Across the Life Span: Prevention, Treatment, and Policy Issues,* ed. JS Baer, GA Marlatt, RJ McMahon, pp. 69–87. Newbury Park, CA: Sage

83. Pentz MA, Dwyer JH, MacKinnon DP, Flay BR, Hansen WB, et al. 1989. A multicommunity trial for primary prevention of adolescent drug abuse: effects on drug use prevalence. *JAMA* 261:3259–66

84. Perry CL, Kelder SH. 1992. Models of effective prevention. *J. Adolesc. Health* 13:355–63

85. Perry CL, Williams CL, Forster JL, Wolfson M, Wagenaar AC, et al. 1993. Background, conceptualization and design of a community-wide research program on adolescent alcohol use: Project Northland. *Health Ed. Res.* 8:125–36

86. Peterson DE, Zeger SL, Remington PL, Anderson HA. 1992. The effects of state cigarette tax increases on cigarette sales, 1955 to 1988. *Am. J. Public Health* 82:94–96

87. Pisani RG. 1995. Advertising industry. In *Handbook of Drug Abuse Prevention*, ed. RH Coombs, D Ziedonis, pp. 217–48. Boston, MA: Allyn & Bacon

88. Pollay RW, Lee JS, Carter-Whitney D. 1995. Separate but not equal—racial segmentation in cigarette advertising. In *Gender, Race and Class in Media*, ed. G Dines, JM Humez, pp. 109–11. Thousand Oaks, CA: Sage

89. Preusser DF, Williams AF. 1992. Sales of alcohol to underage purchasers in three New York counties and Washington, D.C. *J. Public Health Pol.* 13:306–17

90. Resnick H, Gardner SE, Lorion RP, Marcus CE, eds. 1990. *Youth and Drugs: Society's Mixed Messages.* Rockville, MD: OSAP Prev. Monogr. 6

91. Rohrbach LA, Hodgson CS, Broder BI, Montgomery SB, Flay BR, et al. 1994. Parental participation in drug abuse prevention: results from the Midwestern Prevention Project. *J. Res. Adolesc.* 4: 295–317

92. Room R. 1990. Community action and alcohol problems: the demonstration project as an unstable mixture. See Ref. 35a, pp. 1–21

93. Rosen G. 1958. *A History of Public Health.* New York: MD Publ.

94. Rosen G. 1975. *Preventive Medicine in the United States 1900–1975.* New York: Sci. Hist. Publ.

95. Rosenbaum DP, Lurigio AJ. 1994. An inside look at community policing reform: definitions, organizational changes, and evaluation findings. *Crime Delinq.* 40:299–314

96. Rossi PH. 1965. *Community.* New York: Free Press

97. Sampson RJ. 1992. Family management and child development: insights from social disorganization theory. In *Facts, Frameworks, and Forecasts: Advances in Criminological Theory*, ed. J McCord, 3:63–93. New Brunswick, NJ: Transaction

98. Schinke SP, Orlandi MA, Cole KC. 1992. Boys & Girls Clubs in public housing developments: prevention services for youth at risk. *J. Comp. Psychol.* 20:118–28. OSAP Spec. Issue

99. Selik RM, Chu SY, Buehler JW. 1993. HIV infection as leading cause of death among young adults in US cities and states. *JAMA* 269:2991–94

100. Shea S, Basch CE. 1990. A review of five major community-based cardiovascular disease prevention programs. Part I: Rationale, design, and theoretical framework. *Am. J. Health Promot.* 4: 203–13

101. Shea S, Basch CE. 1990. A review of five major community-based cardiovascular disease prevention programs. Part II: Intervention strategies, evaluation methods, and results. *Am. J. Health Promot.* 4:279–87

102. Sims C. 1992. Community groups attack the industry's rich franchise at the corner store. *NY Times*, Nov. 29, Sect. 3:1, 6

103. Single E. 1994. The impact of social and regulatory policy on drinking behavior. In *The Development of Alcohol Problems: Exploring the Biopsychosocial Matrix of Risk*, pp. 205–48. Rockville, MD: NIAAA. Res. Monogr. 26

104. Skogan WG. 1990. *Disorder and Decline: Crime and the Spiral of Decay in American Neighborhoods.* Berkeley: Univ. Calif. Press

105. Skogan WG. 1994. The impact of community policing on neighborhood residents: a cross-site analysis. In *The Challenge of Community Policing: Testing the Promise*, ed. DP Rosenbaum, pp. 167–81. Thousand Oaks, CA: Sage

106. Skogan WG, Annan S. 1993. Drug enforcement in public housing. See Ref. 19a, pp. 162–74

107. Skogan WG, Lurigio AJ. 1992. The correlates of community antidrug activism. *Crime Delinq.* 38:510–21

108. Stokols D, 1992. Establishing and maintaining healthy environments: toward a social ecology of health promotion. *Am. Psychol.* 47:6–22

109. St. Pierre TL, Kaltreider DL, Mark MM, Aikin KJ. 1992. Drug prevention in a community setting: a longitudinal study of the relative effectiveness of a three-year primary prevention program in Boys & Girls Clubs across the nation. *Am. J. Comp. Psychol.* 20:673–706

110. The COMMIT Research Group. 1995. Community Intervention Trial for Smoking Cessation (COMMIT): I. Cohort results from a four-year community intervention. *Am. J. Publ. Health* 85: 183–92

110a. Tonry M, Wilson JQ, eds. 1990. *Drugs and Crime.* Chicago: Univ. Chicago Press

111. Toomey L, Jones-Webb R, Wagenaar A. 1993. Recent research on alcohol beverage control policy: a review of the literature. *Annu. Rev. Addict. Res. Treat.* 3:279–92

112. Wagenaar AC, Murray DM, Wolfson M, Forster JL, Finnegan JR. 1994. Communities Mobilizing for Change on Alcohol: design of a randomized com-

munity trial. *J. Comp. Psychol.* 22:79–101. OSAP Spec. Issue.

113. Wagenaar AC, Perry CL. 1994. Community strategies for the reduction of youth drinking: theory and application. *J. Res. Adolesc.* 4:319–45

114. Wallace R. 1990. Urban decertification, public health and public disorder: "Planned shrinkage", violent death, substance abuse and AIDS in the Bronx. *Soc. Sci. Med.* 31:801–13

115. Wallack L. 1990. Two approaches to health promotion in the mass media. *World Health Forum* 11:143–54

116. Wallack L. 1994. Media advocacy: a strategy for empowering people and communities. *J. Public Health Pol.* 15: 420–36

117. Wallack L, Corbett K. 1990. Illicit drug, tobacco, and alcohol use among youth: trends and promising approaches in prevention. See Ref. 90, pp. 5–29

118. Wallack L, Dorfman L, Jernigan D, Themba M. 1993. *Media Advocacy and Public Health: Power for Prevention.* Newbury Park, CA: Sage

119. Wallerstein N, Bernstein E. 1988. Empowerment education: Friere's ideas adapted to health education. *Health Ed. Q..* 15:379–94

120. Wallerstein N, Bernstein E. 1994. Introduction to community empowerment, participatory education, and health. *Health Ed. Q.* 21:141–48

121. Wilson WJ. 1987. *The Truly Disadvantaged: The Inner City, the Underclass, and Public Policy.* Chicago: Univ. Chicago Press

Annu. Rev. Public Health. 1996. 17:359–82

POPULATION AND WOMEN'S REPRODUCTIVE HEALTH: An International Perspective

Kate Miller and Allan Rosenfield

Columbia University School of Public Health, New York, NY 10032

KEY WORDS: gender issues, sexually transmitted diseases, maternal mortality, abortion, adolescent pregnancy

ABSTRACT

This paper gives a brief overview of current world population or demographic issues, followed by a discussion of the ICPD proceedings and various notable aspects of the ICPD Programme of Action. It then focuses on six of the most pressing reproductive health concerns facing women today: gender inequalities, access to contraceptive services, sexually transmitted diseases (including HIV), maternal mortality, unsafe abortion, and adolescent pregnancy. Because the ICPD Programme of Action is intended to have far-reaching consequences for each of these issues, it is taken as a focal point of analysis.

INTRODUCTION

This has been an outstandingly successful conference.

On September 13, 1994, with these words, Dr. Nafis Sadik, executive director of the United Nations Population Fund, officially closed the United Nations' decennial International Conference on Population and Development (ICPD). As the secretary-general of the conference, she may have been tempted to overplay the success of the event, but in fact her closing words are more than rhetoric. The goal of the ICPD, an eight-day event that drew over 14,000 people to Cairo and generated extensive international press, was to adopt a unified Programme of Action on population and development, intended to guide policy-making over the next 20 years among the 179 countries represented at the conference. The final Programme of Action does indeed constitute, in Sadik's words, a "quantum leap" over previous efforts, particularly in its attitude toward individual reproductive rights and the central role of women.

359

POPULATION GROWTH

The United Nations' population conferences have all been motivated by concerns about the effects of the rapid population growth of roughly the last 150 years. It took all of known history to reach the first one billion people in the early 1800s. We are now adding one billion people every 11 years. Between 1950 and 1992, the population of the world more than doubled, from 2.5 billion to 5.5 billion (63). The total world population was estimated to be 5.7 billion in mid-1995 (44) and to reach 6 billion by 1998.

Currently, the annual world growth rate is 1.6%, with large regional differences. The most developed nations are growing at about 0.6% per year, the less developed at about 2% per year, and the least developed at 3% or more. The growth rates in Africa are the highest in the world, and will continue to be so through 2025 according to United Nations projections, notwithstanding the effects of the AIDS epidemic (63).

In the period from 1985 to 1990, the world total fertility rate (TFR) was estimated at 3.4 children per woman at the end of the childbearing years, which represented a 10% decrease from the previous decade, with the fastest regional decline (15%) achieved by the less developed countries. However, the rates remained high: for less developed countries, 4.2 births per woman; for the least developed countries it is 6.4; and in the most developed nations, 1.9, which is below the replacement level of 2.1 births per woman, a level in which two parents are replaced by two children (63). Populations with high TFRs will continue to grow for many years because the numbers of young people are so large. With time, these young cohorts will move into their reproductive years and begin bearing children. Even if the TFRs have declined by that time, the sheer number of people reproducing will still result in significant population growth. In other words, populations have a certain "momentum"; they keep expanding even after fertility rates decline. Alarm over these demographic circumstances has motivated many of the international and national population policies of the past few decades, especially with the evidence of adverse consequences of high population growth rates for the social and physical environment (41, 77). This is the demographic backdrop against which the ICPD took place, coupled with a complex array of social and political issues, discussed below.

THE INTERNATIONAL CONFERENCE ON POPULATION AND DEVELOPMENT

The ICPD was by no means an isolated event. The conference was preceded by several years of preparations, including three official UN Preparatory Committee (PrepCom) conferences, charged with drafting the Programme of Action. These PrepComs were paralleled by several regional conferences designed to gain local consensus on a range of issues, as well as by six Expert Group Meetings on Population Policies and Programmes, hosted by the United Nations. Perhaps more important than these formal preparations, however, were innumerable nongovernmental organization (NGO) conferences, of various sizes and on myriad issues, that eventually had significant impact on the final conference and document. In addition, many official delegations to Cairo (including the US) included NGO representation.

The ICPD itself was accompanied by a large NGO forum, which attracted almost 4000 people representing 1500 organizations from 133 countries, and which significantly influenced Programme language. The NGO forum was divided into several caucuses, the largest and most powerful of which was the women's caucus, which focused on lobbying the ICPD daily (45).

The ICPD in the Context of Previous Decennial Population Conferences

The first conference, held in 1974 in Bucharest, Romania, was characterized by a relatively unproductive standoff between Western industrialized nations and an ideological alliance of "Third World" nations and the Communist Bloc. The industrialized nations were interested in the demographic consequences of high birthrates, and were mainly prepared to discuss direct governmental interventions in the form of family planning programs. The Third World and Communist Bloc nations, however, viewed demographic effects as secondary to (and emergent from) economic conditions, and focused their discussions on a proposed "new international economic order." As a result, the discussion devolved to an entrenched North/South dialogue with cold war undertones, and little was accomplished in terms of productive population policy (21).

The second conference, held in Mexico City in 1984, witnessed a surprising reversal of roles since Bucharest (22). Many southern nations had severe economic problems and were in the midst of strenuous "Situation Adjustment" programs mandated by the World Bank. Under these conditions, the consequences of high birthrates and young age structures were distressingly apparent. By 1984, these nations generally had already initiated (or were prepared to initiate) directed family planning programs.

Meanwhile, the Reagan Administration had completely changed the United States' position. Its official statement to the conference declared that "The relationship between population growth and economic development is not necessarily a negative one... . . population control programs alone cannot substitute for the economic reforms that put a society on the road toward growth and, as an after effect, toward slower population increase as well." In addition, the United States, allied with the Vatican, had adopted a strict antiabortion stance, which later resulted in the "Mexico City" clause prohibiting USAID funding support for any NGO programs that provided or referred for abortions. As in Bucharest, but now for very different reasons, there was much conflict between the US and the less developed nations.

By 1994, however, this dramatic ideological schism had all but disappeared. Since 1984, many LDCs had adopted directed population policies, some with stated demographic targets (59); fully 82% of all member states provided family planning services as a matter of course in public health care systems. The estimated contraceptive prevalence rate in the developing world had grown from less than 9% in 1960–1965 to 50% by 1990 (74). Moreover, by 1994, 61% of countries in less developed regions considered their population growth rates to be too high (63).

Meanwhile, the Clinton Administration, elected in 1992, had once again altered the United States' population policies, this time in full support of family planning programs and with recognition of the importance of safe abortion services. The "Mexico City" clause and several domestic regulations were overturned by the President in his first week in office. The US statement at the third PrepCom declared that "a determined cooperative effort must be launched to make good quality voluntary family planning and the full range of reproductive health services universally available.....(and) in the interest of public health and as a matter of principle, women should have access to safe abortion services and to humane services for complications due to unsafe abortions" (68). President Clinton was quoted as suggesting that abortion should be safe, legal, and rare (68).

This ideological congruence between most of the more and less developed nations set the stage for unprecedented cooperation at the 1994 ICPD. Although economic issues were generally recognized as crucial to any development effort, the focus on population and reproductive health was not significantly diluted by economic-based debates. Instead, the major points of contention were on approaches to population issues themselves. Specifically, the disputed text of the draft Programme of Action focused on six issues: reproductive freedom and the wide availability of family planning methods without coercion, access to reproductive health services, the right to reproductive and sexual health, adolescent sexual health, human reproductive rights, and voluntary choice (1). Also, for the first time, high priority was given to the empowerment of women and gender equity.

The debates on reproductive health were drawn mainly along religious lines, since the most vocal opponents to the Programme were the Holy See, a handful of mostly Catholic states, and several Islamic nations. In particular, the Holy See took issue with the use of the phrases "family planning," "unsafe abortion," "safe motherhood," "reproductive health," "reproductive rights," and "sexual health," as well as references to confidentiality of adolescent services, increased condom distribution for HIV prevention, and the "various concepts of the family," all of which the Holy See viewed as virtual endorsements of abortion services on demand and homosexual activity. In the end, however, even the Vatican managed to sign on to the Programme of Action, and only the Vatican and 16 countries formally registered objections to particular chapters of the document, mostly on reproductive health issues (11).

Major Innovations of the Programme

In terms of reproductive issues, this Programme of Action is remarkable on three overarching points. First, it places the primary emphasis on women as responsible agents of change who are deserving of full reproductive health and reproductive rights, empowerment, and equity. Second, it shifts the focus of population policies from broad demographic targets to meeting individual reproductive intentions. Third, it envisions family planning services as only one part of a larger goal of providing comprehensive reproductive health services to individuals. Each of these three points is discussed individually below.

THE ROLE OF WOMEN   In her closing remarks, Nafis Sadik quoted the British journalist Maggie Brown's description of the ICPD: "Where else has the fundamental condition of all women, whatever their status or the state of their personal freedom, been so intensely debated, or seen to be so relevant to the next century?" (55) Clearly, since only women become pregnant and bear children, the crux of the Programme of Action is women, as agents of change, as individuals deserving of reproductive health and rights, and as the ultimate determinants of fertility behavior.

Chapter four of the Programme deals with gender equality. It first recognizes that "The empowerment and autonomy of women and the improvement of their political, social, economic and health status is a highly important end in itself," and goes on to describe the range of power relations and inequities that impede women's progress globally. It further states that "population and development programmes are most effective when steps have simultaneously been taken to improve the status of women" (46, paragraph 4.1). In response to this, the Programme places a significant emphasis on education so as to empower women with the necessary knowledge and skills needed for participation in development and related activities (46).

INDIVIDUAL VS DEMOGRAPHIC FOCUS   At the Bucharest and Mexico City conferences, when the debate addressed population issues, it focused on broad demographic effects. That is, fertility was analyzed on the level of populations rather than individuals, an attitude that led, especially in the 1970s, to population policies in some nations that set specific demographic targets without sufficient consideration of individual fertility intentions. As previously noted, these policies were largely driven by concerns about high population growth rates.

The current view is that populations need not be coerced into lowering their fertility, but that with accessible family planning and reproductive health services, fertility will be lowered as an expression of individual desires. In fact, one study compared unmet need for family planning, as measured by various Demographic and Health Surveys (DHS), with the demographic targets set in several countries. The results show that simply meeting unmet need for family planning among individual women would meet or exceed the stated demographic targets in these countries (59). Thus, programs that respect individual fertility intentions can meet unmet need to space or limit births and can meet demographic targets, without creating an ethically questionable atmosphere of compulsory family planning.

The ICPD was infused with this individualist perspective. While accepting that demographic goals can be a component of governmental development strategies, the Programme states that family planning goals should only be set in terms of unmet needs; targets and quotas, on the other hand, should not be used or imposed on individuals (46). In the section on gender inequality, the Programme recognizes that "improving the status of women also enhances their decision-making capacity at all levels in all spheres of life, especially in the area of sexuality and reproduction. This, in turn, is essential for the long-term success of population programmes" (46, paragraph 4.1). Hence, instead of population programs determining women's behavior, individual women are seen as determining the success of population programs.

REPRODUCTIVE HEALTH SERVICES   The third significant conceptual shift in the Programme of Action is the view that family planning services should not be provided in a vertical program, but as one part of a broad range of reproductive health services. The argument for providing family planning in a reproductive health context largely emerges from the recognition of a complete picture of women's health. For example, the connection between reproductive health and general female morbidity (and mortality, as discussed below) is undeniably clear. A survey of maternal morbidity in five countries found that 70% of the 16,000 subjects reported a health problem related to maternity or chronic conditions arising from pregnancy or childbirth (20). Similarly, there were many women who had contraceptive-related complaints. These results are echoed in regional studies throughout the world. To take one example, a study of two villages in Egypt found that only 15% of the women were free of gynecological and related conditions (79). Data such as these suggest the need to develop programming in broader reproductive health areas, but the

Programme did not answer the serious concerns as to how to find the additional financial support for such activities.

Directed family planning programs can inadvertently exclude large segments of the female population, which is important not only for reasons of equity—a nonsexually active woman may be in need of reproductive health care but excluded from programs focused on family planning—but also for medical reasons. That is, childhood health problems, such as malnutrition resulting in an underdeveloped pelvis, can lead to serious maternal health consequences. In general, it is difficult to draw a clear, workable distinction between sexual health, maternal health, and women's health (56). This all argues for an integrated approach that includes all these reproductive health issues (for further discussion, see 17).

In light of these arguments, the Programme contains a remarkable definition of reproductive health that recognizes the vast social and medical consequences of women's reproductive behavior:

> Reproductive health is a state of complete physical, mental, and social well-being and not merely the absence of disease or infirmity, in all matters relating to the reproductive system and to its functions and processes. Reproductive health therefore implies that people are able to have a satisfying and safe sex life and that they have the capability to reproduce and the freedom to decide if, when, and how to do so......In line with the above definition of reproductive health, reproductive health care is defined as the constellation of methods, techniques, and services that contribute to reproductive health and well-being through preventing and solving reproductive health problems. It also includes sexual health, the purpose of which is the enhancement of life and personal relations, and not merely counseling and care related to reproduction and sexually transmitted diseases (paragraph 7.2).

This broad definition of reproductive health constitutes a major conceptual advance, but the ICPD did not solve the serious logistical and financial problems associated with providing such comprehensive care. Many countries have remarkably limited health budgets (53) as well as significant unmet need for contraceptive services, as measured by the DHS (67). In these constrained contexts, difficult priority decisions must be made about which reproductive health services to provide. At Cairo, a priority was given to access to contraceptive services, and it was recommended that significant fiscal resources be allocated to these services (see Access to Contraceptive Services, below).

The ICPD Process

In addition to these conceptual innovations reflected in the Programme, the ICPD achieved several procedural milestones. First, the role of NGOs, as mentioned above, cannot be overestimated. The formal delegations of many countries included NGO representatives in addition to governmental officers--half of the United States delegation of 43 was from the nongovernmental sector. Moreover, the role of women's NGOs was particularly strong. The women's caucus at the NGO Forum exerted tremendous influence over the wording of the final Programme. Most important, however, was the attendance of thousands of women representatives of NGOs from every region of the world, and the inclusion of their voices in the process. One expected result of this focus on women is that some percentage of donor money for reproductive health will probably shift from governmental programs to local women's NGOs (13).

Second, the role of the Holy See and fundamentalism in general was highlighted in Cairo. The Vatican, from the start of the PrepComs, strongly opposed the reproductive health agenda, a stance that was strengthened by the growing world consensus around family planning and abortion. This was a posture the Holy See did not face in the first two conferences. At first, the Vatican was allied with several Islamic states against the Programme due to the issues of abortion and homosexuality, and Saudi Arabia, Sudan, Iraq, and Lebanon eventually boycotted the conference over these issues. The Vatican's strong stance, fueled by fundamentalism, particularly in Egypt, led to much tension at the Conference and also generated an unofficial debate about the appropriateness of the Holy See's status as an official observer to the United Nations, which is granted to no other religion.

The most obvious result of the Vatican's activities was the abortion debate, the longest, most intractable discussion at the ICPD, one that generated by far the most press coverage. The fact that the public health consequences of unsafe abortion were recognized at all at such a large international forum was a point of celebration for many delegates and particularly women's NGOs; this issue had not been fully and openly addressed in previous conferences (12). But the Vatican took issue with every instance of the phrase "unsafe abortion" in the Programme because it implied the existence of "safe abortion," which the Vatican does not feel exists (from the perspective of the fetus). After three days of stubborn debate, the Holy See finally abandoned its campaign, claiming that it did not wish to "prolong the present discussion" (12). The Vatican was partially appeased by the inclusion of the statement that "Abortion is in no case a form of family planning" (46, paragraph 8.25). At that point, the Vatican agreed to remove the brackets around "family planning," which until then it had felt included abortion (see the discussion of unsafe abortion, below).

SIX ISSUES IN WOMEN'S REPRODUCTIVE HEALTH

The ICPD was an extraordinary forum for the discussion of global reproductive health issues. Imbued with importance by the sheer number of participants as well as by the large number of senior governmental officials, the conference covered a vast array of reproductive health topics. Of these, six major concerns—gender inequality, access to contraceptive services, sexually transmitted diseases (including HIV/AIDS), maternal mortality, unsafe abortion, and adolescent pregnancy—are addressed here. Isolating each of these issues is difficult because, as discussed above, almost all aspects of women's reproductive health are inseparably intertwined. The issues presented below are all intricately linked along biological and social lines, and should be considered not as isolated concerns but as different facets of the same challenge.

Gender Inequality

Perhaps the most powerful adverse determinant of women's overall reproductive health—as well as the most historically overlooked—is gender inequality. Nafis Sadik wrote that "Women's educational attainment, work patterns, income levels, access to and control of resources and social roles—all have considerable impact on their health and the well-being of their children, in general, and on their reproductive health, practice of family planning and involvement in fertility decisions, in particular" (54).

One of the most important gender inequalities, as recognized in the Programme of Action, is education levels. Literacy rates, which are fairly strong predictors of infant mortality rates and other health indices (72, 74), are frequently lower for women than for men in less developed settings (29). Educated women are also more likely to have some measure of control over household roles and fertility decisions (9). (Education also strongly interacts with adolescent fertility—see below.)

Violence against women is another strong adverse determinant of reproductive health, and occurs in all societies and classes, virtually without exception (7, 16, 26, 27, 40). Within the household, untold morbidity is caused by battery from husbands or partners, and the simple threat of battery often maintains the decision-making inequities in a household. Women who cannot deny their partners intercourse or decide to use contraception on their own are virtually powerless to prevent conception and exposure to sexually transmitted diseases. The practice of female genital mutilation, which the World Health Organization estimates has been carried out on 85 to 114 million women worldwide (62), is another important expression of gender-specific violence that has severe reproductive health consequences for women (27).

Finally, economic inequities have a broad impact on women's health. "Women's work," namely child rearing, household upkeep, and often agricultural labor, is almost universally undervalued as a contribution to the national economy. The resulting poverty leads to less access to health care and education, and can force women into prostitution, which carries obvious reproductive and mental health risks.

Conversely, access to financial resources can positively impact women's reproductive health, as demonstrated by the Grameen Bank in Bangladesh, a credit agency established in 1976 that makes small loans to women in rural areas. The loans are mainly used for small scale income-generating activities such as processing paddies, keeping livestock, or selling crafts, and the repayment rates are generally excellent. Women who participate in this program generally increase their mobility, financial resources, and standing in their families, all of which has been shown to have a strong positive effect on contraceptive use (57).

With its emphasis on women, the Programme of Action was designed to recognize these issues as strongly as possible, and it dedicates an entire chapter to this topic. It directly recognizes, in Principle 4, that "advancing gender equality and equity and the empowerment of women, the elimination of all kinds of violence against women, and ensuring women's ability to control their own fertility, are cornerstones of population and development-related programmes."

It is certainly a positive development that the intimate connection between gender inequality and population growth has been established on a prominent international stage. However, these issues of gender relations are some of the most intractable in every society, and this is by no means the first international document to recommend gender equality. In fact, it is precisely because unequal gender relations are such a fundamental underpinning of society that they so strongly impair reproductive health and behavior and that they are so difficult to change. Probably for this reason, the recommendations in this section of the Programme of Action appear the least specific and most rhetorical of all.

Access to Contraceptive Services

Contraceptive services are often inaccessible to couples due to financial constraints, physical distance from outlets, legal barriers, or psycho-social unacceptability of methods. There has certainly been a dramatic increase in access to and use of contraception since the 1960s, when family planning programs were first developed. During these years, clinic-based programming was supplemented by the use of auxiliary personnel to distribute contraceptives, coupled with creative village-based social marketing programs, such as those organized by PSI and other organizations. Despite these dramatic changes in prevalence of contraceptive use, DHS surveys have revealed that currently as many as 100 million women worldwide do not desire any more children, yet are not practicing effective contraception with their partners (67). This situation is exaggerated by the increasing number of young women entering reproductive age each year. Thus there is still much to be done to meet the stated needs of women in this area.

The delegates at the ICPD generally agreed that women and men should have ready access to contraceptive services as a particularly crucial part of the larger reproductive health agenda. As a result of this concern, the Programme of Action recommends that by the year 2000, $17 billion (in 1993 US dollars) be allocated to family planning, increasing to $21.7 billion in 2015. These figures constitute 60% of the total budget for the reproductive health agenda, a fact that generated considerable debate from some governments that felt other components of the agenda warranted more attention. Discussions at the conference generated agreement that further study was necessary to be able to estimate more accurately the costs of the other components of the Programme.

Sexually Transmitted Diseases (Including HIV/AIDS)

Sexually transmitted diseases (STDs) include chlamydia, gonorrhea, trichomoniasis, syphilis, and human papilloma virus (HPV), as well as HIV/AIDS, which is often addressed separately due to the gravity of the epidemic.

PREVALENCE OF STDS   Leaving aside HIV for the moment, it is difficult to get an exact estimate of the general prevalence of STDs, especially in asymptomatic populations. One review of 13 STD prevalence studies in less developed countries found that among high-risk groups, the prevalence was as high as 50% for gonorrhea, 12% for chancroid, 23% for syphilis, 25% for chlamydia, and 20% for trichomoniasis. A review of 19 surveys among low-risk groups in less developed countries (mainly antenatal patients) showed that with the exception of gonorrhea, these rates were not much lower (6). In 1990, the most prevalent STDs in industrialized countries were human papilloma virus (HPV or genital warts) and chlamydia. Genital herpes is also an important and common problem (14).

As for HIV, paragraph 8.28 of the Programme of Action contains a concise summary of recent statistics: "WHO estimates that the cumulative number of AIDS cases in the world amounted to 2.5 million persons by mid-1993 and that more than 14 million people had been infected with HIV since the pandemic began, a number that is projected to rise to between 30 million and 40 million by the end of the decade, if effective prevention strategies are not pursued. As of mid-1993, about four-fifths of all persons ever infected with HIV lived in developing countries where the infection was being transmitted mainly through heterosexual intercourse and the number of new cases was rising most rapidly among women."

DETERMINANTS OF STD PREVALENCE   The impact of STDs on women arises from both biological and social factors. Generally, STDs have two biological characteristics that put women at a particular disadvantage: First, the risk of transmission from a man to a woman during vaginal intercourse is generally much higher than the reverse; and, second, symptoms tend to be less apparent in women, so they are not recognized until later in the course of the disease.

Several social factors exacerbate this situation. The generally low status of women in many developing contexts decreases their ability to obtain knowledge about their own symptoms or to seek health care when necessary (66). Commonly, a general reluctance to speak openly about sexual matters, even among health care personnel, further inhibits proper health care, particularly among women (31). As discussed above, social, familial, or economic dependence on partners, as well as the threat of violence, decreases a woman's ability to refuse intercourse or protect herself from STDs (2, 25). In addition, in many parts of Africa, preference for intercourse with a "dry, tight" vagina leads women to insert drying substances in themselves, which causes skin irritation and probably increases vulnerability to STDs (5). The inequitable effects of poverty among women, in combination with male demand for commercial sex, generates a population of commercial sex workers who are among the highest risk groups in the world, and are mainly women.

Societal attitudes toward male sexual behavior also aggravates women's susceptibility. Polygamy, acceptance of male infidelity, and male license to patronize commercial sex workers all generally increase women's exposure to STDs. In addition, strong social stigmas against seeking STD treatment keep both men and women from effective health care. In some settings, however, there is no social stigma around STDs for men, and they are accepted as a rite of passage (3).

HEALTH EFFECTS OF STDS   The health effects of STDs among women, especially in the developing world, are severe. One of the most common complications of STDs is acute and chronic pelvic inflammatory disease (PID). The risk may be increased when the cervix, a natural barrier between the upper and lower genital tracts, is breached due to IUD insertion, abortion, or childbirth. Among the complications of PID are chronic pelvic pain, recurrent infection, tuboovarian abscesses, ectopic pregnancy (which contributes substantially to maternal mortality rates), and death. PID also leads to infertility: About 25% of PID cases become sterile, an occurrence that often has drastic social and economic consequences for women. PID prevalence is difficult to determine, but some information can be gained from hospital admission data. In India, 3–10% of gynecological hospital admissions are estimated to be women with complications of acute PID, in Southeast Asia this figure is 15–37%, and in Africa it is 17–40% (39, 66).

STD infection can also lead to poor pregnancy outcomes in the form of spontaneous abortion, stillbirth, low birth weight, and congenital or perinatal infection (66). A series of studies in Nairobi have shown that STDs determine fetal and maternal morbidity rates, and are expressed among the infants most commonly as blindness, chlamydial pneumonia, premature birth, stillbirth, and congenital syphilis, and among the mothers as postpartum pelvic infection and ensuing infertility (6).

Moreover, HPV is a suspected causal agent of cervical cancer, the most common form of cancer among women in developing countries. This form of cancer is almost always fatal if not found and treated early, and it strikes in a younger cohort than most cancers (under 50), so it kills women in their more productive years. Of the incident cases of cervical cancer, 77% occur in developing regions, but screening and treatment facilities, which are effective and taken for granted in developing countries, are costly and quite rare in developing countries (66). And, while it is feasible in some countries to establish a Pap smear screening program, these are of little help if the clinical services are not available to manage the positive results of such a screening program.

Finally, not least among the consequences of STDs is increased susceptibility to HIV infection (64, 65). This may also work in reverse, in that HIV infection possibly "prolongs or augments the infectiousness of individuals with STDs" (66).

INTERACTION WITH FAMILY PLANNING   Various family planning methods alter a woman's risk of STD infection. Condoms, diaphragms, and spermicide generally offer some protection against STDs in that they provide a physical or chemical barrier against biological materials; of these, condoms clearly offer the strongest protection. Despite some misconceptions, IUDs themselves are not associated with higher STD rates, but among women whose sexual practices place them at increased risk of STDs, the IUD can increase the risk of acute PID when an STD develops. Hormonal methods do not protect against STDs, nor are they responsible for an increase in risk. While the mechanism is still not entirely understood, however, these hormonal methods do appear to protect against acute PID (42). Thus, unfortunately, the family planning methods that provide the best protection against pregnancy are the least effective against STDs, and vice versa. STD symptoms are at times mistaken for side effects of family planning, creating a motive to discontinue family planning use, as well as a disincentive to seek STD care (8).

THE PROGRAMME OF ACTION AND STDs   The Programme's chapter on reproductive rights and health includes a section on STDs and HIV/AIDS that gives full recognition to the particular vulnerabilities faced by women in this arena.

One important recommendation is the inclusion of STD and HIV/AIDS services in all reproductive and sexual health services. This point has been contested by various groups because many societies have a strong stigma against seeking STD care, so its integration with other kinds of health care could deter clients. However, the immense morbidity associated with STDs as well as the fatality of the HIV/AIDS epidemic weigh heavily against this argument, and the recommendation for integration of services stands (46, paragraph 7.32). Condoms are also strongly recommended for inclusion in all reproductive health services, and the World Health Organization and UNICEF are urged to increase their procurement (46, paragraph 7.33). Again, this is a strong recognition of the importance of STD protection to all reproductive health clients, and was recommended over the vociferous objections of the Vatican.

The health impact of these recommendations is bound to be positive, but the financial impact is troubling. Many states simply cannot afford to launch national STD screening and treatment programs, particularly for HIV/AIDS, which is exceedingly expensive to treat. To make matters worse, some strains of STD pathogens are becoming resistant to treatment, thereby requiring newer and costlier medicines (75). Moreover, because contraceptive services were given priority in the Programme of Action, only about 8% of the Programme's reproductive health budget is allocated to STD/HIV/AIDS services. Of course, the provision of condoms is an important component of both contraceptive and STD programs.

Maternal Mortality

The magnitude of maternal mortality in the developing world is overwhelming. Almost half a million women are estimated to die as a result of pregnancy-related complications every year, and 99% of those deaths occur in developing countries (70). The disparity in maternal mortality ratios (number of deaths per 100,000 live births)[1] between less and more developed countries is the largest of any health indicator, including infant mortality rates, which are often used as a proxy for general health status (78).

Maternal mortality ratios in more developed countries range between 8 and 25 deaths per 100,000 live births, whereas for developing countries the ratio varies between 100 and 1000 deaths per 100,000 live births (50). The lifetime maternal mortality risk of a woman in North America is 1 in 4000, whereas in Western Africa the risk is 1 in 18 (71). A look at the causes of maternal mortality reveals the reason behind this massive disparity.

The five major causes of maternal deaths are obstructed labor and ruptured uterus, postpartum hemorrhage, hypertensive disease of pregnancy (toxemia)

[1]Maternal mortality rates are the number of deaths per 100,000 women.

leading to eclampsia (or convulsions), postpartum infection, and complications of a botched unsafe abortion (51). The percentage for each varies in different societies, but hemorrhage and abortion complications are often the most common causes.

In the less developed nations, several specific conditions contribute to these high maternal mortality ratios. First, developing areas with high fertility rates tend to have young age structures and a young average age at first birth; two well-established characteristics of maternal mortality are that it strikes young women and high parity women. For example, a study in Matlab, Bangladesh, found that girls aged 10 to 14 have five times the risk of women 20 to 24 years old, and girls 15 to 19 have twice the risk of the older cohort. Interestingly, this relationship persists across several more and less developed countries. Moreover, regardless of age, the second and third births tend to be the safest, with increasing risk thereafter. Maternal mortality strikes high-fertility countries so forcefully not only because women are exposed to the risks of childbirth more often, but also because they are exposed to a higher risk more often (78).

Second, the endemic levels of various infectious diseases can be quite high, with serious consequences for pregnant women. For reasons that are not quite understood, childhood resistance to malaria begins to break down around the fourteenth week of pregnancy, which can contribute to maternal mortality. Similarly, viral hepatitis appears to strike pregnant women more often than other women in high endemic areas, possibly as a result of poor nutrition. Third, girls in developing countries often suffer from poor nutrition, which may result in underdeveloped pelvic bones. This, in turn, can lead directly to obstructed labor, one of the major causes of maternal mortality (78).

More important than these factors, however, are the low levels of family planning use and the general lack of emergency obstetric care in developing countries. Family planning and emergency obstetric care have been identified as two of the most effective means of reducing maternal mortality (23, 51).

Family planning reduces maternal mortality in two ways. First, family planning averts pregnancies, thereby removing women from the risks of the puerperium. Data from DHS studies have shown as many as 100 million women stating that they do not wish more children than they already have, but are not currently using any form of contraception. One analysis showed that if all this unmet need for family planning were met, total births would be reduced by about 35% in Latin America, 33% in Asia, and 17% in Africa. The maternal mortality ratios would be reduced by even larger amounts since the averted births would tend to be high parity/high risk (37).

The second major effect of these averted pregnancies would be a reduction in unsafe abortions. Worldwide, unsafe abortions are estimated to account for 25 to 33% of maternal mortality (30). This figure has been estimated as 20% in India (58), and as high as 50% in Latin America (35), Sub-Saharan Africa

(49), and Albania (48). In general, the demographic results of restrictive abortion laws are expressed in higher maternal mortality, and not in a decline in total abortions (28). Clearly, maternal mortality would be substantially reduced if these abortions could be averted (See "Unsafe Abortion," below).

Family planning is the best response to unwanted fertility in a population. Once pregnant, however, emergency obstetric care is essential to the management of the five major causes of maternal mortality. A look at the five most common causes of maternal mortality listed above reveals that most can be treated with well-established, fairly simple procedures: caesarean section, blood transfusion, IV antibiotics, or vacuum aspiration. Moreover, these procedures need not be performed only by a physician, but can be safely provided by well-trained nurses or midwives (51). Because most obstetric emergencies do not cause death immediately (but within a matter of hours or days), and because it would be an impossible challenge to the health budgets of developing countries, these services need not be located in every village, but rather at appropriately spaced district or regional locations. They would have to be staffed 24 h per day, and would rely on a well-trained referral network involving local traditional birth attendants and midwives (23, 60).

That such a system would reduce maternal mortality is apparent from several observations. First, it is remarkably difficult to predict which pregnancies will lead to major complications. There are certainly groups of women who are at higher risk than others (young, hypertensive, or high parity women, for example), but these rough screening measures have poor predictive values. The only way to adequately cover all the complicated births that will arise in a population is to assure access to emergency obstetric care to everyone (23, 51).

Furthermore, the fact that in all socioeconomic contexts maternal mortality is lower in urban areas than rural areas (78) reflects the higher availability of emergency care in cities. On a larger scale, the enormous discrepancy in maternal mortality between the more and less developed regions of the world is due more to the accessibility of this kind of care in industrialized settings than to differences in the risk factors listed above (51).

Interestingly, this quality of maternal mortality—that it responds most dramatically to emergency obstetric care—sharply differentiates it from most other reproductive health concerns. On a population level, many health indicators (such as STD prevalence, infant mortality rates, and child survival) are affected by broad-based and diffuse improvements in health, through primary health care campaigns at village level, for example, or improvements in nutrition. Maternal mortality, on the other hand, does not strongly respond to these kinds of interventions, nor is it directly correlated to literacy rates, employment status, or other socioeconomic measures. Rather, among those women who conceive and give birth, access to emergency obstetric care is a strong determinant of maternal mortality (23).

The ICPD Programme of Action sets specific targets for maternal mortality. Countries should reduce their maternal mortality ratios "by one half of the 1990 levels by the year 2000 and a further one half by 2015." In addition, no country should have a maternal mortality ratio above 75 per 100,000 live births by the year 2015 (46, paragraph 8.21).

The Programme takes a broad approach in its recommendations for actions to reduce maternal mortality. Health systems "should include education on safe motherhood, prenatal care that is focused and effective, maternal nutrition programmes, adequate delivery assistance that avoids excessive recourse to caesarean sections and provides for obstetric emergencies; referral services for pregnancy, childbirth and abortion complications; post-natal care and family planning" (46, paragraph 8.22). However, improving access to emergency obstetrical care is only the first step. Providing all the other components without such an emergency system in place will do little to reduce maternal mortality ratios.

Unsafe Abortion

Abortion is perhaps the single most controversial issue in society today, yet the World Health Organization estimates that 25% of all pregnancies end in abortion, for a total of about 45 million abortions per year (73). Most serious, however, is the fact that an estimated 20 million of these abortions are performed under unsafe and septic conditions, 88% of which occur in the developing world (73).

The health consequences of unsafe abortion are drastic. Anywhere from 50,000 to 100,000 deaths result from these abortions every year (73), and untold morbidity is caused, in the form of sepsis, hemorrhage, uterine perforation, cervical trauma, pelvic peritonitis, pelvic abscess, jaundice, septicemia, and an almost endless litany of less dire conditions. The long-term sequelae can include chronic pelvic pain, PID, tubal occlusion, infertility, and eventual hysterectomy (10, 73) and, as noted above, further degradation of the status of women.

In contrast, first trimester abortion performed under aseptic, skilled conditions is a remarkably safe procedure, far safer than childbirth. In the United States, the death rate for legal abortions is 0.6 per 100,000 procedures, similar to a penicillin injection. Illegal abortions in less developed countries have estimated mortality risks of between 100 to 1000 per 100,000 procedures (63).

One of the largest determinants of the mortality associated with abortion is its legal status. Abortion remains illegal in many nations, and its legality is increasingly threatened in others (32). A survey of abortion policies in 186 countries showed that, in general, the less developed nations are the most restrictive; as of 1993, in 50 countries abortion was either completely banned or allowed only to save the life of the woman (63).

That abortion is least safe in the developing world interacts poorly with the demographic profile of those regions. Measured between 1980–85 and 1985–90, the worldwide TFR displayed an overall decline, and the TFR in all developing areas was stagnant or declining (with the exception of East Africa). Moreover, desired fertility—as measured by the DHS—is declining even faster, which portends further fertility decline (63). Already, abortion is estimated to account for 10 to 20% of deliberate fertility regulation in Africa and 25% of fertility regulation in Latin America (24). If these regions maintain their restrictive abortion policies in the face of a general decline in desired fertility, the negative consequences of unsafe abortions will only become more prevalent.

The abortion situation in Central and Eastern Europe is particularly noteworthy. Since the breakup of the Soviet Union at the turn of the decade, demographic and health data from this region has become increasingly available. Central and Eastern European countries have maintained posttransition fertility rates for decades, but it was not clear until recently that this fertility control was heavily based on abortion. In fact, 60% of all fertility regulation in the region is estimated to be due to abortion (24). A recent survey in St. Petersburg revealed that women over 25 have had an average of three abortions. Only 14% of the sample of 650 women had never had an abortion, and a "small minority" had over 20 procedures. Thirty-two percent had self-aborted (15).

Thus, the health consequences of unsafe abortion are seen to a greater or lesser extent worldwide. These effects may be mitigated in part, however, if the anti-progestin, RU-486, becomes widely available. The drug, a nonsurgical abortifacient, has been available in France and the UK for several years, and after years of pressure its manufacturer, Roussel-Uclaf, has recently given toxicological and chemical data to the FDA and the rights to the drug to the Population Council. RU-486 may be approved for use in the United States by 1996 (51).

RU-486 does not require surgical equipment, so it avoids the risk of sepsis and of most sequelae of unsafe abortion listed above, and it is not as dependent on the skill of medical personnel. However, RU-486 could only be used in states that already have legal abortion, such as India, China, Vietnam, Togo, and Zambia (36). Moreover, the clinical trials of RU-486 were run on relatively healthy populations; it is not clear what effectiveness or side effects the drug displays among anemic or malnourished women (36, 52). However, RU-486 is a promising intervention to help alleviate the effects of unsafe abortion, especially if China or India produce and make available this drug.

To return to the Programme of Action, the paragraph addressing abortion contains the most debated language in the document. The entire text of paragraph 8.25 reads as follows:

> In no case should abortion be promoted as a method of family planning. All Governments and relevant intergovernmental and non-governmental organizations are urged to strengthen their commitment to women's health, to deal with the health impact of unsafe abortion[2] as a major public health concern and to reduce the recourse to abortion through expanded and improved family planning services. Prevention of unwanted pregnancies must always be given the highest priority and all attempts should be made to eliminate the need for abortion. Women who have unwanted pregnancies should have ready access to reliable information and compassionate counseling. Any measures or changes related to abortion within the health system can only be determined at the national or local level according to the national legislative process. In circumstances in which abortion is not against the law, such abortion should be safe. In all cases women should have access to quality services for the management of complications arising from abortion. Post-abortion counselling, education and family planning services should be offered promptly, which will also help to avoid repeat abortions.

Given the grave effects of unsafe abortion, the language of paragraph 8.25 is a relatively weak response. However, to recognize abortion as a major public health concern and to recommend services for the sequelae of abortion regardless of its legal status constitute significant steps forward from previous conferences.

Adolescent Pregnancy

Adolescent pregnancy, whether it occurs within or outside the bounds of a socially sanctioned relationship, has tremendous physical and social consequences for the woman, in many cases more so than adult pregnancy. Early childbearing is associated with high fertility over the entire lifespan (18, 76), and some evidence suggests that the earlier the first birth, the shorter the ensuing birth intervals (76). In all economic settings, adolescent mothers have consistently higher maternal and infant mortality rates because their access to care is often limited, and because for younger adolescents (less than 15 years of age) their pelvic bones may not be fully developed, which can lead to obstructed labor.

Adolescents are seeking abortion in rising numbers around the world, although the abortion rate for older teenagers (17–19) has stabilized in more developed countries. These young women are at particular risk for unsafe abortions, since many medical systems will not give reproductive health care

---

[2]Unsafe abortion is defined as a procedure for terminating an unwanted pregnancy either by persons lacking the necessary skills or in an environment lacking the minimal medical standards or both (World Health Organization, WHO/MSM/92.5).

to unmarried women, and adolescents in general tend to seek health care later than adults, leading to later-term abortions (61).

Adolescent pregnancy can take place within or outside a formal union. For those countries with young average age at first marriage, adolescent pregnancy is a sanctioned, even encouraged, process. This is particularly marked in India, where about 13 million girls under 18 are married (43), and the births associated with these young women are especially plagued by low birth weight and high maternal and infant mortality (34). In general, women under twenty are less likely than their older counterparts to seek prenatal care when it is available, and are less equipped to recognize the normal or abnormal signs of pregnancy (76).

Adolescents who give birth within a marriage usually enjoy emotional and economic support from their society; the other face of adolescent pregnancy is that outside of a sanctioned relationship. Nonetheless, sexual activity before marriage is common worldwide and for both married and unmarried adolescents, contraceptive use is quite low (33, 47, 76). Combined with a declining age at menarche in many areas (4) and, frequently, a lack of sexual education or family planning knowledge, this low level of contraceptive use leads to a high risk of adolescent pregnancy outside of marriage.

One of the most telling social aspects of adolescent pregnancy is its effect on school enrollment. Childbearing and education are often seen as mutually exclusive activities: If an adolescent bears a child, she usually cancels or defers her education, which leads to fewer employment opportunities and an increased risk of poverty (69). Conversely, women who continue with their education have later and more widely spaced births (18, 76).

However, increased education levels, along with increased urbanization, are often connected to modern (or Westernized) attitudes. In Sub-Saharan Africa in particular, the transition from traditional to modern cultures is having a significantly detrimental effect on adolescent fertility (4, 19). In most traditional societies, a girl would be protected by her family until her marriage, which would often take place early. As the general level of education is rising, however, adolescents are resisting early marriage, but girls in these societies are still expected to maintain their virginity until the end of their schooling. Meanwhile, the age at first intercourse is declining in some regions, echoing the industrialized nations.

Despite this range of strong societal reactions to adolescent fertility, policy makers the world over have a long history of ignoring the issue of adolescent sexuality (33, 38, 76). Thus again, the fact that this issue was openly addressed at ICPD and recognized for its public health consequences, both within and outside marriage, is a remarkable achievement. The Programme of Action states that "information and services should be made available to adolescents that can help them understand their sexuality and protect them from unwanted pregnancies, sexually transmitted diseases and subsequent risk of infertility" (46, paragraph 7.41).

CONCLUSION

The 1994 International Conference on Population and Development was of great significance as it dealt with issues of enormous importance and complexity. The topics it addressed are some of the most intractable and controversial in the world, yet overall the event enjoyed an unprecedented level of international consensus. In the field of reproductive health, the discussion at the ICPD was notable for its openness on matters that have been historically overlooked at public conferences, particularly equity for women, unsafe abortion, and adolescent sexuality. The ICPD also was marked by the significant input of women, and by ample collaboration between governments and nongovernmental organizations, to a far larger extent than at previous conferences.

The Programme of Action is the tangible result of these proceedings. It is most notable for its recognition of the pivotal role of women in population programs, and dedicates an entire chapter to broad gender issues. Indeed, the social structures that enforce unequal division of resources among men and women—as reflected in education levels, violence against women, and economic inequities—have potent consequences for reproductive health.

The Programme also addresses the specifics of the other five pressing reproductive health issues discussed here. It places a priority on improving access to contraceptive services in light of the unmet need for contraception worldwide, estimated at 100 million or more women in developing countries alone. The urgency of other issues—STDs including HIV/AIDS, maternal mortality, unsafe abortion, and adolescent pregnancy—also is reflected in the Programme. Taken together, these four reproductive health crises result in high rates of morbidity and mortality in the world today, most of which is avoidable.

The Programme's major drawback is that it is simply a document; its actual effect ultimately depends on governments' political and financial will. Because the United States is the single largest donor to international population programs (11), its political climate influences the strength of many programs throughout the world. The elections of November 1994 deeply altered the makeup of the Congress, which now stands at the brink of reversing the government's supportive stance on population issues and abortion. Moreover, on the eve of the United Nations Conference on Women in Beijing, the Vatican has returned to its aggressive posture and seems intent on reversing the advances gained in Cairo. Finally, the Programme's recommendations require a tremendous financial commitment, which some nations may be unwilling or unable to fulfill.

Ultimately, the Programme stands as a mirror of the most pressing population issues of the decade and the attendant international consensus. It undoubtedly reflects those issues with more accuracy and potential than any other comparable document, and in that sense the ICPD was indeed "outstandingly successful."

Literature Cited

1. Aslam A. 1994. The Cairo Programme of Action. *Populi* 21(5):8–10
2. Awusabo-Asare K, Anarfi J, Agyeman D. 1993. Women's control over their sexuality and the spread of STDs and HIV/AIDS in Ghana. *Health Transition Rev.* 3:69–84 (Suppl.)
3. Bassett M, Mhloyi M. 1993. AIDS and sexually transmitted diseases: an important connection. In *Women and HIV/AIDS: An International Resource Book*, ed. M Berer, S Ray. London: Pandora. 383 pp.
4. Bledsoe C, Cohen B. 1993. *Social Dynamics of Adolescent Fertility in Sub-Saharan Africa, Population Dynamics in Sub-Saharan Africa Series*. Washington: Natl. Acad. Press. 208 pp.
5. Brown R, Brown J, Ayowa O. 1993. The use and physical effects of intravaginal substances in Zairan women. *Sex. Transm. Dis.* 20:96–99
6. Brunham R, Embree J. 1992. Sexually transmitted diseases: current and future dimensions of the problem in the third world. See Ref. 24a, pp. 35–58
7. Carrillo R. 1992. Battered dreams: gender, violence, and development. *Populi* 19:7–9
8. Cates W, Stone K. 1992. Family Planning: The Responsibility to Prevent Both Pregnancy and Reproductive Tract Infections. See Ref. 24a, pp.93–129
9. Chowdhury KP. 1992. *Education, work, and women's lives: does education provide women with power and autonomy?* Ann Arbor: Univ. Microfilms Int. 307 pp.
10. Coeytaux F. 1990. *Abortion, sexually transmitted diseases, and infertility: Reproductive health problems family planning programs can no longer ignore.* Presented at Natl. Counc. Int. Health Conf., 17th, Arlington, VA
11. Cohen SA, Richards CL. 1994. The Cairo Consensus: population, develop-ment and women. *Int. Fam. Plan. Perspect.* 4(20):150–55
12. Crossette B. 1994. Vatican drops fight against UN population document. *NY Times,* Sept. 10
13. Crossette B. 1994. Population debate: The premises are changed. *NY Times,* Sept. 14
14. De Schryver A, Meheus A. 1990. Epidemiology of sexually transmitted diseases: the global picture. *Bull. WHO* 68:639–54
15. Dorman S. 1993. More access to contraception? Russian city surveyed. *Popul. Today* 21:5–10
16. El-Bushra J, Piza-Lopez E. 1993. Gender-related violence: its scope and relevance. *Focus Gend.* 1:1–9
17. Eschen A, Whittaker M. 1993. Family planning: a base to build on for women's reproductive health services. See Ref. 31a, pp. 105–31
18. Ferrando D. 1993. Adolescent pregnancy and its implications. In *Int. Popul. Conf., Montreal, 24 Aug.–1 Sept.* Liege, Belgium: Int. Union Sci. Stud. Popul., pp. 353–55
19. Feyisetan B, Pebley AR. 1989. Premarital sexuality in urban Nigeria. *Stud. Fam. Plan.* 20:343–54
20. Finger W. 1994. Maternal morbidities affect tens of millions. *Network* 14:8–11
21. Finkle J, Crane B. 1975. The politics of Bucharest: population, development, and the new international economic order. *Pop. Dev. Rev.* 1:87–114
22. Finkle J, Crane B. 1985. Ideology and Politics at Mexico City: The United States at the 1984 International Conference on Population. *Pop. Dev. Rev.* 11:1–28
23. Freedman L, Maine D. 1993. Women's mortality: a legacy of neglect. See Ref. 31a, pp. 147–70
24. Frejka T. 1993. The role of induced abortion in contemporary fertility regu-

lation: overview. In *Int. Popul. Conf., Montreal, 24 Aug.–1 Sept.*. Liege, Belgium: Int. Union Sci. Stud. Pop. 355 pp.

24a. Germain A, Holmes K, Piot P, Wasserheit J. eds. 1992. *Reproductive Tract Infections: Global Impact and Priorities for Women's Reproductive Health*, New York: Plenum. 395 pp.

25. Goyal R. 1993. AIDS and youth: an Indian perspective. *Development* 2:43–46

26. Heise L. 1993. Gender violence and reproductive choice: freedom close to home. *Populi* 20:7–11

27. Heise L. 1993. Violence against women. See Ref. 31a, pp. 171–95

28. Jacobson J. 1990. The global politics of abortion. *Worldwatch Pap.* 97

29. Jacobson J. 1993. Women's health: the price of poverty. See Ref. 31a, pp. 3–31

30. Ketting E. 1993. Global overview of abortion. *Plan. Parent. Chall.* 1:27–29

31. Ketting E. 1993. A global picture: overview. *Plan. Parent. Chall.* 2:28–30

31a. Koblinsky M, Timyan J, Gay J. 1993. *The Health of Women: A Global Perspective*. Boulder: Westview Press. 291 pp.

32. Kunins H, Rosenfield A. 1991. Abortion: a legal and public health perspective. *Annu. Rev. Public Health* 10: 361–82

33. Koontz SL, Conly SR. 1994. *Youth at risk: meeting the sexual health needs of adolescents*. Popul. Action Int. Washington, DC. 8 pp.

34. Kushwaha KP, Rai AK, Rathi AK, Singh YD, Sirohi R. 1993. Pregnancies in adolescents: fetal, neonatal, and maternal outcomes. *Indian Pediatr.* 30: 501–5

35. Kwast B. 1992. Abortion: its contribution to maternal mortality. *Midwifery* 8:8–11

36. leGrand A. 1992. The abortion pill: a solution for unsafe abortions in developing countries? *Soc. Sci. Med.* 35:767–76

37. Maine D, Rosenfield A, Wallace M, Kimball A, Kwast B, et al. 1987. *Prevention of maternal deaths in developing countries: program options and practical considerations*. Presented at Int. Safe Motherhood Conf. Nairobi. WHO 1528

38. Marques M, Paxman J, Bruce J. 1993. *Gente joven/young people: a dialogue on sexuality with adolescents in Mexico*. Popul. Counc. Qual. No. 5. New York. 28 pp.

39. Meheus A. 1992. Women's Health: importance of reproductive tract infections,

pelvic inflammatory disease and cervical cancer. See Ref. 24a, pp. 61–91

40. O'Connell H. 1993. Editorial. *Focus Gend.* 1:ii–vi

41. Omenn, GS. 1993. Population and environment: core issues for PSR's agenda on peace and security. *PSR Q.* 3:8–11

42. Ory HW, Forrest JD, Lincoln R. 1983. *Making Choices: Evaluating the Health Risks and Benefits of Birth Control Methods*. New York: Alan Guttmacher Inst.

43. Pathak K, Ram F. 1993. Adolescent motherhood: problems and consequences. *J. Fam. Welfare* 39:17–23

44. Population Reference Bureau. 1995. *World Population Data Sheet, 1995*. Washington, DC: Popul. Ref. Bur.

45. ICPD 94. *Newsl. Int. Conf. Pop. Dev.* No. 19

46. Program of Action 1994 Int. Conf. Popul. Dev. 1995. *Pop. Dev. Rev.* 21: 187–213

47. Recio R, Villegas M, Trujillo A, Moran J, Bassol S. 1993. Contraceptive practice and pregnancy in Mexican adolescent mothers. *Br. J. Fam. Plan.* 19:198–200

48. Rich V. 1992. Albania: family planning available. *Lancet* 340(8825):964

49. Rogo K. 1993. Induced abortion in Sub-Saharan Africa. *East Afr. Med. J.* 70: 386–95

50. Rosenfield A. 1989. Maternal mortality in developing countries: an on-going, but neglected "epidemic". *JAMA* 262: 376–79

51. Rosenfield A. 1992. Maternal mortality: community-based interventions. *Int. J. Gynecol. Obstetr.* 38:S17–22 (Suppl.)

52. Rosenfield A. 1993. Mifepristone (RU-486) in the United States: What does the future hold? *N. Engl. J. Med.* 328: 1560–61

53. Ross JA, Mauldin WP, Miller VC. 1993. *Family Planning and Population: A Compendium of Int. Statistics*. New York: Popul. Counc. UN Popul. Fund. 202 pp.

54. Sadik N, ed. 1991. *Population Policies and Programmes: Lessons Learned from Two Decades of Experience*. UN Popul. Fund. New York: New York Univ. Press. 464 pp.

55. Sadik N. 1994. Dr. Sadik: ICPD was a 'Quantam Leap'. *Newsl. Int. Conf. Popul. Develop.* No. 19

56. Sai F, Nassim J. 1989. The need for a reproductive health approach. *Int. J. Gynecol. Obstetr.* 3:103–13 (Suppl.)

57. Schuler SR, Hashemi SM. 1994. Credit programs, women's empowerment, and contraceptive use in rural Bangladesh. *Stud. Fam. Plan.* 25:65–76

58. Shiva M. 1991. Of human rights and women's health. *Health Millions* 17:34–36
59. Sinding SW, Ross JA, Rosenfield AG. 1994. Seeking common ground: unmet need and demographic goals. *Int. Fam. Plan. Perspect.* 20:23–27
60. Thaddeus S, Maine D. 1994. Too far to walk: maternal mortality in context. *Soc. Sci. Med.* 38:1091–110
61. Tietze C, Henshaw S. 1986. *Induced Abortion, A World Review.* New York: Alan Guttmacher Inst. 6th ed.
62. Tradition of Harm. 1994. *Populi* 21:4–5
63. United Nations Dep. Econ. Soc. Inf. Policy Anal., Popul. Div. 1994. *Concise Report on the World Population Situation in 1993.* ST/ESA/SER.A/138. New York: United Nations
64. Wald A, Corey H, Handsfield HH, Holmes KK. 1993. Influence of HIV infection on manifestations and natural history of other sexually transmitted diseases. *Annu. Rev. Public Health* 14:19–42
65. Wasserheit J. 1992. Epidemiological synergy: interrelationships between HIV infection and other sexually transmitted diseases. *Sex. Transm. Disease* 9:61–77
66. Wasserheit J, Holmes K. 1992. Reproductive tract infections: challenges for international health policy, programs, and research. See Ref. 24a, pp. 7–33
67. Westoff CF, Ochoa LH. 1991. Unmet need and the demand for family planning. *Demogr. Health Surv. Comp. Stud. No. 5.* Columbia, MD: Inst. Resource Dev./Macro Int., Inc. 37 pp.
68. Wirth TE. 1994. *Statement of the Honorable Timothy E. Wirth on Behalf of the United States of America.* Int. Conf. Popul. Dev. Prep. Meet., 2nd. Press Release USUN #39-(94). 5 pp.
69. Witwer M. 1993. Poverty risk for families of Chilean teenage mothers determined by woman's education, father's support. *Int. Fam. Plan. Perspect.* 19:75–76
70. World Health Organization. 1986. *Prevention of Maternal Mortality: Report of a World Health Organization Interregional Meeting.* FHE/86.1. Geneva
71. World Health Organization Division of Family Health, Maternal Health and Safe Motherhood Programme. 1991. *Maternal Mortality Ratios and Rates: A Tabulation of Available Information..* Geneva: WHO. 100 pp. 3rd ed.
72. World Health Organization. 1992. *Women's Health: Across Age and Frontier.* Geneva: WHO. 107 pp.
73. World Health Organization Maternal Health and Safe Motherhood Programme, Division of Family Health. 1993. *Abortion: A Tabulation of Available Data on the Frequency and Mortality of Unsafe Abortion, 2nd Edition.* WHO/FHE/MSM/93.13. Geneva: WHO. 114 pp.
74. World Health Organization. 1993. *Implementation of the Global Strategy for Health for All by the Year 2000: Second Evaluation, Eighth Report on the World Health Situation.* Geneva: WHO. 178 pp.
75. World Health Organization. 1993. *Recommendations for the management of sexually transmitted diseases. WHO Advis. Group Meet. Sex. Transm. Dis. Treat., Geneva, 18–19 Feb..* WHO/GPA/STD/93.1. Geneva: WHO
76. World Health Organization. 1993. *The Health of Young People: A Challenge and A Promise.* Geneva: WHO. 106 pp.
77. World Resources Institute. 1994. *World Resources 1994–1995.* Washington DC: World Resourc. Inst. 400 pp.
78. Zahr C, Royston E. 1991. *Maternal Mortality: A Global Factbook.* Geneva: WHO Div. Fam. Health. 598 pp.
79. Zurayk H, Younis N, Khattab H. 1994. Rethinking family planning policy in light of reproductive health research. *Policy Ser. Reprod. Health.* New York: Popul. Counc. 23 pp.

Annu. Rev. Public Health. 1996. 17:383–409

THE ROLE OF MEDICAL EXAMINERS AND CORONERS IN PUBLIC HEALTH SURVEILLANCE AND EPIDEMIOLOGIC RESEARCH[1]

Randy Hanzlick

Emory University School of Medicine, Atlanta, Georgia 30322

R. Gibson Parrish

Surveillance and Programs Branch, Division of Environmental Hazards and Health Effects, National Center for Environmental Health, Centers for Disease Control and Prevention, Atlanta, Georgia 30341

KEY WORDS: death investigation, mortality statistics, autopsy, postmortem examination, cause of death, surveillance, epidemiology

ABSTRACT

The role of medical examiners and coroners (ME/Cs) in public health surveillance and epidemiologic research is reviewed. Definitions are offered, and discussion centers on the advantages of, and obstacles to the use of ME/C data; existing surveillance systems relevant to ME/Cs; studies assessing the usefulness of ME/C data; newly emerging tools for ME/C surveillance and epidemiologic research; and recommendations for the future. ME/C data have been used quite successfully in some settings and are potentially very useful for surveillance and epidemiologic research on a large scale, but the data have limitations that need to be addressed in the future.

INTRODUCTION

Medical examiners and coroners (ME/Cs) investigate and certify the cause of approximately 20% of the more than 2 million deaths that occur annually in

---

the United States, including homicides and suicides, most deaths related to unintentional injuries, and many sudden, unexplained deaths (56). As a result, data collected by ME/Cs may be a valuable source of information on some deaths of public health interest (56).

For more than a century, public health and death investigation by ME/Cs have been entwined—cholera and other epidemics in the 19th century resulted in the formation of boards of health, which laid the structural framework for improved death investigation, registration of deaths, and a working relationship between ME/Cs and the public health community (15, 61). This fundamental relationship between ME/Cs and public health was personified by the late Roger Fossum, Chief Medical Examiner of the State of New Hampshire, who was two-time president of the New Hampshire State Public Health Association (49).

Although medical examiner databases may be uniquely suited for use in epidemiologic investigations because autopsies are often performed, toxicologic data are frequently analyzed, police reports are available, and many types of deaths are included (23), such characteristics are not universal. In this article, we critically review the role of ME/C records and data in public health surveillance and epidemiologic research.

DEFINITIONS

Coroner and *Medical Examiner* are titles assigned to an official, usually elected or appointed, respectively, who on behalf of a county, a group of counties, or a state conducts investigations of specific types of death. Qualifications and duties are usually described in state or local law. In 24 of 28 states with coroners, most coroners are lay individuals, but states usually require that medical examiners be physicians and may require some training in anatomic or forensic pathology (12). Only seven states with coroners have mandatory training requirements (CDC-MECISP, unpublished).

Investigator is a title for a person who, under the authority of the ME/C, assists with death investigations (60, 68, 80).

Jurisdiction is a state, district or region within a state, or county for which a medical examiner or coroner conducts official death investigations. Among the 3137 counties in the United States, there are approximately 2185 death investigation jurisdictions—21 are statewide; 97 are regions or districts composed of two or more counties; and 2068 are counties (27). There are 218 medical examiner and 1967 coroner jurisdictions in the United States, although 58% of the U.S. population lives in areas served by medical examiners (12, 27). Some states have a coroner in every county; some have no coroners; and some have medical examiners in some counties and coroners in others (12). Often, coroners rely on a local or regional medical examiner (or pathologist) to conduct autopsies, and the coroner serves as the primary death investigator and completes the death certificate based on the medical examiner's findings. Figure 1 shows the type of system(s) for each state.

Official Death Investigations are conducted under the authority of state or local laws by a medical examiner, coroner, or similar official on behalf of the state or local government. The types of deaths generally include homicides; suicides; accidental traumatic deaths (e.g. deaths from falls, burns, drownings); deaths caused by drugs and toxic agents or agents that threaten public health; deaths that occur during employment or while in custody or confinement; and sudden, unexplained deaths. The scope of each investigation, depending on the circumstances of death, may include an investigation of the scene of injury or death, collection of evidence and death-related historical and circumstantial information, an external examination of the body, the performance of an autopsy, tests of body tissues or fluids for the presence of drugs or other substances, and the completion of the death certificate on which the cause and circumstances of death are indicated. Most states give the ME/C discretion regarding the extent of investigation and whether or not to accept a case for investigation. The ME/C often "declines" reported cases if a physician can be located to sign the death certificate and can explain the death with reasonable certainty, and the death does not involve injury or poisoning. Even in these cases, useful data may be collected by the ME/C about the place, time, cause, and circumstances of death.

Epidemiologic Research consists of *describing* the health status of populations by enumerating the occurrence of conditions (disease or injury), obtaining the relative frequencies within groups, and discovering important trends; *explaining* the etiology of conditions by determining factors that "cause" specific diseases or trends; and *predicting* the number of occurrences and the distribution of health status within populations with the goal of controlling the distributions of conditions in the population (44).

Public Health Surveillance is the ongoing systematic collection, analysis, and interpretation of outcome-specific data for use in the planning, implementation, and evaluation of public health practice. Surveillance includes prompt dissemination of results to those who need to know in order to take action. Surveillance does not include epidemiologic research and or implementation of delivery programs, but can be used to portray the natural history of selected conditions, to detect epidemics, to document the distribution and spread of selected conditions, to test hypotheses, to evaluate control and prevention measures, and to monitor changes in selected conditions (77–79).

ADVANTAGES OF USING ME/CS FOR SURVEILLANCE

ME/C jurisdictions are defined geographically; thus, ME/C jurisdictions are population based and conducive to surveillance and epidemiologic research.

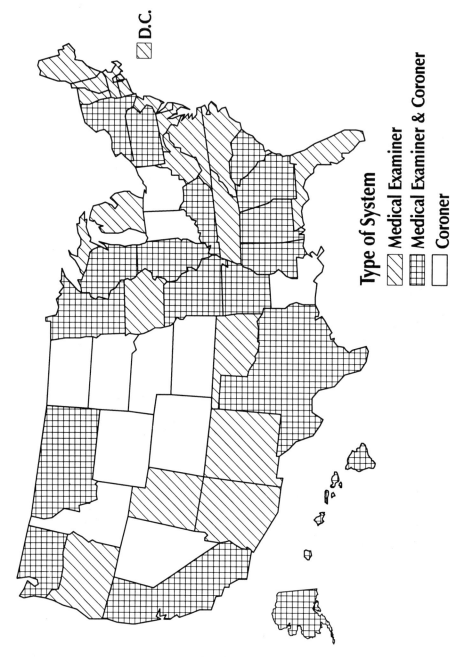

Figure 1   Death investigation system by state, 1995.

Because investigations by ME/Cs are initiated immediately after the ME/Cs are notified of a death, data collected by ME/Cs are ideal for the timely monitoring and study of reportable deaths (13).

Depending on the nature and scope of the investigation, an ME/C record may contain a police report, an autopsy or postmortem examination report, the results of toxicologic or other laboratory testing, and reports from other consultants such as forensic anthropologists and odontologists. Some ME/C jurisdictions keep electronic (computer) records that contain some, though usually not all, of the information on each case. Manner of death (homicide, suicide, accident, natural, or undetermined) is the information item most commonly kept in ME/C databases, followed by toxicology results, a description of how a fatal injury occurred, and a narrative description of circumstances, in descending order of frequency (26). Most offices include the cause of death in their database, but usually in coded form or in language other than that on the death certificate (26). Thus, although potentially very valuable, the content and format of both written and electronic records are not standardized.

In general, ME/C records (but not necessarily the databases) contain much more information about a death than do death certificates. One study found that ME/C records were much more useful for identifying deaths of homeless persons than were death certificates (10, 31). ME/C autopsy reports are amenable to the coding of injuries and application of injury scales for research purposes (13). Reporting of toxicologic and injury information is more consistent in ME/C records than on death certificates (55, 58). While death certificates only contain information about the usual occupation of the decedent, ME/C records may contain information about occupation at the time of death (13).

ME/Cs AND SURVEILLANCE

Stroup et al identify the following routine "sources" of data for surveillance: notifiable disease reporting systems, vital statistics, sentinel surveillance, registries, surveys, and administrative data collection systems (75). These sources are actually an assortment of data collection systems for specific outcomes [vital statistics and notifiable disease reporting systems]; methods for collecting data [sentinel surveillance, registries, and surveys]; general purpose data systems [administrative data collection systems]; and miscellaneous surveillance systems. We next discuss the involvement of ME/Cs with each of these data sources.

Vital statistics   ME/Cs certify approximately 20% of the deaths in the United States (9, 56). Of the deaths certified by a ME/C, about one half to two thirds, depending on the jurisdiction, are deaths due to natural causes; the remainder are deaths resulting from intentional and unintentional injuries (CDC-Medical Examiner/Coroner Information Sharing Program (MECISP), unpublished).

Notifiable disease reporting   In most states, ME/Cs should have the same legal obligation to report "notifiable" conditions (e.g. infectious diseases, occupational fatalities) to local or state agencies as do other health care providers. We are unaware, however, of any studies concerning the reliability of ME/Cs in reporting these conditions. No national surveillance system collects reports of notifiable conditions directly from ME/Cs.

Sentinel surveillance   This term describes the monitoring of sentinel health events including "preventable disease, disability, or untimely death whose occurrence serves as a warning signal that the quality of preventive and/or therapeutic medical care may need to be improved," as proposed and refined by Rutstein in 1976 and 1983 (66, 75). Three programs already use ME/C data for the surveillance of preventable or untimely deaths from drug abuse, consumer products, and medical products and devices, respectively (see below).

Registries   In the 1980s, a registry of "unusual" cases was established, but specific criteria for reporting were not published and the registry was not widely used (18). In 1985, the National Association of Medical Examiners established a Pediatric Toxicology Registry for reports from ME/Cs of deaths from drugs and poisons among children (28). No other registries exist that rely exclusively on reports from ME/Cs, although the establishment of national registries of anesthesia deaths and exercise- and sports-related asthma deaths has been discussed (82; H Mirchandani, personal communication).

Surveys   ME/Cs served as an important source of information on injury-related deaths for the 1993 National Mortality Follow-Back Survey (45). Surveys have evaluated the approach taken by ME/Cs in certifying specific types of death such as those due to Russian roulette, cocaine, sudden infant death syndrome, or work-related injury (41, 46, 64, 85); the extent of computerization of ME/C offices; and the usefulness of ME/C data for surveillance of HIV positive individuals (26, 38).

Administrative data collection systems   Some ME/C offices have established their own electronic data systems to provide easy access to case data for research, to respond to inquiries, or to facilitate administrative activities such as overseeing personnel, billing, or tracking inventory. There is, however, no formal, national system for collecting and using these data directly that would be analogous to the emergency room–based National Electronic Injury Surveillance System (NEISS). There are enough similarities among ME/C practices to provide the basis for the development of such systems, like the concept of a National Coronial Information System (NCIS) in Australia (2).

OBSTACLES TO SURVEILLANCE

With the exception of deaths that occur on Indian reservations or federal military facilities, the investigation of deaths in the United States is governed by state rather than federal law. These states laws are extremely varied. Although the Model Postmortem Examinations Act was written in 1954, it has been adopted by few states and is in need of revision (12, 32). Thus, certain types of deaths may not be investigated in all states and national surveillance using ME/Cs would be hampered. For example, some states (e.g. Delaware) require investigation of anesthetic deaths by the ME/C, whereas other states (e.g. Georgia) do not.

Even within a state, death investigation practices may vary because different ME/Cs may interpret and apply the same statute in different ways (32). For example, one ME/C may decline to investigate deaths of stillborn infants because there was, legally, no life and, therefore, no death. Another ME/C may interpret the statute more loosely and investigate such "deaths." To address such problems, standard language in death investigation laws has been advocated (32).

The presence of 2185 separate death investigation jurisdictions in the United States is good in the sense that services are often local, but the large number of jurisdictions poses an obstacle to surveillance system coordination, communication, education, and training.

Medical examiners and coroners each have their own organizations with relatively little overlapping membership. Membership in the National Association of Medical Examiners is not open to nonphysician coroners. The International Association of Coroners and Medical Examiners is a small group of predominantly lay coroners. The American Academy of Forensic Sciences (AAFS) is a diverse group of more than 4000 members representing all forensic science disciplines, of which only about 700 are ME/Cs, and many coroners do not qualify for membership. Lack of organizational cohesiveness makes discussion of, and uniformity among ME/C viewpoints and practices difficult to achieve.

The budgets and available support services for various ME/C offices vary substantially. As a result, the extent and quality of investigations vary. For example, some offices routinely perform a "complete" toxicologic analysis whereas other offices selectively perform toxicologic testing (CDC-MECISP, unpublished).

There is a shortage of trained manpower. According to the American Board of Pathology, fewer than 750 physicians have been certified in forensic pathology since the American Board of Pathology first offered the certification examination in 1959, yet an estimated 900 full-time forensic pathologists would be needed in the United States if they were to oversee all official death investigations (CDC-MECISP, unpublished). Training programs produce only about 40 forensic pathologists per year, and only 200–300 practice forensic pathology on a full-time basis (National Association of Medical Examiners, unpublished). Thus, other persons must perform death investigations who may not possess adequate training or experience.

The ME/C is asked by many agencies and organizations, or is required by law, to refer selected types of cases for follow-up, research, or other purposes. Each agency may require reporting in a different format, on a different form, or through different media, and such reporting can be cumbersome and time consuming. Thus, ME/Cs may be reluctant to participate in additional data collection or reporting projects for surveillance and epidemiologic research. One medical examiner's office in Canada hired an epidemiologist to coordinate reporting to various agencies (J Butt, personal communication), perhaps an indication of trends to come.

Some investigators may consider the collection of information for public health purposes beyond their scope of duty, as may some ME/Cs. Although some medical examiners have academic appointments in medical schools and some ME/C offices are operated within academic medical centers, most ME/C offices are branches of county or state government, which may not foster or give priority to academic or public health interests (27, 60).

There are no standardized, universally accepted procedures for investigating various types of deaths in the United States (37). For example, many ME/Cs do not adhere to the definition of sudden infant death syndrome, which requires a review of the deceased infant's clinical history, a scene investigation, and a complete autopsy (41). The extent of histologic, toxicologic, metabolic, and radiologic investigation in such cases also varies substantially (41).

Using death certificate data, Pollock et al found that ME/C autopsy rates in 1989 for deaths due to nonhomicidal blunt and penetrating trauma deaths ranged from 10% in Oklahoma to 95% in Hawaii; were higher in metropolitan (58%) than in nonmetropolitan (30%) counties; and were higher in jurisdictions served by medical examiners (64%) than in those served by coroners (52%) (59). Furthermore, current autopsy practices do not usually conform to the concept of the epidemiologic necropsy with a protocol geared to consistently evaluate a given set of parameters (67). An autopsy may consist of very limited dissection such as removal of a bullet. Such factors may limit the use of ME/C-performed autopsies for surveillance and epidemiologic research.

Studies have shown that the wording used in the cause-of-death statement varies considerably among ME/Cs, and that the variation may affect the ultimate nosologic classification. For example, cocaine-related deaths are under-reported on death certificates (85). The manner of death may also be assigned differently by ME/Cs for the same case scenario (25). ME/Cs in some areas routinely write the blood alcohol concentration on the death certificate, whereas other ME/Cs never do, and still others include it only if it is above the legal limit as defined in the state (CDC MECISP, unpublished). Some ME/Cs certify Russian roulette deaths as suicides, whereas others certify them as accidents (46).

The National Association of Medical Examiners has developed "Standards for Inspection and Accreditation of a Modern Medicolegal Investigative System" (49). However, the standards are somewhat general, only about 25 of the more than 200 ME systems have been inspected and accredited, and no similar inspection or accreditation process exists for coroner systems.

Some data are stored electronically by ME/Cs for approximately 25% of ME/C death investigations in the United States (26). Although several commercial, electronic database products exist for ME/Cs, most automated offices have developed their own data systems using personal computers and local area networks with customized off-the-shelf database packages, causing variability in data formats (26, 34). Many studies in nonautomated offices require searching and abstracting information from paper records.

The linkage of ME/C investigative data and autopsy reports with other sources of data, such as police reports, can improve their usefulness, but such data may be difficult to link because they are often collected and stored by various agencies that use different tracking and data management systems (13, 71). In fact, many ME/C offices process their autopsy reports in one computer system and their case-investigation data in another, with no linkage of the two databases (CDC-MECISP, unpublished).

ME/Cs investigate deaths of both residents and nonresidents that occur in their jurisdiction, and they may investigate deaths of people who were injured or who died in other jurisdictions (13). In a North Carolina study of occupational injury deaths, for example, Sniezek & Horiagon found that 12% of the deaths involved out-of-state residents (71). Such factors may complicate comparisons of data from different jurisdictions, as well as the calculation of mortality rates from ME/C data.

ME/Cs are responsible for completing the medical certification portion of the death certificate for cases they investigate, but the funeral director often completes the demographic portion after the ME/C completes the medical certification. This may lead to discrepancies between the demographic information contained in ME/C records and that contained in vital records (CDC—MECISP, unpublished).

The obstacles just described tell us that people using ME/C data for surveillance or epidemiologic research data should be thoroughly familiar with the applicable local statutes, the training and qualifications of the personnel conducting the investigations, autopsy performance practices, and other procedures, traditions, and practices of the ME/C office where the data were collected, so that limitations of the data will be understood (30).

EXISTING SURVEILLANCE SYSTEMS

Drug Abuse Warning Network (DAWN)

The Office of Applied Studies (OAS) in the Substance Abuse and Mental Health Services Administration (SAMHSA) is responsible for the operation of DAWN, a large-scale, ongoing, drug-abuse data-collection system (76). Started in the early 1970s and based on systematic reporting from DAWN-affiliated emergency rooms and medical examiner offices, drug abuse is defined by DAWN as the nonmedical use of substances for psychic effect, dependence, or suicide attempt/gesture. ME/Cs report data on paper forms or electronically using a standardized report format. ME/C data are tabulated separately from emergency room data and are published quarterly and yearly for 76 drugs that receive more than 10 "mentions" (i.e. references to drugs that may or may not have contributed to morbidity or mortality). In 1993, 145 ME/C jurisdictions in 43 metropolitan areas in 40 states consistently reported data to the DAWN system. However, reporting procedures vary because some ME/Cs may include cases based on circumstantial evidence, whereas others require confirmation with toxicologic analyses. Deaths involving AIDS and those in which the only drug mention is "drug unknown" are excluded from the data. Reports of opiates of unspecified type are included in the "heroin/morphine" category. Homicidal drug deaths are also not included. The manner of death for a case is assigned to each drug mentioned in the case, necessitating some caution when the motive for drug use is analyzed in the context of drug mention patterns (76). Two studies of the DAWN emergency room system showed that DAWN surveillance methods for drug-related morbidity result in systematic undercounts (3, 4). Pollock et al showed that 75% more cocaine-related deaths occurring from 1983 through 1988 were reported to DAWN than were ascertained from national death certificate data, and stressed the importance of improving the capacity of public health surveillance systems to measure the impact of drug deaths and to evaluate the effectiveness of prevention programs (58).

Medical Examiners and Coroners Alert Project (MECAP)

The Directorate of Epidemiology of the Consumer Product Safety Commission (CPSC) is responsible for the Medical Examiners and Coroners Alert Project, which is designed to promptly collect reports of deaths involving consumer products. An analogous Emergency Physicians Reporting System exists for nonfatal injuries (14). Reporting by ME/Cs is voluntary and is not standardized in report content or reporting base. Reports are solicited for deaths caused by asphyxiation, poisoning, drowning, fires and burns, falls, electricity, and inhalation, and for other miscellaneous deaths related to consumer products. In March and April 1995, 423 cases were reported to MECAP. Selected cases are published by CPSC in a bimonthly newsletter entitled MECAP NEWS. Apart from the newsletter, MECAP reports and data are not readily available. A major limitation is that there is no published analysis of the relationship between the cause of death and the consumer product, and specific brand names and design features of involved products are usually not published for the individual case reports. We could not find a published study reporting the usefulness or limitations of the MECAP.

FDA MedWatch Medical Products Reporting Program

In June 1993, the Food and Drug Administration (FDA) implemented Med-Watch—a streamlined and consolidated medical products and adverse drug reaction reporting program that replaced five prior forms and programs (21). Because MedWatch solicits case reports of fatal incidents involving all types of medical products (including drugs), ME/Cs are an excellent potential source of information. Case report criteria are contained in a published reporting guide, but reporting and adherence to the criteria vary. Unfortunately, data obtained from MedWatch are not routinely published or readily accessible, and as many as 50% of physicians are not aware of the reporting system (21). The FDA Medical Bulletin contains reports of specific product problems identified through the reporting system; however, we could not find a published study that analyzes the usefulness or limitations of the system regarding ME/C reporting of device-related problems. Of 14 recent articles concerning Med-Watch, 11 dealt with announcing the new program and 2 with specific problems reported through the system (83, 84). Letters have expressed concern that the data are expensive to obtain and not readily accessible by physicians; that reports discussing the results of follow-up investigations are lacking; that further database development is needed; and that emerging problems detected through MedWatch need additional epidemiologic investigations (20, 81).

The Fatal Accident Reporting System (FARS)   In the mid-1970s, the National Highway Traffic Safety Administration established the Fatal Accident Reporting System (FARS). FARS gathers data on all motor vehicle crashes occurring on public roadways that are not caused by natural disasters and that result in the death of a person within 30 days of the crash. Under contract with FARS, states collect data from police, hospitals, selected ME/C offices, emergency medical services, state vehicle registration, driver licensing agencies, highway department files, vital statistics documents, and death certificates. FARS publishes a statistical report annually summarizing the results of its data collection activities (53).

The Medical Examiner and Coroner Information Sharing Program (MECISP)

In 1986, the Centers for Disease Control and Prevention (CDC) established the Medical Examiner and Coroner Information Sharing Program to improve the quality of death investigations; promote standardized practices; facilitate communication among the death investigation community, the public health community, federal agencies, and other groups; improve the quality, completeness, management, and dissemination of information; and promote the sharing and use of ME/C death investigation data (8). The MECISP annually collects electronic death investigation records from approximately 12 ME/C offices in the United States in the data format used by the offices themselves, and nearly 750,000 death investigation cases are on file electronically. Efforts are under way to convert the data from individual ME/C offices into a standardized format that is more easily queried, but data are not yet accessible on-line. The MECISP is developing a strategy to implement a Medical Examiner and Coroner Mortality, Epidemiology, and Surveillance System (McMESS) for receiving reports from ME/Cs on specific types of death.

MECISP has made an effort to standardize ME/C data collection through the publication of generic death investigation report forms (DIRFS); a manual describing a model ME/C death investigation data set (McDIDS); and publication of articles concerning the automation of ME/C offices (26, 33, 34).

Surveillance for Work-Related Deaths

Regulations require that certain occupation-related deaths be reported to the Occupational Safety and Health Administration (OSHA), and ME/Cs are obliged to ensure that deaths meeting the OSHA criteria are reported. However, only deaths of employees are reportable to OSHA, and not all workers are under OSHA jurisdiction; recent studies suggest considerable underreporting of fatalities that do fall under OSHA jurisdiction (74). The potential ME/C contribution to surveillance of work-related injuries may exceed that enabled through OSHA reporting system because ME/Cs investigate work-related deaths not subject to OSHA reporting.

Information on occupational injury deaths is also collected by the National Institute of Occupational Safety and Health through its National Traumatic Occupational Fatalities (NTOF) surveillance system and by the Bureau of Labor Statistics through its Census of Fatal Occupational Injuries (CFOI) (5, 54). NTOF does not receive reports of individual deaths from ME/Cs; instead, information for NTOF is taken from death certificates. Only certificates with a positive response to the "injury at work" item are collected, which may result in some undercounting of deaths. The CFOI was developed by the Bureau of Labor Statistics and state agencies with the goal of collecting information on all fatal occupational injuries (5). Presently, CFOI relies on multiple data sources including death certificates, worker's compensation reports and claims, and other Federal and State administrative records, but does not capture data for all occupational injury deaths. ME/Cs do not report directly to CFOI officials, but ME/C records are used by CFOI as a source to verify occupational fatalities in about 61% of cases reported by CFOI (5). We found no recent studies comparing the usefulness of ME/C data with that of CFOI data. CFOI data are published each year with selected relevant articles (5).

Pediatric Toxicology Registry

In 1985, the National Association of Medical Examiners established a Pediatric Toxicology Registry for the voluntary reporting of information on drugs and poisons found in fetuses, infants, and children aged 15 years or younger (28). Criteria for reporting are the presence (confirmed by laboratory testing) of one or more drugs or poisons. The registry was created to provide data to better differentiate "normal," "toxic," and "lethal" levels of commonly detected drugs, and to gather cases that involve unusual or rarely detected substances. More than 1000 case reports involving more than 100 different substances have been submitted. Periodic data summaries are published in NAME's bimonthly newsletter, *NAME NEWS*. Because the validity of the submitted data cannot be ensured, the raw data are not generally accessible in printed or electronic form. Data are published only after careful review, and are released only in response to specific inquiries after a NAME pathologist personally discusses the data with the inquirer.

STUDIES ASSESSING THE USE OF ME/C DATA FOR SURVEILLANCE

Natural Deaths

Graitcer et al compared the noninjury-related deaths that occurred in Fulton County, Georgia, in 1984 and had been reported to the medical examiner with all of the noninjury-related deaths that occurred in the same county jurisdiction, as determined from vital statistics (23). The authors categorized the disease conditions into major International Classification of Disease (ICD) categories (e.g. 240–279 endocrine system; 140–239 neoplasms; etc) and concluded that ME/C data are of limited usefulness for the surveillance of natural disease conditions. For example, 25.5% of deaths in the vital statistics series were attributed to neoplasms, whereas only 6.0% of deaths in the ME/C series were.

They also concluded that black males accounted for a higher percentage of ME/C cases than they did as measured by vital statistics data, and that ME/Cs are more likely than an attending physician to attribute death to alcoholism—a statement supported by another report from the same county showing that 79% of all deaths attributed to alcoholism were certified by the medical examiner (24). Graitcer et al claimed that ME data are sensitive and representative for the surveillance of sudden and unexpected conditions, but they did not specify those conditions. A weakness of the report is that data were presented only for major disease categories. Closer analysis, for example, might have shown that ME/C data are sensitive for detecting some specific natural conditions (e.g. congenital anomalous coronary artery) even though ME/C data may not be useful for surveillance of cardiovascular deaths in general.

Injury Deaths

Smith & Middaugh assessed various sources of data for injury surveillance in Alaska by their ability to identify deaths and nonfatal injuries caused by the use of all-terrain vehicles (ATVs) in 1983 and 1984 (69). They used death certificates; a survey of all coroners; data tapes from the Alaska Department of Transportation (DOT); records from emergency medical services, the Indian Health Service, and the military medical bases; and four reporting systems operated by the Consumer Product Safety Commission (CPSC). No single source of data included all deaths. Seventeen of the 20 ATV-related deaths were detected from death certificates, 17 from ME reports, 16 from DOT records, and 9 from CPSC reports. ME records identified two cases that were not identified by the death certificates. The other sources provided few or no additional reports. Together, death certificates and ME records identified 95% of ATV deaths. The authors concluded that linking death certificate and ME data was the best approach for surveillance of ATV-related deaths, but cautioned that this approach might not be applicable to other types of injuries. The authors also emphasized that ME and DOT data, as well as other such data, were extremely helpful in providing descriptive information that could be used to detail the specific injuries sustained in the ATV fatalities (70). A major weakness in their study was the small number of ATV fatalities available for study.

Dijkhuis et al showed the fallacy in the widely held assumption that ME/C databases contain information for all deaths due to injury (16). By analyzing all deaths of Iowa residents caused by injuries that occurred in Iowa during 1990 and 1991, they were the first to assess the completeness of ME/C data for the study of deaths from all types of injuries. Using death certificates filed with the state registrar and ME reports filed in the Iowa State Medical Examiner's office, the authors took extensive measures to ensure that all injury deaths had been identified. They found that the ME reports underestimated the actual number of injury deaths; ME reports were available for only 69% of people with fatal injuries, 57% of women with fatal injuries, 80% of people who died as a result of transportation crashes, 37% of people who died of a fall, and 57% of people who died of other unintentional injuries. The authors concluded that ME/C data for women, the elderly, and those dying of unintentional falls should be viewed with caution, and that linkage of ME/C data and vital records was necessary to identify all injury deaths. Because deaths are investigated locally in Iowa and finalized reports are submitted to a state office for filing, the results of the Iowa study may not be comparable with data from jurisdictions in which all ME/C cases are investigated and filed within a single office.

In North Carolina, Rainey & Runyon found that newspaper accounts could be used to detect 91% of childhood fire deaths and 72% of the childhood drownings reported in ME records in 1988–1989 (62). Newspaper accounts were less useful than ME records for determining race and alcohol involvement but were more complete in terms of information about the suspected cause of fires and the presence or absence of protective factors for both fires and drownings. The study illustrates how an analysis of ME/C data can lead to an improvement in ME/C data collection procedures: After the study, the ME office added items to its investigative forms to document in greater detail information about the presence of smoke detectors, life preservers, and other relevant items. A weakness of the study is that a newspaper clipping service was needed to review the more than 200 newspapers in the state, and the costs and methods of the clipping service were not detailed.

In Northern Ireland, Gaffney studied childhood injury deaths that had been registered in the Coroner Information System for 1984 through 1988 (22). The author concluded that lack of standardized reporting formats posed a significant obstacle to effective surveillance and that coroners' reports had insufficient detail to provide consistent, useful information for assessing the effectiveness of prevention strategies. Coroner reports of pedestrian, passenger, bicycle, fire, crush, and railway deaths were all noted to lack detailed information. The study did not address the sensitivity of coroner data for detecting such deaths.

Work-Related Injury Deaths

Sniezek & Horiagon noted that ME data from North Carolina yielded a fatal occupational injury rate of 6.0/100,000 employed-person years compared with a rate of 8.8/100,000 reported in a study performed by the National Institute of Occupational Safety and Health during a similar time period (71). The authors attributed the discrepancy to differences in reporting sources and inclusion criteria but did not investigate the discrepancy further. Centralized ME data collection, such as that in the state ME office in North Carolina, may facilitate statewide studies. However, although 21 states have state medical examiner systems, not all of them have centralized record keeping (12, 26).

Stanbury & Goldloft studied occupational injuries that occurred in New Jersey during 1984 and 1985 by comparing OSHA data with death certificate data and medical examiner data (73). OSHA data indicated 77 fatalities, whereas all three sources together indicated 204 fatalities. The authors concluded that OSHA data were not a good sole source for surveillance of fatal occupational injuries but that they should be included in any injury surveillance system because they did capture some cases not in other data sources. They also concluded that death certificate and ME data are needed for adequate surveillance of work-injury deaths because 43% of such deaths fall outside of OSHA's jurisdiction. A limitation of this report was that data were not presented separately for death certificates and ME cases, precluding an analysis of the relative usefulness of each data source.

Studies in Maryland, Oklahoma, and Pennsylvania have shown that ME/C data were more sensitive for ascertaining externally caused occupational deaths than were death certificates (13). Russell & Conroy also showed that in Oklahoma, during 1985 and 1986, occupational deaths involving transportation, farming, and agriculture were underestimated by all data sources, particularly death certificates, and emphasized that a combination of data sources were required to maximize case ascertainment (65). They also noted a wide variation in estimates of work-related fatalities derived from Bureau of Labor Statistics data, NIOSH data, and National Safety Council data. Each of these studies was conducted in the 1980s, however, before a standard set of criteria was published for defining a work-related injury for death certificate purposes (50).

In 1991, Stout & Bell performed a meta-analysis of ten studies to evaluate the ability of different source documents to identify fatal occupational injuries (74). The average ascertainment rates for the various data sources were 81% for death certificates; 68% for medical examiner records; 57% for workers compensation data; 32% for OSHA fatality reports; and 27% for state health or labor department records. Sole sources included death certificates (36%), workers compensation records (17%), ME/C records (12%), state health and labor records (5%), and OSHA fatality reports (1%). ME/C data showed the greatest state-to-state variation in the percentage of work-related deaths identified. The authors recommended ME office computerization and more consistent data collection practices among ME/Cs.

A few states (AZ, AK, CA, CT, DE, DC, FL, KY, MA, NJ) have statutes that require "industrial" or occupational deaths to be reported to the ME/C even when an injury may not be involved (13). Such statutes may facilitate surveillance and epidemiologic research of deaths that occur while working.

Lerer & Meyers studied occupational deaths in South Africa during 18 months in 1990 and 1991 (47). Using medical examiner records as the standard, they found that 28% of such deaths had not been reported to the Department of Manpower (DOM) as required by statute. The authors did not indicate how many occupational deaths had not been investigated by a medical examiner.

Maternal Deaths

Allen et al studied the usefulness of ME data for ascertaining maternal deaths during 1983 and 1984 in New York City (1). ME/C records proved to be the most useful source for uniquely ascertaining maternal deaths, adding 10.5% of cases, while death certificates added 6.3%. The authors did not report how often the ME failed to indicate recent pregnancy on the death certificate, although a special item on the death certificate for such an entry was omitted on 40% of all applicable death certificates. The authors had to perform an extensive manual search of ME records in order to identify maternal deaths, serving as an indicator that ME records may not be amenable to routine maternal mortality surveillance. Another study found that 8 of 12 maternal deaths had been reported to the ME and that autopsies had been performed on these decedents, but the authors did not indicate the ascertainment methods or rates for the various data sources (35).

Poisoning Deaths

Linakis & Frederick ascertained 369 drug-, poison-, and toxin-related deaths from Rhode Island State Medical Examiner records but only 45 from poison control center records during the same time period (48). The authors attributed this difference to two factors: Many poison deaths occurred at home or among people who were pronounced dead on arrival at a hospital, and poisoning was often not suspected until an autopsy was performed by the ME. They concluded that ME records were a good source for deaths due to poisoning. In a similar study in Massachusetts, Soslow & Woolf compared the completeness with which deaths due to poisoning were reported by poison control center records, death certificates, and state medical examiner records (72). They found that the concordance of the three data sets was only 17% and concluded that ME/C records were an underappreciated, rich source of data for deaths from poisoning, even though 15% of deaths found in the records of poison control centers were not contained in ME/C records.

Medical examiner records played a critical role in evaluating the epidemic and emerging patterns of cocaine deaths in Dade County, Florida, where a 20-fold increase in cocaine overdose deaths occurred from 1971 through 1987 (19). Another study of medical examiner data showed that the rate of cocaine use among homicide victims in Atlanta increased from 1985 through 1989 and that cocaine or its metabolites were detected in 33% of homicide victims in 1989 (29). Many descriptive studies of drug detection among ME/C cases have been published.

Other Studies Of The Usefulness Of Me/c Data

Most publications based on ME/C data consist of case reports of unusual or previously unrecognized or undocumented causes and circumstances of death, or descriptive case series targeted at a specific problem in a given jurisdiction. A sample of such publications is shown in the Appendix, which also includes a list of publications based on ME/C data from one office to illustrate the variety of ME/C information that may be available for public health planning and practice.

Pearson compared suicides as determined from coroners' reports in North and West Devon (England) and found differences in the patterns of suicide, which the author attributed to local factors, concluding that the variability in the local coroners' verdicts had an important influence on reported suicide rates (57).

Runyon et al sent 57 county medical examiners a set of 22 case scenarios and asked them which were work related (64). Deaths involving transportation, nonpaid workers, farming, or a job other than the decedent's usual job were classified most inconsistently. They concluded that the lack of standard definitions for job, work, and on-the-job contributed to the inconsistencies. The recently published operational guidelines for determining injury at work may help to reduce such inconsistency (50).

Jordan & Bass analyzed death certificates for a variety of errors in the stated cause(s) of death for hospital deaths and coroner cases in Ontario, Canada (39). They concluded that error rates in the stated cause(s) of death were no lower among coroner cases than among hospital cases. To improve the error rate of coroners, they advocated ongoing education and feedback for certifiers of death.

Kendall et al reviewed 179 coroners' autopsies in England that were performed on patients who died in the emergency room and found the information of potential use for evaluating iatrogenic trauma induced during resuscitation and for conducting departmental audits aimed at improving clinical skills (42).

Romano & McLoughlin analyzed death certificates from ME/Cs in the San Francisco area and concluded that lack of detailed injury information on death certificates seriously hampers the use of death certificate data for prevention research (63). They did show that ME/C diagnoses were valuable for injury research but that such information was often not transferred from the ME/C case record to the death certificate.

IDENTIFICATION OF EMERGING PROBLEMS BY ME/Cs

ME/Cs have served as "sentinels" in recognizing and describing a number of emerging public health problems such as legionnaire's disease, hantavirus pulmonary syndrome, and over-the-counter medications intentionally adulterated with cyanide, to name just three (6, 11). The dangers of inhaled hydrocarbons (such as typewriter correction fluid), five-gallon buckets in which toddlers drown, and commonly aspirated foods and objects are just a few of the everyday hazards brought to light by ME/Cs (36, 40, 43). After Hurricane Hugo in Puerto Rico and South Carolina, several fatal electrocutions were caused by electrical hazards that resulted from the storm. These problems were identified from ME/C data and were heavily publicized in South Florida prior to Hurricane Andrew several years later, after which no such electrocutions were reported (7).

NEW TOOLS FOR SURVEILLANCE AND EPIDEMIOLOGIC RESEARCH

NAME NEWS is the newsletter of the National Association of Medical Examiners (NAME) mailed bimonthly to the more than 800 ME/C NAME members and administrative and investigative affiliates in the United States and abroad. It is within the scope of the newsletter's mission to publish survey and case-report forms. The newsletter, however, does not reach most coroners. NAME also maintains an Internet Listserv, "NAME-L," to which NAME members and affiliates may subscribe. This electronic mode of communication may eventually play an important role in the collection and dissemination of ME/C information that can be used for surveillance or epidemiologic research.

The CDC is developing an Internet home page for ME/Cs that will be accessible through the World Wide Web (WWW); the home page title will be the "Information Resources Guide (IRG) for Medical Examiners, Coroners, and Medicolegal Death Investigators" (52). The IRG home page will be linked to the CDC home page under environmental health and will serve the traditional functions of newsletter, bulletin board, directory, archive, and database, and will also provide training materials.

More than 40 states now have multidisciplinary child fatality review teams (CFRTs) to review children's deaths in a systematic fashion (17). Usually, these teams include ME/Cs and use information from their reports, and are designed with the goal of preventing childhood deaths and correcting system process problems. Thus, CFRTs may eventually be a good source of multidisciplinary records and ME/C data with coverage of a substantial portion of childhood deaths in the United States.

DIFFICULTIES IN SEARCHING ME/C LITERATURE

Using Medline, we located 133 articles published from 1991 through mid-1995 that were categorized under the medical entities subject heading (MeSH) of "coroner and medical examiners." Using a title search for the same period, we found only 34 articles with the words "medical examiner" or "coroner" in the title. Using an abstract search for the same words, we detected 169 articles. Under the MeSH heading of "forensic medicine," we found 1270 articles. For a similar time period, using a text word search of Medline titles and abstracts that included various words and proximity operators in the search strategy, we found 106 to 372 articles. For example, we did not locate an article concerning heat-related deaths in Philadelphia that was based substantially on ME/C data when we searched for the MeSH category "coroners and medical examiners," but we did locate it by searching for "epidemiologic methods." Researchers should be aware of the possible need to use nonroutine search strategies when querying for ME/C publications of potential interest.

CONCLUSIONS

ME/Cs and the data that they collect are potentially valuable for surveillance and epidemiologic research. ME/C data have been used most often in the surveillance and study of occupational and injury-related deaths, although ME/C data are also being used in studies of other types of death. The ME/C literature also contains many case reports and descriptive studies that may have public health importance. Because ME/C practices and data collection are not standardized, the usefulness of ME/C data for surveillance and epidemiologic research depends largely on the characteristics of the ME/C office from which the information is obtained. Variations in statutes, funding, staffing, training and experience, practices, automation, and methods of managing records and data each affect the quality and usefulness of ME/C records and data. Efforts are needed to standardize and improve the quality of investigations and related data-collection and management practices, and to facilitate the dissemination of data electronically in an organized and planned manner. At present, linkage of ME/C data with other data sources is often needed to identify all selected deaths of interest.

RECOMMENDATIONS

We recommend that the following steps be taken to improve the usefulness of ME/C data for surveillance, epidemiologic research, and public health pro- grams:

1. Increase recognition of the importance of high-quality death investigations and the data derived from them among the public and those responsible for making public health and public safety policy at the local, state, and federal levels.
2. Educate ME/Cs about the potential uses of their data for surveillance and epidemiologic research.
3. Revise the Model Postmortem Examinations Act and standardize the death investigation laws among states.
4. Develop and disseminate guidelines, protocols, procedures, and forms for conducting high quality investigations of deaths.
5. Promote more uniform procedures for collecting, managing, storing, and reporting data on investigated deaths.
6. Automate individual ME/C offices and promote the networking and communication among these offices through connection to, and use of, the Internet.
7. Establish a national clearinghouse to collect ME/C data.
8. Establish a ME/C surveillance system for reporting of selected types of death.
9. Improve coordination among the agencies requesting data from ME/Cs.
10. Increase funding of ME/C offices by their parent agencies and provide additional ME/C funding by having data users reimburse ME/Cs for data shared.
11. Encourage academic ties for ME/C offices.

APPENDIX

Sample recent case reports and decriptive studies using ME/C death investigations and data:

Baron RC, Thacker SB, Gorelkin L, Vernon AA, Taylor WR, Choi K. 1983. Sudden death among Southeast Asian refugees: an unexpected nocturnal phenomenon. *JAMA* 250:2947–51

Berkelman RL, Herndon JL, Callaway JL, Stivers R, Howard LB, et al. 1985. Fatal injuries and alcohol. *Am. J. Prev. Med.* 1:21–28

Bern C, Lew J, McFeeley P, Ing D, Ing RT, Glass RI. 1993. Diarrheal deaths in children living in New Mexico: toward a strategy of preventive interventions. *J. Pediatr.* 122:920–22

Blaser MJ, Jason JM, Weniger BG, Elset WR, Finton RJ, et al. 1984. Epidemiologic analysis of a cluster of homicides of children in Atlanta. *JAMA* 251:3255–58

Boglioli LR, Taff ML. 1995. "The Santa Claus Syndrome": entrapment in chimneys. *J. Forensic Sci.* 40:499–500

Brison RJ, Wicklund K, Mueller BA. 1988. Fatal pedestrian injuries in young children: a different pattern of injury. *Am. J. Public Health* 78:793–95

Campbell S, Hood I, Ryan D. 1990. Death as a result of asthma in Wayne County medical examiner cases, 1975–1987. *J. Forensic Sci.* 35:356–64

Chernichko L, Saunders LD, Tough S. 1993. Unintentional house fire deaths in Alberta 1985–1990: a population study. *Can. J. Public Health* 307:1212–13

Cherpitel CJ. 1994. Alcohol and casualties: a comparison of emergency room and coroner data. *Alcohol* 29:211–18

Copeland AR. 1989. Suicide by jumping from buildings. *Am. J. Forensic Med. Pathol.* 10:295–98

Downs JCU, Milling D, Nichold CA. 1995. Suicidal ingestion of barium-sulfide-containing shaving powder. *Am. J. Forensic Med. Pathol.* 16:56–61

Eberhart-Phillips JE, Saunders TM, Robinson AL, Hatch DL, Parrish RG. 1994. Profile of mortality from the 1989 Loma Prieta earthquake using coroner and medical examiner reports. *Disasters* 18:160–70

Emerick SJ, Foster LR, Campbell DT. 1986. Risk factors for traumatic infant death in Orgeon, 1973–1982. *Pediatrics* 77:518–22

Ferrara SD, Tedeschi L, Frison G, Rossi A. 1995. Fatality due to gamma-hydroxy-butyric acid (GHB) and heroin intoxication. *J. Forensic Sci.* 40:501–4

Goodman RA, Mercy JA, Rosenberg ML. 1986. Drug use and interpersonal violence: barbiturates detected in homicide victims. *Am. J. Epidemiol.* 124: 851–55

Graham C, Burvill PW. 1992. A study of coroner's records of suicide in young people, 1986–88 in Western Australia. *Aust. NZ J. Psychiatry* 26:30–39

Greenberger PA, Miller TP, Lifschulz B. 1993. Circumstances surrounding deaths from asthma in Cook County. *Allergy Proc.* 14:321–26

Haberman PW, French JF, Chin J. 1993. HIV infection and intravenous drug use: medical examiner cases in Essex and Hudson Counties, New Jersey. *Am. J. Drug Alcohol Abuse* 19:299–307

Hall JR, Reyes HM, Meller JL, Stein RJ. 1993. Traumatic death in urban children, revisited. *Am. J. Dis. Child.* 147:102–7

Jones ST, Liang, Kilbourne EM, Griffin MR, Patriarca PA, et al. 1982. Morbidity and mortality associated with the July 1980 heat wave in St. Louis and Kansas City, MO. *JAMA* 247:3327–31

Kellerman AL, Reay DT. 1986. Protection or peril? An analysis of firearm-related deaths in the home. *N. Engl. J. Med.* 314:1557–60

Koponen MA, Siegel R. 1995. Hamartomatous malformation of the left ventricle associated with sudden death. *J. Forensic Sci.* 40:495–98

MayoSmith MF, Hirsch PJ, Wodzinski SF, Schiffman FJ. 1986. Acute epiglottitis in adults. An eight-year experience in Rhode Island. *N. Engl. J. Med.* 314:1133–39

McCormick GM, Young DB. 1995. Death caused by an allergic reaction to ethanol. *Am. J. Forensic Med. Pathol.* 16:45–47

Patetta MJ, Cole TB. 1990. A population-based descriptive study of housefire deaths in North Carolina. *Am. J. Public Health* 80:1116–17

Quan L, Gore EJ, Wentz K, Allen J, Novack AH. 1989. Ten-year study of pediatric drownings and near-drownings in King County, Washington: lessons in injury prevention. *Pediatrics* 83:1035–40

Robinson CC, Kuller LH, Perper J. 1988. An epidemiologic study of sudden death at work in an industrial county, 1979–1982. *Am. J. Epidemiol.* 128:806–20

Rogers D. 1995. Accidental fatal monochloroacetic acid poisoning. *Am. J. Forensic Med. Pathol.* 16:115–16

Rutledge R, Messick WJ. 1992. The association of trauma death and alcohol use in a rural state. *J. Trauma* 33:737–42

Ruttenber JA, Luke JL. 1984. Heroin-related deaths: new epidemiologic insights. *Science* 226:14–20

Schierer CL, Hood IC, Mirchandani HG. 1990. Atherosclerotic cardiovascular disease and sudden deaths among young adults in Wayne County. *Am. J. Forensic Med. Pathol.* 11:198–201

Spence LJ, Dykes EH, Bohn DJ, Wesson DE. 1993. Fatal bicycle accidents in children: a plea for prevention. *J. Pediatr. Surg.* 28:214–16

Teo CE. 1993. A study of coroner's cases from hospitals: a comparison of autopsy and clinical diagnoses. *Ann. Acad. Med. Singapore* 22:3–7

Sample studies based on ME/C data from one ME/C office, Fulton County, Georgia:

Cent. Dis. Control. 1993. Enumerating deaths among the homeless. *Morbid. Mortal. Wkly. Rep.* 42:719, 25–26

Cent. Dis. Control. 1993. Characteristics of death certifiers and institutions where death is pronounced—Fulton County, Georgia, 1991. *Morbid. Mortal. Wkly. Rep.* 42:683–84

Cent. Dis. Control. 1994. Homicides of persons aged less than 18 years—Fulton County, Georgia. 1988–1992. *Morbid. Mortal. Wkly. Rep.* 43:254–61

Cent. Dis. Control. 1994. Adolescent homicide—Fulton County, Georgia, 1988–1992. *Morbid. Mortal. Wkly. Rep.* 43:728–30

Early A, Hanzlick R. 1987. Fire deaths in Fulton County, 1983–85. *J. Med. Assoc. Georgia* 76:494–97

Frost R, Hanzlick R. 1988. Deaths in custody: Atlanta City Jail and Fulton County Jail, 1974–1985. *Am. J. Forensic Med. Pathol.* 9:207–11

Gowitt G, Hanzlick R. 1986. Suicide in Fulton County, Georgia (1975–1984). *J. Forensic Sci.* 31:1029–38

Gowitt GT, Hanzlick R. 1992. Atypical autoerotic deaths. *Am. J. Forensic Med. Pathol.* 13:115–19

Guarner J, Hanzlick R. 1987. Suicide by hanging: a review of 56 cases. *Am. J. Forensic Med. Pathol.* 8:23–26

Hanzlick R. 1988. Death certificates, natural death, and alcohol. *Am. J. Forensic Med. Pathol.* 9:149–50

Hanzlick R. 1989. Postmortem tricyclic antidepressant concentrations: lethal versus nonlethal levels. *Am. J. Forensic Med. Pathol.* 10:326–29

Hanzlick R, Gowitt G. 1991. Cocaine metabolite detection in homicide victims. *JAMA* 265:760–61

Hanzlick R, Hawkins C, Hammami A. 1988. A "back-door" approach to analysis of ethanol-associated risks and behavior. *Am. J. Forensic Med. Pathol.* 9:322–30

Hanzlick R, Jarret D, Birdsong G. 1987. Demographics of Atlanta's homicide epicenter, 1984. *J. Med. Assoc. Georgia* 76:825–32

Hanzlick R, Koponen M. 1994. Murder suicide in Fulton County, Georgia, 1988–1991. *Am. J. Forensic Med. Pathol.* 15:168–73

Hanzlick R, Lazarchick J. 1989. Health care history and utilization for Atlantans who died homeless. *J. Med. Assoc. Georgia* 78:205–8

Hanzlick R, Masterson K, Walker B. 1990. Suicide by jumping from high-rise hotels: Fulton County, Georgia, 1967–1986. *Am. J. Forensic Med. Pathol.* 11:294–97

Hanzlick R, Parrish RG. 1993. Deaths among the homeless in Fulton County, Georgia, 1988–90. *Public Health Rep.* 108:488–91

Hanzlick R, Ross W. 1986. Automobile passenger deaths in children less than five years of age. *J. Med. Assoc. Georgia* 75:209–11

Hanzlick R, Ross WK. 1987. Suicide far from home: the concept of transjurisdictional suicide. *J. Forensic Sci.* 32:189–91

Hanzlick R, Rydzewski D. 1990. Heart weights of white men 20 to 39 years of age: an analysis of 218 autopsy cases. *Am. J. Forensic Med. Pathol.* 11:202–4

Hanzlick R, Sperry K. 1990. Maternal deaths in Fulton County, Georgia 1988–89. *Atlanta Med.* 64:19–23

Renz B, Hanzlick R. 1992. Penetrating wounds of the female breast. *Emory Univ. J. Med.* 6:29–32

Walker G, Hanzlick R. 1986. Traffic fatalities and drinking teens: how big is the problem in Fulton County? *J. Med. Assoc. Georgia.* 75:606–62

Any *Annual Review* chapter, as well as any article cited in an *Annual Review* chapter, may be purchased from the Annual Reviews Preprints and Reprints service. 1-800-347-8007; 415-259-5017; email: arpr@class.org

---

Literature Cited

1. Allen MH, Chavkin W, Marinoff J. 1991. Ascertainment of maternal deaths in New York City. *Am. J. Public Health* 81:380–82
2. Australian Institute of Health and Welfare. 1994. National Coronial Information System. *Injury Issues Monit.*, Dec.
3. Blanc PD, Jones MR, Olson KR. 1993. Surveillance of poisoning and drug overdose through hospital discharge coding, poison control center reporting, and the Drug Abuse Warning Network. *Am. J. Emerg. Med.* 11:14–19
4. Brookoff D, Campbell EA, Shaw LM. 1993. The under reporting of cocaine-related trauma: drug abuse warning network reports versus hospital toxicology test. *Am. J. Public Health* 83:369–71
5. Bureau of Labor Statistics. 1994. *Fatal Workplace Injuries in 1992: A Collection of Data and Analysis.* Washington DC: US Dep. Labor
6. Cent. Dis. Control Prev. 1991. Cyanide poisoning associated with over-the-counter medication—Washington State, 1991. *Morbid. Mortal. Wkly. Rep.* 40:161–68
7. Cent. Dis. Control Prev. 1992. Preliminary report: medical examiner reports of deaths associated with Hurricane Andrew—Florida, August 1992. *Morbid. Mortal. Wkly. Rep.* 41:641–44
8. Cent. Dis. Control Prev. 1993. *The Medical Examiner and Coroner Information Sharing Program.* Atlanta: CDC
9. Cent. Dis. Control Prev. 1993. Characteristics of death certifiers and institu-

tions where death is pronounced—Fulton County, Georgia, 1991. *Morbid. Mortal. Wkly. Rep.* 42:683–84

10. Cent. Dis. Control Prev. 1993. Enumerating deaths among the homeless. *Morbid. Mortal. Wkly. Rep.* 42:719, 725–26

11. Cent. Dis. Control Prev. 1994. *Addressing Emerging Disease Threats: A Prevention Strategy for the United States.* Atlanta: PHS

12. Combs DL, Parrish RG, Ing RT. 1992. *Death Investigation in the United States and Canada, 1992.* Atlanta: CDC

13. Conroy C, Russell JC. 1990. Medical examiner/coroner records: uses and limitations in occupational injury epidemiologic research. *J. Forensic Sci.* 35:932–37

14. Consumer Product Safety Commission. 1995. *MECAP NEWS* 20:1–4

15. Cordner SM, Loff B. 1994. 800 years of coroners: have they a future? *Lancet* 344:799–801

16. Dijkhuis H, Zwerling C, Parrish G, Bennett T, Kemper HCG. 1994. Medical examiner data in injury surveillance: a comparison with death certificates. *Am. J. Epidemiol.* 139:637–43

17. Durfee MJ, Gellert GA, Tilton-Durfee D. 1992. Origins and clinical relevance of child death review teams. *JAMA* 267:3172–75

18. Eckert WG. 1981. International Registry of Unusual Cases: gunshot wound of the chest with five intrathoracic foreign bodies. *Am. J. Forensic Med. Pathol.* 2:163–74

19. Escobedo LG, Ruttenber J, Agoes MM, Anda RF, Wetli CV. 1991. Emerging patterns of cocaine use and the epidemic of cocaine overdose deaths in Dade County, Florida. *Arch. Pathol. Lab. Med.* 115:900–5

20. Falch GA. 1993. Postmarketing surveillance: beyond MedWatch. *JAMA* 270:2180

21. Food and Drug Admin. 1993. MedWatch: the FDA Medical Products Reporting Program. *FDA Med. Bull.* 23. Rockville, MD: FDA

22. Gaffney BP. 1993. Use of coroner's reports for surveillance of accidental death. *J. Public Health Med.* 15:272–76

23. Graitcer PL, Williams WW, Finton RJ, Goodman RA, Thacker SB, Hanzlick R. 1987. An evaluation of the use of medical examiner data for epidemiologic surveillance. *Am. J. Public Health* 77:1212–14

24. Hanzlick R. 1988. Death certificates, natural death, and alcohol. *Am. J. Forensic Med. Pathol.* 9:149–50

25. Hanzlick R. 1993. Misclassification of deaths caused by cocaine: further discussion and possible solution for death certification. *Am. J. Forensic Med. Pathol.* 14:351–52

26. Hanzlick R. 1994. Survey of medical examiner office computerization. *Am. J. Forensic Med. Pathol.* 15:110–17

27. Hanzlick R, Combs D, Parrish RG, Ing RT. 1993. Death investigation in the United States, 1990: a survey of statutes, systems, and educational requirements. *J. Forensic Sci.* 38:628–32

28. Hanzlick R, Frost J, Bennett T. 1986. Pediatric toxicology registry. *Am. J. Forensic Med. Pathol.* 7:256–57

29. Hanzlick R, Gowitt G. 1991. Cocaine metabolite detection in homicide victims. *JAMA* 265:760–61

30. Hanzlick R, Parrish RG. 1993. Classifying unspecified and/or unexplained causes of death [letter]. *Am. J. Public Health* 83:1490–91

31. Hanzlick R, Parrish RG. 1993. Deaths among the homeless in Fulton County, Georgia 1988–90. *Public Health Rep.* 108:488–91

32. Hanzlick R, Parrish RG. 1994. Standard language in death investigation laws. *J. Forensic Sci.* 38:628–32

33. Hanzlick R, Parrish RG. 1994. Death investigation report forms (DIRFs): generic forms for investigators (IDIRFs) and certifiers (CDIRFs). *J. Forensic Sci.* 39:629–36

34. Hanzlick R, Parrish RG, Ing RT. 1993. Features of commercial computer software systems for medical examiners and coroners. *Am. J. Forensic Med. Pathol.* 14:334–39

35. Hanzlick R, Sperry K. 1990. Maternal deaths in Fulton County, Georgia. 1988–89. *Atlanta Med.* 64:19–23

36. Harris CS, Baker SP, Smith GA, Harris RM. 1984. Childhood asphyxiation by food: a national analysis and overview. *JAMA* 251:2231–35

37. Iyasu S, Hanzlick R, Rowley D, Willinger M. 1994. Proc. Workshop Guidel. Scene Invest. Sudden Unexplained Infant Deaths—July 12–13, 1993. *J. Forensic Sci.* 39:1126–36

38. Jason D. 1994. *A survey of medical examiner/coroner HIV testing.* Presented at Annu. Meet. Natl. Assoc. Med. Exam., 27th, Charleston

39. Jordan JM, Bass MJ. 1993. Errors in death certificate completion in a teaching hospital. *Clin. Invest. Med.* 16:249–55

40. Jumbelic MI, Chambliss M. 1990. Accidental toddler drowning in 5-gallon buckets. *JAMA* 263:1952–53

41. Kaplan JA, Hanzlick R. 1995. The di-

agnosis of sudden infant death syndrome: medical examiner practices and attitudes. *Proc. Am. Acad. Forensic Sci., 47th, Seattle,* pp. 135–36. Colorado Springs: Am. Acad. Forensic Sci.

42. Kendall IG, Wynn SM, Quinton DN. 1993. A study of patients referred from A&E for coroner's postmortem. *Arch. Emerg. Med.* 10:86–90

43. King GS, Smialek JE, Troutman WG. 1985. Sudden death in adolescents resulting from the inhalation of typewriter correction fluid. *JAMA* 253:1604–6

44. Kleinbaum DG, Kupper LL, Morgenstein H. 1982. *Epidemiologic Research,* p. 21. New York: Van Nostrand

45. Kung HC, Spitler J. 1995. Contributing factors and methods of violent death. *Proc. Am. Acad. Forensic Sci., 47th, Seattle,* p. 126. Colorado Springs: Am. Acad. Forensic Sci.

46. Lantz PE, McFeeley PJ, Parrish RG, Maes EF. 1993. *Manner of death certification in Russian Roulette deaths.* Presented at Annu. Meet. Am. Acad. Forensic Sci., 45th, Boston

47. Lerer LB, Meyers JE. 1994. Application of two secondary documentary sources to identify the under reporting of fatal occupational injuries in Cape Town, South Africa. *Am. J. Ind. Med.* 26:521–27

48. Linakis JG, Frederick KA. 1993. Poisoning deaths not reported to the regional poison control center. *Ann. Emerg. Med.* 22:1822–28

49. Natl. Assoc. Med. Exam. 1987. *Standards for Inspection and Accreditation of a Modern Medicolegal Investigative System.* St. Louis, MO. 28 pp.

50. Natl. Assoc. Med. Exam. 1994. Operational guidelines for determination of injury at work. *NAME NEWS,* 2:3:3. St. Louis, MO

51. Natl. Assoc. Med. Exam. 1994. The medical examiner and public health: an example. *NAME NEWS* 2:6. St. Louis, MO

52. Natl. Assoc. Med. Exam. 1994. Information Resources Guide for Medical Examiners, Coroners, and Medicolegal Death Investigators. *NAME NEWS* 2 (6):2. St. Louis, MO

53. Natl. Highway Traffic Safety Admin. 1991. *Fatal Accident Reporting System 1989.* Washington, DC: US DOT. DOT Doc. HS 807 693

54. Natl. Inst. Occup. Safety & Health. 1993. *Fatal Occupational Injuries to Workers in the United States, 1980–1989: A Decade of Surveillance.* Cincinnati, OH. DHHS (NIOSH) No. 93–108

55. Nelson DE, Sacks JJ, Parrish RG, Sosin DM, McFeeley P, Smith SM. 1993. *Sensitivity of Multiple-Cause Mortality Data for Surveillance of Deaths Associated with Head or Neck Injuries.* Morbid. Mortal. Wkly. Rep. CDC Surveill. Summ. 42 (SS-5):29–35

56. Parrish RG. 1995. Assessing and improving the quality of data from medical examiners and coroners. *Proc. Int. Collab. Effort Injury Stat., Vol. 1.* Bethesda, MD: Natl. Cent. Health Stat. (DHHS Publ. No. PHS 95–1252)

57. Pearson VA. 1993. Suicide in North and West Devon: a comparative study using coroner's inquest records. *J. Public Health Med.* 15:320–26

58. Pollock DA, Holmgreen P, Lui KJ, Kirk ML. 1991. Discrepancies in the reported frequency of cocaine-related deaths, United States, 1983 through 1988. *JAMA* 266:2233–37

59. Pollock DA, O'Neil JM, Parrish RG, Combs DL, Annest JL. 1993. Temporal and geographic trends in the autopsy frequency of blunt and penetrating trauma deaths in the United States. *JAMA* 269:1525–31

60. Prahlow JA, Lantz PE. 1995. Medical examiner/death investigator training requirements in state medical examiner systems. *J. Forensic Sci.* 40:55–58

61. Public Health Service. 1950. History and organization of the vital statistics system. *Vital Stat. US* 1:1–19

62. Rainey DY, Runyon CW. 1992. Newspapers: a source for injury surveillance? *Am. J. Public Health* 82:745–46

63. Romano PS, McLoughlin E. 1992. Unspecified injuries on death certificates: a source of bias in injury research. *Am. J. Epidemiol.* 136:863–72

64. Runyan CW, Loomis D, Butts J. 1994. Practices of county medical examiners in classifying deaths as on the job. *J. Occup. Med.* 36:36–41

65. Russell J, Conroy C. 1991. Representativeness of deaths identified through the injury-at-work item on the death certificate: implications for surveillance. *Am. J. Public Health* 81:1613–18

66. Rutstein DD, Mullan RJ, Frazier TM, Halperin WE, Melius JM, Sestito JP. 1983. Sentinel health events (occupational): a basis for physician recognition and public health surveillance. *Am. J. Public Health* 73:1054–62

67. Siminovis NJ, Wells CK, Feinstein AR. 1991. In-vivo and post-mortem gallstones: support for validity of the epidemiologic necropsy screening technique. *Am. J. Epidemiol.* 133:922–31

68. Smith S. 1995. The need for death investigator training. *Am. J. Forensic Med. Pathol.* 16:181
69. Smith SM, Middaugh JP. 1986. Injuries associated with three-wheeled all-terrain vehicles Alaska, 1983–1984. *JAMA* 255:2454–58
70. Smith SM, Middaugh JP. 1989. An assessment of potential injury surveillance data sources in Alaska using an emerging problem: all-terrain vehicle-associated injuries. *Public Health Rep.* 104:493–98
71. Sniezek JE, Horiagon TM. 1989. Medical-examiner-reported fatal occupational injuries, North Carolina, 1978–1984. *Am. J. Ind. Med.* 15:669–78
72. Soslow AR, Woolf AD. 1992. Reliability of data sources for poisoning deaths in Massachusetts. *Am. J. Emerg. Med.* 10:124–27
73. Stanbury M, Goldloft M. 1990. Use of OSHA inspections data for fatal occupational injury surveillance in New Jersey. *Am. J. Public Health* 80:200–2
74. Stout N, Bell N. 1991. Effectiveness of source documents for identifying fatal occupational injuries: a synthesis of studies. *Am. J. Public Health* 81:725–28
75. Stroup NE, Zack MM, Wharton M. 1994. Sources of routinely collected data for surveillance. See Ref. 78, 3:31–85
76. Substance Abuse and Mental Health Serv. Admin. 1995. *Annual Medical Examiner Data, 1993*, p. 82. DHHS Publ. No. (SMA) 95–3019. Rockville, MD: Substance Abuse Mental Health Serv. Admin.
77. Teutsch SM. 1994. Considerations in planning a surveillance system. See Ref. 78, 2:18–30
78. Teutsch SM, Churchill RE, eds. 1994. *Principles and Practice of Public Health Surveillance.* New York/Oxford: Oxford Univ. Press. 274 pp.
79. Thacker SB. 1994. Historical development. See Ref. 78, pp. 1:3–17
80. Voelker R. 1995. More expertise needed in death investigations. *JAMA* 273:1164–65
81. Vogt CL. 1994. Adverse drug reactions: getting information back from MedWatch [letter]. *JAMA* 272:590
82. Ward R. 1988. *The registry of anesthesia deaths: started and in first gear.* Presented at Annu. Meet. Natl. Assoc. Med. Exam., 21st, Boston
83. White RD. 1993. Maintenance of defibrillators in a state of readiness. *Ann. Emerg. Med.* 22:302–6
84. Wysowski DK, Green L. 1995. Serious adverse events in Norplant users reported to the Food and Drug Administration's MedWatch Spontaneous Reporting System. *Obstet. Gynecol.* 85:538–42
85. Young TW, Pollock DA. 1993. Misclassification of deaths caused by cocaine: an assessment by survey. *Am. J. Forensic Med. Pathol.* 14:43–47

Annu. Rev. Public Health. 1996. 17:411–48

RACIAL DIFFERENCES IN HEALTH: Not Just Black and White, But Shades of Gray[1]

Marsha Lillie-Blanton[1,2], P. Ellen Parsons[1,3], Helene Gayle[4], and Anne Dievler[1]

[1]School of Hygiene and Public Health, The Johns Hopkins University, 624 North Broadway, Baltimore, Maryland 21205; [2]Kaiser Commission on the Future of Medicaid, 1450 G Street, N.W., Suite 250, Washington, D.C. 20005,[3]National Center for Health Statistics, 3700 East-West Highway, Hyattsville, Maryland 20782; [4]National Center for HIV, STD, and TB Prevention, Centers for Disease Prevention and Control, 1600 Clifton Road NE, E07, Atlanta, Georgia 30333

ABSTRACT

Explanations for racial/ethnic disparities in health are varied and complex. This paper reviews the literature to assess the extent to which current disparities are a consequence of racial differences in the social class composition of the US population. We focus this review on African Americans and examine studies that provide information on the effects of race on four outcome measures: infant mortality, hypertension, substance use, and mortality from all-causes. Twenty-three studies were identified that met criteria for inclusion in this review. As expected, most studies provide evidence that socioeconomic conditions are a major factor explaining racial differences in health. Findings, however, vary for the different health indices. Research in the area of substance abuse provides the most consistent evidence that socioeconomic conditions account for observed racial differences. In contrast, studies on infant mortality and hypertension provide a compelling case that the effects of socioeconomic status are important, but not sufficient to explain racial differences. Evidence on mortality from all-causes is equally divided between studies showing no significant race effect and those in which racial differences persist after adjusting for social class. The paper offers possible explanations for the seemingly divergent results and identifies conceptual and methodologic issues for future research seeking to disentangle the complex relations between race, social class, and health.

Introduction

Despite substantial gains in the health of racial and ethnic minority populations in the United States, large disparities persist in morbidity and mortality

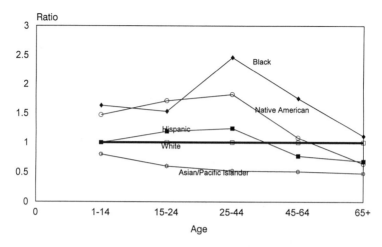

SOURCE: DHHS. Health United States, 1990.

Figure 1   Ratio of minority-white death rates, 1988

(USDHHS 1985). More disturbing is the fact that for some health indicators, the magnitude of the disparity has changed little or has widened in the last decade (20, 41). The most recently available mortality data by race and ethnicity provide evidence that three of the four largest U.S. racial/ethnic minority groups (i.e. African-Americans, Hispanics, and Native Americans) continue to experience poorer health outcomes when compared to whites under age 45 (see Figure 1 above).[2] Explanations for racial/ethnic disparities in health are varied and complex. Among the more frequently advanced hypotheses are that there are racial differences in life-style behaviors, use of medical care, and exposure to socio-environmental risk factors such as poverty.

This paper reviews evidence about the extent to which two factors—racial/ethnic status and social class—influence the poorer health outcomes of minority populations. Disentangling the influence of race/ethnic status and social class on health outcomes is a challenge for many reasons. Health statistics are routinely presented by race and ethnicity without adjustments for social class differences that could affect the comparisons. These comparisons (sometimes called descriptive statistics) provide insight on a population group

[2]In U.S. Census and survey data, individuals are generally asked to report their race as: white; black; Asian or Pacific Islander; Aleut, Eskimo, American Indian; or other. In another question information on Hispanic ethnic origin is asked. Persons of Hispanic origin may be of any of the racial categories.

as a whole. They are particularly useful in answering the question: "What is occurring?" Descriptive statistics, however, can be misleading if the primary question of interest is: "Why are the observed patterns occurring?"

The practice of reporting unadjusted descriptive statistics by race is commonplace and has led many to question whether current racial disparities in health are a consequence of higher poverty rates among minority populations rather than race-specific barriers in society. To some extent, this distinction may be artificial since racial/ethnic barriers have contributed to economic inequalities that have had implications from generation to generation. Nonetheless, more precise knowledge of the specific role played by inequalities related to race/ethnicity and economic circumstances should help in directing resources to target particular factors that contribute to disparities in health.

Scope of This Review: What is the Question?

This review evaluates current research to assess whether racial/ethnic disparities in health are explained by social class differences in the population groups. We examine the literature on "health outcomes" rather than "health care use." As such, the intent is to assess measures of functioning and quality of life. It is recognized that a population's health is related to health care use, particularly for those conditions in which effective preventive techniques or treatments are available. However, an assessment that includes health care use as an outcome or as a mediating factor is a distinct subject of inquiry that is beyond the scope of this review.

By the 1960s, national and international research had begun to focus attention on economic status and its relation to health (13, 17). Moreover, there is now a considerable body of evidence that social class position (as variously defined by measures of income, education, or occupation) is inversely related to health[3]. In the landmark study by Kitagawa & Hauser (17), the association between socioeconomic status and mortality was found to be as consistent for nonwhites as for whites. However, the authors acknowledge that at this point in history, there was barely sufficient variation in the social strata of minority populations to adequately assess the effects of social class differences among nonwhites. The study also did not disaggregate data for specific nonwhite population groups, resulting in conclusions about all nonwhites who, even then, were a heterogenous mix.[4]

---

[3]Although much of the research does not provide evidence of a causal relationship, there is ample evidence of a strong association. Stated in the extremes, persons in the lower social class groups have higher mortality rates and those in the upper social class groups have lower mortality rates.

[4]It is, however, known that about 75% of nonwhites during that era of U.S. history were black Americans.

This article begins with two basic assumptions. First, the authors acknowledge that social class and health status are inversely related. Second, the authors recognize that African Americans, Hispanics, and Native Americans are disproportionately represented among the poor and near-poor[5]. It is, therefore, not only conceivable but highly probable that a larger share of minority than nonminority Americans are in poorer health.

Thus, the question is *not whether* social class is related to the health of minority populations but *how much* of the poorer health of minority populations is attributable to an individual's social class position. Sometimes the question is framed in the extremes of is the problem one of race *or* class. Conceptualization of the question in the absolute fails to acknowledge the link between two factors that, throughout American history, have been very much intertwined. It also does not consider the gradients that may occur depending on factors such as age cohort, geographic place of residence, or family social support systems.

From an assessment of prior reviews on the subject (10, 28, 30, 32, 50), we also concluded that a study approach is needed that permits an appraisal of the evidence for specific population groups and health conditions. The diversity within and across U.S. racial/ethnic population groups and the multiple factors that affect a population's health make it difficult to summarize the current state of knowledge without a more focused approach. Focusing the scope of this review also helps to avoid forming conclusions that apply to one but not the other minority group or health condition.

Methods

This paper examines evidence from studies that compare the risk of certain outcomes for persons exposed to similar social conditions (as measured by social class) but who differ by race. The term risk is used broadly to include studies of incidence or prevalence of the outcome. The review focuses on an assessment of evidence for African Americans, a choice reflecting the experience of the authors as well as the limited data and research on the other minority populations. In addition, the review is limited to studies of overall mortality and several selected health conditions—hypertension, infant mortality, and substance abuse. The three conditions were selected because they contribute substantially to excess premature mortality among African Americans and they are conditions for which the authors perceived themselves to be sufficiently knowledgeable to evaluate the literature. Two of the conditions, hypertension and substance abuse, are health outcomes as well as risk factors

[5]Racial/ethnic status, however, is not synonymous with social class even though researchers sometimes use race as a proxy for lower socioeconomic status.

for several leading causes of death. They are included in this review as outcome measures with the intent of identifying studies that have assessed whether race-specific factors influence their prevalence.

Findings were selected for inclusion in the review if the study (*a*) analyzed person-specific data collected after 1970 on a predominantly nonelderly sample population; (*b*) explicitly stated intent to examine the health outcomes of at least whites and African Americans; and (*c*) methodologically or statistically controlled for social class differences of the population groups. Although recent literature has criticized the measurement of both race/ethnicity and social class in health-related studies (16, 38, 50), an assessment of how well these variables were measured was not a selection criterion. Social class could have been defined using commonly used indicators of socioeconomic status or by indices such as the Hollingshead's Four Factor Index of Social Status (13). Race could have been defined as self-report or observation of racial identity using any of the commonly accepted identifiers for blacks and whites. As a consequence, reported classifications of race and social class are similar but not necessarily identical. This review reports on the study findings using the varying terminology of the studies' authors.

To identify published articles on the subject, several approaches were used. First, the references of frequently cited articles were reviewed (10, 31, 49). Second, we searched for articles in the Medline (1976–1995) database that addressed race/ethnicity, socioeconomic status (SES), and health status (including mortality and morbidity)[6]. A total of 1204 articles were retrieved in this search. Many of these articles examined the impact of race and SES on health status separately. A much smaller subset were articles where the authors examined the impact of race on health status, controlling for socioeconomic status. This smaller subset of articles was included in our review.

A Review and Critique of the Empirical Evidence

Few studies have empirically examined the influence of both race and class on health outcomes in the United States. Studies meeting criteria for this review are briefly described in Appendices 1–4, with an appendix devoted to each outcome measure. Twenty-three studies were identified: Eight provide information on infant mortality; four on hypertension; five on substance abuse; and six on mortality from all causes. A synthesis of key findings from these studies is presented in the following sections of the paper along with tables presenting data from selected studies that help illuminate key or unexpected findings.

---

[6]Medline gives references to more than 4000 professional and scholarly journals. Compiled by the National Library of Medicine, it is the electronic version of the print Index Medicus, the Index to Dental Literature, and the International Nursing Index.

rtality

__.cial disparities in pregnancy outcomes are the most well documented and troubling of disparities in health. Concerns have prompted research by leading maternal and child health epidemiologists and health services researchers in the nation (37). Despite an extensive body of research, factors contributing to twofold differences in the infant mortality rates of African Americans and whites remain poorly understood. Particularly disturbing is that after comparable declines in black and white infant mortality rates between 1966 and 1981, evidence is now emerging that the racial gap is widening (41).

Much of the excess in infant mortality among African Americans has been attributed to higher rates of low birthweight (LBW) infants and premature births. This review article, therefore, identified studies of racial differences in either infant mortality, LBW, or prematurity. Appendix 1 includes eight studies that investigated one or a combination of pregnancy outcomes while holding constant socioeconomic characteristics of the study population. Five of the studies examined racial differences in infant mortality and three focused on LBW and/or prematurity. The studies represent a diversity of national and local sample populations, including two of military populations, and one of college graduates.

Four of the five studies of infant mortality (1a, 22, 39, 41) found higher mortality rates among African American than white women of a similar social strata. Krieger et al (22) and Singh & Yu (41) analyzed vital records using national linked birth and infant death files. Schoendorf et al (39) examined pregnancy outcomes of college graduates while also holding constant sociodemographic factors (maternal age, marital status, and parity) and prenatal care. Alexander et al (1a) compared infant outcomes of military personnel stationed in Hawaii. It is worthwhile to note that while the study by Alexander et al (1a) found racial differences in infant mortality, it did not find racial differences in neonatal (first 28 days) mortality. Similar mortality rates of infants during the neonatal period may reflect comparable access to hospital care shared by military personnel. Only the study by Rawlings & Weir (35) found no significant difference in the infant mortality rate for blacks and whites of comparable social position. Blacks, however, had a higher incidence of low birthweight infants. Rawlings & Weir (35) examined the birth outcomes of dependents of military personnel stationed in Washington state between 1985 and 1990.

Studies in Appendix 1, which report findings on low birthweight and prematurity, offer convincing but conflicting evidence on the extent to which racial differences in social class account for racial disparities. Analyses by Starfield et al (43) and by Kleinman & Kessel (19) provide evidence from national data sources that racial differences in LBW infants persist among

Table 1 Relative likelihood of low birth weight by race and poverty status using three poverty measures: 1979–1988[a]

	Odds ratios (blacks vs whites)[b]		
	Poverty status in year of sample selection	Poverty status in year pregnancy began	Poverty pattern
Poor	1.12	1.33	1.50
Non poor	2.03*	2.29*	1.96*

* 95% confidence interval showed a statistically significant effect.

[a] As reported in Starfield et al (43).

[b] Based on logistic regression analysis. Adjusted for mother's education, age of mother (continuous), age of mother by poverty (categorical), marital status, smoking, and interaction of race and poverty.

Data Source: National Longitudinal Survey of Labor Market Experience of Youth, 1979–1988.

women of a similar social strata. Moreover, and contrary to what one might predict, these studies provide evidence that racial differences are larger among women perceived to be at lower risk for poor outcomes.

Starfield et al's (43) study is unique in its assessment of the impact of three measures of poverty on birth outcomes using a longitudinal data set. Outcomes were assessed for women who were poor: (a) in the year of the selection of the sample, an indicator of the women's economic status when almost all were teenagers; (b) in the year the pregnancy began; and (c) over a pattern of years, an indicator of their economic status during most of the years of the study (1979–1988). For poor women, there was no statistically significant racial difference in the likelihood of a low birthweight infant regardless of the poverty measure (see Table 1). Among the nonpoor, however, the likelihood of a low birthweight infant was significantly higher for black compared to white women.

In contrast, analyzing a hospital-based cohort of women in Boston, Lieberman et al (24) provide compelling evidence that socioeconomic and medical risk factors explain racial differences in premature birth. The study makes an important contribution to the field, in part because of its systematic assessment of the effects of known medical as well as socioeconomic risk factors. Lieberman et al (24) found that maternal anemia (or some related factor) accounted for 60% of the racial difference in LBW and that 40% of the racial difference was a result of socioeconomic factors (see Table 2).

Although racial disparities were reduced when stratifying by a measure of social class, significant racial differences persisted in most of the studies cited in this review. Some would argue that the literature on pregnancy outcomes is, at best, inconclusive. Nonetheless, it is noteworthy that several

Table 2 Relative likelihood of prematurity by race, the economic, demographic and behavioral (EDB) variable, and hematocrit[a]

Model	Odds ratio for prematurity
Race[b]	1.94
Model	
Race	1.38
Hematocrit (1 point change)[c]	1.23
Model	
Race	1.22
EDB Variable[d]	1.52
Model	
Race	1.03
EDB Variable	1.31
Hematocrit (1 point change)	1.22

[a] As reported in Lieberman et al (24)

[b] Reference category: white

[c] Hematocrit was used as a continuous variable in the model.

[d] The EDB variable is defined as the number (zero, one, or two or more) of the following factors present: age <20 years, single marital status, having less than a high school education, and receiving welfare support.

Data source: originally collected data from women giving birth in a Boston, MA, hospital.

well-designed studies provide strong evidence that socioeconomic position, as currently measured, does not fully explain higher rates of problematic birth outcomes among African American compared to white women.

Hypertension

Race differences in the prevalence of hypertension have been well-documented in the public health literature (2, 14, 18, 40, 48). Results from the Third National Health and Nutrition Examination Survey conducted from 1988–1991 confirm these long-standing disparities. According to these data, which are presented in Table 3, the age-adjusted prevalence of hypertension among non-Hispanic African Americans is nearly 10 percentage points higher than among non-Hispanic white Americans (5). The magnitude of the differential is similar for both men and women, though rates are higher for men generally.

The four studies cited in Appendix 2 include both racial groups in their study samples and consider the contribution of at least one measure of social class to race differences in hypertension. One of the studies is limited to men (46), one includes only women (1), and two include both men and women (15, 47).

Table 3 Prevalence of hypertension in US adult population by race and sex[a]

	Age-adjusted percent (SE)[b]	Estimated population (SE)
		(000s)
<u>Non-Hispanic black</u>	32.4 (1.1)	5672 (427)
Men	34.0 (1.6)	2664 (209)
Women	31.0 (1.0)	3008 (252)
<u>Non-Hispanic white</u>	23.3 (0.7)	34,697 (2746)
Men	25.4 (1.2)	17,259 (1642)
Woman	21.0 (0.9)	17,438 (1334)

[a] As reported in Burt et al (5)
[b] Age-adjusted to the 1990 US civilian, noninstitutionalized population.
Data source: Third National Health and Nutrition Examination Survey (NHANES III) conducted during 1988 to 1991.

In an effort to replicate earlier findings among a sample of African-American men only (14), James et al (15) determined that socioeconomic status[7] and John Henryism[8] interact to influence the risk for hypertension among blacks (both men and women). James et al studied adults in one county in North Carolina who participated in an evaluation of a community-based high blood pressure control program. The strongest association between socioeconomic status and the prevalence of hypertension was found among black men of lower socioeconomic status and high levels of John Henryism. Black men with high levels of John Henryism and high socioeconomic status exhibited low prevalence of hypertension, as shown in Table 4. Although white men scored higher on the John Henryism scale than did white women, no relationship was found between higher levels of John Henryism and higher rates of hypertension.

These findings illustrate how socially distributed personal characteristics, like John Henryism, interact with social attributes, such as race, class, and gender, to influence the prevalence of disease (hypertension) in different racial groups. The existence of such socially distributed characteristics that affect health may be but one of many mechanisms through which the health effects of race and social class are expressed.

[7]In this study, socioeconomic status was measured separately for the two racial groups using race-specific categories constructed by combining measures of education (years) and occupation. The construction of race-specific categories represents an innovative approach to measuring social class that takes into account differences in the historical experience of whites and blacks in the United States as well as contemporary differences in the practical meaning of social class gradations in black vs white communities.

[8]John Henryism refers to "strong personality predisposition to cope actively with psychosocial stressors in one's environment" and is measured by The John Henryism Scale for Active Coping, a 12-item Likert scale.

Table 4 Adjusted[a] prevalence of hypertension[b] for four socioeconomic status (SES)[c] John Henryism[d] groups, by race, Edgecombe County, NC, 1983[e]

	Blacks	Whites
	Percent hypertensive	
Low John Henryism		
Low SES	25.0	13.4
High SES	23.4	8.7
High John Henryism		
Low SES	31.4	10.1
High SES	11.5	17.8

[a] Adjusted for age, sex, age*sex, and Quetelet index (weight/height²).

[b] Hypertension = mean of the diastolic pressure ≥ 90mm Hg or currently taking antihypertensive medication.

[c] Low SES, blacks: < 9 years of education or low blue-collar job; high SES, blacks: ≥ 9 years of education and high blue-collar or white-collar job; low SES, whites: <12 years of education or blue-collar job; high SES, whites: ≥12 years of education and white-collar job.

[d] Low John Henryism ≤ 53; high John Henryism ≥ 54.

[e] As reported by James et al (15).

Data Source: originally collected data on adults in 5 townships of Edgecomb Co., NC.

The higher prevalence of hypertension among blacks in the United States leads to increased risk for more serious conditions subsequent to hypertension. Whittle et al (47) address these racial disparities in a study of end-stage renal disease (ESRD). They report that ESRD and renal failure secondary to

Table 5 Hypertensive status of women in Massachusetts by education and race[a]

	Blacks	Whites
	Percent hypertensive	
Education in years		
Less than 12	54.8	23.5
12	32.9	19.0
More than 12	19.0	16.3

[a] As reported in Adams-Campbell et al (1).

Note: Hypertension was self-reported and included both treated and untreated hypertension.

Data Source: originally collected data from women selected randomly from 38 cities/towns in Massachusetts.

hypertension (HT-ESRD) are nearly fourfold and eightfold higher, respectively, among blacks than among whites. The purpose of their study was to determine whether the association between race and the incidence of HT-ESRD persists after adjusting for a number of risk factors, including socioeconomic status.

Using population-based mean group estimates, the incidence of HT-ESRD was 58% higher in areas where less than two thirds of the residents had completed high school compared with areas with a similar, but more educated population. However, the overall relative risk of HT-ESRD remained 4.5 even when controlling for all the risk factors, including education. The study concluded that higher rates of HT-ESRD in black populations are not explained by other risk factors, though socioeconomic factors were considered important.

The deliberate study of racial differences in hypertension among women as well as men has become more common in the past 15 years (2, 9, 21, 52). The study by Adams-Campbell et al (1) included here specifically addresses socioeconomic status differences, as measured by years of education, and the independent and joint effects of race and social class on the prevalence of self-reported hypertension among middle-aged women. In this statewide study in Massachusetts, black women were twice as likely as white women to report being hypertensive. However, the prevalence of hypertension varies inversely with education for both racial groups. Although race differentials persist after controlling for education, as Table 5 indicates, the prevalence gap narrows as educational attainment increases.

In contrast to the other studies reviewed here, which seek to understand race differences in hypertension by addressing a variety of risk factors that include at least one measure of social class, Waitzman & Smith (46) specifically sought to examine how the interaction between occupational class transitions and race affects the incidence of hypertension. Using a longitudinal follow-up linked to a nationally representative sample to study the impact of different occupational behavior patterns over time, Waitzman & Smith characterized black and white men according to the relationship between their occupational class positions at baseline vs that at follow-up, a period of about ten years. The incidence of hypertension was found to be significantly associated with occupational class position and transition for both black and white men. Black and white men who remained in the lower occupational classes over the study period experienced higher rates of hypertension relative to white men who remained in the top occupational class over the same period. Blacks were more concentrated in the lower occupational classes and were less likely to move out of the lower end of the occupational matrix. Generally, the relative risk of hypertension was higher among blacks and among those in the lower occupational classes, as noted in Table 6. No significant race difference was found

Table 6 The effect of occupational class[a] transitions on the likelihood of hypertension[b] at follow-up[c]

	Black		White	
	OR[d]	95% CI	OR	95% CI
Stayed in class				
1	2.55	0.75, 8.69	1.00	. . .
2	16.31	4.18, 63.64	1.25	0.82, 1.89
3	4.91	1.83, 13.16	1.87	1.30, 268
4	4.62	2.33, 9.15	1.30	0.88, 1.92
Moved down to class				
2	**		0.75	0.39, 1.45
3	1.67[e]	0.29, 9.62	1.64	1.04, 2.60
4	9.47	2.06, 43.45	1.33	0.87, 2.03
Moved up to class				
1	6.36	0.96, 42.27	1.67	1.12, 2.47
2	1.07	0.16, 7.27	1.56	0.83, 2.91
3	14.57	2.75, 77.32	0.89	0.42, 187

Note: OR: odds ratio; Cl: confidence interval.

[a] In general, jobs in class 1 rank high in educational requirements and/or decision-making authority; jobs in class 2 rank high with respect to vocational training; jobs in class 3 rank low with respect to vocational training and/or high repetitive operations; jobs in class 4 rank very low with respect to training requirements.

[b] Includes controlled and uncontrolled hypertension. Follow-up systolic $\geq$ 140mm Hg or diastolic $\geq$ 90 mm Hg or respondent takes blood pressure medication at follow-up.

[c] As reported by Waitzman & Smith (46).

[d] Odds ratios were derived from logistic regression models that also included age, aging between baseline and follow-up exams, body mass index, alcohol use, urban residence, and hypertension. All covariate measurements were taken at baseline unless otherwise noted.

[e] Only one case in this category.

Data Source: NHANES I baseline conducted 1971–1975 and the National Health Examination Follow-up Survey (NHEFUS) conducted 1982–1984.

for blacks and whites who remained in the top occupational class over the study period.

These four studies address the question of racial differences in hypertension rates using a variety of study designs, sample populations, measures of socioeconomic status, and underlying models of the relationships among race, class, and hypertension. Nevertheless, each of these studies concludes that, although the effect of socioeconomic status is important, it is not sufficient to explain racial disparities in hypertension rates. The joint effects of socioeconomic status and race appear to be strongest among the lowest socioeconomic categories, and gaps between the races tend to be larger at the low end of the socioeconomic scale. These findings suggest that race and class interact to increase the likelihood of being hypertensive among blacks who occupy lower

Table 7 Percentage of black and white respondents reporting use of
alcohol, cigarettes, and illicit drugs: Ages 18 and older, 1991[a]

Drug measure	Race/Ethnicity	
	Blacks	Whites
Alcohol		
Nonheavy use in past month	41.3	50.2
Heavy use in past month[b]	6.0	5.7
Cigarettes		
Non heavy use in past month	19.6	10.4
Heavy use in past month[c]	11.9	18.3
Marijuana		
Non frequent use in past month	7.4	6.9
Frequent use in past month[d]	5.1	2.2
Cocaine		
Non frequent use in past year	1.9	2.3
Frequent use in past year[e]	2.3	0.6
Crack		
Any use in past year	1.5	0.3
Poly-illicit drug use		
Use of 3 or more illicit drugs in past year	1.5	1.8

[a] As reported in Flewelling et al (7).
[b] Five or more drinks on 5 or more days in the past month.
[c] Smoked a pack or more of cigarettes a day in the past month.
[d] Use once a week or more often in the past year.
[e] Use once a month or more often in the past year.
Data Source: 1991 National Household Survey of Drug Abuse.

class positions. The various directions taken by these researchers provide us
with guidance for fruitful research in the future.

Substance Abuse

Data on the use and misuse of tobacco, alcohol, and illicit drugs are routinely
collected and reported by race/ethnicity. Table 7, for example, shows that a
higher proportion of blacks than whites reported nonheavy use of cigarettes,
frequent use of marijuana and cocaine, and use of crack cocaine. Mortality
rates from alcohol-related conditions such as cirrhosis of the liver or tobacco-
related conditions such as lung cancer also are higher for African Americans
than whites. These descriptive comparisons along with arrest records, news
reports of drug-related criminal activity, and statistics on the use of publicly
financed treatment services have resulted in public perceptions that substance
use is more common among African Americans than whites.

The presentation of race-associated differences in substance use and related
problems, without adjusting for differences in socioeconomic factors that could
influence the comparison, furthers the belief that patterns of substance use are
a function of characteristics inherent to the individual or population group.

Table 8   Relative likelihood of using alcohol, cigarettes, and illicit drugs for blacks vs whites: Ages 18 to 49, 1991[a]

Drug measure	Odds ratios[b]
Alcohol	
Non heavy	0.72***
Heavy use	0.55***
Cigarettes	
Non heavy	1.21*
Heavy use	0.36***
Marijuana	
Non heavy	0.68**
Heavy use	1.29
Cocaine	
Non heavy	0.55
Heavy use	1.87*
Crack	1.87
Poly-illicit drug use	0.43***

[a] As reported in Flewelling et al (7)
[b] Adjusted for demographic, SES and social variables.
*Data Source: 1991 National Household Survey of Drug Abuse.

Theories explaining patterns of substance use generally include biomedical (e.g. genetic predisposition), social environmental factors (e.g. economic resources, availability of drugs), as well as personal behavioral characteristics (e.g. skills for coping with life stressors). Few studies, however, have controlled for differences in factors such as these when exploring racial differences in substance use and related problems.

Cited in Appendix 3 are studies that examined the association of race with measures of substance use after adjusting for the socioeconomic conditions or other factors associated with patterns of use such as age and gender. Investigating these factors individually and when combined with race provide some evidence that patterns of use are not consistent across racial groups. Three studies show a combined effect of race with a sociodemographic factor. Lillie-Blanton et al (27) found that while a similar percentage of black and white women who had not completed high school were heavy drinkers, black women with four or more years of college were less likely to be heavy drinkers than their white counterparts. Chilcoat et al (6) found crack cocaine use to be higher among African American than white males aged 30 and older. Montgomery & Carter-Pokras (30) found that black women who are pregnant are more likely to drink than white women who are pregnant.

Two of the studies (7, 25), when comparing blacks and whites of similar social conditions, provide evidence that racial identity was not independently associated with an increased risk of substance use. Flewelling et al (7) provide the most current information on racial differences in use of alcohol and other drugs based on analysis of the 1991 National Household Survey of Drug Abuse. Table 8 shows that African Americans, aged 18 to 49, generally had odds of alcohol and other drug use that were equal to or no higher than whites, after statistically controlling for demographic and socioeconomic characteristics. Of the measures of drug use examined, only the likelihood of nonfrequent cigarette use and frequent cocaine use were higher among African Americans than whites. Socio-economic variables included in the analysis were education, occupation of chief household wage earner, and household income.

All-Cause Mortality

In four of the five age groups shown in Figure 1, African Americans compared to whites had a higher risk of mortality in 1988. Studies cited in Appendix 4 provide convincing but conflicting evidence regarding the influence of race-specific factors on the higher mortality rates of African Americans. Several of the studies support theories that race-specific factors still account for some of the higher mortality; others provide evidence to the contrary.

Studies by Sorlie et al (42), Pappas et al (34), and Otten et al (33) provide evidence that race differentials are greatly reduced but *not* eliminated when controlling for a measure of social class. Both Sorlie et al (42) and Otten et al (33) test whether the differences observed between blacks and whites are statistically significant. As such, both studies provide credible evidence on the effects of race-specific factors while controlling for social class. The study undertaken by Pappas et al (34) focused on the influence of economic rather than racial inequalities on health. Thus it provides less definitive but useful information on racial differences in health.

Otten et al's (33) research is particularly noteworthy because it quantified how much of the racial difference in mortality was explained by income and several behavioral risk factors including smoking and alcohol use. Otten et al (33) found that about a third of the racial differential in mortality was left unexplained by the measures of social class or risk factors examined. This study is important because it assessed racial differences while statistically controlling the two factors most frequently cited as accounting for racial disparities in health.

Although the primary aim of the study by Pappas et al (34) was not to assess the influence of race on health, the study provided insightful information in its computation of race-specific mortality rates by two frequently used measures of social class[9]. Tables 9 and 10, derived from the study by Pappas and

---

[9]Pappas et al's (34) principal finding was that disparities by income and education persisted in the 1980s and have widened since the 1960s, for blacks and whites. For example, black males with the least income had a three- to fourfold higher risk of mortality than black males with the most income.

Table 9 Ratio of mortality rates by education and income: Women ages 25 – 64, 1986[a]

Socioeconomic indicator	Deaths per 1000		Ratio B:W
	Blacks	Whites	
Education (years)			
0 –11	6.2	3.4	1.82
12	3.9	2.5	1.56
13 –15	3.2	2.1	1.52
>16	2.2	1.8	1.22
Income ($)			
< 9000	7.6	6.5	1.17
9000 –14,999	4.5	3.4	1.32
15,000 –18,999	3.7	3.3	1.12
19,000 –24,999	2.8	3.0	.93
>25,000	2.3	1.6	1.44

[a] As reported in Pappas et al (34).
Data Source: National Mortality Followback Survey, 1986.

colleagues, present the black/white ratio of age-adjusted mortality for men and women by level of education and income. For women, there is some evidence of increasing parity at higher levels of education. Surprisingly, mortality ratios by income show that the greatest racial disparity occurs at the upper income levels ($25,000 or higher). This finding, as well as the inconsistency between

Table 10 Ratio of mortality rates by education and income: Men ages 25 – 64, 1986[a]

Socioeconomic indicator	Deaths per 1000		Ratio B:W
	Blacks	Whites	
Education (years)			
0 –11	13.4	7.6	1.76
12	8.0	4.3	1.86
13 –15	5.0	4.3	1.16
>16	6.0	2.8	2.14
Income ($)			
< 9000	19.5	16.0	1.22
9000 –14,999	10.8	10.2	1.06
15,000 –18,999	9.8	5.7	1.72
19,000 –24,999	4.7	4.6	1.02
>25,000	3.6	2.4	1.50

[a] As reported in Pappas et al (34).
Data Source: National Mortality Followback Survey, 1986.

Table 11 Relative likelihood of mortality by sociodemographic characteristics: US adults, 1986[a]

Sociodemographic		Odds Ratios		
characteristic	Model 1	Model 2	Model 3	Model 4
Demographic				
Race				
Black	1.48***	1.29***	1.17***	1.01
White	1.0	1.0	1.0	1.0
Age[b]	1.55***	1.54***	1.46***	1.48***
Sex				
Male	1.76***	2.10***	1.95***	2.16***
Female	1.0	1.0	1.0	1.0
Family status				
Marital status				
Not Married	—	1.80***	—	1.54***
Married	—	1.0	—	1.0
Family size[b]	—	1.12***	—	1.21***
Socioeconomic status				
Income[b]	—	—	0.71***	0.70***

*** $p \leq 0.001$
[a] As reported in Rogers (36).
[b] Categorical variable
— Variable not included in model
Data Source: National Institute of Health Interview Survey, 1986 and the National
Mortality Followback Survey, 1986.

the findings for two measures—income and education—that generally have
similar effects, deserve to be probed further.

In contrast, three of the studies reviewed (4a, 10, 36) provide evidence that
race differentials are eliminated when controlling for a measure of social class.
Rogers (36) assessed the influence of race within a nationally representative
sample of deaths that occurred in 1986. Studies by Haan et al (11) and by
Berkman & Breslow (4a) provide race-specific mortality rates for a cohort of
7000 adults in Alameda County, California, who were followed between 1965
and 1982. Of the three studies, Rogers' (36) findings are significant because
they can be generalized to the US population.

Using the 1986 NHIS and the 1987 NMFS, Rogers (36) assessed determinants of racial disparities in overall mortality and cause-specific mortality
(see Table 11). In four different statistical models, Rogers explored the effects
of race on overall mortality. Race-specific effects were observed in the first
three models that include varying combinations of gender, age, income, and
family characteristics (size and marital status). When both income and family
characteristics were in the same model, race ceased to have an independent
effect on overall mortality. The 48% higher odds of mortality for blacks

compared to whites, which was found when holding only age and gender constant, was reduced to near equal odds of mortality. Race, however, continued to be associated with several cause-specific mortality rates when adjusting for socioeconomic status[10].

Studies of all-cause mortality give qualitatively different results on the effects of race—a perplexing but understandable finding given the limited research in this area. The opposite findings may, in part, be a consequence of studies varying in their definitions and precision of measuring race and social class. They may also be due to differences in the study populations (e.g. age distributions) or analytic techniques. Further research is needed to disentangle the influence of these and other factors. It is therefore fair to conclude that despite the existence of a number of well-designed studies, the effects of race on overall mortality remain unclear.

Discussion

A small, but growing, number of researchers are now investigating and providing insight on the complex relationships between race, social class, and health. Disproportionately high rates of poverty among minority Americans have led many to assume that racial differences in social class account for persistent racial disparities in health. Empirical research examining this explanation as well as other hypotheses, however, has been limited to date. From this review of selected studies and health indices, several observations can be drawn.

Summary and Analysis of Key Findings

Most of the studies in this review provided strong evidence that socioeconomic conditions are a major factor explaining racial differentials in the health indices examined. When comparing African Americans and whites of a similar social stratum, differentials are less than when data are not stratified or adjusted for social class position. However, the extent to which social class indicators explain racial disparities apparently varies for specific health outcomes. This suggests that generalizations across health conditions as well as racial/ethnic groups should be made cautiously. Evidence that racial differences are explained primarily by socioeconomic conditions is strongest for substance use and abuse. In contrast, studies of infant mortality and hypertension provide compelling evidence that racial disparities are *not* primarily explained by social class indicators. Evidence on all-cause mortality was equally divided between

---

[10]Blacks had higher mortality risk from infectious diseases, homicide, and diabetes; lower mortality risk from respiratory disease, accidents, and suicide; and same mortality risk from circulatory diseases and cancer.

studies that found that racial differences were eliminated and those showing that racial differences remained when adjusting for social class indicators.

Studies that examined racial disparities in pregnancy outcomes and hypertension are perplexing, but consistent in several aspects. Most of the studies do not conclude that racial disparities are fully explained by differences in socioeconomic status. Rather, the studies maintain that race differences persist when social class is taken into account. Studies provide evidence that racial differences in the rate of hypertension are greater among those in lower socioeconomic positions, whether measured by education and/or occupation. Studies of infant outcomes provide evidence that racial disparities persist within each social stratum, but are most pronounced for women in higher socioeconomic positions.

Several studies cited in this review provide evidence that, in the current historical period, the effects of race are not consistent across social strata. In the early part of the 20th century, the effect of race on one's quality of life was fairly uniform, resulting in the vast majority of African Americans being impoverished and in poorer health. Today, one would expect that discrimination based on income and race would translate into low-income African Americans having worse health outcomes relative to low-income whites. Surprisingly, however, racial disparities were found to be less dramatic among the poor than the nonpoor when examining data for all causes (34) and infant outcomes (22, 43). If an accurate reflection of racial disparities in these outcomes, it is an indication that this nation may have achieved greater progress in reducing inequalities among lower income than higher income individuals. It suggests that social welfare programs in health and income maintenance, at minimum, may have prevented poor blacks from doing any worse than poor whites.

For those studies finding a persistence of racial disparities, some possible explanations are explored. For example, it is suggested that racial differences in hypertension may be related to stressors (e.g. at work, home, family) that are not captured well by existing measurement tools. Racial differences in nutritional intake, sexual activity, and intergenerational factors (e.g. the accumulation of wealth or health deficits) are among the factors noted as deserving to be explored as determinants of racial differences in pregnancy outcomes. Research by LaVeist (23), which showed that the black-white gap in infant mortality was greater in more highly segregated cities, broadens the framework of conceivable explanatory variables to the social context of people's lives and neighborhoods.

Of concern is that most of the studies examined for this review have sought to explain differential rates by race mainly in terms of differences in biological, psychosocial, or socioeconomic risk factors at the individual level. In recent years, these risk factors are coming to be understood in the context of the larger social structure and the physical environment engendered by that structure (4, 22, 26, 50). The studies reviewed here confirm that racial differences both modify and are modified by social class differences. It is, therefore, important to develop an approach to studying racial differences that examines the broader social environment from which the meaning and implication of one's race and social class are derived. Taken together, these studies suggest that there are many mechanisms through which the health effects of race and social class are expressed.

Directions for Future Research

The development of knowledge on the effects of race and social class on health has been hampered by the limited pool of researchers interested in the area and the underdevelopment of the methodologic tools for research in this area. While it is generally assumed that peer-reviewed research findings are accurate and not primarily a function of how variables are measured or analyzed, this is not a wise assumption to make when examining studies on the health effects of race and social class. The methods and analytic tools used in research on these issues are relatively young in development and there is little agreement on the "gold standards."

The paucity of research in this area is related to the complexity of the issues as well as historical differences about the meaning and implications of the terms race and social class. Perceptions of racial classifications as primarily measures of biologic or innate characteristics have resulted in the exclusion of minority populations from epidemiologic studies because race was viewed as a confounding factor. Other researchers presume that minority status can be equated with lower socioeconomic status and fail to undertake analyses to disentangle the independent effects of each factor. Finally, few researchers systematically investigate the social dimensions of race, which for minority Americans include subtle and overt forms of racial discrimination and their implications for health.

Measurement of social class has been similarly affected by conflicting perceptions of the meaning and interpretation of the term. Perceptions of the United States as a "classless society" or as a society where there is considerable mobility across economic strata have resulted in a predominant research culture that gives little thought to the influence of social class divisions on health. Epidemiologic studies typically include measures of income, education, and occupation as indicators of social class position. While there are general concerns about the use of these measures to define an individual's social class position in society, there are specific concerns about how well these indicators measure the social class position of African Americans. For example, there is considerable evidence that racial differences in family wealth are not captured well by measures of family income. Krieger et al (22) also criticized some of the assumptions that undergird the most commonly used approaches to studying the effects of race and social class. One assumption criticized by Krieger et al (22) is that blacks and whites overlap sufficiently in socioeconomic positions to permit use of statistical adjustment techniques.

Quantifying the independent and combined influence of race and social class on health is a challenge. Nonetheless, it is important to acknowledge the complexity of the issue and to develop a study approach that allows for evaluating the many factors that potentially interact to influence the relationship between race, social class, and health. For example, researchers studying racial/ethnic disparities in health should:

- Collect data or develop methodologic approaches that will permit an assessment of factors for which racial/ethnic status commonly is used as a proxy (such as social class, culture, attitudes, biomedical factors);
- Develop conceptual models for studying the influence of race that are interactive with other social factors (e.g. consider race as a marker for exposure to racism or to social conditions at work or in one's neighborhood; consider links between occupation and the dynamic qualities of one's work experience);
- Develop the methodologic tools for studying measures of social class that extend beyond individual indicators of social status to measures of social environmental conditions of life (e.g. access to good schools, employment in satisfying jobs, opportunities, and choices) and of family wealth (such as home ownership, savings, and other assets).

Additionally, when race-associated differences are observed, researchers should vigorously investigate potential explanations. This will require seeking out expertise knowledgeable of the racial/ethnic population studied and others skilled in using sophisticated analytic strategies. For example, researchers should consider:

- statistically testing whether the effects of race are consistent across demographic and socioeconomic categories, when the sample size is adequate; and
- using analytic strategies such as geocoding of census tracts and neighborhood blocks (22) and alternating logistic regression (51) that permit more careful measurement of social environmental context variables.

One frequently asked question is whether data should be collected and analyzed by race, particularly for conditions in which socioeconomic conditions are known to contribute the greatest explanatory power. There are many reasons for studies to present and undertake analysis of the population classified by racial and ethnic heritage. While there are risks that some researchers or policymakers will misinterpret the meaning of racial classifications, the data are important for monitoring progress and setbacks in reducing racial/ethnic disparities. The challenge is to undertake these analyses with greater methodologic sophistication and rigor.

Conclusion

Causal pathways by which race and social class may affect health are complex and require thoughtful attention to the conceptual framework, the measurement, and the analytic strategies. The model for studying the influence of race and social class is not likely to flow from a conceptual framework in which an individual's race and social class are defined by distinct variables. Instead, the framework will need to consider that the two variables are very much interconnected and have been shaped from a long history of racial inequalities in the United States. Measures of race capture a social experience that is not simply black or white, but an experience that has been modified by a family's class position as well as other innate characteristics. Research efforts, therefore, are needed that explore the mechanisms that provide the links between race, social class, and health. Investigations to disentangle these complex relations will require cross-disciplinary collaboration between researchers in the social sciences and public health—linkages that are in their infancy—but that are essential for advancing knowledge about the underlying causes of racial disparities in health.

Appendix 1 Infant mortality: Key studies on the effects of race and social class

Num-ber	Author (year)	Study purpose related to review article	Data source (Year)	Scope (National vs Local)	Description of population	Study methods	Key findings
1	Alexander et al (1993)	To determine the relative impact of ethnicity on birth outcomes among dependents of active military personnel. Outcome (LBW and neonatal Mortality)	Hawaii vital records for 1979–1989	State of Hawaii	33,812 births of military dependents residing in Hawaii from 1979–1989, included non-Hispanic whites (24,674), African Americans (4617), and Filipinos (4521)	Significance tests of bivariate relationships. Multiple logistic regression used to calculate odds ratios for the independent effects of maternal factors (age, parity, prenatal care, hospital utilization, maternal and paternal education) on LBW, neonatal, and infant mortality.	Controlling for maternal risk factors, blacks had a higher risk of LBW and VLBW than whites. There were no significant differences in neonatal and infant mortality between ethnic groups. Within low and normal birthweight categories, no significant difference was found in infant mortality.
2	Kleinman & Kessel (1987)	To determine the separate effects of maternal risk factors on low birthweight for blacks and whites. Outcome (LBW)	Birth certificates for 1973 and 1983	28 states	713,061 births in 1973 (83% white; 17% black) and 1,331,008 births in 1983 (84% white; 16% black)	Multinomial logistic regression models to determine the effects of education, marital status, age and parity.	Births of infants with very LBW increased among blacks and decreased among whites. Fifteen percent of the decline in moderate LBW among whites could be attributed to positive changes in maternal characteristics (primarily improvement in education); 35 percent of the increase in very LBW among blacks could be attributed to negative changes in maternal characteristics (primarily an increase in births to unmarried women).

Appendix 1 *(continued)*

Num-ber	Author (year)	Study purpose related to review article	Data source (Year)	Scope (National vs Local)	Description of population	Study methods	Key findings
3	Lieberman et al (1987)	To investigate risk factors associated with increased rate of premature birth to black women versus white women Outcome (Prematurity)	Personal interviews with women and review of hospital medical records	Hospital in Boston, MA	8903 women (15% black; 85% white)	Logistic regression used to determine whether medical factors or socio-demographic factors (education, single marital status, receiving welfare, age <19) were associated with increased risk of premature births	When hematocrit level and the sociodemographic factors were controlled for, there was no significant racial variation in prematurity
4	Rawlings & Weir (1992)	To investigate race and rank differences in infant mortality rates among dependents of military officers and soldiers Outcome (IMR)	Medical records for births between 1985 and 1990	Madigan Army Medical Center in Tacoma, WA	15,495 live births (75.8% white; 16.9% black)	Chi square analysis was used to determine differences in infant mortality, prematurity, LBW, and neonatal hospital stays for whites and blacks. Stepwise logistic regression was used to determine differences in infant mortality by race and pay grade	There was no significant difference in black/white infant mortality; but blacks had higher rates of prematurity, a higher incidence of LBW, and longer neonatal hospital stays than whites. Neither rank nor race was significantly associated with infant mortality

Appendix 1 (*continued*)

Number	Author (year)	Study purpose related to review article	Scope (National vs Local)	Data source (Year)	Description of population	Study methods	Key findings
5	Schoendorf et al (1992)	To determine whether differences in infant mortality rates between whites and blacks would remain after adjustment for sociodemographic factors. Outcome (IMR)	National	National Linked Birth and Infant Death Files for 1983–1985	907,358 infants born to college graduates (95% white; 5% black)	Logistic regression was used to determine differences in infant mortality, controlling for maternal age, marital status, parity, and prenatal care	After adjusting for the sociodemographic factors, the likelihood of death for a black infant was still much higher than that for a white infant (odds ratio: 1.82). The observed differences in mortality among black infants was attributable to a higher incidence of low birthweight
6	Singh & Yu (1995)	To examine long-term trends and differentials in infant, neonatal, and postneonatal mortality in the U.S. from 1950 to 1991 by race, ethnicity, education, and family income. Outcome (IMR)	National	National Vital Statistics System (1950–1991); National Linked Birth and Infant Death data sets (1985–1987); 1988 National Maternal and Infant Health Survey; National Natality Survey & National Infant Mortality Survey (1964–1966)		Infant mortality rates were calculated over time by maternal race/ethnicity, maternal education, family or household income, and cause of death	Blacks had significantly higher IMR than whites at all levels of maternal education. In 1988, the black-white disparity in infant mortality was greater at higher levels of education and higher levels of income

Appendix 1 (*continued*)

Num-ber	Author (year)	Study purpose related to review article	Data source (Year)	Scope (National vs Local)	Description of population	Study methods	Key findings
7	Starfield et al (1991)	To determine the relative impact of race and family income on risk of LBW, examining the impact of factors antecedent to the pregnancy as well as concurrently with it Outcome (LBW)	National Longitudinal Survey of Labor Market Experience of Youth (1979–1988)	National	1396 black infants, 2440 white infants, weighted to represent national population	Used logistic regression, to determine the effects of poverty and race on LBW, controlling for maternal education, maternal age, age/parity risk, marital status, smoking, family income and family size	The risk of LBW among poor black infants was not significantly greater than that among poor white infants; but the risk of LBW was more common among nonpoor black infants than among nonpoor white infants. In the logistic regression analysis, blacks had a significantly increased risk of LBW, regardless of the measure of poverty, even after controlling for other risk factors
8	Krieger et al (1993)	To review key findings and methods used in studying the relationship between race, social class and health Outcome (LBW and IMR)	National linked birth and infant death files (1983–1985)	National		Computed relative risks (and 95% confidence interval) of infant mortality by race/ethnicity and education of mother	Infant mortality rates were twice as high among Blacks as whites across the educational levels. The disparity was lowest among women who had not completed high school (rate ratio = 1.70) and highest among college graduates (rate ratio = 2.20)

Appendix 2 Hypertension: Key studies on the effects of race and social class

Number	Author (year)	Study purpose related to review article	Data source (Year)	Scope (National vs Local)	Description of population	Study methods	Key findings
1	Waitzman & Smith (1994)	To examine how interaction between occupational class transitions and race affects incidence of HT	1982–84 NHEFUS (linked to 1971–75 NHANES)	National	Black and white males 25–55 at baseline. N = 1982 (183 black). SES = 4 occupational classes based on education and training requirements and ratings of decision-making latitude & requirement for repetitious work	Logistic regression on 2 measures of HT at follow-up. Males classified by relationship of occupational class at baseline vs follow-up. Included interactions between race and occupational class transitions	Incidence of HT was significantly associated with occupational class position and transition among both black and white men. Relative to white men who remained in top class, black and white men who remained in lower classes had signifiantly higher incidence rates of HT. Differences were greater among blacks, who are more concentrated in & less likely to move upward from the lower end of the occupational matrix
2	Whittle et al (1991)	To determine whether association between race and HT-ESRD incidence persists after adjusting for risk factors, including SES	1980–85 Maryland Network 31 ESRD Regional Registry; HCFA Chronic Renal Disease Medical evidence Report; 1981–82 Maryland Statewide Household Hypertension Survey	State of Maryland (except DC metro counties)	4427 MSHHS participants living in Network 31 divided into 26 geographic areas (13 black, 13 white); SES = % of persons in each area with high school education, household income of $10,000 or more	For each study area, incidence of HT-ESRD = Network 31 Registry cases/ 1980 census; HT prevalence & risk factors estimated from MSHHS; regression analyses to determine log of relative risk associated with putative risk factors, included race and interactions	Higher HT-ESRD incidence for blacks than for whites; estimated prevalence of HT & severe HT higher for blacks than for whites; relative risk of HT-ESRD for blacks vs whites remained 4.5 when controlling for other variables; lower education group had 58% higher incidence of HT-ESRD; authors conclude that, although important, differences in SES do not explain excess risk of HT-ESRD in blacks

Appendix 2 *(Continued)*

Number	Author (year)	Study purpose related to review article	Data source (Year)	Scope (National vs Local)	Description of population	Study methods	Key findings
3	James et al (1987)	To replicate findings from James et al (1983) (Black male graduates had lower BP than nongraduates, but the difference was limited to men who scored high on John Henryism scale) and extend findings to women and whites	1983 survey; evaluation of effectiveness of 5-year community-based high BP control program	5 townships of Edgecombe Co., NC	1548 adults (18+) in 800 randomly selected households; 50% black; SES = separate measures for black and white— white: < high school or blue collar = low SES, high school graduate or white collar = high SES; black: < 9 yrs. education or low blue collar = low SES, 9 yrs. or more & high blue collar = high SES	Multiple-linear regression used to describe correlates of John Henryism for black & white; race-specific models constructed to assess independent contributions of age, sex, marital status, SES, life satisfaction, self-perceived health status	SES inversely related to John Henryism among blacks, but not whites; SES and John Henryism interact to influence risk for HT in blacks; no SES or SES*John Henryism effect for whites; stronger association between SES and prevalence of HT observed at higher levels of John Henryism among blacks

Appendix 2 *(Continued)*

Number	Author (year)	Study purpose related to review article	Data source (Year)	Scope (National vs Local)	Description of population	Study methods	Key findings
4	Adams-Campbell et al (1993)	To examine prevalence of self-reported HT in black and white middle-aged women in MA; assess association between self-reported HT and risk factors—including education; explore roles of risk factors in accounting for race differences	1981–82 survey of MA women	State of Massachusetts	8050 women aged 45–55 selected randomly from city/town census in 38 cities/towns selected with probabilities proportional to size within 10 strata defined by city/town size, per capita income, & % black. 7705 were white, 220 black, & 123 other. Analysis includes only the 5344 whites who live in towns that include blacks. SES = education: less than 12 years, 12 years, & more than 12 years.	Prevalence of HT compared; risk factors identified; step-wise logistic regression, including race* risk factor interactions	Among middle-aged women in MA, risk of HT among black women about twice that of white women; prevalence of HT varied with education in both races, with HT most prevalent among least educated; race differences in prevalence of self-reported HT persist after controlling for SES (education); difference in prevalence of HT between blacks and whites declines with increasing education; relative odds that a black woman was hypertensive varied inversely with education

Appendix 3 Substance use: key studies on the effects of race and social class

Number	Author (year)	Study purpose related to review article	Data source (year)	Scope (National vs Local)	Description of population	Study methods	Key findings
1	Chilcoat & Schutz (1995)	To examine racial/ethnic differences in the odds of ever using crack/cocaine within age strata and over a two year time period	National Household Survey of Drug Abuse (NHSDA), 1988 & 1990	National	9259 respondents 12 years of age or older from the US civilian population	Employed a post-stratification procedure, grouping respondents into risk sets or neighborhood strata, to examine racial/ethnic differences in crack/cocaine use while holding constant neighborhood-specific factors. Used generalized additive models to examine trends in age-specific prevalence of ever using crack cocaine	African Americans 30–34 years old had significantly higher odds of ever using crack than White Americans in the same age strata (Relative Odds = 2.51). The overall increase in lifetime crack use among African Americans was explained by an increase in prevalence for African Americans who are approximately 30 years old from 5% in 1988 to 8% in 1990

Appendix 3 *(continued)*

Number	Author (year)	Study purpose related to review article	Data source (year)	Scope (National vs Local)	Description of population	Study methods	Key findings
2	Flewelling et al (1993)	To examine the extent to which racial/ethnic differences in drug use prevalence may be influenced by differences in other sociodemographic characteristics	NHSDA, 1991	National	32,594 individuals from the US civilian population.	Developed weighted populated based estimates of the prevalence of drug use by demographic and by socioeconomic status variables. Multiple logistic regression was used to examine the independent effects of race/ethnicity and other sociodemographic variables	Among drug use measures that exhibited a significantly higher initial likelihood of use among blacks, controls for SES and other social characteristics substantially reduced the disparities. The odds of use for three of the five measures, including crack were statistically nonsignificant. Only nonheavy use of cigarettes and frequent use of cocaine remained significantly more likely among blacks than whites.
3	Lillie-Blanton et al 1991	Compares racial differences in alcohol use and abuse and assess factors associated with patterns of drinking	Baltimore Epidemiologic Catchment Area Survey, 1981–83	Baltimore, MD	2,100 women from Baltimore	Linear and logistic regression models were used to examine the extent to which race was associated with alcohol use while holding constant soiodemographic characteristics of age, education, income, marital status, and employment status.	Black women were found to be at no greater risk than whites for heavy drinking or for suffering from alcohol abuse or dependence than whites.

Appendix 3 (*continued*)

Num-ber	Author (year)	Study purpose related to review article	Data source (year)	Scope (National vs Local)	Description of population	Study methods	Key findings
4	Lillie-Blanton et al 1993	To probe the meaning of reported racial/ethnic group differences in the crack cocaine smoking and to estimate the degree to which crack use is associated with personal factors specific to race/ethnicity	NHSDA, 1988	Interviews were held with 8,814 individuals ages 12 and older from the U.S. civilian population	National	Employed a post-stratification procedure, grouping respondents into risk sets or neighborhood strata, to examine racial/ethnic differences in crack/cocaine use while holding constant neighborhood-specific factors. A conditional logistic regression model was used to estimate the relative odds of crack cocaine use by race/ethnicity.	The relative odds of crack cocaine use did not differ significantly for African Americans or for Hispanic Americans compared to White Americans

Appendix 3 *(continued)*

Number	Author (year)	Study purpose related to review article	Data source (year)	Scope (National vs Local)	Description of population	Study methods	Key findings
5	Montgomery & Carter-Pokras 1993	Reviews studies and data sources to asses racial/ethnic differences in four areas of health status: mortality, health of women of reproductive age, infant and child health and adult mortality	National Maternal and Infant Health Survey, 1988	Survey of 18,594 women, 46% of whom were Black	National	Analysis of cigarette and alcohol use among pregnant women stratified by level of education (<high school; high school graduate; and >high school).	White women with fewer than 12 years of education were more likely to smoke than black women or other minority women. Black women were more likely to report drinking 3 or more drinks per week during pregnancy than white women. The racial difference was greatest among women with less than 12 years of education with 12.8% of blacks compared to 3.9% of whites reporting 3 or more drinks

Appendix 4 All cause mortality: Key studies on the effects of race and social class

Num-ber	Author (year)	Study purpose related to review article	Data source (year)	Scope (National vs Local)	Description of population	Study methods	Key findings
1	Berkman & Breslow (1983)	To examine the 23-year mortality experience of a random sample of adults	Originally collected longitudinal data source. Sample selected in 1965	Alameda County, CA	Representative sample of 7000 adults	Mortality experience of a 1965 cohort assessed through 1982. Used a measure of income adjusted for family size as primary socioeconomic indicator	Before adjustment, blacks had 34% higher mortality rate than whites. After adjustment, the difference between black and white survival was no longer significant
2	Sorlie et al (1995)	To estimate the effects of race, employment status, income, education, occupation, marital status, and house-hold size on mortality.	Selected Current Population Surveys (CPS) between 1979 –1985; National Death Index (NDI) 1979 – 1989	National	530,000 persons 25 years of age or older	Individuals identified in CPS were fol-lowed for mortality through the NDI. The Cox propor-tional hazards model was used to estimate the relative risk of mortality in terms of various social and economic variables	After adjustment for socio-economic characteristics, the excess risk of blacks 25 to 65 years of age was reduced but still significantly higher than that of whites

Appendix 4 *(continued)*

Num-ber	Author (year)	Study purpose related to review article	Data source (year)	Scope (National vs Local)	Description of population	Study methods	Key findings
3	Otten et al (1990)	To investigate risk factors for excess black mortality	National Health and Nutrition Examination Survey I Epidemiologic Follow-up Survey	National	8806 persons 35 to 77	Cause-specific mortality rates were calculated for blacks and whites. Cox proportional hazards model was used to estimate the mortality RR before and after adjusting for income and the six risk factors (smoking, blood pressure, cholesterol, body-mass index, alcohol intake, and diabetes)	About a third of the mortality differential by race was left unexplained after adjusting for income and six risk factors. For persons 35 to 54 years old, the rate ratio of mortality for blacks vs whites decreased from 2.3 (unadjusted) to 1.4 when adjusted for the six risk factors and income
4	Pappas et al (1993)	To examine changes in mortality rate from 1960 through 1986 according to income and level of education among persons 25 to 64 years of age in the U.S.	National Mortality Followback Study (NMFS) & 1986 National Health Interview Survey (NHIS)	National	NMFS is a sample of 18,733 people 25 years of age or older, who died in 1986. 13,491 records were analyzed. NHIS includes 30,725 persons 25 – 64	Calculated direct standardized mortality rates and indirect standardized mortality ratios for persons 25 to 64 according to race, sex, income, and family status	Principal finding was that disparities by income and education persisted in the 1980s and have widened since the 1960s, for blacks and whites. Black males with the least income and education had a 3 – 4 times higher risk of mortality than black males with the most income and education

Appendix 4 (continued)

Num-ber	Author (year)	Study purpose related to review article	Data source (year)	Scope (National vs Local)	Description of population	Study methods	Key findings
5	Haan (1987)	To examine association between SES and poor health	Original (1965–74)	Oakland, CA	Random sample of adults 35+. This analysis is restricted to 1811 Oakland residents; R = w/nw, SES = income, education, employment	A 19 year study of Alameda County, CA residents. The analysis compares the 1965–1974 mortality experience of Oakland residents living in a federally designated "poverty" area with the mortality experience of those who lived elsewhere in Oakland	Nonwhite males and females had lower age adjusted mortality rates than whites in poor and nonpoor neighborhoods. (race difference was significant)
6	Rogers (1992)	To examine the demographic and social factors associated with black and white differences in life expectancy	Linked 1986 NHIS with 1986 NMFS	National	Representative sample of 1986 deaths in the civilian non-institution (N = 14,471) age 25+. Social class measures included in the analysis were family income and size	Multiple logistic regression was used to examine the relationship between race and mortality, holding constant demographic, family and socioeconomic characteristics	Racial differences in mortality were eliminated after adjusting for age, gender, income, marital status and family size. Blacks, however, had higher risk than whites of mortality from several specific causes (infectious diseases, homicide and diabetes)

Literature Cited

1. Adams-Campbell LL, Brambilla DJ, McKinlay SM. 1993. Correlates of the prevalence of self-reported hypertension among African-American and white women. *Ethn. Dis.* 3:119–25
1a. Alexander G, Baruffi G, Mor J, Kieffer E, Hulsey T. 1993. Multiethnic variations in pregnancy outcomes of military dependents. *Am. J. Public Health* 83:1721–25
2. Anastos K, Charney P, Charon RA, Cohen E, Jones CY, Marte C, Swiderski DM, Wheat ME, illiams S. 1991. Hypertension in women: What is really known? *Ann. Intern. Med.* 115:287–93
3. Anderson NB, Myers HF, Pickering T, Jackson JS. 1989. Hypertension in blacks: psychosocial and biological perspectives. *J. Hypertens.* 7:161–72
4. Anthony JC. 1992. The scope of epidemiologic research on drug use: a rationale for change. In *Proc. Brasil-United States Binatl. Meet. Drug Abuse Res. Sao Paulo, Brasil,* May, ed. MG Monteiro, JA Inciardi, pp. 213–23, Wilmington: Univ. Delaware
4a. Berkman L, Breslow L. 1983. *Health and Ways of Living: The Alameda County Study.* Cambridge, MA: Oxford Univ. Press
5. Burt VL, Whelton P, Roccella EJ, Brown C, Cutler JA, et al. 1995. Prevalence of hypertension in the US adult population: results from the Third National Health and Nutrition Examination Survey, 1988–1991. *Hypertension* 25:305–13
6. Chilcoat HD, Schultz CG. 1995. Racial/ethnic differences in crack use within neighborhoods. *Addict. Res.* In press
7. Flewelling RL, Ennett ST, Rachal JV, Theisen AC. 1993. *National Household Survey on Drug Abuse: Race/Ethnicity, Socioeconomic Status, and Drug Abuse 1991.* 1–81, Washington.
8. Deleted in proof
9. Geronimus AT, Andersen HF, Bound J. 1991. Differences in hypertension prevalence among U.S. black and white women of childbearing age. *Public Health Rep.* 106:393–99
10. Haan M, Kaplan G. 1985. The contribution of socioeconomic position to minority health. In *Rep. Secretary's Task Force on Black and Minority Health,* 2:69–103. Washington, DC: US DHHS
11. Haan M, Kaplan G. Camacho T. 1987. Poverty and health. *Am. J. Epidemiol.* 125:989–98
12. Deleted in proof
13. Hollingshead A, Redlich F. 1958. *Social Class and Mental Illness.* New York: Wiley
14. James SA, Hartnett SA, Kalsbeek WD. 1983. John Henryism and blood pressure differences among black men. *J. Behav. Med.* 6:259–78
15. James SA, Strogratz DS, Wing SB, Ramsey DL. 1987. Socioeconomic status, John Henryism, and hypertension in blacks and whites. *Am. J. Epidemiol.* 126:664–73
16. Jones CP, LaVeist TA, Lillie-Blanton M. 1991. Race in the epidemiologic literature: an examination of the *American Journal of Epidemiology,* 1921–1990. *Am. J. Epidemiol.* 134:1079–84
17. Kitagawa E, Hauser P. 1973. *Differential Mortality in the United States: A Study in Socioeconomic Epidemiology.* Cambridge: Harvard Univ. Press
18. Klag MJ, Whelton PK, Coresh J, Grim CE, Kuller LH. 1991. The association of skin color with blood pressure in US blacks with low socioeconomic status. *JAMA* 265:599–602
19. Kleinman JC, Kessel SS. 1987. Racial differences in low birthweight. *N. Engl. J. Med.* 317:749–53
20. Kochanek KD, Maurer JD, Rosenberg HM. 1994. Why did black life expectancy decline from 1984 through 1989 in the United States? *Am. J. Public Health* 84:938–44
21. Krieger N. 1990. Racial and gender discrimination: risk factors for high blood pressure? *Soc. Sci. Med.* 30:1273–81
22. Krieger N, Rowley DL, Herman AA, Avery B, Phillips MT. 1993. Racism, sexism, and social class: implications for studies of health, disease, and well-being. *Am. J. Prev. Med.* 9(Suppl.):82–122
23. LaVeist T. 1993. Segregation, poverty, and empowerment: health consequences for African Americans. *Milbank Mem. Fund* 1:(1)
24. Lieberman E, Ryan KJ, Monson RR, Schoenbaum SC. 1987. Risk factors accounting for racial differences in the rate of premature birth. *N. Engl. J. Med.* 317:743–48
25. Lillie-Blanton M, Anthony J, Schuster C. 1993. Probing the meaning of racial/ethnic differences in crack cocaine. *JAMA* 269:993–97
26. Lillie-Blanton M, LaVeist T. 1995. Race/ethnicity, the social environment, and health. *J. Soc. Sci. Med.* In press

27. Lillie-Blanton M, MacKenzie E, Anthony JC. 1991. Black-white differences in alcohol use by women: Baltimore Survey findings. *Public Health Rep.* 106: 124–33

28. Lillie-Blanton M, Martinez R, Taylor A, Robinson B. 1993. Latino and African American women: continuing disparities in health. *Int. J. Health Serv.* 23:555–83

29. Deleted in proof

30. Montgomery LE, Carter-Pokras O. 1993. Health status by social class and/or minority status: implications for environmental equity research. *Toxicol. Ind. Health* 9:729–73

31. Navarro V. 1990. Race or class or race and class: growing mortality differentials in the United States. *Lancet* 336: 1238–40

32. Nickens HW. 1995. The role of race/ethnicity and social class in minority health status. *J. Health Serv. Res.* 30: 151–62

33. Otten Jr. M, Teutsch S, Williamson D, et al. 1990. The effect of known risk factors on the excess mortality of black adults in the United States. *JAMA* 263: 845–50

34. Pappas G, Queen S, Hadden W, Fisher G. 1993. The increasing disparity in mortality between socioeconomic groups in the United States, 1960 and 1986. *N. Engl. J. Med.* 329:103–9

35. Rawlings JS, Weir MR. 1992. Race and rank-specific infant mortality in a U.S. military population. *Am. J. Dis. Child.* 146:313–16

36. Rogers R. 1992. Living and dying in the USA: sociodemographic determinants of death among blacks and whites. *Demography* 29, May

37. Rowley D, Tosteson H. 1993. Racial differences in preterm delivery: developing a new research paradigm. *Am. J. Prev. Med.* 9:1–123

38. Schneider J. 1986. Rewriting the SES: demographic patterns and divorcing families. *Soc. Sci. Med.* 23:211–22

39. Schoendorf KC, Hogue CJR, Kleinman JC, Rowley D. 1992. Mortality among infants of black as compared with white college-educated parents. *N. Engl. J. Med.* 326:1522–26

40. Seedat YK. 1990. Perspectives of hypertension in black patients: black vs. white differences. *J. Cardiovasc. Pharmacol.* 16:S67–70 (Suppl. 7)

41. Singh GK, Yu SM. 1995. Infant mortality in the United States: trends, differentials and projections, 1950 through 2010. *Am. J. Public Health* 85:957–64

42. Sorlie PD, Backlund E, Keller JB. 1995. US mortality by economic, demographic, and social characteristics: the National Longitudinal Mortality Study. *Am. J. Public Health* 85:949–56

43. Starfield B, Shapiro S, Weiss J, Kung-Yee L, Knut R, et al. 1991. Race, family income and low birthweight. *Am. J. Epidemiol.* 134:1167–11

44. Deleted in proof

45. Deleted in proof

46. Waitzman N, Smith K. 1994. The effects of occupational class transitions on hypertension: racial disparities among working-age men. *Am. J. Public Health* 84:945–50

47. Whittle JC, Whelton PK, Seidler AJ, Klag MJ. 1991. Does racial variation in risk factors explain black-white differences in the incidence of hypertensive end-stage renal disease? *Arch. Intern. Med.* 151:1359–64

48. Wiist WH, Flack JM. 1992. A test of the John Henryism hypothesis: cholesterol and blood pressure. *J. Behav. Med.* 15:15–29

49. Williams D. 1990. Socioeconomic differentials in health: a review and redirection. *Soc. Psychol.Q.* 53:81

50. Williams DR, Lavizzo-Mourey R, Warren RC. 1994. The concept of race and health status in America. *Public Health Rep.* 109:26–41

51. Zeger SL, Carey VJ, Diggie P. 1995. Modeling multivariate history data with alternating logistic regressions. *Biometrika.* In press

52. Zimmerman MK, Hartley WS. 1982. High blood pressure among employed women: a multi-factor discriminant analysis. *J. Health Soc. Behav.* 23:205–20

Annu. Rev. Public Health. 1996. 17:449–65

HEALTH AND UNEMPLOYMENT

David Dooley[1], Jonathan Fielding[2], and Lennart Levi[3]

[1]School of Social Ecology, University of California, Irvine, California 92717;
[2]Schools of Public Health and Medicine, University of California, Los Angeles,
California 90095; [3]Karolinska Institutet, Solna, Sweden

KEY WORDS: unemployment, underemployment, health, mental health, health behaviors

ABSTRACT

This paper reviews the relationship between health and inadequate employment,
especially unemployment. Poor physical or mental health can lead, via poor work
performance, to job loss; however, studies that control for such selection effects
are still scarce except for a few health outcomes. For example, aggregate-level
studies typically find a positive association between unemployment and suicide
rates over time. At the individual level of analysis, panel surveys of laid-off
workers tend to find increased psychiatric problems such as depression and
substance abuse. Few studies have evaluated interventions to prevent or reduce
the adverse health effects of job loss. There have been even fewer studies of the
health effects of other types of inadequate employment such as the increasingly
prevalent forms of underemployment.

INTRODUCTION

This paper is intended to review the relationship of health and unemployment,
and possible initiatives to promote the health of workers who have lost jobs
or who experience various kinds of underemployment.

The present restructuring of the world economy has given many American
employees reason to fear the loss of their jobs in the next few years. The health
consequences of unemployment and resulting special health needs have received little attention.

According to recent OECD analyses, over 33 million people were unemployed in the developed countries in 1993, with an increase to 35 million in
1994 (84, 101). As of August 1995, in the United States, there were 7,457,000
unemployed people (5.6% unemployment rate), down somewhat from a year
earlier (104). Unemployment falls unevenly on different population subgroups.
Typically, young people and ethnic minorities face the highest rates, with those

449

of black youth being chronically extremely high (103). Data on underemployment are less widely available, in part because of the lack of standardization of the term. One of several categories of underemployment is that of involuntary part-time employment. In June 1994, there were 8.6 million Americans who regarded themselves as full-time workers but who were working less than 35 hours per week for economic or noneconomic reasons (103).

KEY TERMS

Unemployment

Unemployment may refer either to a community's aggregate unemployment rate or an individual's personal unemployment experience. According to the official measure used in the United States, the unemployment rate is the number of people who have recently been seeking work divided by the number of people who are in the labor force, i.e. either employed or seeking work. Some analysts consider this definition flawed because individuals who want work but who have given up seeking work, the so-called discouraged workers, are not counted as officially unemployed. Sometimes called the "subunemployed," they are grouped in official labor statistics with others such as full-time students and certain groups of retirees as out of the labor force (OLF). Paradoxically, the official unemployment rate could decrease even in bad times if many job seekers became discouraged. Another unemployment measure, the number of people receiving unemployment compensation, is an even poorer indicator. It underestimates the number of people who are unemployed since not every worker has unemployment insurance and because unemployment insurance runs out after a period of time whether new employment is found or not. Neither of these measures reliably discriminates the unemployed who cannot find work at their preferred wage level (called the reservation wage) from those who can find no work at any wage.

Individual-level personal unemployment may result from losing a job or from entering the workforce but failing to find a job. Job loss usually includes a sequence of stressful events from anticipation of job loss (e.g. after the announcement of plant closure), through the layoff itself, to job search and training and finally, to reemployment. The link between aggregate and personal unemployment is seldom studied but appears to be complex and warrants further research (13). Moreover, the new job found after job loss may well be one of the increasingly common variety termed underemployment.

Health

Just as the presumed stressor of employment status is complex, so the presumed outcome of health has been categorized in a variety of ways: physical health, mental health, and well-being or role functioning. Suspected physical health responses to unemployment have ranged from self-reported physical illness (61) to mortality, especially suicide (9). Suspected mental health effects of unemployment have included admissions to mental hospitals (7) and incidence of surveyed clinical mental disorders (32).

The category of well-being and role functioning is an umbrella term for other psychosocial outcomes. Well-being includes measures of psychological and psychophysiological or somatic symptoms (e.g. the General Health Questionnaire, or GHQ) (107) that reflect distress short of psychiatric diagnosis. The distinction between a symptom score reflecting subclinical demoralization and a score that meets the criterion for a clinical case (e.g. anxiety disorder) may be only one symptom above an arbitrary cut-point. However, ordinary symptom counts and the risk of having clinically high symptom levels appear to move together in response to unemployment (33, 62). The other element of this third type of outcome measure, role functioning, includes behaviors that are considered disruptive or antisocial behaviors such as child abuse.

Such different kinds of health outcomes probably involve varying etiologic and pathogenic processes, and some may be strongly influenced by sociocultural factors. Unemployment may also affect some illness processes indirectly by causing loss of health insurance, but this mechanism goes beyond the scope of the present analysis.

Mechanisms

There exist a number of pathways by which a downturn in the economy might produce this variety of potential outcomes (30). One mechanism is a direct effect of aggregate unemployment on people regardless of employment status (13, 81). A downturn in the economy may lead to restructured job routines that bring increased stress (41). Decreased job opportunities may force people to stay in or move to unsatisfying and insecure jobs, at too few hours, at too low wages, or with a too heavy work load ("lean production," or more overtime work).

Most of the unemployment research, at the individual level, has focused on the indirect effect of aggregate unemployment via personal unemployment on the health of the job loser. Personal unemployment is usually viewed as a stressor that involves loss of financial resources and possibly of psychosocial assets such as goal and meaning in life, time structure, status, and social support (57). Whether adverse psychosocial outcomes of unemployment can only be remedied by reemployment is of practical significance because it could guide interventions other than the obvious, i.e. finding and/or creating new jobs—either income maintenance alone or additional assistance targeted at replacing the psychosocial functions of employment. The answer to this question probably varies across social contexts and different types of people. For example, controlling for financial loss, unemployment is more difficult for people with high employment commitment than those with low psychological orientation to work (107). On the other hand, providing a social safety net of unemployment benefits has been credited with reducing the adverse effects of job loss (94).

Although most studies of personal unemployment have limited their assessment of health consequences to the job loser, several studies report social contagion from the job loser to dependents, particularly the spouse (75, 91). Less is known about the social contagion effects on the children of job losers, and virtually nothing is known about the social contagion from underemployment, but the total impact of unemployment surely goes beyond directly affected workers. Finally, a host of variables may moderate the effect of personal unemployment, including both personal characteristics such as coping repertoire, hardiness, social support, education, or ethnicity, and social environmental factors such as the prevailing economic climate in which the unemployed live.

INFERENTIAL PROBLEMS AND RESEARCH DESIGN

The varying strength of association in research studies on the health effects of unemployment may be due in part to the instability of the unemployment/health relationship across eras, locales, and types of people. Studies may show no adverse outcomes from unemployment because of a generous social safety net. Some studies actually show improvement following job loss for especially proactive people (45). Different findings may also reflect the variable nature of occupations and work environments. Employment imposes health risks in its own right, including job stress (63, 71, 72), worksite pollution, and occupational accidents (82). Leaving an especially stressful job may bring relief (110). Interventions to return the unemployed to the workplace must balance the potential gains and health risks from reemployment, especially of the underemployment type.

Aggregate-Level Methods

The aggregate method studies the effect of community level unemployment on community level pathology over time, e.g. correlating annual psychiatric admissions with manufacturing employment (7). Such methods risk the ecological fallacy of drawing incorrect individual-level interpretations from aggregate-level data (90). They have also provoked a statistical debate about the proper way to model time series (15, 26, 47).

Individual-Level Methods

Relying on the cross-sectional, individual approach risks the danger of reverse causation (43). In contrast, the various longitudinal, individual or panel approaches avoid such reverse causation by controlling for the health status of people before they experience joblessness. The closing-factory method follows workers beginning when they learn that their plant will close, continuing through their actual layoff and beyond (3, 25, 73, 74). Another panel method surveys a general population over time and thus requires a large initial sample in order to yield enough unemployed people (76). A related method begins with high school students and follows them into the workforce to determine the effects of finding or not finding employment (49, 111). Each of these approaches has found adverse effects of unemployment, but most of these individual-only studies omit the effect of community economic conditions.

Cross-Level Methods

Cross-level studies combine measures of the economic climate with personal economic stressors and health outcomes and thus can explore the direct and moderating effects of the aggregate economy simultaneously with the indirect effect of the economy via the personal unemployment of individuals. There are some indications of both direct effects (33) and interaction effects (27) of the aggregate economy, but other studies have not replicated these effects (32).

FINDINGS ON UNEMPLOYMENT AND HEALTH

Reviews of the unemployment and health literature are numerous. These include the school-leaver unemployment literature (40, 87, 111) and reviews of unemployment among adults (3, 16, 35, 42, 46, 50, 51, 53, 57, 58, 60, 88, 96, 108). One of the key features of the unemployment literature is the association of research design type with the outcome studied (31). Such low-incidence phenomena as suicide and mental hospitalization have been studied mainly through archival records giving aggregate rates, but these time-series analyses risk the ecological fallacy and controversy about statistical procedure. On the other hand, self-reported symptoms of physical illness or psychological well-being are usually studied at the individual level using sample survey questionnaires. The resulting literature has produced only a few areas with numerous replications using similar designs and measures. Because of the risks of type I error and nonpublication of valid nonsignificant results (92), small numbers of studies reporting an adverse effect of unemployment on a health outcome may be considered insufficient evidence on which to base policy decisions. The present paper tries to characterize those subareas of the literature with a substantial body of work rather than noting every health outcome appearing in an unemployment study. However, the relationship between health and unemployment occurs in both directions. That people in mental or physical ill health are at more risk for selection into the ranks of the unemployed has been well documented (43). As just one example, among people who were employed at the first interview of one large-scale epidemiological survey, those who had ever been diagnosed with alcohol disorder were over twice as likely as those not so diagnosed to become unemployed a year later (32). As a result, the best-designed studies of the social costs of unemployment adjust for the confounding effects of preexisting health status.

Physical Health

Most evidence supports the generally assumed negative effects of unemployment on physical and mental health and well-being. In one of the best studies of effects of job loss on biochemical factors, a longitudinal Swedish plant closure study reported evidence for consistent significant increases in cortisol, prolactin, growth hormone, cholesterol, and HDL-cholesterol, and decreased immune reactions (3, 4, 10, 74). However, there have been few efforts to replicate these and other biochemical outcomes. Most individual-level studies rely on self-reported symptoms or events linked to stress associated with job loss or chronic unemployment. One cross-level study found that self-reported incidence of illness or accident was related indirectly to the aggregate economy via the incidence of personal job and financial life events (19). There have been relatively few studies of specific medical diagnoses or other objective health outcomes, e.g. dyspepsia and joint swelling (59) and corticoid production (99).

Unemployment has been shown to lead to an increase in unhealthy behaviors such as alcohol (32, 48) and tobacco consumption (68), diet, exercise, and other health-related behaviors, which, in turn, might lead to subsequently increased risk for disease or mortality. Unfortunately, there have been rather few replications to establish with confidence the net impact of unemployment on such risk factors, and the effect is likely to be highly moderated. For example, naturally active persons might take advantage of their unemployment to increase their exercise, while their more sedentary counterparts might well decrease their exercise. The literature does offer some aggregate studies correlating unemployment rates with overall (56) and cardiovascular-renal disease mortality (9), infant mortality (8, 22, 112), low birthweight (23), highway fatalities (69), and ischemic heart disease mortality (6, 12). Aside from the small number of their replications, these mortality studies share the problems common to all aggregate-only analyses. Even the interpretation that recession—unless it is extreme, as in the former USSR (93, 100)—causes added mortality is debatable, albeit likely.

Of all of the physical health outcomes, suicide has produced the largest literature, consisting mainly of aggregate time-series studies [see Platt (88) for the most detailed review including parasuicide or nonfatal suicide attempts]. By 1986, at least 20 such studies (31) had appeared, most of which came to the conclusion that unemployment and suicide were positively correlated over time. One exception was Pierce's (86) finding that economic change per se (i.e. either up or down, following Durkheim) (39) led to increases in suicide, but that conclusion was challenged on reanalysis (80). Another exception occurred in the United Kingdom where the suicide rate fell while unemployment was rising between 1962 and 1971, but this pattern was attributed to the coincident detoxification of domestic gas during that time period (65). These and other negative findings (34) point up the importance of making interpretations only on the basis of well-designed and replicated studies.

Mental Health and Behavior

As a "life change" event, job loss might be expected to provoke both other kinds of life change events and certain kinds of mental health disorders such as adjustment disorder. Some early research measured the association between recently experienced unemployment and other types of life events of the kind included on such scales as the social readjustment rating scale of Holmes & Rahe (52). In one such study, elevated unemployment rates in the community were associated with elevated risk of undesirable job or financial life events in middle socioeconomic status respondents more than for either high or low status respondents. Those respondents who experienced such undesirable job or financial events were in turn more likely to report recent illness or injury health events (19). Such job and nonjob stressful life events are in turn associated with elevated psychological symptoms such as demoralization (37). The magnitude of the effect of unemployment on mental health measures varies from report to report, depending on the population under study and the disorder being measured. For example, in analyses based on the NIMH Epidemiologic Catchment Area project, becoming unemployed was associated with a doubling of the risk of increased symptoms of depression (36), but with no increased risk of symptoms of anxiety disorder. In contrast, in the same data set, unemployment was associated with a ninefold increase in the risk of having clinical alcohol disorder (32). Individual- and cross-level studies have seldom been able to survey enough respondents to study low-incidence psychiatric admissions regardless of diagnosis. However, a study of 677 bricklayer union members found that the risk of admission to a psychiatric facility was significantly higher for those unemployed more than half the time in the past year (67). One problem with admissions studies is that it is possible that community-level economic stress leads to increased use of mental health services by uncovering or revealing existing cases of disorder rather than by provoking or triggering new cases (17). An alternative is to study self-reported help-seeking with controls for actual symptoms, and one such cross-level survey found multiple pathways between the aggregate economy and help-seeking (20).

The largest part of the unemployment-mental health literature consists of time-series studies of aggregate economic change and mental hospitalization rates (at least 15 such reports by 1986) (31). One potential problem with such aggregate admissions studies is that community economic change can lead to changes in the supply of public psychiatric services that, in turn, might moderate the covariation between unemployment and admission rates (95). Although many of these studies report the expected positive correlation of unemployment and admissions, there are numerous exceptions. In one of the earliest studies of this type, Brenner (7) reported both positive coefficients for some subgroups and negative coefficients for others. While he found, in general, that inpatient admissions increased with worsening economic times, others found just the opposite (28) or a mixture of a few significant associations among numerous nonsignificant ones (5). Efforts to replicate Brenner's work have succeeded sometimes (79) but failed other times (20, 38, 78). The net effect in these aggregate studies of psychiatric admissions is one of great complexity, with patterns that seem highly time- and place-specific rather than robustly stable.

A few studies have also found links between unemployment and such behaviors as increased drinking (32), aggression (21), divorce (97), and child abuse (98). Other studies have dealt with behaviors that have an indirect bearing on health such as criminal deviance (9), and at least one such study has linked community underemployment to high arrest rates for young adults (1).

Well-Being and Behavior

Most of the individual- and cross-level unemployment literature and virtually all of the minuscule underemployment literature focuses on self-reported subclinical symptoms such as depression, anxiety, self-esteem, and demoralization. Among adults, factory-closing studies have reported the lowest level of well-being in the anticipation phase before the job loss itself (3, 4, 25, 74), suggesting a multistage model in which symptoms rise and fall at different times in the unemployment process. Panel surveys of adults tend to find that becoming unemployed is associated with a worsening in psychological symptoms such as depression, somatization, and anxiety (76). In contrast, school-leaver studies tend to find that young people who fail to find satisfactory jobs (111) do not experience decreases in self-esteem but rather fail to gain as much as their more happily employed counterparts [however, see (49)]. Seven relatively recent studies from the Nordic countries (2, 49, 54, 55, 58, 66, 109) all find evidence of adverse effects on well-being.

In sum, most individual-level studies have detected a statistically significant adverse effect of unemployment on psychological symptoms, but the magnitude of this effect has tended to be relatively modest, consistent with an adjustment of many job losers to their unemployment.

DIRECTIONS FOR RESEARCH TO GUIDE INTERVENTIONS

Stress Buffering Mechanisms

Research could usefully identify those types of persons who are most and least vulnerable to economic stress, as well as causal processes that transmit or moderate their stress reactions. While there are hints as to the kinds of people who are more vulnerable (e.g. those with a psychological commitment to work) (107), the literature has not established a well-replicated set of such risk factors.

Social Contagion

A few studies have documented the adverse effects of the wage earner's unemployment on the spouse or children within a family system (29), but very little work has followed up the research hints that unemployment may play a role in child abuse (98) or infant mortality (22, 23). Findings from such research could target unemployment interventions, not just at the job loser but also at other family members.

Underemployment and Reemployment

The majority of job leavers do so to move to a better job or to relocate geographically. Involuntary joblessness can, as indicated above, have adverse health effects. Although some studies report that finding a new job is an antidote to the toxic experience of this type of unemployment (62), for some proportion of the employed the new job that follows unemployment (particularly involuntary unemployment) may be hazardous, unsatisfactory, insecure, low-paid, or stressful (83). Interventions predicated on reemployment may need to be reconsidered in light of the new research on underemployment and its potentially adverse effects. What facets of a job are restorative to the newly reemployed—the salary, the security, the psychological satisfaction of the work itself—and how shall we assure that new jobs include these characteristics (84, 85)?

School-Leavers

If one were to target unemployment interventions based on unemployment rates, the most vulnerable age segment would certainly be recent school-leavers, especially drop-outs from school and minority youth. Interventions in this area will need to deal with such complexities as the interface of secondary education and the job market as well as the culture of poverty, but there may be useful guidance in European approaches to the school-to-work transition.

Immigrant Unemployment

Often drawn by or pushed to low-pay, low-benefit jobs, undocumented workers may have the least employment security and the least-developed social safety net in case of job loss. Research on the occupational risks of employed immigrants is scarce (105), and research on the health impact of their unemployment or underemployment is virtually nonexistent.

Interventions to Reduce Adverse Effects of Unemployment

An appropriate extension of interest in the health effects of unemployment is what interventions can reduce adverse consequences for the small but important job terminations that are involuntary. The unemployment intervention literature has been summarized mainly in program descriptions (89) or bibliographies (RH Price & L Bronfman, unpublished paper), and it has not received a comprehensive review in recent years [the closest approximation being Koziowski et al (64)]. Interventions are usually expensive and lengthy, infrequently funded, and when they do take place, often described in unpublished technical reports. Unemployment programs may be categorized along various dimensions including the time of intervention (before or after job loss) and the level of intervention (macro versus individual) (18). However, there is no consensus among economists on the advisability of public policy interventions to prevent unwanted job loss or the effectiveness of localized efforts to stimulate employment, including many targeted to the newly unemployed. More constructive approaches may include attempts by the social parties on the labor market to enhance lifelong employability by promoting lifelong learning at the workplace or outside it.

Rising unemployment rates usually entail massive economic costs in the form of lost income taxes and depleted unemployment insurance accounts and social welfare funds. On the other hand, unemployment increases are sometimes regarded as a means of preventing inflation, which explains why the stock and bond markets sometimes react bullishly to rising joblessness. Proposals to lower unemployment by raising government spending are typically challenged as aggravating the federal deficit and imposing an unfair debt on future generations. The economics of unemployment are complex; age and social class groups of the population are affected differently by the same employment policies.

Health and social researchers have usually contributed indirectly to the unemployment policy debate through basic epidemiologic research document-ing the health effects of economic stress (14). This strategy was attempted in the 1970s in the United States when scholarly support for federally guaranteed full-employment legislation was mustered by research (commissioned by the Joint Economic Committee of Congress) showing the social costs of unem-ployment (9). Although endorsing full employment in principle, Congress never provided the budgetary support to implement the policy. Perhaps the basic research on the adverse effects of unemployment has not been convinc-ing. Or perhaps some of the actors on the labor market were unwilling to listen, in spite of strong evidence.

Helping Workers Cope

Most developed countries have some form of safety net of public assistance such as unemployment insurance and access to health care. These programs vary in their coverage of the population and the duration and type of assistance provided. Many western European countries provide a more comprehensive safety net than does the United States. Some studies that have found no association between unemployment and well-being have attributed this result to the effectiveness of such national programs [e.g. for Dutch school-leavers, see (94)].

Some unemployed workers manage to cope effectively on their own or with the help of friends and family. This may explain, in part, the low utilization rates reported by many unemployment counseling programs, and the natural coping processes of the most resilient workers could give clues to improving more formal, participative, interventions (44). The less resilient unemployed can seek professional services at any time, including those of clergy, marriage counselors, psychiatrists, psychologists, general practice medical doctors, or others. One recent study capitalized on the closing of a number of General Motors plants to survey a panel of 1597 workers (11). Controlling for prior use of mental health service, unemployment status did not predict increased usage of specialty mental health services, although depression and nonfinancial stressful events did. Surprisingly, the use of mental health services was asso-ciated with a decrease in mental well-being. This perplexing finding warrants further research, but it does not necessarily address the effectiveness of mental health interventions custom-tailored to the needs of dislocated workers. In Norway, attempts have been made to encourage primary health workers to help unemployed people both to regain health and reenter the labor market (24).

One such program was offered to the workers at the closing General Motors plant in Southgate, California (77). The dislocated workers who voluntarily participated reported elevated levels of distress. Those in retraining felt higher levels of worry (39 vs 2%), depression (27 vs 15%), and anger (20 vs 7%) than those not in training (i.e. seeking only job placement), suggesting that stress may come with training. However, common to most such programs, emotional support was offered without complementary tangible support or empowerment. This may explain why so relatively few of those offered psychosocial assistance accepted such help. Just 112 individual and family therapy clients received treatment on an ongoing basis out of 2000 workers over a one-year period, and the outcome of this treatment was not evaluated. More workers accepted other kinds of assistance such as screening for hypertension [407], job search workshops that included health promotion techniques [302], and support groups dealing with the stress of relocation [126]. These utilization findings highlight the resistance of blue-collar workers to potentially stigmatizing purely mental health–oriented interventions.

Another type of intervention was offered to a group of women workers as part of a Swedish plant closing study (10, 74). The aim of this program was to stimulate structured daily activities such as various courses, and coffee meetings to serve as substitutes for the latent functions lost through unemployment such as time structure and social engagement. Unfortunately, there were no statistically significant benefits of this program on mental or physical well-being, possibly because unemployment is best dealt with by creating or finding a new and satisfactory job.

The best-designed American unemployment intervention in recent years was conducted by the Michigan Prevention Research Center (106). Unemployed workers were recruited while waiting in line at state employment offices, and those interested in receiving an intervention were randomly assigned to a two-week, eight-session experimental program or a self-guided booklet control condition. Of the 752 persons assigned to the experimental condition, 440 (59%) never came. Participants were those who attended at least one session (mean sessions attended = 6.2). The experimental program covered such topics as preparing resumes, using social networks to find jobs, learning problem-solving processes, and accepting social support. The outcomes included benefits both in becoming reemployed and on mental health variables such as anxiety and depression. When the participants' outcomes were compared with those estimated for the controls who would have participated, the results showed significant benefits for the participants in reemployment and mental health, and follow-up analyses suggested that the persons who most needed the program self-selected themselves into it (106).

CONCLUSION

Workers can experience the economy in a variety of employment roles ranging on a continuum from unemployment through underemployment to adequate or even overemployment. This paper summarized the adverse health effects of the various less-than-adequate employment conditions and the kinds of health promotion interventions that might be initiated in response to these conditions.

Although its serious economic and social consequences are known, unemployment's health effects are not yet fully understood despite over a century of research. Aggregate-level studies have typically found significant positive associations over time between unemployment and suicide, the most frequently studied physical health outcome. Aggregate-level studies of mental health have produced mixed findings for the most commonly studied outcome of psychiatric treatment rates. But such aggregate-level studies cannot be interpreted at the individual level as evidence that personal unemployment raises the risk of suicide or mental disorder, and some of these time-series analyses have used controversial statistical methods. Most individual- and cross-level studies have focused on measures of well-being such as symptoms of physical and/or mental distress or dysfunctional behaviors, and typically find adverse effects of personal unemployment on the job loser. However, many questions remain unanswered about the mechanisms of the unemployment-health relationship, the restorative effects of reemployment in the restructured workforce with its rising underemployment, and the impact of unemployment on special groups such as school-leavers, dependents of job losers, and immigrants.

Most studies on the relation between unemployment status and health have contrasted just two conditions—employment vs unemployment. But in recent years, increasing numbers of American workers have found themselves in various types of underemployment, including involuntary part-time employment, poverty-wage employment, and insecure employment (i.e. intermittent unemployment). For example, the rate of involuntary part-time employment increased from 2.8% in 1967 to 4.8% in 1985 (70), and the share of full-time workers making poverty wages increased from 12% in 1979 to 18% in 1992 (102). Because these underemployment statuses share some of the more stressful features of unemployment (e.g. decreased income, status, or time structure), it seems plausible that they could produce adverse effects on health similar to those reported above for unemployment. It follows that future research in this area might usefully explore the health correlates of these increasingly common statuses that fall between adequate employment and unemployment on the employment continuum.

Literature Cited

1. Allan EA, Steffensmeier DJ. 1989. Youth, underemployment, and property crime: differential effects of job availability and job quality on juvenile and young adult arrest rates. *Am. Sociol. Rev.* 54:107–23
2. Angelöw B. 1988. *Att Berövas Sitt Arbete (To Be Deprived of One's Job)*. Räviunda/Stockholm: Fri Press/Symp.
3. Arnetz B, Brenner S, Hjelm H, Levi L, Petterson, et al. 1988. *Stress reactions in relation to threat of job loss and actual unemployment: physiological, psychological, and economic effects of job loss and unemployment.* Stress Res. Rep. No. 206. Stockhom: Karolinska Inst.
4. Arnetz B, Brenner S-O, Levi L, Hjelm R, Petterson I-L, et al. 1991. Neuroendocrine and immunologic effects of unemployment and job insecurity. *Psychother. Psychosom.* 55:76–80
5. Barling P, Handal P. 1980. Incidence of utilization of public mental health facilities as a function of short term economic decline. *Am. J. Community Psychol.* 8:31–39
6. Brenner MH. 1971. Economic changes and heart disease mortality. *Am. J. Public Health* 59:1154–68
7. Brenner MH. 1973. *Mental Illness and the Economy.* Cambridge, MA: Harvard Univ. Press
8. Brenner MH. 1973. Fetal, infant, and maternity mortality during periods of economic stress. *Int. J. Health Serv.* 3:145–59
9. Brenner MH. 1976. *Estimating the social costs of economic policy: implications for mental and physical health, and criminal aggression.* Pap. No. 5, Rep. Congr. Res. Serv. Libr. Congr. Joint Econ. Comm. Congr. Washington, DC: US GPO
10. Brenner S-0, Starrin B. 1988. Unemployment and health in Sweden: public issues and private troubles. *J. Soc. Issues* 4:125–44
11. Broman CL, Hoffman WS, Hamilton VL. 1994. Impact of mental health services on subsequent mental health of autoworkers. *J. Health Soc. Behav.* 35:80–94
12. Bunn AR. 1979. Ischaemic heart disease mortality and the business cycle in Australia. *Am. J. Public Health* 69:772–81
13. Burchell B. 1992. Towards a social psychology of the labour market: Or why we need to understand the labour market before we can understand unemployment. *J. Occup. Organ. Psychol.* 65:345–54
14. Cahill J. 1983. Structural characteristics of the macroeconomy and mental health: implications for primary prevention research. *Am. J. Community Psychol.* 11:553–71
15. Catalano R. 1981. Contending with rival hypotheses in correlation of aggregate time-series (CATS): an overview for community psychologists. *Am. J. Community Psychol.* 9:67–79
16. Catalano R. 1991. The health effects of economic security. *Am. J. Public Health* 81:1148–52
17. Catalano R, Dooley D. 1979. Does economic change provoke or uncover behavioral disorder? A preliminary test. In *Mental Health and the Economy*, ed. L Ferman, J Gordus, pp. 321–41. Kalamazoo, MI: Upjohn Inst.
18. Catalano R, Dooley D. 1980. Economic change in primary prevention. In *Prevention in Mental Health: Research, Policy, and Practice*, ed. RH Price, RF Ketterer, BC Bader, J Monohan, pp. 21–40. Beverly Hills, CA: Sage
19. Catalano R, Dooley D. 1983. Health effects of economic instability: a test of economic stress hypothesis. *J. Health Soc. Behav.* 24:46–60
20. Catalano R, Dooley D, Jackson R. 1985. Economic antecedents of help seeking: reformulation of time-series tests. *J. Health Soc. Behav.* 26:141–52
21. Catalano R, Dooley D, Novaco R, Wilson G, Hough R. 1993. Using ECA survey data to examine the effect of job layoffs on violent behavior. *Hosp. Community Psychiatr.* 44:874–79
22. Catalano R, Serxner S. 1992. Neonatal mortality and the economy revisited. *Int. J. Health Serv.* 22:275–86
23. Catalano R, Serxner S. 1992. The effect of ambient threats to employment on low birthweight. *J. Health Soc. Behav.* 33:363–77
24. Claussen B. 1992. *Arbeidsledighet og Helse. (Unemployment and Health)*. Oslo: Helsedirektoratet
25. Cobb S, Kasi SV. 1977. *Termination: the consequences of job loss*. Rep. No. 76–1261. Cincinnati, OH: DHEW (NIOSH)
26. Cohen LE, Felson M. 1979. On estimating the social costs of national economic policy: a critical examination of the Brenner study. *Soc. Indicators Res.* 6:251–59

27. Cohn RM. 1978. The effect of employment status change on self-attitudes. *Soc. Psychol.* 41:81–93
28. Dear M, Clark G, Clark S. 1979. Economic cycles and mental health care policy: an examination of the macrocontext for social service planning. *Soc. Sci. Med.* 13:43–53
29. Dew MA, Penkower L, Bromet EJ. 1991. Effects of unemployment on mental health in the contemporary family. *Behav. Modif.* 15:501–42
30. Dooley D, Catalano R. 1980. Economic change as a cause of behavioral disorder. *Psychol. Bull.* 87:450–68
31. Dooley D, Catalano R. 1986. Do economic variables generate psychological problems? Different methods, different answers. In *Economic Psychology: Intersection in Theory and Application*, ed. AJ MacFadyen, HW MacFadyen, pp. 503–46. Amsterdam: Elsevier
32. Dooley D, Catalano R, Hough R. 1992. Unemployment and alcohol disorder in 1910 and 1990: drift versus social causation. *J. Occup. Organ. Psychol.* 65: 277–90
33. Dooley D, Catalano R, Rook KS. 1988. Personal and aggregate unemployment and psychological symptoms. *J. Soc. Issues* 44:107–23
34. Dooley D, Catalano R, Rook KS, Serxner S. 1989. Economic stress and suicide: multilevel analyses. Part 1: Aggregate time-series analyses of economic stress and suicide. *Suicide Life Threat. Behav.* 19:321–36
35. Dooley D, Catalano R, Serxner S. 1988. The economy as stressor. In *Location and Stigma: Contemporary Perspectives on Mental Health and Mental Health Care*, ed. CJ Smith, JHA Giggs, pp. 134–51. Boston: Unwin Hyman
36. Dooley D, Catalano R, Wilson G. 1994. Depression and unemployment: panel findings from the Epidemiologic Catchment Area Study. *Am. J. Community Psychol.* 22:745–65
37. Dooley D, Rook K, Catalano R. 1987. Job and non-job stressors and their moderators. *J. Occup. Psychol.* 60:115–32
38. Dowdall GW, Marshall JR, Morra WA. 1990. Economic antecedents of mental hospitalization: a nineteenth-century time-series test. *J. Health Soc. Behav.* 31: 141–47
39. Durkheim E. 1897. *Suicide: A Study in Sociology*. Transl. J Spaulding, G Simpson, 1966. New York: Free Press
40. Feather NT. 1990. *The Psychological Impact of Unemployment*. New York: Springer-Verlag
41. Fenwick R, Tausig M. 1994. The macro-

economic context of job stress. *J. Health Soc. Behav.* 35:266–82
42. Fineman S. 1983. *White Collar Unemployment: Impact and Stress*. New York: Wiley
43. Fruensgaard K, Benjaminsen S, Joensen S, Heistrup K. 1983. Psychosocial characteristics of a group of unemployed patients consecutively admitted to a psychiatric emergency department. *Soc. Psychiatr.* 18:137–44
44. Fryer D, Fagan R. 1993. Coping with unemployment. *Int. J. Polit. Econ.* 23: 95–120
45. Fryer D, Payne R. 1984. Proactive behaviour in unemployment: findings and implications. *Leis. Stud.* 3:273–95
46. Gordus JP, McAlinden SP. 1984. *Economic change, physical illness, mental illness, and social deviance*. A study for the Subcomm. Econ. Goals Intergov. Policy Joint Econ. Comm. Congr. Washington, DC: US GPO
47. Gravelle HS E., Hutchinson G, Stern J. 1981. Mortality and unemployment. A critique of Brenner's time-series analyses. *Lancet* ii:675–79
48. Halford WK, Learner E. 1984. Correlates of coping with unemployment in young Australians. *Aust. Psychol.* 19: 333–44
49. Hammarström A. 1986. *Youth unemployment and ill health. Results from a two-year follow-up study*. Doctoral diss. Stockholm: Karolinska Inst.
50. Hartley J, Fryer D. 1984. The psychology of unemployment: a critical appraisal. *Prog. Appl. Soc. Psychol.* 2: 3–30
51. Hayes J, Nutman P. 1981. *Understanding the Unemployed: The Psychological Effects of Unemployment*. New York: Tavistock
52. Holmes TH, Rahe RH. 1967. The social readjustment rating scale. *J. Psychosom. Res.* 11:213–18
53. Horwitz AV. 1984. The economy and social pathology. *Annu. Rev. Sociol.* 10: 95–119
54. Isaksson K. 1990. *Arbetslöshetoch Mental Hälsa Bland Unga Manliga Socialtjänstklienter. (Life Without Work. Unemployment and Mental Health in Young Male Clients of Social Welfare)*. Stockholm: Univ. Stockholm
55. Iversen L. 1990. *Virksomhedslukninger, Arbeodslöshed og helbred. (Closures of Enterprises, Unemployment and Health.* Copenhagen: FADL's Forlag
56. Iversen L, Andersen O, Andersen PK, Christoffersen K, Keiding N. 1987. Unemployment and mortality in Denmark 1970–80. *Br. Med. J.* 295:879–84

57. Jahoda M. 1982. *Employment and Unemployment: A Social Psychological Analysis.* New York: Cambridge Univ. Press

58. Janlert U. 1991. *Work deprivation and health: consequences of job loss and unemployment.* Doctoral diss. Luleå/Sundbyberg: Karolinska Inst.

59. Kasl SV, Gore S, Cobb S. 1975. The experience of losing a job: repeated changes in health, symptoms, and illness behavior. *Psychosom. Med.* 37:106–22

60. Kaufman HG. 1982. *Professionals in Search of Work. Coping with the Stress of Job Loss and Underemployment.* New York: Wiley

61. Kessler RC, House JS, Turner JB. 1987. Unemployment and health in a community sample. *J. Health Soc. Behav.* 28: 51–59

62. Kessler RC, Turner JB, House JS. 1988. Effects of unemployment on health in a community survey: main, modifying, and mediating effects. *J. Soc. Issues* 44:69–85

63. Kompier M, Levi L. 1994. *Stress at Work: Causes, Effects, and Prevention.* Dublin: Eur. Found.

64. Kozlowski SWJ, Chao GT, Smith EM, Hedlund J. 1993. Organizational downsizing: strategies, interventions, and research implications. *International Review of Industrial and Organizational Psychology: 1993.* New York: Wiley

65. Kreitman N, Platt S. 1984. Suicide, unemployment and domestic gas detoxification in Britain. *J. Epidemiol. Community Health* 38:1–6

66. Laheima E. 1989. Unemployment, reemployment and mental well-being. A panel survey of industrial jobseekers in Finland. *Scand. J. Soc. Med.* 43 (Suppl.)

67. Lajer M. 1982. Unemployment and hospitalization among bricklayers. *Scand. J. Soc. Med.* 10:3–10

68. Lee AJ, Crombie IK, Smith WCS, Tunstall-Pedoe HD. 1991. Cigarette smoking and employment status. *Soc. Sci. Med.* 33:1309–12

69. Leigh JP, Waldon HM. 1991. Unemployment and highway fatalities. *J. Health Policy* 16:135–56

70. Leppel K, Cain SH. 1988. The growth in involuntary part-time employment of men and women. *Appl. Econ.* 20:1155–66

71. Levi L, ed. 1981. *Society, Stress and Disease: Working Life.* Oxford/New York/Toronto: Oxford Univ. Press

72. Levi L. 1984. *Stress in Industry: Causes, Effects and Prevention.* Geneva: ILO

73. Levi L. 1992. Intervening in social systems to promote health. In *Aging, Health, and Behavior,* ed. MG Ory, RP Abeles, PD Lipman, pp. 276–95. Newbury Park, CA: Sage

74. Levi L, Brenner S-O, Hall EM, Hjelm R, Salovaara H, et al. 1984. The psychological, social, and biochemical impacts of unemployment in Sweden. *Int. J. Ment. Health* 13:18–34

75. Liem R, Liem JH. 1988. Psychological effects of unemployment on workers and their families. *J. Soc. Issues* 44:87–105

76. Linn MW, Sandifer R, Stein S. 1985. Effects of unemployment on mental and physical health. *Am. J. Public Health* 75:502–06

77. Maida CA, Gordon NS, Farberow NL. 1989. *The Crisis of Competence: Transitional Stress and the Displaced Worker.* New York: Brunner/Mazel

78. Marshall JR, Dowdall GW. 1982. Employment and mental hospitalization: the case of Buffalo, New York, 1914–1955. *Soc. Forces* 60:843–53

79. Marshall JR, Funch DP. 1979. Mental illness and the economy: a critique and partial replication. *J. Health Soc. Behav.* 20:282–89

80. Marshall JR, Hodge RW. 1981. Durkheim and Pierce on suicide and economic change. *Soc. Sci. Res.* 10:101–14

81. Martin R. 1987. The effect of unemployment upon the employed: a new realism in industrial relations. In *Unemployment: Personal and Social Consequences,* ed. S. Fineman, pp. 219–34. London: Tavistock

82. McKenna SP, McEwen J. 1987. Employment and health. In *Unemployed People: Social and Psychological Perspectives,* ed. D Fryer, P Ullah, pp. 174–93. Philadelphia: Open Univ. Press

83. OECD. 1993. *OECD Employment Outlook.* Paris: OECD

84. OECD. 1994. The OECD Jobs Study. *OECD Econ. Outl.* 55:1–4

85. OECD. 1994. *The OECD Jobs Study. Facts, Analysis, Strategies.* Paris: OECD

86. Pierce A. 1967. The economic cycle and the social suicide rate. *Am. Sociol. Rev.* 32:457–62

87. Petersen AC, Mortimer JT, eds. 1994. *Youth Unemployment and Society.* New York: Cambridge Univ. Press

88. Platt S. 1984. Unemployment and suicidal behavior: a review of the literature. *Soc. Sci. Med.* 19:93–115

89. Popay J. 1985. Responding to unemployment at a local level. In *Health Policy Implications of Unemployment,* ed. G. Westcott, PG Svensson HFK

Zollner, pp. 383–99. Copenhagen: WHO, Reg. Off. Eur.

90. Robinson WS. 1950. Ecological correlations and the behavior of individuals. *Am. Soc. Rev.* 15:352–57

91. Rook K, Dooley D, Catalano R. 1991. Stress transmission: the effects of husbands' job stressors on the emotional health of their wives. *J. Marriage Fam.* 53:165–77

92. Rosenthal R. 1979. The "file drawer problem" and tolerance for null results. *Psychol. Bull.* 86:638–41

93. Russian Ministry of Health. 1994. *Towards a Healthy Russia. Policy for Health Promotion and Disease Prevention: Focus on Major Noncommunicable Diseases.* State Res. Cent. Prevent. Med., Moscow (From Russian)

94. Schaufeli WB, VanYperen NW. 1992. Unemployment and psychological distress among graduates: a longitudinal study. *J. Occup. Organ. Psychol.* 65: 291–305

95. Searight HR, Handal PJ, McCauliffe TM. 1989. The relationship between public mental health admission rates, institutional constraints, and unemployment. *Admin. Policy Ment. Health* 17: 33–42

96. Seidman E, Rapkin B. 1983. Economics and psychological dysfunction: toward a conceptual framework and prevention strategies. In *Preventive Psychology: Theory, Research and Practice*, ed. RD Felner, LA Jason, JN Moritsugu, SS Faber. New York: Pergamon

97. Stack S. 1981. Divorce and suicide: a time series analysis, 1933–1970. *J. Fam. Issues* 2:77–90

98. Steinberg L, Catalano R, Dooley D. 1981. Economic antecedents of child abuse and neglect. *Child Dev.* 52:260–67

99. Theorell T. 1974. Life events before and after the onset of premature myocardial infarction. In *Stressful Life Events: Their Nature and Effect*, ed. BS Dohrenwend, BP Dohrenwend, pp. 101-17. New York: Wiley

100. UNICEF. 1994. *Crisis in Mortality, Health and Nutrition.* Florence: UNICEF Int. Child Dev. Cent.

101. United Nations. 1995. *Draft Declaration of Heads of States and Governments, World Summit for Social Development (revised Oct. 26, 1994).* Copenhagen: UN Inf. Cent. Nord. Ctries.

102. US Bur. Census. 1994. The earnings ladder: Who's at the bottom: Who's at the top? *Stat. Brief,* SB/94–3. Washington, DC: US GPO

103. US Dep. Labor 1994. *Employment and Earnings* 41:7

104. US Dep. Labor 1995. *Employment and Earnings* 42:9

105. Vaughan E. 1993. Chronic exposure to an environmental hazard: risk perceptions and self-protective behavior. *Health Psychol.* 12:74–85

106. Vinokur AD, Price RH, Caplan RD. 1991. From field experiments to program implementation: assessing the potential outcomes of an experimental intervention program for unemployed persons. *Am. J. Community Psychol.* 19:543–62

107. Warr P, Jackson P, Banks M. 1988. Unemployment and mental health: some British studies. *J. Soc. Issues* 44:47–68

108. Warr P, Parry G. 1982. Paid employment and women's psychological well-being. *Psychol. Bull.* 19:498–516

109. Westin S. 1990. *Unemployment and Health: Medical and Social Consequences of a Factory Closure in a Ten-Year Controlled Follow-Up Study: A Study from General Practice.* Trondheim: Tapir

110. Wheaton B. 1990. Life transitions, role histories, and mental health. *Am. Sociol. Rev.* 55:209–23

111. Winefield AH, Tiggemann M, Winefield HR, Goldney RD. 1993. *Growing Up with Unemployment: A Longitudinal Study of Its Psychological Impact.* London: Routledge

112. Winter JM. 1983. Unemployment, nutrition and infant mortality in Britain: 1920–1950. In *Influence of Economic Instability on Health,* ed. J John, D Schwefel, H Zollner, pp. 169–99. Berlin: Springer-Verlag

Annu. Rev. Public Health. 1996. 17:467–88

ECONOMIC EVALUATION OF HIV PREVENTION PROGRAMS[1]

David R. Holtgrave

Center for AIDS Intervention Research, Medical College of Wisconsin, Milwaukee, Wisconsin 53202

Noreen L. Qualls

Division of HIV/AIDS Prevention, Centers for Disease Control and Prevention, Atlanta, Georgia 30333

John D. Graham

Center for Risk Analysis, Harvard School of Public Health, Boston, Massachusetts 02115

KEY WORDS: HIV, AIDS, prevention, cost, evaluation

ABSTRACT

Program managers and policy makers need to balance the costs and benefits of various interventions when planning and evaluating HIV prevention programs. Resources to fund these programs are limited and must be used judiciously to maximize the number of HIV infections averted. Economic evaluation studies of HIV prevention interventions, which we review and critique here, can provide some of the needed information. Special emphasis is given to studies dealing with interventions to reduce or avoid HIV-related risk behaviors. Ninety-three cost-benefit, cost-effectiveness and cost-utility analyses were identified overall. However, only 28 dealt with domestic, behavior change interventions; the remainder focused on screening and testing without prevention counseling, and on care and treatment services. There are compelling demonstrations that behavioral interventions can be cost-effective and even cost-saving. The threshold conditions under which these programs can be considered cost-effective or cost-saving are well defined. However, several important intervention types and multiple key populations have gone unstudied. Research in these areas is urgently needed.

INTRODUCTION AND OVERVIEW

One and a half decades into the HIV (human immunodeficiency virus) epidemic, the overall impact is just beginning to be realized. In the United States in 1993, HIV infection became the leading cause of death for persons age 25–44 (10). As of December 1994, more than 441,000 cases of acquired immunodeficiency syndrome (AIDS) had been reported, and over 270,000 people had died of AIDS (22). The cumulative economic costs to society for the care and treatment of HIV/AIDS patients was estimated to be over $15 billion by 1995 (39).

Primary routes of HIV transmission are via sex and injection drug–use behaviors. Modifying HIV-related risk behaviors alters the probability of HIV infection for HIV-seronegative persons, and reduces the number of HIV transmissions from persons living with HIV and AIDS. To be considered efficacious, HIV prevention interventions must be shown to directly reduce numbers of HIV infections, or to avert or decrease HIV-related risk behaviors. Fortunately, there are clear empirical demonstrations that these sex and drug-use behaviors can be modified (13, 44, 59).

However, this information alone is not sufficient for persons implementing HIV prevention programs. To plan and implement effective programs, HIV prevention community planning groups (CPGs), program managers, and policy makers need scientifically sound yet relevant evaluation information. These decision makers must know what types of interventions are available, which have been shown to be effective, how much they cost, and whether they can be custom-tailored to local circumstances (42). These decision makers need to balance the resources consumed by various HIV prevention programs with the resultant benefits, prevent the maximum number of HIV infections given a limited budget, and consider other important factors (e.g. access and equity).

Here, we review the current state of the HIV prevention *economic evaluation* literature (which considers both resources consumed by, and benefits accrued from various programs), and address three central questions. First, do the economic benefits of HIV prevention programs outweigh the costs? Second, compared to each other, which HIV prevention programs are most cost-effective? Third, relative to other health service programs, how cost-effective are HIV prevention programs?

Our public health experience suggests that these questions are frequently asked by decision makers at the federal, state, and local level. All three questions deal with resource allocation. If a particular HIV prevention program does not meet a funding agency's "standard of success" (e.g. cost-saving or cost-effective), then it is likely to go without resources. The last two questions raise the challenge of demonstrating that HIV prevention programs are "relatively" cost-effective even if they do not necessarily save society money.

Here, we summarize the current state of the economic evaluation literature of HIV prevention programs, provide the best available answers to each of the questions, describe the practical relevance of the literature assembled to date, and discuss areas of needed research. Because behavior change is the primary viable means for slowing the epidemic at this time, our focus is on domestic HIV prevention programs designed to induce changes in HIV-related risk behaviors among specified populations.

LITERATURE REVIEW METHODS

In 1993, a review (46) assessed the size of the HIV/AIDS economic evaluation literature and found 47 published abstracts or papers that met four basic inclusion criteria: (a) a clear identification of a domestic or international prevention or care and treatment program; (b) a quantitative estimate of program costs; (c) a quantitative estimate of program outcomes (benefits, effects, or utilities); and (d) a quantitative comparison of costs and outcomes. Of the 47 references, 21 related to HIV/AIDS antibody screening/testing services, 16 to care and treatment, and only 10 to primary prevention. This previous review paper did not address the three questions described above or assess in detail the methodological rigor of the studies.

For this review, we began by including the 47 references identified through the earlier work and adopting its four broad, basic inclusion criteria. We searched the literature extensively from 1990 through early 1995, which over-lapped with the earlier paper but guarded against omitting relevant citations. We excluded unpublished manuscripts, news articles, and editorials. If there was a question about a particular reference, we erred on the side of inclusive-ness.

Whenever two or more citations dealt with the same study (e.g. an abstract and an article), the more inclusive one was selected. If a particular study used more than one economic evaluation method, the method with the greater emphasis in the discussion was used for classifying the study in Tables 1–4.

MAGNITUDE OF THE LITERATURE

This review identified 93 citations meeting the four basic inclusion criteria (1–9, 11, 12, 14–21, 25–35, 37, 38, 45, 47–52, 54–58, 60–62, 65–68, 70–84, 86–89, 91–102, 104–114), which represents a near doubling of the literature in the last two years. As presented in Table 1, 78% of the citations deal with domestic as opposed to international HIV/AIDS programs. Studies evaluating "behavior change" interventions (very broadly defined to include all studies quantifying behavior change in any way) just outnumber analyses of "antibody screening/testing" programs that do not analytically include consideration of

Table 1 Size and scope of the HIV/AIDS economic evaluation literature

	Program analyzed		
Focus employed	Behavior change	Antibody screening/testing only	Care and treatment
Domestic			
CBAs[a]	5[d]	4	1
CEAs[b]	22	21	13
CUAs[c]	1	4	2
International			
CBAs	3	4	1
CEAs	6	3	2
CUAs	0	0	1

[a] Cost-benefit analyses
[b] Cost-effectiveness analyses
[c] Cost-utility analyses
[d] Cell entries are numerical counts only.

behavior change. Cost-effectiveness analyses (CEAs) far outnumber cost-benefit and cost-utility analyses (CBAs and CUAs).

Table 2 provides more information about those studies focusing on domestic, behavior change, and antibody screening/testing only programs, which are cross-classified as to type of intervention employed and primary population served. The pattern is striking. Counseling, testing, referral, and partner notification (CTRPN) has received the most study of the behavior change interventions. This intervention is usually brief in its delivery, and its potential for inducing behavior change is *relatively* limited compared to other, more intensive interventions.

Table 2 also shows that several economic evaluation studies have been completed for other, non-CTRPN interventions, but primarily for only one population—injection drug users (IDUs). A number of key populations have received very limited or no attention in this literature. Thus, numerous important knowledge gaps are readily apparent.

COSTS AND BENEFITS OF HIV PREVENTION

There are two basic variants of the first question for our review: (*a*) Under what conditions are HIV prevention programs cost-saving?; and (*b*) have economic evaluation studies shown that HIV prevention programs are cost-saving? Both variants are best addressed via cost-benefit analyses.

Table 2 Economic evaluation method used by target population and intervention type for domestic HIV/AIDS prevention programs

Target population	CTRPN[a]	Drug treatment	IEC[b]	Occupational exposure	Outreach[c]	Antibody screening/testing only
			Intervention type Behavior change			
Adolescents						
Young adults						
Adults[d]	2 CBAs					2 CBAs
	7 CEAs					9 CEAs
	1 CUA					
Health care patients[e]	1 CEA					5 CEAs
						4 CUAs
Health care workers						1 CBA
				2 CEAs		5 CEAs
Injection drug users		1 CBA			1 CBA	
	3 CEAs	1 CEA	2 CEAs		5 CEAs	
Men who have sex with men	1 CEA					
Women of child-bearing age/pregnant	1 CBA					1 CBA
						2 CEAs

[a] Counseling, testing, referral, and partner notification services
[b] Information, education, and counseling services (individual-/group-level)
[c] Community-level, needle and syringe exchange, or street
[d] Includes general/multiple and heterosexual populations
[e] Clinic/hospital

The conditions under which HIV prevention programs are cost-saving can be identified, at least partially, by combining cost-benefit and threshold (i.e. "break-even") analyses. If the costs of an HIV prevention program are less than the number of HIV infections averted by the program multiplied by the dollar value of each infection averted (i.e. the economic benefits), then the program is cost-saving. Guinan et al (36) calculated [based on Hellinger's undiscounted cost data (40)] the present value of medical treatment costs avoided when an HIV infection is averted to be approximately $56,000–$80,000 (in 1992 and 1991 dollars, respectively). Medical treatment costs avoided can be considered one monetary valuation of an HIV infection averted. However, other factors—such as lost productivity—may be considered as well. For instance, lost productivity (in terms of an HIV-infected individual's foregone wages) was approximated at just over $430,000 (in 1990 dollars) by Holtgrave et al (45), based on McKay & Phillips' earlier calculations (75). Therefore, using a cost-benefit analysis framework and assuming a societal perspective, an HIV prevention program is cost-saving if the cost per HIV infection averted is less than roughly $485,000–$515,000 (an approximate range given the inherent imprecision in such calculations). Clearly, other intangible factors (e.g. pain and suffering) would raise this monetary valuation if they could be quantified. Also, survey methods used to assess persons' willingness-to-pay to avoid certain health hazards have generally yielded much higher valuations of human life (75).

To determine whether studies have shown that HIV prevention programs are cost-saving, one must refer to cost-benefit analyses of specific HIV prevention programs. Table 3 lists five cost-benefit analyses of behavior change interventions and indicates the population served, methods employed, and base case conclusions. While some studies employed highly rigorous and comprehensive methods, this was not universally true. Reports of cost-benefit analyses should contain, at a minimum, descriptions of the following: (*a*) perspective employed (e.g. societal, individual, or governmental); (*b*) time horizon used; (*c*) index year for dollar values (e.g. costs expressed in 1992 dollars); (*d*) comparison program or policy; (*e*) primary outcome measure; and (*f*) sensitivity analyses performed. It was not possible to assess this minimal information for all studies in Table 3.

It is extremely important to resist directly comparing the five studies' quantitative results as very different situations were analyzed, and varying methods used. Therefore, we discuss each study separately, and provide base case results for the most rigorous and comprehensive studies. Table 3 should be consulted for the index year of dollar values. We further caution the reader to return to the original sources when making consequential programmatic decisions using cost-benefit information. Such decision making is done under conditions of uncertainty—not all of the desired information is known. Carefully conducted economic evaluation studies recognize this fact, and include sensitivity analyses to gauge the robustness of study results to changes in model parameters and assumptions. Space limitations prohibit our describing all sensitivity analyses from the original papers; the base case results for the more rigorous studies provided below should not be taken out of context from the sensitivity analyses performed by the authors.

Holtgrave et al assessed the 1990 national HIV CTRPN program, using its publicly funded budget for cost data. They valued each HIV infection averted at just over $515,000, and estimated the number of HIV infections averted by the program from various estimates of the behavioral impact of counseling and testing (CT) services reported in the literature. In the base case, they assumed *no* behavior change for persons testing HIV seronegative, and for every 100 persons testing HIV seropositive CTRPN services lead to 20 HIV infections averted. They found the HIV CTRPN program to be substantially cost-saving under the base case assumptions ($3,781,918,000 in benefits compared with $188,217,600 in costs). Sensitivity analysis showed that even if

Table 3 Summary of five cost-benefit analyses of domestic, behavior-change HIV/AIDS prevention interventions

Intervention	Reference	Population size and composition	Methods	Summary (base case) results[a]
Counseling, testing, referral, and partner notification (CTRPN)	45	674,590 clients of publicly funded HIV CTRPN	Societal;[b] 12 years;[c] 6%;[d] 1990 $;[e] no CTRPN;[f] HIV-related risks;[g] empirical[h]	Base case ratio;[i] cost beneficial;[j] yes/yes[k]
Counseling and testing (CT)	5	10,000 California women of child-bearing age (high-risk only)	Societal; 1992–2000; 4%; 1988 $; existing levels w/ no new CT; child-bearing, needle-sharing, sexual; illustrative	Total savings per woman screened; cost saving if screening medium and/or high-risk women and preventing HIV infection in adult contacts; yes/no
Partner notification (PN)	50	768 Colorado needle-sharing of sex partners of HIV+ persons	Program; NR;[l] NR; NR; no PN; needle-sharing, sexual; illustrative	NR; cost beneficial; no/yes
Drug treatment (DT)	58	3000 (city A) and 30,000 (city B) injection drug users	Societal; 5 years; NR; 1992 $; no DT; drug use; illustrative	Monetary savings; cost saving; yes (city A only)/no
Needle and syringe exchange (NSE)	14	800,000 injection drug users	Societal; 1 year; NA;[m] NR; no NSE; needle/syringe-sharing; illustrative	Monetary savings; cost saving; no/yes

[a] As reported in the original article
[b] Perspective
[c] Time horizon
[d] Discount rate
[e] Costs expressed in 19__$
[f] Comparison condition
[g] Behavior change(s) assessed
[h] Empirical vs illustrative economic analysis
[i] Base case result expressed as . . .
[j] Determination
[k] Sensitivity/threshold analyses completed
[l] Not reported
[m] Not applicable

only 1 HIV infection was averted for every 100 persons testing HIV seropositive, the economic benefits still (just) outweighed the costs.

Brandeau et al analyzed an illustrative program of voluntary CT services for women of child-bearing age in California, and used a dynamic, compartmental model to convert possible behavior changes to number of HIV infections averted. Their results indicated that a one-time screening program would be cost-saving if offered to "medium-" to "high-risk" women only, saving approximately $4300 per woman screened. The authors conducted numerous sensitivity analyses. Most of the benefits accrued are from avoiding HIV infection transmission to adult sex partners rather than to infants perinatally.

Kahn et al (54–58) undertook a novel set of illustrative, economic analyses for five different behavior change interventions for IDUs, one of which was a CBA of drug treatment (DT) (58). Based on their results, DT services yielded HIV-related economic benefits to society of $5000 to $7000 per year per treatment slot.

Hence, there are compelling analyses to show that HIV prevention efforts can be cost-saving to society; at least this is true for some interventions in some settings.

COMPARING HIV PREVENTION PROGRAMS TO EACH OTHER

Cost-effectiveness analyses (CEAs) are directly relevant for determining which HIV prevention programs are most cost-effective compared to each other. However, it is useful to begin by describing an ideal literature for answering this second question. Decision makers must set priorities among various HIV prevention interventions that comprise the prevention portfolio of, for instance, state health departments. Therefore, it would be desirable to have access to a volume of published literature in which CEAs of numerous types of HIV prevention interventions for various populations were described (i.e. a literature for which Table 2 would be nearly complete). It is also important for the CEA results to be compared meaningfully. Thus, at a minimum, these studies should possess a common approach to: (a) identifying comparison conditions (e.g. comparing all interventions against a "no intervention" condition); (b) choosing an economic evaluation measure (such as cost per HIV infection averted); (c) measuring program costs; (d) assessing program effects; (e) deriving a cost-effectiveness ratio (e.g. use of the same perspective, time horizon, and discount rate); and (e) dealing with multiple, uncertain estimates. Unfortunately, the set of CEA studies summarized in Table 4 do not possess these common methodological attributes. Further, it was not possible to extract certain, basic information from all studies (see Table 4). Therefore, at best, only partial answers to this second policy question can be provided.

Table 4 Summary of 22 cost-effectiveness analyses of domestic, behavior-change HIV/AIDS prevention interventions

Intervention	Reference	Population size and composition	Methods	Summary (base case) results[a]
Counseling and testing (CT)	35	1053 Connecticut and Massachusetts injection drug users	Program;[b] 18 months;[c] NR;[d] 1991 \$;[e] no CT;[f] drug use, sexual;[g] empirical[h]	Cost per client made aware of HIV serostatus;[i] cost-effective;[j] no/yes[k]
Counseling and testing (CT)	55	3000 (city A) and 30,000 (city B) injection drug users	Program; 5 years; NR;[l] 1992 \$; no CT; drug, sexual; illustrative	Cost per adult HIV infection averted; cost-effective; yes (city A only)/no
Counseling and testing (CT)	75	9700 HIV+ marriage license applicants nationwide	Societal; NR; 8%; 1988 \$; no CT; practicing safe sex; illustrative	Cost per case of HIV infection prevented; cost-effective; yes/no
Counseling and testing (CT)	79	100,000 general population members	NR; NR; NR; NR; no CT; HIV-related risks; illustrative	Cost per detected case of HIV infection; cost-effective for high-risk populations only; yes/no
Counseling and testing (CT)	83	90,000 men who have sex with men	Societal; 5 years; NR; NR; no CT & ZDV therapy; number of sex partners; illustrative	Cost per AIDS case prevented; cost-effective; no/no
Counseling and testing (CT)	84	Acute-care hospital patients	NR; NR; NR; NR; no CT; HIV-related risks; illustrative	Cost per life year gained for HIV+ person; cost-effective with sustainable risk-taking reductions or higher HIV prevalence in target population; yes/no
Partner notification (PN)	19	218 New Jersey needle-sharing or sex partners of HIV+ persons	Program; 1 year; NA;[m] 1988–89 \$; no PN; needle-sharing, condom use; empirical	Cost per contact unaware of being HIV+ or at high risk; not cost-effective; no/no
Partner notification (PN)	57	2009 (city A) and 15,465 (city B) drug or sex partners of HIV+ injection drug users	Program; 5 years; NR; 1992 \$; no PN; drug, sexual; illustrative	Cost per adult HIV infection averted; cost-effective; no/no

Table 4 (*Continued*)

Intervention	Reference	Population size and composition	Methods	Summary (base case) results[a]
Partner notification (PN)	86	807 Utah needle-sharing or sex partners of HIV+ persons	Program; 2 years; NR; 1988–90 $; no PN; needle-sharing, sexual; empirical	Cost per partner identified and newly testing HIV+ cost-effective; no/yes
Partner notification (PN)	95	135 San Francisco opposite-sex sex partners of AIDS patients	Program; 27 months; NR; 1985–87 $; no PN; sexual; empirical	Cost per sero-positive partner identified; cost-effective if targeted toward women of child-bearing age to prevent vertical transmission of HIV infection; no/no
Information, education, and counseling (IEC)	56	3000 (city A) and 30,000 (city B) injection drug users	Program; 5 years; NR; 1992 $; CT only; drug, sexual; illustrative	Cost per adult HIV infection averted; cost-effective; yes (city A only)/no
Needle and syringe exchange (NSE)	51	>1500 injection drug users	Program; 5 years; NR; 1992 $; no NSE; needle-/syringe-sharing, sexual; illustrative	Cost per HIV infection averted; cost-effective; yes, (city B only)/no
Needle and syringe exchange (NSE)	52	Injection drug users	Program; 1 year; NA; 1992 $; bleach distribution, CT, IE; needle-/syringe-sharing; empirical	Cost per client contact; cost-effective; no/no
Occupational exposure (OE)	62	1 health care worker	Hospital; 1 year; NA; 1992 $; no needlestick prevention devices; occupational exposure; illustrative	Cost per needlestick injury prevented; cost-effective; yes (hospital A only)/no
Partner notification (PN)	100	239 Colorado needle-sharing or sex partners of HIV+ persons	Program; 1 year; NA; 1988 $; no PN; needle-sharing, sexual; empirical	Cost per newly identified HIV+ partner; cost-effective; no/no
Partner notification (PN)	112	90 South Carolina sex partners of HIV+ persons	Program; <1 year; NA; 1987 $; no PN; number of sexual contacts, condom use; empirical	Cost per HIV+ man identified; cost-effective; no/no

Table 4 *(Continued)*

Intervention	Reference	Population size and composition	Methods	Summary (base case) results[a]
Drug treatment (DT)	61	Injection drug users	Program; 1 year; NA; NR; outreach risk-reduction education; drug use; illustrative	Cost per prevented HIV-1 infection; not cost-effective; no/no
Information, education, and counseling (IEC)	16	253 injection drug users	Program; 18 months; NR; NR; no IEC; sharing injection equipment, condom use; empirical	Cost per 1 percentage point change in behavior; cost-effective for drug-related behaviors; no/no
Occupational exposure (OE)	70	Health care workers (HCWs)	Societal; 1 year; NA; NR; no CT of acute-care hospital patients; medical/ surgical needlestick exposure; illustrative	Cost per HCW HIV infection averted; not cost-effective; yes/no
Outreach	54	3000 (city A) & 30,000 (city B) injection drug users	Program; 5 years; NR; 1992 $; no bleach distribution; drug; illustrative	Cost per adult HIV infection averted; cost-effective; no/no
Outreach	109	641 HIV–injection drug users	Societal; 1 year; NA; 1992 $; methadone maintenance; needle-/ syringe-sharing; empirical	Cost per prevented HIV-1 infection; cost-effective; no/yes
Outreach	111	349,892 injection drug users and youths in high-risk situations	Program; 1 year; NA; 1991–92 $; no outreach; HIV-related risks; empirical	Cost per contact; cost-effective; yes/yes

[a] As reported in the original article
[b] Perspective
[c] Time horizon
[d] Discount rate
[e] Costs expressed in 19__$
[f] Comparison condition
[g] Behavior change(s) assessed
[h] Empirical vs illustrative economic analysis
[i] Base case result expressed as . . .
[j] Determination
[k] Sensitivity/threshold analyses completed
[l] Not reported
[m] Not applicable

Table 4 displays six CEAs that evaluated counseling and testing (CT) interventions. Some studies used "cost per HIV infection averted" as their main economic evaluation measure, others "cost per HIV infection identified," and another "cost per life year gained." Perhaps this indicates varying philosophies as to whether the authors believe the purpose of counseling and testing is infection identification or behavior change. In addition, relatively little information was given in some of the papers as to what "counseling" entailed, making the interventions, and thereby the analyses, difficult to compare. One general finding emerged from these cost-effectiveness studies: Counseling and testing services were more likely to have lower estimates of cost per HIV infection prevented in specified populations or areas with elevated HIV seroprevalence rates. For example, a study of mandatory premarital testing for HIV antibody (75) found that under two different assumptions about HIV seroprevalence among the pool of marriage license applicants, the cost per HIV infection prevented differed by a factor of roughly three (e.g. $98,000, assuming 2600 HIV seropositive applicants, compared to $26,000, assuming 9700 HIV seropositive applicants). While the general population should have access to counseling and testing services, providing these services to very low seroprevalence populations could be an expensive proposition.

Table 4 displays six CEAs that dealt with partner notification (PN) services. Five examined "cost per HIV positive partner identified," and reported base case values of roughly between $800 and $3200. PN services seemed to be viewed as valuable to the extent they reach populations with a likely high seroprevalence (i.e. needle-sharing or sex partners of HIV seropositive persons) and recruit them for CT. Four of the five studies reported that PN services were "cost-effective" compared to the intervention's absence; a typical argument used to support this assertion is that only a few HIV infections have to be averted by the program in order for society to save money by avoiding HIV-related medical care and treatment costs. However, this argument requires that a quantitative linkage be made between number of HIV seropositive partners identified and number of HIV infections averted, and this linkage is generally absent in the partner notification literature. The sixth study, by Kahn et al, used cost per HIV infection averted as the outcome measure and is discussed in more detail below.

Two CEA studies (see Table 4) examined occupational exposure interventions to prevent HIV infection in health care workers (HCWs). One study described an illustrative analysis of using various needlestick prevention devices in hospital settings. It argued that the program was cost-effective because needlestick injuries could be prevented for roughly $1000 to $2000 each under base case assumptions. The other study examined HIV antibody testing of acute care hospital patients as a strategy for facilitating adoption of more rigorous infection control procedures by HCWs. The economic evaluation measure was "cost per HCW HIV infection averted." The authors concluded that the costs were extremely high (in the hundreds of millions of dollars per infection averted) and, thus, not cost-effective.

Table 4 describes eight CEAs of behavior change interventions primarily for IDUs: One study examined drug treatment services; two discussed information, education, and counseling (IEC); two dealt with needle and syringe exchange (NSE) services; and three assessed street outreach (one outreach study also included data for youth in high-risk situations). Different methods and measures are readily apparent. Although most of these studies examined "cost per HIV infection averted," one NSE and one street outreach study assessed "cost per client contact." Seven of the eight CEAs purported the intervention to be cost-effective relative to various comparison conditions.

Although it is difficult to directly compare the results of these CEA studies, there is an important exception. Kahn et al (54–58) used a common methodological framework to assess five interventions for IDUs, four of which employed cost-effectiveness analysis (54–57). The four interventions were examined for the cases of two different cities. The interventions were (a) counseling and testing services; (b) information, education and counseling (here, extended post-test counseling); (c) partner notification services; and (d) street outreach (especially bleach distribution). The cost per HIV infection averted for the four interventions ranged from $3000 to $32,000 in one city, and from $4000 to $66,000 in the other city. Among the interventions, the most cost-effective was information, education, and counseling at roughly $3500 to $4100 per infection averted.

One other study of an intervention for injection drug users is especially noteworthy. Wiebel et al found that a street outreach program in the Chicago area prevented 82 new HIV infections among 641 injection drug users during a four-year period. The cost per infection prevented ranged from approximately $150–$300.

COMPARING HIV PREVENTION TO OTHER HEALTH SERVICES

Before considering the empirical studies that answer the third question of our review, we address the conditions under which HIV prevention programs would be cost-effective relative to non-HIV–related health service programs. To compare HIV prevention programs to, say, cancer prevention programs, a common economic evaluation measure must be utilized. Some alternatives include "cost per life saved," "cost per year of life saved," or "cost per quality adjusted life year (QALY) gained." CUAs often utilize the latter measure, which takes into consideration both morbidity and mortality. However, quality of life can be especially difficult to measure (85).

There is no one specific "cost per QALY gained" figure above which society is unwilling to pay for a particular program. However, some general statements can be made about a cutoff point. For example, a Canadian pharmacoeconomics group (63, 64) suggested that a threshold probably exists in the range of $20,000–$100,000 (in 1990 Canadian dollars) per QALY gained. Other researchers have been more specific; Owens et al (81) used $45,000 per QALY saved in a CUA of HIV antibody screening in clinical settings. Other benchmarks may also be considered, such as those based on surveys of persons' willingness-to-pay to avoid certain health risks.

Holtgrave & Qualls (43) combined a CUA framework with threshold analysis. The authors first estimated the number of QALYs gained each time an HIV infection was averted, deriving both undiscounted and discounted figures (28.85 and 9.26, respectively), and then identified in the literature various dollar amounts society seemed willing to pay to "buy" one QALY. Although under base case assumptions the authors adopted Owens et al's $45,000 per QALY saved cutpoint, they varied this figure widely to account for its inherent uncertainty. They arrived at a base case monetary threshold above which society would likely be unwilling to pay to avert an HIV infection; the threshold is $417,000 (1993 dollars, and is derived by multiplying $45,000 by 9.26 and then rounding to the nearest thousand). This figure ranged from $185,000 to $648,000, depending upon what society would be willing to pay per QALY gained. Therefore, if any HIV prevention program can avert one HIV infection at a cost of $417,000 or less, then it can be argued the program is cost-effective relative to other health service programs readily accepted by society.

However, do HIV prevention programs meet these conditions? Ideally, the literature would contain several cost-utility analyses spread across various types of interventions and populations, with each study reporting a "cost per QALY gained." Unfortunately, we identified only one cost-utility analysis of a domestic HIV prevention program that involved behavior change in some way. Weinstein et al (108) described an illustrative cost-utility analysis of mandatory, premarital counseling and testing and tentatively concluded that it was cost-effective relative to other health service programs. One important reason for the lack of cost-utility analyses is that the quality-of-life literature for persons living with HIV and AIDS is just beginning to mature and to be utilized in economic evaluation and other policy analysis studies (43, 46, 85).

Although cost-utility analyses of HIV behavior change interventions are scarce, cost-benefit analyses can be used to partially answer this third question. For example, in cost-benefit analysis, all costs and benefits are valued in monetary units (e.g. dollars). If common methodologies are used across health service programs, then one could at least categorize the five cost-saving HIV prevention services listed in Table 3 with other health service programs identified as cost-saving.

Cost-effectiveness analysis can also be used to partially answer this third question in two ways. First, some cost-effectiveness analyses report economic evaluation measures that can be compared across health service programs, but do not consider quality adjustments. For example, Paltiel & Kaplan's (84) illustrative CEA of voluntary CT for acute-care hospital inpatients utilized a "cost per life year gained" measure that can be compared to other health service programs. Second, cost-effectiveness analyses utilizing HIV-specific economic evaluation measures can be modified to address this third question. If a cost-effectiveness study reports on the "cost per HIV infection averted" but not on the "cost per QALY gained," the reader can make the translation with some quick yet rough calculations. For instance, if a study reports $150,000 per HIV infection averted, the reader can note that Holtgrave & Qualls (43) estimated the discounted number of QALYs gained on average for each HIV infection averted to be 9.26. Therefore, a crude calculation of $150,000/9.26 yields $16,200 per QALY gained. Although this does not take into account specific characteristics of the study cohort (such as mean age), it provides a rough approximation of the "cost per QALY gained." This figure, in turn, can be compared *very tentatively* to other health service programs.

PRACTICAL IMPLICATIONS AND CONCLUSIONS

This literature review has direct implications for policy analysts, intervention researchers, and decision makers, which we discuss in turn below.

Policy Analysts

There are three major implications for policy analysts. First, broader thinking is needed when selecting HIV prevention programs for economic evaluation studies. Services for several important populations in the HIV epidemic have gone unstudied, and several especially promising types of interventions have been understudied. Further, essentially no research has been done on "bundles" of interventions that taken together comprise an HIV prevention program, nor on incremental analyses of components of these bundles.

Second, analysts should make every effort to use common methodologies whenever possible, allowing for much more meaningful comparisons among studies (103). Of course, standardization can be constraining, and each study aims to answer a somewhat different research question that may require modifying standard methods. However, a mutually agreeable set of methodologies could serve as the base case for each study, and be altered in the sensitivity analyses to satisfy each analyst's interests and preferences (69). Readily available economic evaluation methodological guides and primers (23, 24, 90) could serve as a basis for such standardization. The Public Health Service is currently working on methods standardization (69). Analysts should report clearly and completely on the methods used in their studies so that others can easily assess the methodological quality.

Third, analysts should render economic evaluation studies as policy relevant as possible. Kahn & Washington (53) described several strategies for making policy analyses as relevant as possible to decision makers. We underscore the notion that analysts need to (a) help others use their models; and (b) make it as easy as possible for others to judge the model's suitability for local circumstances and general technical quality. The format in which economic evaluations of HIV prevention programs are presented can greatly assist with this determination. For example, Drummond et al (24) published a list of ten key questions to ask to determine the merit of any economic evaluation study, which analysts could easily address in their published papers. Policy analysts can also structure their sensitivity analyses to include a broad array of situations facing decision makers.

Intervention Researchers

The literature on the behavioral effectiveness of HIV prevention programs is much better developed than that of economic evaluations. Intervention researchers can help develop policy relevant, economic evaluation studies even if they do not undertake formal CBAs, CEAs, or CUAs themselves. For example, it has been (41) suggested that intervention researchers present detailed descriptions of the components of their interventions and cost information for each component, as feasible. They can also foster economic evaluations by selecting those behavioral outcome measures needed as inputs for models that link behavioral and health outcomes. These models often require data on the number of sex partners and acts per partner, condom use, drug use, and so on. For practical reasons, intervention researchers usually collect data for a subset of these variables, but not all. Still, the most meaningful variables should be assessed to help link behavioral and health outcomes.

Decision Makers

Decision makers can derive several important lessons from the HIV prevention economic evaluation literature. First, the conditions under which HIV prevention programs can be considered cost-saving or cost-effective relative to each other are quite well defined and are useful criteria by which to gauge the success of an already planned or implemented program. These conditions may appear astonishingly easy to attain. Unfortunately, believing it is possible to save an HIV infection is not the same as actually averting one. In order to assert an HIV infection has or will be averted, decision makers need behavioral data, biological evidence, or expert judgment that this infection avoidance is feasible and likely.

Second, as presented in Tables 3 and 4, several economic evaluation studies of HIV prevention programs have documented sufficient evidence of infection avoidance so that they can be considered cost-saving or cost-effective. Yet, decision makers must consider the external validity of these studies when extrapolating their results to local circumstances.

Third, decision makers must recognize that the current state of the art of the economic evaluation literature does not offer easy-to-access, ready answers to all of their pressing policy-related questions. For example, decision makers who must allocate limited HIV prevention funds may wish to know which HIV prevention interventions or combinations thereof are most cost-effective relative to each other for a particular population. Although they cannot simply look up these answers in the literature, partial responses can be found in the studies reviewed here. Thus, decision makers should make use of the best available data while articulating their information needs to policy analysts and intervention researchers, and commissioning custom-tailored analyses to address specific policy questions of local relevance.

With someone in the United States becoming HIV-infected every few minutes, and given the study results reviewed here, it is worthwhile for society to continue to invest in HIV prevention programs. The remaining challenge is to determine with the aid of well-defined economic analyses the optimal allocation of HIV prevention resources among promising types and portfolios of behavioral interventions.

ACKNOWLEDGMENTS

DR Holtgrave was supported in part by grant P30-MH52776 from the National Institute of Mental Health during the preparation of this chapter. NL Qualls was supported by a Visiting Fellowship from the Prevention Effectiveness Activity in CDC's Epidemiology Program Office. The authors are grateful to Lynda Doll, Peter Drotman, Paul Farnham, Steve Teutsch, Linda Wright-DeAguero, and Ralph Resenhoeft for helpful reviews of an earlier draft of this chapter.

Literature Cited

1. Allen UD, Read S, Gafni A. 1992. Zidovudine for chemoprophylaxis after occupational exposure to HIV-infected blood: an economic evaluation. *Clin. Infect. Dis.* 14:822–30

2. Altman R, Shahied SI, Pizzuti W, Brandon DN, Anderson L, Freund C. 1992. Premarital HIV-1 testing in New Jersey. *J. Acquired Immune Defic. Syndr.* 5:7–11

3. Arno PS, Green J, Mofenson L, Bonuck K, Futterman D, Shenson D. 1991. Early intervention in pediatric HIV disease: the economic impact. *Int. Conf. AIDS* 7:72 (Abstr. No. TU.D.62)
4. Bloom DE, Glied S. 1991. Benefits and costs of HIV testing. *Science* 252:1798–804
5. Brandeau ML, Owens DK, Sox CH, Wachter RM. 1993. Screening women of childbearing age for human immunodeficiency virus: a model-based policy analysis. *Manage. Sci.* 39:72–92
6. Buxton MJ, Dubois DJ, Turner RR, Sculpher MJ, Robinson PA, Searcy C. 1991. Cost implications of alternative treatments for AIDS patients with cryptococcal meningitis. Comparison of fluconazole and amphotericin B-based therapies. *J. Infect.* 23:17–31
7. Caceres CF, Rosasco AM, Mandel JS, Hearst N. 1994. Evaluating a school-based intervention for STD/AIDS prevention in Peru. *J. Adolesc. Health* 15:582–91
8. Cameron C, Shepard J, Mann J, Somaini B, Dubois JA, et al. 1990. Prevention scenarios: Swiss AIDS programme. *Int. Conf. AIDS* 6:290 (Abstr. No. F.D.834)
9. Castellano AR, Nettleman MD. 1991. Cost and benefit of secondary prophylaxis for pneumocystis carinii pneumonia. *JAMA* 266:820–24
10. Cent. Dis. Control Prev. 1995. Update: acquired immunodeficiency syndrome—United States, 1994. *Morbid. Mortal. Wkly. Rep.* 44:64–67
11. Chavey WE, Cantor SB, Clover RD, Reinarz JA, Spann SJ. 1994. Cost-effectiveness analysis of screening health care workers for HIV. *J. Fam. Pract.* 38:249–57
12. Cheung TW, Fahs M, Sacks HS. 1990. Cost-effectiveness analysis of early treatment of HIV disease with zidovudine (AZT). *Int. Conf. AIDS* 6:473 (Abstr. No. 4078)
13. Choi KH, Coates TJ. 1994. Prevention of HIV infection. *AIDS* 8:1371–89
14. Clark HW, Corbett JM. 1993. Needle exchange programs and social policy. *J. Ment. Health Admin.* 20:66–71
15. Cleary PD, Barry MJ, Mayer KH, Brandt AM, Gostin L, Fineberg HV. 1987. Compulsory premarital screening for the human immunodeficiency virus: technical and public health considerations. *JAMA* 258:1757–62
16. Cole G, Gorsky R, MacGowan R, Collier C. 1993. Costs and cost-effectiveness of HIV prevention activities in methadone treatment clinics. *Int. Conf. AIDS* 9:749 (Abstr. No. PO-C24–3191)
17. Cowley P. 1993. Preliminary cost-effectiveness analysis of an AIDS vaccine in Abidjan, Ivory Coast. *Health Policy* 24:145–53
18. Cowper P, Oddone EZ, Matchar D, Hamilton J, Hartigan P, et al. 1992. Factors influencing the cost-effectiveness of early versus later zidovudine (AZT) treatment of symptomatic human immunodeficiency virus infection. *Med. Decis. Making* 12:340 (Abstr.)
19. Crystal S, Dengelegi L, Beck P, Dejowski E. 1990. AIDS contact notification: initial program results in New Jersey. *AIDS Educ. Prev.* 2:284–95
20. DeCiantis ML, DeBuono B, Scott HD, Carpenter C. 1990. Routine HIV testing in an acute care hospital inpatient setting. *Int. Conf. AIDS* 6:332 (Abstr. No. Th.D.826)
21. de Moya EA, Peguera CP, Charles W, Adams KG, Gomes MF, et al. 1992. Measuring the costs and benefits of HIV screening systems in Trinidad and Tobago, the Dominican Republic and the Philippines. *Int. Conf. AIDS* 8:D454 (Abstr. No. PoD5402)
22. Div. HIV/AIDS Prev. 1994. *HIV/AIDS Surveillance Report: US HIV and AIDS Cases Reported through December 1994* (Year-end ed.) 6:7,19. CDC, Natl. Cent. Prev. Serv., Atlanta
23. Drummond M, Davies L. 1990. Economic evaluation of programmes for AIDS and HIV infection: methodological issues. In *Economic Aspects of AIDS and HIV Infection*, ed. D Schwefel, R Leidl, J Rovira, MF Drummond, pp. 107–17. Berlin: Springer-Verlag
24. Drummond MF, Stoddart GL, Torrance GW. 1987. *Methods for the Economic Evaluation of Health Care Programmes.* Oxford: Oxford Univ. Press
25. Eisenstaedt RS, Getzen TE. 1988. Screening blood donors for human immunodeficiency virus antibody: cost-benefit analysis. *Am. J. Public Health* 78:450–54
26. Etchason J, Petz L, Keeler E, Calhoun L, Kleinman S, et al. 1995. The cost effectiveness of preoperative autologous blood donations. *N. Engl. J. Med.* 332:719–24
27. Forsythe S, Schvartz E, Janowitz B, Suarez E, de Moya T, et al. 1992. Measuring costs and benefits of target condom distribution programs in Latin American and Caribbean countries. *Int. Conf. AIDS* 8:D454 (Abstr. No. PoD5403)
28. Freedberg KA, Cohen CJ, Barber TW. 1992. Preventing mycobacterium avium complex infection in patients with

AIDS: a cost-effectiveness analysis. *Med. Decis. Making* 12:339 (Abstr.)

29. Freedberg KA, Tosteson ANA, Cohen CJ, Cotton DJ. 1991. Primary prophylaxis for pneumocystis carinii pneumonia in HIV-infected people with CD4 counts below 200/mm3: a cost-effectiveness analysis. *J. Acquired Immune Defic. Syndr.* 4:521–31

30. Freedberg KA, Tosteson ANA, Cotton DJ, Goldman L. 1992. Optimal management strategies for HIV-infected patients who present with cough or dyspnea: a cost-effectiveness analysis. *J. Gen. Intern. Med.* 7:261–72

31. Fulop G, Strain J, Fahs M, Sacks H. 1989. Scatter bed versus cluster unit treatment of AIDS inpatients. *Int. Conf. AIDS* 5:1045 (Abstr. No. T.H.P.7)

32. Gail MH, Preston D, Piantadosi S. 1989. Disease prevention models of voluntary confidential screening for human immunodeficiency virus (HIV). *Stat. Med.* 8:59–81

33. Gelles GM. 1993. Costs and benefits of HIV-1 antibody testing of donated blood. *J. Policy Anal. Manage.* 12:512–31

34. Giesecke J, Ramstedt K, Granath F, Ripa T, Rado G, Westrell M. 1991. Efficacy of partner notification for HIV infection. *Lancet* 338:1096–100

35. Gorsky RD, MacGowan RJ, Swanson NM, DelGado BP. 1995. Prevention of HIV infection in drug abusers: a cost analysis. *Prev. Med.* 24:3–8

36. Guinan ME, Farnham PG, Holtgrave DR. 1994. Estimating the value of preventing a human immunodeficiency virus infection. *Am. J. Prev. Med.* 10:1–4

37. Harris RL, Boisaubin EV, Salyer PD, Semands DF. 1990. Evaluation of a hospital admission HIV antibody voluntary screening program. *Infect. Control Hosp. Epidemiol.* 11:628–34

38. Healy JC, Frankforter SA, Graves BK. 1992. Autologous predeposit in total hip arthroplasty: a cost-effectiveness analysis. *Med. Decis. Making* 12:339 (Abstr.)

39. Hellinger FJ. 1992. Forecasts of the costs of medical care for persons with HIV: 1992–1995. *Inquiry* 29:356–65

40. Hellinger FJ. 1993. The lifetime cost of treating a person with HIV. *JAMA* 270:474–78

41. Holtgrave DR. 1994. Cost analysis and HIV prevention interventions. *Am. Psychol.* 49:1088–89

42. Holtgrave DR, Qualls NL. 1994. HIV prevention programs. *Science* 266:16

43. Holtgrave DR, Qualls NL. 1995. Threshold analysis and HIV prevention programs. *Med. Decis. Making.* In press

44. Holtgrave DR, Qualls NL, Curran JW, Valdiserri RO, Guinan ME, Parra WC. 1995. An overview of the effectiveness and efficiency of HIV prevention programs. *Public Health Rep.* 110:134–46

45. Holtgrave DR, Valdiserri RO, Gerber AR, Hinman AR. 1993. Human immunodeficiency virus counseling, testing, referral, and partner notification services: a cost-benefit analysis. *Arch. Intern. Med.* 153:1225–30

46. Holtgrave DR, Valdiserri RO, West GA. 1994. Quantitative economic evaluations of HIV-related prevention and treatment services: a review. *Risk* 5:29–47

47. Houshyar A. 1991. Screening pregnant women for HIV antibody: cost-benefit analysis. *AIDS Public Policy J.* 6:98–103

48. Janssen RS, Gorsky R, Raimondi V. 1994. Costs of strategies for routine HIV counseling and testing of U.S. hospital patients. *Int. Conf. AIDS* 10:300 (Abstr. No. PC0586)

49. Johanson JF, Sonnenberg A. 1990. Efficient management of diarrhea in the acquired immunodeficiency syndrome (AIDS): a medical decision analysis. *Ann. Intern. Med.* 112:942–48

50. Judson FN. 1990. Partner notification for HIV control. *Hosp. Pract.* 25:63–73

51. Kahn JG. 1993. Are NEPs cost-effective in preventing HIV infection? In *The Public Health Impact of Needle Exchange Programs in the United States and Abroad*, ed. P Lurie, AL Reingold, 18:473–509. Univ. Calif., Sch. Public Health, Berkeley/Univ. Calif., Inst. Health Policy Stud., San Francisco

52. Kahn JG. 1993. How much does it cost to operate NEPs? See Ref. 51, pp. 243–59

53. Kahn JG, Washington AE. 1994. Optimizing the policy impact of HIV modeling. In *Modeling the AIDS Epidemic: Planning, Policy, and Prediction*, ed. EH Kaplan, ML Brandeau, 12:217–35. New York: Raven

54. Kahn JG, Washington AE, Showstack JA, Berlin M, Phillips K. 1992. Bleach distribution. In *Updated Estimates of the Impact and Cost of HIV Prevention in Injection Drug Users*, 7:95–103. Univ. Calif., Inst. Health Policy Stud., San Francisco

55. Kahn JG, Washington AE, Showstack JA, Berlin M, Phillips K. 1992. Counseling and testing. See Ref. 54, pp. 47–66

56. Kahn JG, Washington AE, Showstack JA, Berlin M, Phillips K. 1992. Ex-

tended counseling/education. See Ref. 54, pp. 67–77

57. Kahn JG, Washington AE, Showstack JA, Berlin M, Phillips K. 1992. Partner notification. See Ref. 54, pp. 78–94

58. Kahn JG, Washington AE, Showstack JA, Berlin M, Phillips K. 1992. Treatment of drug dependency. See Ref. 54, pp. 104–22

59. Kelly JA, Murphy DA, Sikkema KJ, Kalichman SC. 1993. Psychological interventions to prevent HIV infection are urgently needed: new priorities for behavioral research in the second decade of AIDS. Am. Psychol. 48:1023–34

60. Kongsin S, Dhiratayakinant K. 1994. Cost benefit analysis of screening HIV antibody (AIDS) in venereal disease patients. Int. Conf. AIDS 10:385 (Abstr. No. PD0720)

61. Lampinen TM. 1991. Cost-effectiveness of drug abuse treatment for primary prevention of acquired immunodeficiency syndrome: epidemiologic considerations. In Economic Costs, Cost-Effectiveness, Financing, and Community-Based Drug Treatment, Res. Monogr. 113, ed. WS Cartwright, JM Kaple, pp. 114–28. Rockville, MD: Natl. Inst. Drug Abuse

62. Laufer FN, Chiarello LA. 1994. Application of cost-effectiveness methodology to the consideration of needle-stick-prevention technology. Am. J. Infect. Control 22.75–82

63. Laupacis A, Feeny D, Detsky AS, Tugwell PX. 1992. How attractive does a new technology have to be to warrant adoption and utilization? Tentative guidelines for using clinical and economic evaluations. Can. Med. Assoc. J. 146:473–81

64. Laupacis A, Feeny D, Detsky AS, Tugwell PX. 1993. Tentative guidelines for using clinical and economic evaluations revisited. Can. Med. Assoc. J. 148:927–29

65. Lawrence VA, Gafni A, Kroenke K. 1993. Preoperative HIV testing: Is it less expensive than universal precautions? J. Clin. Epidemiol. 46:1219–27

66. Le Gales C, Moatti JP, Paris-Tours Study Group of Antenatal Transmission of HIV, Group '9 Maternités.' 1990. Cost-effectiveness of HIV screening of pregnant women in hospitals of the Paris area. Eur. J. Obstet. Gynecol. Reprod. Biol. 37:25–33

67. Le Gales C, Seror V, Courpotin C, Tricoire J, Reynert P, Diakate F. 1992. Cost-benefit analysis of HIV prenatal screening in France. Int. Conf. AIDS 8:C380 (Abstr. No. PoC4824)

68. Levine AA, Sandler RS. 1994. Screening for human immunodeficiency virus in physicians: Who should we test and what will it cost? NC Med. J. 55:136–40

69. Luce BR, Simpson K. 1995. Methods of cost-effectiveness analysis: areas of consensus and debate. Clin. Ther. 17:109–25

70. Lurie P, Avins AL, Phillips KA, Kahn JG, Lowe RA, Ciccarone D. 1994. The cost-effectiveness of voluntary counseling and testing of hospital inpatients for HIV infection. JAMA 272:1832–38

71. Mathews WC, Fenton C, Fullerton S, Abramson I, Coley E, La Belle J. 1990. Cost-effectiveness of secondary PCP prophylaxis using aerosolized pentamidine: evaluation of a hospital-based program. Int. Conf. AIDS 6:376 (Abstr. No. 2088)

72. McCarthy BD, Schreiber MB, Ward RE, Saravolatz LD. 1994. Should all pregnant women be screened for HIV infection? Med. Decis. Making 14:437 (Abstr.)

73. McCarthy BD, Wong JB, Munoz A, Sonnenberg FA. 1993. Who should be screened for HIV infection? A cost-effectiveness analysis. Arch. Intern. Med. 153:1107–16

74. McFarland W, Kahn JG, Katzenstein D, Mvere D, Shamu R. 1994. Blood donor deferral by HIV risk factors is cost-effective in Zimbabwe. Int. Conf. AIDS 10:8 (Abstr. No. 326C)

75. McKay NL, Phillips KM. 1991. An economic evaluation of mandatory premarital testing for HIV. Inquiry 28:236–48

76. Mendelson DN, Sandler SG. 1990. A model for estimating incremental benefits and costs of testing donated blood for human immunodeficiency virus antigen (HIV-Ag). Transfusion 30:73–75

77. Moses S, Plummer FA, Ngugi EN, Nagelkerke NJD, Anzala AO, Ndinya-Achola JO. 1991. Controlling HIV in Africa: effectiveness and cost of an intervention in a high-frequency STD transmitter core group. AIDS 5:407–11

78. Mullins JR, Harrison PB. 1993. The questionable utility of mandatory screening for the human immunodeficiency virus. Am. J. Surg. 166:676–79

79. Nahmias S, Feinstein CD. 1990. Screening strategies to inhibit the spread of AIDS. Socio-Econ. Plan. Sci. 24:249–60

80. Owens DK, Harris RA, Scott PM, Nease RF Jr. 1995. Screening surgeons for HIV infection: a cost-effectiveness analysis. Ann. Intern. Med. 122:641–52

81. Owens DK, Nease RF, Harris R. 1993.

Use of cost-effectiveness and value of information analyses to customize guidelines for specific clinical practice settings. *Med. Decis. Making* 13:395 (Abstr.)

82. Owens DK, Nease RF, Harris RA. 1993. Screening for HIV infection in acute-care settings: determinants of cost-effectiveness. *Med. Decis. Making* 13:395 (Abstr.)

83. Paltiel AD, Kaplan EH. 1991. Modeling zidovudine therapy: a cost-effectiveness analysis. *J. Acquired Immune Defic. Syndr.* 4:795–804

84. Paltiel AD, Kaplan EH. 1994. Cost-effectiveness of voluntary HIV testing in acute-care hospitals. *Med. Decis. Making* 14:439 (Abstr.)

85. Patrick DL, Erickson P. 1993. *Health Status and Health Policy: Quality of Life in Health Care Evaluation and Resource Allocation* New York: Oxford Univ. Press

86. Pavia AT, Benyo M, Niler L, Risk I. 1993. Partner notification for control of HIV: results after 2 years of a statewide program in Utah. *Am. J. Public Health* 83:1418–24

87. Petersen LR, White CR, Premarital Screening Study Group. 1990. Premarital screening for antibodies to human immunodeficiency virus type 1 in the United States. *Am. J. Public Health* 80:1087–90

88. Phillips KA, Lowe RA, Kahn JG, Lurie P, Avins AL, Ciccarone D. 1994. The cost-effectiveness of HIV testing of physicians and dentists in the United States. *JAMA* 271:851–58

89. Posen AS, Turvey J, Goldstone I. 1992. Economic implications of Vancouver's needle exchange. *Int. Conf. AIDS* 8:D454 (Abstr. No. PoD5406)

90. Prev. Effectiveness Activity. 1994. *A Practical Guide to Prevention Effectiveness: Decision and Economic Analyses.* CDC, Epidemiol. Program Off., Atlanta

91. Ramsey SD, Nettleman MD. 1992. Cost-effectiveness of prophylactic AZT following needlestick injury in health care workers. *Med. Decis. Making* 12:142–48

92. Revicki D, Simpson KN, LaVallee R, Palmer C. 1993. Cost-utility of adding ddC to AZT treatment for AIDS patients in the United States. *Int. Conf. AIDS* 9:920 (Abstr. No. PO-D28–4216)

93. Rose DN, Schechter CB, Sacks HS. 1993. Influenza and pneumococcal vaccination of HIV-infected patients: a policy analysis. *Am. J. Med.* 94:160–68

94. Russo G, La Croix SJ. 1992. A second look at the cost of mandatory human immunodeficiency virus and hepatitis B virus testing for healthcare workers performing invasive procedures. *Infect. Control Hosp. Epidemiol.* 13:107–10

95. Rutherford GW, Woo JM, Neal DP, Rauch KJ, Geoghegan C, et al. 1991. Partner notification and the control of human immunodeficiency virus infection: two years of experience in San Francisco. *Sex. Transm. Dis.* 18:107–10

96. Schopper D, Auvert B. 1994. Estimating the global impact of interventions to decrease the spread of HIV in developing countries by the year 2000. *Int. Conf. AIDS* 10:330 (Abstr. No. PC0253)

97. Schulman KA, Lynn LA, Glick HA, Eisenberg JM. 1991. Cost effectiveness of low-dose zidovudine therapy for asymptomatic patients with human immunodeficiency virus (HIV) infection. *Ann. Intern. Med.* 114:798–802

98. Sell RL, Jovell AJ, Siegel JE. 1994. HIV screening of surgeons and dentists - a cost-effectiveness analysis. *Infect. Control Hosp. Epidemiol.* 15(10):635–45

99. Smith MD, Murray RB, McAvinue S, Suldan M, Chaisson RE. 1990. Cost-effectiveness of aerosolized pentamidine (AP) prophylaxis against pneumocystis carinii pneumonia. *Int. Conf. AIDS* 6:289 (Abstr. No. F.D.830)

100. Spencer NE, Hoffman RE, Raevsky CA, Wolf FC, Vernon TM. 1993. Partner notification for human immunodeficiency virus infection in Colorado: results across index case groups and costs. *Int. J. STD AIDS* 4:26–32

101. Stock SR, Gafni A, Bloch RF. 1990. Universal precautions to prevent HIV transmission to health care workers: an economic analysis. *Can. Med. Assoc. J.* 142:937–46

102. Sweat M, Siegel G, de Zoysa I, Coates T. 1994. Identifying goals for behavior change programs in urban African settings: high effectiveness and moderate coverage maximize impact and cost-effectiveness. *Int. Conf. AIDS* 10:300 (Abstr. No. PC0589)

103. Tengs TO, Adams M, Pliskin JS, Safran DG, Siegel JE, et al. 1994. *Five-Hundred Life-Saving Interventions and their Cost-Effectiveness.* Boston: Harvard Sch. Public Health, Cent. Risk Anal.

104. Tramarin A, Milocchi F, Tolley K, Vaglia A, Marcolini F, et al. 1992. An economic evaluation of home-care assistance for AIDS patients: a pilot study in a town in northern Italy. *AIDS* 6:1377–83

105. Turnock BJ, Kelly CJ. 1989. Mandatory premarital testing for human immunode-

ficiency virus: the Illinois experience. *JAMA* 261:3415–18

106. Wachter RM, Luce JM, Safrin S, Berrios DC, Charlebois E, Scitovsky AA. 1995. Cost and outcome of intensive care for patients with AIDS, pneumocystis carinii pneumonia, and severe respiratory failure. *JAMA* 273:230–35

107. Watson-Williams EJ, Kataaha P, Senyonga P, Kyeyune D. 1994. Cost-effectiveness of Uganda blood programme. *Int. Conf. AIDS* 10:8 (Abstr. No. 325C)

108. Weinstein MC, Graham JD, Siegel JE, Fineberg HV. 1989. Cost-effectiveness analysis of AIDS prevention programs: concepts, complications, and illustrations. In *AIDS: Sexual Behavior and Intravenous Drug Use*, ed. CF Turner, HG Miller, LE Moses, pp. 471–99. Washington, DC: Natl. Acad. Sci.

109. Wiebel W, Jimenez A, Johnson W, Ouellet L, Murray J, O'Brien M. 1993. Positive effect on HIV seroconversion of street outreach intervention with IDU

in Chicago, 1988–1992. *Int. Conf. AIDS* 1:96 (Abstr. No. WS-C15–2)

110. Wilfert CM. 1994. Mandatory screening of pregnant women for the human immunodeficiency virus. *Clin. Infect. Dis.* 19:664–66

111. Wright-De Aguero LK, Gorsky RD, Seeman GM. 1995. Cost of outreach for HIV prevention among drug users and youth at risk. *Drugs Soc.* In press

112. Wykoff RF, Heath CW, Hollis SL, Leonard ST, Quiller CB, et al. 1988. Contact tracing to identify human immunodeficiency virus infection in a rural community. *JAMA* 259:3563–66

113. Yawn BP. 1992. Clinical decision analysis of HIV screening. *Fam. Med.* 24:355–61

114. Zowall H, Fraser RD, Gilmore N, Deutsch A, Grover S. 1990. HIV antibody screening among immigrants: a cost-benefit analysis. *Can. Med. Assoc. J.* 143:101–7

Annu. Rev. Public Health. 1996. 17:489–509

PREVENTION AND THE REFORMING U.S. HEALTH CARE SYSTEM: Changing Roles and Responsibilities for Public Health[1]

Randolph L. Gordon[1][2], Edward L. Baker[1], William L. Roper[2], and Gilbert S. Omenn[3]

[1]Public Health Practice Program Office, Centers for Disease Control and Prevention, 1600 Clifton Road, Atlanta, Georgia; [2]Prudential HealthCare, Roseland, New Jersey 07068; [3]School of Public Health and Community Medicine, University of Washington, Seattle, Washington 98195

KEY WORDS: public health practice, prevention, health care reform, managed care, financing

ABSTRACT

This review presents historical and cost-effectiveness perspectives of prevention in health care; discusses the nature, extent, and determinants of health system change, particularly the transition to managed care with large integrated health care corporations; and identifies implications for public health agencies and opportunities for prevention within the reforming health system.

INTRODUCTION

The overarching goal of health care reform, whether led by the private sector or by state or federal government, should be to improve the health and quality of life of the American people (3, 50), while constraining costs. A comprehensive system to prevent diseases and injuries, promote more healthful behaviors, and assure a healthier environment is a necessary component of any health care system. Such a system can provide a base for sustained, widespread

---

[1]The US Government has the right to retain a nonexclusive, royalty-free license in and to any copyright covering this paper.

[2]Current address: Virginia Department of Health, 1500 East Main Street, Richmond, Virginia 23219

Table 1 Causes of death, U.S., 1990

Listed causes		"Real causes"	
Heart disease	720,000	Tobacco	400,000
Cancers	505,000	Diet/activity patterns	300,000
Cerebrovascular	144,000	Alcohol	100,000
"Accidents"	92,000	Microbial agents	90,000
Chronic lung disease	87,000	Toxic agents	60,000
Pneumonia/influenza	80,000	Firearms	35,000
Diabetes mellitus	48,000	Sexual behavior	30,000
Suicide	31,000	Motor vehicles	25,000
Chronic liver disease	26,000	Illicit use of drugs	20,000
HIV infection	25,000		
TOTAL U.S. 1990	2,148,000	SUBTOTAL	1,060,000

Reference (42)

improvement in health and quality of life. Three highly cost-effective, mutually reinforcing components are required (51):

- community-based essential public health services: monitoring health indicators; educating the public about health risks and promoting healthy behaviors; and reducing health risks from air, water, food, consumer products, work place, and recreational hazards;
- clinical preventive services: immunizations, screening tests, and counseling by physicians and other health professionals; and
- social, economic, and regulatory policies that promote healthy behaviors, reduce hazardous exposures, and promote healthy standards of living including access to medical care.

We are accustomed to lists of the leading causes of death for two million Americans each year. Although the lists are useful in identifying the specific manifestation of the terminal disease or injury process (heart disease, cancers, etc), such lists fail to elucidate the underlying, often preventable factors responsible for premature death. The "real causes" of death relate to these underlying behaviors and environmental agents (42); such potentially preventable conditions account for at least half of all the deaths in this country (see Table 1). Poverty and associated deficiencies in education, jobs, housing and medical care are important co-variates.

HISTORY OF PREVENTION

The earliest prevention programs in this country were in the rapidly growing port cities of the eastern seaboard, with a primary aim of protecting the population from the introduction of epidemic diseases, such as the yellow fever epidemic that crippled Philadelphia in 1793 and later cholera pandemics (15). There emerged a struggle between those who relied on the police function of quarantines and those who believed that diseases could be prevented by cleaning up the filthy conditions of food, water, workplaces, docks, alleys, and streets that placed local residents at risk. The endemic conditions of typhoid, typhus, measles, diphtheria, influenza, tuberculosis, and malaria were "met with a stolid indifference born of familiarity and a sense of helplessness" (15, p. 3). We can recognize an all-too-familiar analogy in our current societal indifference (or ineffectiveness) in the face of drug abuse, violence, teen pregnancy, STDs, and alcoholism.

Lemuel Shattuck, in his 1850 report to the Massachusetts Legislature, argued for investment in prevention. He stated that thousands of lives are lost that might have been saved, that the resulting preventable evils require an enormous expenditure, and that measures for prevention would be more effective than remedies for the cure of the disease (70, p. 10). Shattuck advocated a "comprehensive plan of sanitary reform, by which ... the greatest possible amount of physical suffering may be prevented, and the greatest possible amount of physical, social and moral enjoyment may be attained" (70, p. 306). This prescription is remarkably close to the World Health Organization's contemporary definition of health as a state of complete physical, mental, and social well-being, not merely the absence of infirmity. The Massachusetts Legislature subsequently created boards of health with the responsibility for prevention and quarantine.

In the late 19th century, social reform movements spread across the country and such organizations as the American Public Health Association (1872), the American Red Cross (1882), and the American Tuberculosis Association (1904) emerged. The Committee of One Hundred on National Health (including Jane Addams, Andrew Carnegie, William H. Welch, and Booker T. Washington) campaigned for federal regulation of public health. In response, just before World War I, the federal government expanded the Marine Hospital Service (established in 1798) into the US Public Health Service (46). In 1920, Welch of Johns Hopkins would proclaim to an audience of philanthropists, "merely from a mercenary and commercial point of view it is for the interest of the community to take care of the health of the poor. Philanthropy assumes a totally different aspect in the eyes of the world when it is able to demonstrate that it pays to keep people healthy" (15, p. 5). As noted elsewhere (52), this speech may have marked the beginning of "health promotion and disease prevention," of academic health center fundraising, and of cost-effectiveness analysis of public health, all wrapped into one message!

The practice of prevention was greatly advanced by the development of academic centers that trained practitioners and developed a scientific base for public health practice. The Rockefeller Foundation was instrumental in the early twentieth century in stimulating and funding the development of schools of public health at leading universities in this country (Johns Hopkins, Harvard, Yale, Columbia) and abroad (London, Toronto, Sao Paolo) to meet the need for individuals trained in public health to direct local, state, and national programs on a full-time, professional basis. Public health students were often older physicians who had worked in public health positions without specialist qualifications or young scientists interested in the new fields of bacteriology, epidemiology, and statistics. From the beginning there was the dilemma we face today: Few young physicians chose to take public health training after earning the medical degree, thus contributing to the disjunction between public health and clinical practice.

Prevention as the responsibility of governmental public health agencies was firmly endorsed by resolutions passed in 1942 by the American Medical Association (AMA) and the American Public Health Association (APHA). The AMA urged the establishment of "complete coverage of the nation's area and population by local, county, district or regional full-time modern health services" to address the lack of "even minimum necessary sanitary and other preventive services for health" (14, p. 5). The APHA stated, "Whereas the most effective state and national health services can be provided only when all communities have accepted the responsibility of applying the science and art of preventive medicine as a permanent function of local civil government, therefore be it resolved that ... collaboration be sought to obtain total coverage of the nation by local health units at the earliest practicable date" (14, p. 6).

The separation of public health services (both community-based and individual preventive services) from clinical medical practice was accentuated during the mid-twentieth century by the advent of private health insurance as the dominant means of financing personal health care delivery in the United States. Typically, clinical preventive services were excluded from the package of covered services, due to reasoning related to life insurance theory. The notion was that insurance should apply to events that occur unpredictably with regard to specific individuals and infrequently within any given population and are difficult for individuals to pay for due to large costs. Thus, such insurance would not be used for events or services that are predictable and universal. This logic assumes, for example, that it would be more efficient and less costly for everyone to pay for his or her own family's immunizations and avoid the insurance fees and overhead. Such a line of reasoning neglects the central issue: Preventive services are intended to protect against infrequent and unpredicted severe complications of illness or injury. As health insurance evolved to become the central mechanism for financing health services, preventive services were not covered (i.e. not paid for) by the privately funded health system.

Over 95% of our nation's health dollar is consumed by the costs of the personal health system, designed for alleviating pain and suffering, trying to cure disease after it has become manifest (61). In view of the real determinants of death in the United States (Table 1), there is a substantial maldistribution of financial resources within the health system. Further, medical school training is based on a model that diagnoses and treats. Prevention is not traditionally part of mainstream medicine, as evidenced by the small amount of curricular time devoted to it in medical training, the lack of departments of preventive medicine in many medical schools, and the lack of schools of public health in most academic health centers (37).

Over recent decades, responsibility for delivery of preventive services has largely been the responsibility of publicly funded governmental health agencies, which have operated quite separately from the insurance-funded personal health care system. Clinical preventive services, performed in public health clinics or in physicians' offices, include screening for high risk conditions, such as elevated blood lead levels, elevated blood pressure, and elevated serum cholesterol; provision of immunizations; management of certain communicable diseases, especially sexually transmitted diseases and tuberculosis; and counseling to reduce risky behaviors. At long last, private policies and now Medicare have begun to cover some clinical preventive services (mammographic screening; pneumococcal and influenza vaccinations), though they still systematically exclude payment for population-oriented, community-based public health services. Medicaid has long offered clinical preventive services as part of routine care of babies and children and as part of the Early & Periodic Screening Diagnosis & Treatment (EPSDT) Program.

Community-Based Prevention: Essential Public Health Services

Community-based prevention comprises those essential public health services provided to the community as a whole and to specific subpopulations (see Table 2). These services have the potential to benefit everyone in an entire geographic area. Although most public health services have been provided to communities by governmental public health agencies (79), other public and private organizations have, over recent years, become involved in these community-wide efforts. Organizations like the March of Dimes and the American Cancer Society, American Heart Association and American Lung Association supplement community-wide efforts of governmental public health agencies to assess health status, to develop and disseminate appropriate policies, and to assure needed services are available. The mission of all such public health efforts is to promote physical and mental health and prevent disease, injury and disability. Such efforts aim to achieve the vision of public health as "Healthy People in Healthy Communities" (3).

These public and nonprofit agencies perform activities for which no private sector financial incentives are perceived to exist or which transcend the jurisdictions of private businesses (56, 60). Under a fee-for-service health care payment mechanism, in fact, a theoretical disincentive exists: if prevention programs are successful, they may reduce health care utilization and the accompanying reimbursement.

Meanwhile, public health agencies have become responsible for the delivery of personal health services to uninsured and medically indigent individuals. Filling the gaping holes in the medical care system for the poor and for other vulnerable populations has overwhelmed the capacity of many local health departments, and the responsibility to respond to ill patients has tended to claim staffing and funding that might have supported prevention activities. Because of the pressures on public treasuries, the level of funding to health departments for personal health service delivery, let alone community-based prevention programs, has been inadequate. Increasingly, public health departments have turned to billing for patients who do have some kind of coverage.

COST-EFFECTIVENESS OF PREVENTION

The irony of our present situation is that public health agencies are struggling to maintain a focus on prevention while there is increasing pressure to control medical care expenditures and improve quality of life. Prevention can be effective in reducing unnecessary, costly personal health services (53). The people of the United States spent about $1000 billion dollars in 1995, or $4000 per person, on medical care. To effectively reduce the soaring increases in national health care costs, prevention programs that combine community-based services, clinical services, and social policies must become more widely supported.

In recent years, prevention activities have been subjected increasingly to economic assessments using cost-effectiveness analysis or cost-benefit analysis (12, 20, 29, 33, 41, 83). Cost-effectiveness analyses evaluate an intervention in terms of money invested in an intervention to produce a certain outcome, such as cost-per-year of life gained (49, 74). Effectiveness analysis in terms of quality-adjusted-life-years (QALY) gained can compare the results of interventions to decrease morbidity and increase quality of life (17, 73). Cost-benefit analysis compares dollars invested in an intervention to the dollar value of benefits achieved (49).

Just as with medical care, the benefits and costs of various prevention programs vary tremendously (20, 32, 51, 74, 75, 81). Prevention effectiveness research has begun to analyze how effective prevention can be; how big the problem is that is to be prevented; what the prevention programs cost in dollars per life saved, years of life or quality-adjusted life added, or extent of disability

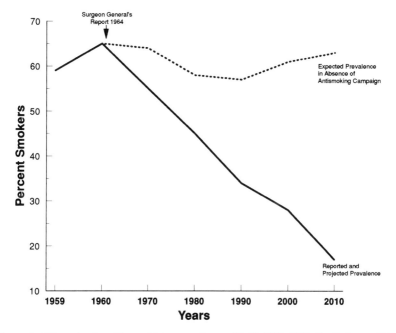

Figure 1   Effect of antismoking activities on males age 40–49, 1950–2010. See Reference 81, p. 15.

averted; whether the prevention program can save so much in medical and social costs that the program would have net savings; and who would get the benefits, who would pay, and who would save. Such research results should be utilized to help integrate prevention into the reform of the medical care system.

Among the most cost-effective interventions are smoking prevention, childhood immunizations, environmental lead reduction, and fluoridation.

Prevention campaigns over the past three decades have dramatically reduced the prevalence of smoking in the U.S. The rate in males has fallen from over 60% in 1960 (shortly before the first Surgeon General's Report on Smoking and Health) to less than 30% today and is projected to continue to decline as shown in Figure 1.

This decline has been attributable to a range of health education and health promotion activities conducted by public health agencies, private organizations (e.g. the American Cancer Society's annual "Great American Smokeout"), schools, hospitals, work sites, and private medical practitioners, as well as tax increases on cigarettes and restrictions on smoking.

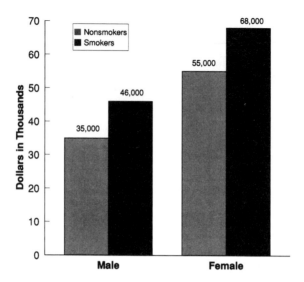

Figure 2   Lifetime medical expenditures for smokers and nonsmokers by gender

Collectively, smoking prevention efforts in the United States over the past three decades have been estimated to have saved 33 million person-years of life. A projected additional four million deaths will be postponed (and millions of additional years of life saved) between 1993 and 2015 as a result of current antismoking activities (81). Medical expenditures for smokers over a lifetime exceed those for nonsmokers by a substantial amount. One estimate of smoking prevention programs put lifetime medical expenditure savings at $11,000 for men and $13,000 for women (81) (see Figure 2).

With vaccine-preventable diseases, notable successes include polio, measles, mumps, rubella, diphtheria, pertussis, and tetanus. In each case, costs are modest and the benefits are dramatic; society saves about $8 in direct medical costs for every $1 spent on childhood immunizations (7, 51, 74, 81, 85).

Excessive lead exposure, a recognized cause of impaired cognitive function in children and adults, has been controlled through the reduction of lead as an additive in gasoline, the prohibition of lead in paint used for internal residential purposes, and abatement of existing lead hazards through targeted public health programs. Blood lead levels in children in the U.S. tested in the NHANES surveys have fallen in parallel with the removal of lead from gasoline. Benefits in improved I.Q. scores and better school and work performance are anticipated as a result of control of exposure to this hazardous environmental neurotoxin. It has been estimated that preventing increase in blood lead levels results in an average increase in lifetime earning of $1147 per mg/dl difference per child

(78). Applying this number to the entire population of children, the economic benefit to society from eliminating leaded gasoline is enormous. In a comparison of 500 life-saving interventions it was estimated that the cost of saving one year of life by reducing the lead in gasoline from 1.1 to 0.1 gram per gallon was less than $50, one of the most cost-effective interventions included in the analysis (74). Furthermore, a cost benefit analysis of a national lead paint abatement program, a much more expensive intervention than removing lead from gasoline, estimated a net benefit of $62 billion (78).

Finally, water fluoridation is another impressive public health success. Decline in dental caries over the past 40 years is such that more than half of children in the U.S. are now free of caries. Over the lifetime of an individual, the cost of restoring a carious tooth may exceed $1000; in contrast, water fluoridation costs about $0.12 per person per year. Thus, fluoridation represents one of the most cost-beneficial of all prevention interventions (9, 74). Nevertheless, 80 million Americans still lack access to a fluoridated water supply (7).

THE REFORMING SYSTEM OF MEDICAL CARE

Two major system changes currently permeating the entire fabric of health care delivery have enormous implications for prevention. These changes are driven by market forces and seem likely to intensify, whether national or state health care reform legislation is enacted, or not.

First, the transition from a fee-for-service to a prepaid capitated form of payment transforms the financial incentives in medical care. Under this arrangement, both comprehensive and specialty services are paid for on a per capita basis through a set payment for a range of services for a specified period of time. In general, financial incentives exist to reduce overall utilization of health services, especially costly services (1, 21). As a result, improving and promoting each person's health should become a high priority for health care providers and their organizations. Although subject to debate (67–69), appropriately targeted prevention strategies and services can reduce utilization and reduce health care costs (51). Decreased utilization can result from fewer patient visits and from less expensive encounters as illnesses are recognized and treated earlier, in some cases after screening of asymptomatic individuals and groups.

The second major system change is integration of primary, secondary, and tertiary medical care services into large corporate organizations. Integration reduces the incentive for cost-shifting, which occurs under more fragmented approaches to health care delivery. The number of persons enrolled in health maintenance organizations (HMOs) has surpassed 50 million and is growing at an accelerating rate (24), while the number of HMOs decreased from 626 in 1986 to 545 in 1993 (24). There is a great variety of managed care, including health maintenance organizations (HMOs), preferred provider organizations (PPOs), independent provider organizations (IPOs), primary care case management (PCCM), and physician hospital organizations (PHOs). Even in rural areas, hospitals and managed care organizations are seeking arrangements with physicians that position them to compete for patients (28). One characteristic of managed care is managing the decisions of health care providers through quality control and utilization review managers, using protocols or clinical guidelines (44, 73). Primary care physicians become more highly valued as gatekeepers and patient advocates (34). Such formalized decision-making and review processes may be a good setting to measure and reinforce the impact of prevention activities.

State-Based Legislative and Regulatory Reform

Reform of the health system is occurring in states throughout the country. Nearly all states have constituted health reform commissions with varying mandates and levels of activity. Comprehensive health reform legislation has been passed in at least six states, while others are considering actions varying from minor changes in health insurance regulations to comprehensive health system change. Here we mention four leading examples.

FLORIDA   The Health Care and Insurance Reform Act of 1993 increased medical insurance regulation and created 11 Community Health Purchasing Alliances to manage the purchasing of health insurance for small employers, individuals, and state employees. Florida received a waiver from the Health Care Financing Administration (HCFA) for its Health Security Plan that will place Medicaid recipients under managed care and use the cost savings to cover the uninsured (30). Some public health agencies formed their own HMOs in order to continue to care for the Medicaid population. Even though the legislature has yet to pass enabling legislation to support all the changes in the waiver, Florida has enrolled 417,000 of its 1.6 million Medicaid beneficiaries into managed care (36).

MINNESOTA   MinnesotaCare—established through comprehensive health reform legislation in 1992, 1993, and 1994—was designed to foster more integration and corporatization of the health care system, laying the groundwork for Integrated Service Networks (45). The goals of reform are increasing access, containing costs, and improving quality. The Department of Health was given the lead role in designing and implementing the reform process. Even though the goal of universal coverage has been modified since the initial legislation, changes central to public health are being implemented. Regional

Coordinating Boards have been established to set public health goals for their regions. The Minnesota Health Data Institute administers a consumer satisfaction survey, and the Department of Health issues report cards on health plans in the state (84).

RHODE ISLAND   RIte Care, the capitated managed care program for Medicaid in Rhode Island, was a result of statewide dialogue on health care reform. It incorporates health improvement goals, a public health data system, quality assurance focused on public health goals, and neighborhood support teams to assist patients in transitioning to the new health care system.

WASHINGTON   In the far-reaching Health Services Act of 1993, the Washington Legislature encouraged further growth of managed care and integration of health services, aiming for universal coverage by 1999. Its employee-based mandate required a federal Employee Retirement Income Security Act (ERISA) waiver for full implementation. An independent, full-time Health Services Commission was given broad authority to establish a uniform benefits package, certify health plans and insurance offerings, and set premium caps to constrain health care expenditures. The Act explicitly acknowledged the goal of improving health status as part of health reform. It assigned a significant role to the state's Department of Health to develop a Public Health Improvement Plan (62) and a data system, and to stimulate integration of medical and public health services. The Public Health Improvement Plan addresses infrastructure and performance of core functions, with outcomes standards, threshold standards for action levels and alarm levels in surveillance programs, and interventions for key problems affecting the health status of state residents, tied to *Healthy People 2000* (4).

After a dramatic shift in the Legislature after the 1994 elections, the Health Services Act reportedly was "repealed." In fact, several major features were retained: portability of health insurance, limitations on restrictions for preexisting conditions, expansion of the Basic Health Plan for working uninsured, community-related insurance pools for individuals and for employees at worksites with fewer than 50 employees, expansion of Medicaid for children, and continuation and enhanced funding for the Public Health Improvement Plan (13). The Commission was reduced to an advisory Policy Forum. Without any prospect of a federal ERISA waiver, other aspects of the reform plan were moot.

MEDICAID MANAGED CARE

As described by Freund & Hurley (18), many of the remaining states are attempting to control the costs of the Medicaid Program by moving eligible patients into systems of managed care, generally without any ties to public health (82). Medicaid beneficiaries enrolled in managed care doubled in one year to 7.8 million in 1994 (80). Forty-five states enroll some of their Medicaid population in managed care and thirty-seven operate freedom-of-choice 1915(b) waivers (65), the regulatory mechanism that allows them to mandate that their Medicaid recipients enroll in a managed care plan (38). Twelve states have received comprehensive research and demonstration 1115 waivers from the Health Care Financing Administration (HCFA). An additional 17 have either submitted an 1115 waiver to HCFA or are in the process of developing one (84).

Medicaid reform offers an opportunity to monitor prevention activities; a case study in Arizona, however, found that neither the Arizona Health Care Cost System (the state Medicaid program) nor the Public Health Department collected data on the use of public health clinics or the provision of clinical preventive services (23). The federal Health Resources and Services Administration (HRSA) is trying to build community-based preventive services into Medicaid reimbursement for federally supported migrant and community health centers.

Business Coalitions for Health

Groups of businesses have formed coalitions to increase the value of the services provided to their employees by health plans and health insurance companies (71). A primary goal is to control costs by curbing, and then preventing, the high rate of increase in health insurance premiums (35). A simultaneous focus on quality of care has resulted in negotiations about benefit packages and expected health outcomes in the enrolled population. The Health Plan Employer Data Information Set (HEDIS) (31) and health plan report cards have been designed to provide accountability measures from the health care industry to businesses purchasing medical services for their employees.

Practice guidelines are being used to improve and assess quality of care. The Agency for Health Care Policy and Research (AHCPR), professional medical and surgical specialty organizations, and various health plans are developing and implementing practice guidelines for therapeutic interventions. Guidelines for clinical preventive interventions were published by the Canadian Task Force on the Periodic Health Examination (CTFPHE), the American College of Physicians (ACP), and the US Preventive Services Task Force (72, 73). The Centers for Disease Control and Prevention (CDC) recently began to assess the effectiveness of community-based guidelines; CDC has collected these guidelines into a Prevention Guidelines Database, available to practitioners through CDC's *PC WONDER*, an on-line electronic communication system (20), and the Internet.

INTEREST IN PREVENTION IN MANAGED CARE AND HOSPITAL ORGANIZATIONS

Managed care organizations are increasing the provision of preventive serv-ices, mostly clinical interventions, including screening, immunizations, and counseling for high-risk conditions (44, 58). Early detection of disease and guidance for personal health–reducing risks are activities in which physicians and other care providers have some training and fit well with the model of office-based health delivery.

Community-based prevention, in contrast, is not usually seen as a respon-sibility of private health care organizations, nor do they consider support of clinical research or access of their patients to cancer treatment protocols a responsibility.

Nevertheless, some leading managed care organizations are now engaged in community-based prevention activities. For example, the Group Health Association of America (GHAA) is collaborating with CDC on a major vaccine initiative. The managed care organizations involved in this project are com-mitting to immunize at least 90% of their enrolled children by approximately two years of age. With over 50 million persons enrolled in HMOs, such cooperative agreements can enhance preventive services.

Group Health Cooperative of Puget Sound, in conjunction with the state and local public health community, the Fred Hutchinson Cancer Research Center, and the University of Washington School of Public Health and Com-munity Medicine, helped pass state legislation that restricts smoking in public places and access for minors, as well as omnibus HIV/AIDS legislation. Group Health sponsors HIV prevention campaigns and youth violence prevention initiatives targeted at high-risk communities in Seattle, not just those enrolled in their plan. With a grant from the CDC, Group Health Cooperative is conducting a study called ENPOWER, Encouraging Preventive Services for Older Women enrolled in Managed Care Plans (A LaCroix, personal commu-nication).

The Harvard Community Health Plan has recognized the importance of violence as a health issue. The Plan's adolescent violence prevention project helps pediatric providers to identify children at risk for being violent and to teach the children alternative methods of expressing their anger (27).

Another traditional function of public health agencies is assessment of the community's health. Hospitals are now performing community health assess-ments in many locales throughout the country, partly or primarily for marketing purposes. The Pennsylvania and Vermont Hospital Associations encouraged their members to perform community needs assessments to determine how best to utilize their resources. The Hospital Association of Pennsylvania de-veloped a five-phase process that begins with a county health profile, sets priorities for community health needs, develops an action plan, offers services, and evaluates the interventions. Not-for-profit hospitals can satisfy their required "community benefit" to maintain their favored tax status by sponsoring community health assessments. California law now requires hospitals to do community health planning to maintain their not-for-profit status. The National Association of County and City Health Officials receives more requests from hospitals than from local health agencies for the *Assessment Protocol for Excellence in Public Health (APEX/PH)*, an assessment tool developed originally for local health departments (2).

Many managed care organizations currently cite the significant turnover among their enrollees as a disincentive for community-based preventive funding, though much of that turnover comes from one to another managed care provider. As these organizations collectively come to serve larger proportions of local and regional populations, we hope that public health agencies and managed care organizations will work together much more closely, sharing expertise to pursue common agendas. Elsewhere, it has been estimated that an additional $3–5/month/person to the present public sector appropriations for public health departments is needed (43, 51, 81).

PUBLIC HEALTH AGENCIES AND PREVENTION: FUTURE DIRECTIONS

As noted above, most public health agencies currently have a dual mission, providing community-based preventive services, including environmental protection, and providing medical care to the disenfranchised (10, 52). Most local and state health departments have their roots in controlling infectious diseases. Clinical preventive services provided by local public health agencies typically include prenatal care, communicable disease control, well child care including immunizations, cancer screening, and family planning. Some, such as Alameda County, California, provide comprehensive health services and are expanding all components of their services.

Public health agencies will continue to provide the community-based essential public health services (Table 2). As public health agencies focus on current public health problems, they will need to work more closely with managed care organizations. By forming partnerships with public health agencies, managed care organizations can realize the benefits of dedicating some resources to community-based prevention programs and garner the expertise of professional public health practitioners (6, 39). Local and state health agencies may become their community's and state's "prevention agencies," like CDC at the national level, hopefully collaborating with schools of public health for training, research, and demonstration projects.

Table 2 Essential public health services

Monitor health status of communities
Investigate health problems and health hazards in the community
Inform, educate, and empower people about health issues
Mobilize community partnerships and action to identify and solve health problems
Develop policies and plans that support individual and community health efforts
Enforce laws and regulations that protect health and ensure safety
Link people to needed personal health services and assure the provision of health care when otherwise unavailable
Assure a competent public health and personal health care workforce
Evaluate effectiveness, accessibility, and quality of personal and population-based health services
Research health problems for new insights and innovative solutions

Reference (8)

Other health departments are forming new public/private partnerships to develop and expand prevention-oriented personal health services through managed care. The Seattle-Kings County Department of Public Health has partnerships with multiple managed care plans that provide revenue that allows for health services expansion. These arrangements also provide increased funding for clinical and population prevention services. The Department has two kinds of partnerships roles—comprehensive health provider (sharing risk) in a managed care system and as a specialized prevention service provider (carve out) under contract for specific interventions such as case management, screening, or health education.

Since the collapse of comprehensive health care reform legislation in 1994, expected improvements in coverage and access for underserved populations have been deferred. Public health agencies will continue to have a role in providing or funding some clinical care, including clinical preventive services, to those unable to pay for medical care, even in the face of cutbacks, as in Los Angeles County in 1995. Some public health leaders fear that with decreased revenue from Medicaid funding for clinical services for medically indigent persons, public health agencies may have less capacity to provide community-based and clinical preventive services in settings where a portion of these primary care revenues has provided base funding for programs in the past.

Federal public health agencies will continue to play the role of maintaining the national capacity for research and research training and of developing programs critical to the nation's public health. Emerging and re-emerging infectious diseases are a prime example of the necessity of a federal role in public health, illustrated by hantavirus, cryptosporidiosis, *Escherichia coli* 0157, and Ebola virus outbreaks in the period 1993–1995. New approaches need to be developed to deal with violence and other behaviorally mediated threats to health. In addition, the health indicators of the nation must continue to be tracked, and national health goals updated. *Healthy People 2000* (77) represents an ongoing process to track and improve the nation's health.

The concept of "A Governmental Presence at the Local Level" is taking on greater significance as solutions for many issues are being found in local communities (60). Public health agencies have convened and mobilized communities to deal with health threats. The Clinton Administration's proposed performance partnerships (40) and Congressional budget cuts both direct more responsibility to the state and local levels.

PARTNERSHIPS AND PREVENTION

In reforming the US health care system, there are increasing examples of private/public efforts to improve and protect the public's health.

The Gaston County, North Carolina, hospital, health department and community leaders formed the Gaston County Community Health Care Commission to develop a workable community-wide agenda to improve health status via a collaborative problem-solving network of organizations and people (6). They are assessing community health needs, identifying interventions and community resources, and evaluating health status improvement. M. D. Health Plan in North Haven, Connecticut, is working with the Department of Health to develop "Working Well Together," a health promotion program utilizing worksite classes, health fairs, and television programming to promote the Governor's wellness priorities (25), to target the community, not just health plan enrollees. The Wellness Plan, an HMO in Detroit, is working with the city government to promote physical fitness and sports activities among senior citizens (26).

Partnerships also have been formed to encourage policy development for prevention. The Partnership for Prevention is a nonprofit organization committed to increase prevention's priority in national health policy and practice (57). The Partnership board of directors—consisting of elected public officials, academicians, executives of private managed care organizations, and public health officials—has produced several important publications (43, 51, 56, 57).

The building of health data systems can reflect the shared interest of the private and public sectors in promoting prevention. As noted above, the Health Plan Employer Data Information Set (HEDIS) is a set of indicators standardized for reporting by managed care organizations, so that employers can compare plans (31, 86). HEDIS 2.0/2.5 uses indicators assessing childhood immunizations; cholesterol, mammography and cervical cancer screening; low birth weight and prenatal care rates; admissions for asthma; diabetic retinal exams; and follow-up of major affective disorders. These HEDIS indicators correspond directly to age-group-related *Healthy People 2000* (77) objectives 20.11, 15.8, 16.11, 16.12, 14.5, 14.11, 11.1, 17.10 and 16.7, respectively.

Combined with existing public health data systems, the data systems supporting the measurement of health plan indicators may generate geographically
coherent surveillance of health status and disease tracking with a single information infrastructure (63).

The training of health care providers in prevention will be a joint effort of
public health and the private sector. The recent *E. coli* outbreak in the state of
Washington provided an opportunity not only to pool resources to address a
health emergency, but also a chance to train practitioners and to link schools
of public health, state and local health departments, the CDC, and providers
of medical care (22, 48). The Group Health Foundation, the educational arm
of the Group Health Association of America, has established a Minority Training Program in HMO management. The steering committee is composed of
representatives from managed care organizations and from the US Public
Health Service (55).

The Pew Charitable Trusts have supported Primary Care 2000: Strategies
for Federal Policy Reform (59). The competencies listed for practitioners for
the year 2005 involve traditional public health skills directed at caring for the
community's health, practicing prevention, and promoting healthy lifestyles.
These recommendations are now being scrutinized and applied to individual
states through initiatives supported by Pew and others. Pew more recently has
convened managed care and academic public health leaders to try to stimulate
research, training, and applications of community-based and plan-based prevention strategies for managed care populations.

The Centers for Disease Control and Prevention are developing a Public
Health Training Network for (re)training health care providers in managed
care, as well as linking them with public health officials (3). The CDC Information Network for Public Health Officials (INPHO) received a National
Information Infrastructure Award and the Association of State and Territorial
Health Officials' Vision Award for outstanding applications of information
technology in the health sector. The Public Health Leadership Institute (66),
sponsored by the Centers for Disease Control and Prevention and the Western
Consortium for Public Health, is presently training its fifth annual cohort of
public health practitioners. Regional leadership institutes have been organized
at the University of Washington (54) and St. Louis University Schools of
Public Health and in the states of Florida, Illinois, Michigan, Missouri, Ohio,
and Texas. These initiatives in training public health leaders can serve as a
model for similar programs of leadership enhancement in the private sector.

CONCLUSIONS

Reform of the health care system in the United States is occurring through
market reforms based on integration of delivery system components and capi-

tation of payment to health care providers. These changes provide incentives to the private system of health care to invest resources in preventing disease and promoting health in their enrolled populations, in persons who may enroll in their plan in the future, and in those whose behaviors may affect the health of their enrollees (64). These incentives should orient activities of managed care organizations to support both clinical and community-based preventive services.

The resulting greater interest in prevention should be matched by an increase in efforts to establish the scientific basis for prevention. Many clinical and community-based preventive services need to be investigated. Just as greater scrutiny is being applied to treatment interventions, recommendations about preventive interventions and programs need to be based on scientifically demonstrated outcomes.

The sharing of some common interests provides reason for public health agencies and managed care organizations to work together. Opportunities for collaboration exist in developing information systems, performing community health assessments, developing policies to promote prevention, implementing prevention programs, developing the science base for prevention, and training health care providers. It is time to heal the schism between public health and curative medicine (19, 85a). As managed care reaches a larger proportion of local and regional populations, payers and providers should find common ground in assuring that an adequate slice of the capitated payment for each covered life is committed to all three elements of the prevention strategy, including funding for community-based prevention programs.

Literature Cited

1. Am. Coll. Physicians. 1992. Universal insurance for American health care. *Ann. Intern. Med.* 117:511–19
2. Assess. Protocol Excellence Public Health (APEX/PH). 1991. Natl. Assoc. County Health Off., Washington, DC
3. Baker EL, Melton RJ, Stange PV, Fields ML, Koplan JP. 1994. Health reform and the health of the public—forging community health partnerships. *JAMA* 272:1276–82
4. Berkowitz B. 1995. Health system reform: a blueprint for the future of public health. *J. Public Health Manage. Policy* 1:1–6
5. Deleted in proof
6. Carroll MC, Shovelin WF. 1994. Collaboration and community health care networks: moving from theory to practice. Presented at Am. Coll. Health Care Exec. Congr. Admin.
7. Cent. Dis. Control Prev. 1994. *An Ounce of Prevention: What are the Returns?* Washington, DC: DHHS
8. Cent. Dis. Control Prev. 1995. Table 1. Public health responsibilities and essential public health services—1994. *Morbid. Mortal. Wkly. Rep.* 44:429
9. Clark RM, Goodrich JA, Ireland JC. 1984. Cost and benefits of drinking water treatment. *J. Environ. Syst.* 14:1–30
10. Comm. Study Future Public Health, Inst. Med. 1988. *The Future of Public*

Health, p. v. Washington, DC: Natl. Acad. Press

11. Deleted in proof
12. Cummings SR, Rubin SM, Oster G. 1989. The cost-effectiveness of counseling smokers to quit. *JAMA* 261:75–79
13. Dyer P. 1995. The re-vision. *Wash. Public Health* 13:28–29
14. Emerson H. 1945. *Local Health Units for the Nation.* New York: Commonw. Fund
15. Fee E. 1991. The origins and development of public health in the United States. In *Oxford Textbook of Public Health,* ed. R Detels, W Holland, J McEwen, GS Omenn, Chap. 1. New York/Toronto: Oxford Univ. Press. 3rd ed.
16. Fielding JE, Lancry PJ. 1993. Lessons from France—'vive la différence'. The French health care system and US health system reform. *JAMA* 270:748–56
17. Foege W. 1994. Preventive medicine and public health. *JAMA* 271:1704–5
18. Freund DA, Hurley RE. 1995. Medicaid managed care contribution to issues of health reform. *Annu. Rev. Public Health* 16:473–95
19. Freyman JG. 1975. Medicine's great schism: prevention vs. cure: an historical interpretation. *Med. Care* 13:525–36
20. Friede A, Taylor WR, Nadelman L. 1993. On-line access to a cost-benefit/cost effectiveness analysis bibliography via CDC WONDER. *Med. Care* 31(7):JS12–17
21. Fries JF, Koop CE, Beadle CE, Cooper PP, England MJ, et al. 1993. Reducing health care costs by reducing the need and demand for medical services. *N. Engl. J. Med.* 329:321–25
22. Goldoft M, Kobayashi J. 1993. Scientific work and epidemiologic vigilance quickly halt *E. coli* epidemic. *Wash. Public Health* 11:1–3
23. Greenberg EL, Atchison CG. 1995. The impact of Medicaid managed care on the public health system in Arizona: a case study. *J. Public Health Manage. Policy* 1:7–15
24. Group Health Assoc. Am. 1994. *1994 National Directory of HMOs.* Washington, DC: Group Health Assoc. Am.
25. Group Health Assoc. Am. 1994. *HMO Managers Lett.* 11(10):6
26. Deleted in proof
27. Group Health Assoc. Am. 1994. HMOs as preventive health pacesetters. *HMO Mag.* 35:105–7
28. Halverson GC. 1993. *Strong Medicine,* pp. 215–17. New York: Random House
29. Hatziandreu EL, Koplan JP, Weinstein MC, Caspersen CJ, Warner KE. 1988.

A cost-effectiveness analysis of exercise as a health promotion activity. *Am. J. Public Health* 78:1417–21
30. Health Care Reform Week. 1994. *Wash. DC* 23:1
31. *Health Plan Employer Data and Information Set and Users' Manual.* 1993. Version 2.0. Natl. Comm. Qual. Assur. Washington, DC
32. Holtgrave DR, Valdiserri RO, Gerber AH, Hinman AH. 1993. Human immunodeficiency virus counseling, testing, referral and partner notification services: a cost-benefit analysis. *Arch. Intern. Med.* 153:1225–30
33. Huntington J, Connell FA. 1994. For every dollar spent, the cost-savings argument for prenatal care. *N. Engl. J. Med.* 331:1303–7
34. Hurley RE, Freund DA, Gage BJ. 1991. Gatekeeper effects on patterns of physician use. *J. Fam. Pract.* 32:167–74
35. Iglehart JK. 1994. The struggle between managed care and fee-for-service practice. Health Policy Report. *N. Engl. J. Med.* 331:63–67
36. Iglehart JK. 1995. Policy report medicaid and managed care. *N. Engl. J. Med.* 332:1727–31
37. Khanna PM. 1992. Preventive care is prescribed to cut costs, but doctor training faces the scalpel. *Wall Street J.,* Nov. 23
38. Ladenheim K, Lipson L, Markus A. 1994. Health care reform: 50 state profiles. *Intergovernmental Health Policy Project.* George Washington Univ., Washington, DC
39. Leaf A. 1993. Preventive medicine for our ailing health care system. *JAMA* 269:616–18
40. Lee P, Weber M, Benjamin T. 1996. Public health policies and strategies in the U.S. See Ref. 15. In press
41. Marks JS, Koplan JP, Hogue CJR, Dalmat ME. 1990. A cost-benefit/cost-effectiveness analysis of smoking cessation for pregnant women. *Am. J. Prev. Med.* 6:282–89
42. McGinnis JM, Foege WH. 1993. Actual causes of death in the United States. *JAMA* 270:2207–12
43. Meyer JA, Regenstein M. 1994. *Prevention is basic to health reform: How to Fund Public Health Activities.* Washington, DC: Partnership Prev.
44. Miller RH, Luft HS. 1994. Managed care plan performance since 1980. *JAMA* 271:1512–19
45. Minn. Health Care Comm. 1993. *Containing Costs in Minnesota's Health Care System.* Minneapolis: Minn. Dep. Health

46. Mullan F. 1989. *Plagues and Politics: The Story of the US Public Health Service.* New York: Basic Books
47. Oberle MW, Baker EL, Magenheim MJ. 1994. Healthy People 2000 and community health planning. *Annu. Rev. Public Health* 15:259–75
48. Oberle MW, Foy HM, Alexander R, Kobayashi J. 1995. Enhancing student practicum opportunities: the outbreak investigation option. *J. Public Health Manage. Pract.* 1:69–73
49. Off. Technol. Assess. 1980. *The Implications of Cost-effectiveness Analysis of Medical Technology.* Washington, DC: GPO
50. Omenn GS. 1994. Don't forget community public health services in the debate on health. Association of Academic Health Centers, Washington, DC. *Washington Post,* Aug. 2, C5
51. Omenn GS. 1994. *Prevention: Benefits, Costs, and Savings.* Washington, DC: Partnership Prev.
52. Omenn GS. 1995. The context for a future school of public health committed to urban health needs. In *The University in the Urban Community: Responsibilities for Public Health,* ed. J Hogness, C McLaughlin, M Osterweis, pp. 93–116. Washington, DC: Assoc. Acad. Health Cent.
53. Omenn GS, Beresford SM, Buchner DM, LaCroix A, Martin M, et al. 1995. Evidence of modifiable risk factors in older adults as a basis for health promotion/disease prevention programs. In *Public Health and Aging,* ed. T Hickey, M Speers. Baltimore: Hopkins Univ. Press. In press
54. Omenn GS, Oberle MW, Gale J, Hoover JJ, Tapp J. 1993. The Northwest Center for Public Health Practice. *Am. J. Public Health* 83:1788–89
55. Packer-Tursman J. 1994. Minorities in managed care. *HMO Mag.* 35:56–61
56. Partnership Prev. 1993. *Prevention is Basic to Health Reform.* Position paper from an expert panel. Washington, DC: Partnersh. Prev.
57. Partnership Prev. 1994. *Prevention is Basic to Health Reform: Model Legislative Language.* Washington, DC: Partnersh. Prev.
58. Pearson TA, Spencer M, Jenkins P. 1995. Who will provide prevention services? The changing relationship between medical care systems and public health agencies in health care reform. *J. Public Health Manage. Policy* 1:16–27
59. Pew Health Professions Comm. 1994. *Primary Care Workforce 2000—Federal Policy Paper.* San Francisco, CA: UCSF Cent. Health Prof. 27 pp.
60. Pickett G. 1980. The future of health departments: the governmental presence. *Annu. Rev. Public Health* 1:297–321
61. Public Health Found. 1994. *State Expenditures for Core Public Health Functions.* Washington, DC: Public Health Found.
62. *Public Health Improvement Plan Working Group Interim Rep.* 1994. Olympia, WA: State Wash., Dep. Health. 262 pp.
63. Quality Letter for Healthcare Leaders. 1994. *Measuring and Improving Community Health* 6(5) June
64. Reidel J, Gibbs J. 1987. *Disease Prevention and Health Promotion: the Blue Cross and Blue Shield Organization Roles.* Chicago Blue Cross and Blue Shield Assoc.
65. Riley T. 1995. Medicaid, the role of states. *JAMA* 274:267–70
66. Roper WL, Baker EL, Dyal WW, Nicola RM. 1992. Strengthening the Public Health System. *Public Health Rep.* 107:609–14
67. Russell LB. 1986. *Is Prevention Better than Cure?* pp. 109–12. Washington, DC: Brookings Inst.
68. Russell LB. 1993. The role of prevention in health reform. *N. Engl. J. Med.* 329:352–54
69. Schauffler HH. 1993. *Health Promotion and Disease Prevention in Health Care Reform.* Univ. Calif., Berkeley
70. Shattuck L. 1850. *Report of the Commission of Massachusetts 1850.* Cambridge, MA: Harvard Univ. Press
71. Sisto D. 1992. The business of health reform. *Rev. Bus.* 14:9–13
72. Sox HC. 1994. Preventive health services in adults. *N. Engl. J. Med.* 330:1589–95
73. Sox HC, Woolf SH. 1993. Evidence-based practice guidelines from US Preventive Services Task Force. *JAMA* 269 (20):2678
74. Tengs TO, Adams ME, Pliskin JS, Safran DG, Siegel JE, et al. 1995. Five-hundred life-saving interventions and their cost-effectiveness. *Risk Anal.* 15:369–90
75. Teutsch SM. 1992. A framework for assessing the effectiveness of disease and injury prevention. *Morbid. Mortal. Wkly. Rep.* 41:RR-3
76. Deleted in proof
77. US Dep. Health Hum. Serv. 1990. *Healthy People 2000: National Health Promotion and Disease Prevention Objectives.* DHHS Publ. No. (PHS) 91–50212

78. US Dep. Health Hum. Serv. 1991. *CDC Strategic Plan for Elimination of Children Level Poisoning.* Washington, DC: US PHS

79. US Dep. Health Hum. Serv. 1994. *Health Care Reform and Public Health: A Paper on Population-Based Core Functions. Public Health Service Core Functions Project.* Washington, DC: DHHS

80. US Dep. Health Hum. Serv. 1994. *Medicaid Managed Care Enrollment Report.* Baltimore, MD: DHHS

81. US Dep. Health Hum. Serv., Off. Dis. Prev. Health Prom., Cent. Dis. Control Prev. 1994. *For a Healthy Nation: Returns on Investment in Public Health.* Washington, DC: DHHS, PHS

82. US Gen. Account. Off. 1993. *Medicaid: States Turn to Managed Care to Improve Access and Control Costs.* Publ. No. GAO/HRD-93-4. Washington, DC

83. US Prev. Serv. Task Force. 1989. *Guide to Clinical Preventive Services: An Assessment of the Effectiveness of 169 Interventions.* Baltimore: Williams & Wilkins

84. Walsh C. 1995. *A Summary of State Health Reforms.* Research Triangle Park, NC: Research Triangle Inst.

85. White CC, Koplan JP, Orenstein WA. 1985. Benefits, risks, and costs of immunization for measles, mumps and rubella. *Am. J. Public Health* 75:739–44

85a. White KL. 1991. *Healing the Schism: Epidemiology/Medicine and the Public's Health.* New York: Springer-Verlag

86. Zaldocki E. 1994. Employer report cards. *HMO Mag.* March/April:27–32

Annu. Rev. Public Health. 1996. 17:511–38

DEVELOPING EVIDENCE-BASED CLINICAL PRACTICE GUIDELINES:
Lessons Learned by the US Preventive Services Task Force*

Steven H. Woolf[1†], Carolyn G. DiGuiseppi[2†], David Atkins[2†], and Douglas B. Kamerow[2†]

[1]Department of Family Practice, Medical College of Virginia, 3712 Charles Stewart Drive, Fairfax, Virginia 22033; [2]Office of the Forum for Quality and Effectiveness in Health Care, Agency for Health Care Policy and Research, 6000 Executive Boulevard, Suite 310, Rockville, Maryland 20852

ABSTRACT

The US Preventive Services Task Force is an expert panel established by the federal government in 1984 to develop evidence-based practice guidelines on screening tests and other preventive services. Its recommendations are published elsewhere. This article explores the lessons learned in the process of developing and disseminating the recommendations. Topics include project organization (analytic philosophy, project sponsorship, panel composition, topic selection); the review of evidence (selecting outcome measures for judging effectiveness, constructing "causal pathways," searching the literature, rating the evidence, synthesizing the results); crafting recommendations (extrapolation, assessing magnitude, balancing risks and benefits, addressing costs, dealing with insufficient data, separating science from policy); peer review; collaboration with other groups; evaluating impact on clinicians' knowledge, attitudes, and behavior; updating recommendations; and defining a research agenda. The lessons learned suggest potential refinements in the future work of the task force and other groups engaged in guideline development.

[†]The authors are former staff of the Office of Disease Prevention and Health Promotion, US Public Health Service, Washington, D.C., where Dr. Kamerow directed the clinical preventive services staff. Drs. Woolf, DiGuiseppi, and Atkins were the science advisors to the US Preventive Services Task Force.

KEY WORDS: preventive services, practice guidelines, health promotion, effectiveness,
              outcomes research

INTRODUCTION

The US Preventive Services Task Force (USPSTF) was established by the US
Public Health Service in 1984. It is a nongovernmental expert panel that
reviews scientific evidence regarding the effectiveness of clinical preventive
services and makes evidence-based recommendations for health professionals
regarding which preventive services to include in the periodic health examination. The clinical preventive services examined by the USPSTF include
screening tests for the early detection of risk factors and preclinical disease,
counseling regarding personal health behaviors, immunizations, and chemoprophylaxis (e.g. hormone replacement therapy). The USPSTF recommendations are published in its book, *Guide to Clinical Preventive Services* (86).

The USPSTF recommendations have played an important role in the evolution of health promotion and disease prevention policy in the United States.
Since its first recommendations appeared in the late 1980s, it has become one
of the most well-accepted authorities on the practice of evidence-based preventive medicine. A growing number of clinicians, public health officials,
health care administrators, and payers are familiar with the *Guide*. The
USPSTF has played a role in health care reform discussions and the prevention
components of managed care programs. The methods used by the USPSTF to
review evidence and make recommendations have been examined by governmental panels and professional societies engaged in developing clinical practice guidelines according to evidence-based methods.

It has been twelve years since the USPSTF was established. This milestone,
and the recent publication of the second edition of the *Guide* (86), provide a
useful opportunity to look back on the project's accomplishments. Although
some of the lessons learned are unique to the USPSTF project, many are
relevant to other expert panels, government agencies, and private organizations
involved in the critical appraisal of scientific evidence, the development of
clinical practice guidelines, or their dissemination and implementation in a
rapidly evolving health care industry.

The evidence-based methodology used by the USPSTF to make recommendations is described in the *Guide* (86). Briefly, the process begins with the
identification of the leading causes of death and disability, and the preventive
services that could potentially reduce morbidity and mortality from these
conditions. The panel then carefully reviews the quality of the supporting
evidence and makes recommendations based on the strength of the data.
Recommendations are generally not based on opinion. Draft guidelines undergo extensive outside review by experts and organizations before final ap-

proval by the panel. USPSTF members, who are empaneled for about five years, consist mainly of clinicians with skills in the analytic sciences, and they examine a wide range of topics encompassing pediatrics, adult medicine, prenatal care, and psychosocial medicine.

This article does not present the USPSTF recommendations, which are available in the *Guide* and are too extensive to summarize here. In general, the USPSTF recommends relatively few clinical preventive services for all asymptomatic patients. The most important recommended services are patient education and counseling about personal health behaviors (e.g. smoking cessation, exercise). Only a few screening tests (e.g. mammography, Papanicolaou smears, fecal occult blood testing) are recommended for routine health maintenance, because most tests lack evidence of effectiveness or may result in more harm than good. Many USPSTF screening recommendations are more conservative than those issued by organizations that do not use an evidence-based approach.

This article focuses less on the content of the USPSTF recommendations than on the lessons it has learned in the process of making them. These lessons may be relevant to other groups and individuals involved in guideline development. Background information is also provided to explain some of the controversial positions the USPSTF has taken over the years. The perspective presented is that of the USPSTF staff, who were responsible for collecting and examining the evidence, writing the *Guide,* and ensuring adherence to the methodology. This "behind the scenes" view may reflect a different perspective than that of panel members or the government body that sponsored the USPSTF. The views expressed in this article are those of the authors and do not necessarily reflect the opinions of USPSTF members or the US Public Health Service.

ORGANIZATION OF THE PROJECT

Analytic Philosophy: The Evidence-Based Approach

A hallmark of the USPSTF has been its commitment to scientific evidence. It was decided from the outset that it would only recommend preventive services meeting predetermined criteria of effectiveness. This approach, inspired by the Canadian Task Force on the Periodic Health Examination (CTFPHE) (11), was adopted at a time (1984) when the prevailing approach to guideline development favored informal consensus development: i.e. most groups developed guidelines based on the personal opinions of an expert panel, rather than by following a predetermined, data-driven methodology (21). An inevitable discrepancy emerged between groups recommending screening tests that they *believed* were appropriate and the more conservative USPSTF recommendations that withheld support until compelling proof became available. Some of the most controversial positions taken by the USPSTF (e.g. not recommending certain cancer screening tests) stem from this difference in philosophy.

There are advantages and disadvantages to the evidence-based approach. The chief advantage is that it places the burden of proof on clinicians and researchers to demonstrate that an intervention results in more good than harm before recommending it to the public. It places appropriate skepticism on the value of opinion as a basis for claiming effectiveness. The burden of proof is even more appropriate for preventive services, which are offered to essentially healthy persons as something "good for them" (73). The explicitness of the evidence-based approach allows guideline developers to define areas of uncertainty in precise terms and to map out a research agenda for acquiring better evidence. It provides a level playing field for comparing the relative effectiveness of different interventions. Most importantly, it provides a clear analytic rationale to defend medical and public health policy.

There are important limitations to the evidence-based approach, however, beginning with the shortage of good data. Proof of effectiveness is lacking for most of what is done in medicine. Clinical practice would come to a halt if practitioners could only perform tests and treatments that had been proven effective in clinical trials. Even when evidence is available, it is often of poor quality, suffering from design flaws that limit its persuasiveness (23). Obtaining evidence for preventive interventions is especially difficult because of the long lag times between interventions and health outcomes. Unreasonably large sample sizes and study durations are often needed to determine whether the lack of an observed benefit is due to ineffectiveness, rather than to inadequate statistical power.

Interest in an evidence-based approach had much to do with the circumstances surrounding the creation of the USPSTF in 1984. Clinicians were performing few recommended preventive services, in part because of skepticism about their effectiveness in preventing disease (91). Similar skepticism dissuaded insurers from paying for preventive care. Most clinicians lacked comprehensive guidelines on exactly what to do. The goals of the USPSTF were designed to address these needs by developing evidence-based guidelines on all aspects of preventive care, compiling them in a book that was accessible and inviting to clincians, and using this information and the governmental imprimatur to motivate providers and payers to strengthen support for prevention. Government, academia, and other organizations were invited to participate as partners in the development and implementation of USPSTF recommendations (JM McGinnis, personal communication).

The Sponsor

The USPSTF was convened by the US Public Health Service (US Department of Health and Human Services). From 1984 to 1995, an office within the US

Public Health Service (Office of Disease Prevention and Health Promotion, Washington, DC) provided staff support for the project, including scientific advisors, meeting planning, and project coordination. In 1995, the USPSTF project was moved to the Agency for Health Care Policy and Research to provide greater resources for implementation and combine it with other federal guideline activities. USPSTF recommendations do not require formal approval from the US Public Health Service.

The governmental home of the USPSTF was selected to address two competing requirements for its success: freedom for the panel to reach independent conclusions and credibility to effect change. The model chosen, federal sponsorship of an independent panel, served a critical role in balancing these needs and ensuring a high-quality product. Governmental resources and imprimatur helped attract the participation of national experts, provide an environment for impartial analysis of the evidence, ensure the product's completion and quality, and facilitate dialogue between the USPSTF and other groups. The governmental setting gave access to specialized experts and databases, and catalyzed the collaboration of public and private groups as committed partners. Most of all, the federal imprimatur signaled the policy importance of the USPSTF to policy makers, payers, providers, and the public (JM McGinnis, personal communication).

Federal, rather than private, sponsorship of an independent panel involves important tradeoffs. It provides both an opportunity and a special obligation to submit draft recommendations for review by relevant US Public Health Service agencies (e.g. National Institutes of Health, Centers for Disease Control and Prevention). Although USPSTF recommendations are not required to conform with official government policy, an effort is made to resolve discrepancies and thereby reduce confusion among the public. When discrepancies are irreconcilable, the USPSTF has firmly maintained its independence; in the late 1980s, for example, discrepancies between the USPSTF and the National Cancer Institute about cancer screening guidelines received attention in the medical literature (70, 71) and lay media (51).

Brokering disagreements between agencies is time-consuming, often tedious, and occasionally an encumbrance to the impartial analysis of evidence, but it almost always improves the product. More often than not, exploring discrepancies with leading federal institutes and national experts has enrichened scientific discourse and disclosed important oversights in the interpretation of data. Bureaucratic interference for political, rather than scientific, reasons has occurred only rarely—the release of the first edition of the *Guide,* for example, was delayed by administration officials concerned about chapters that referred to abortion—but such incidents have been kept to a minimum by governmental diligence in protecting the panel's independence. Indeed, the government's involvement in the USPSTF has probably stimulated scientific debate and accelerated policy developments in ways that would not have been possible under nongovernmental sponsorship.

Panel Composition

The makeup of the panel has evolved over time, illustrating the competing tension between optimal size and multidisciplinary input. The first panel (1984–1989) included 20 members: 14 physicians with backgrounds in primary care and clinical epidemiology, and six nonphysician members (a dentist, nurse, health services researcher, health educator, economist, and sociologist). The multidisciplinary composition provided diverse expertise, but the panel was quite large. Although the panel included two internists (one of whom was the chair) and two family physicians, it had only one pediatrician and no obstetricians. This imbalance was criticized by pediatricians and obstetricians who felt that there was inadequate emphasis on pediatric and prenatal preventive services in the *Guide* (1).

The second USPSTF panel (1990–1995) was restructured to address these concerns. The size was reduced to 10 members, selected to provide equal representation (two members) from internal medicine, family practice, pediatrics, obstetrics-gynecology, and the analytic sciences (epidemiology, decision analysis). Although the second panel lacked the multidisciplinary character of the first group (nine of ten members were physicians), its small size fostered a consistent, cohesive approach to analyzing the issues. The panel lacked nonphysician representation, and specialists criticized the absence of panelists in their area of expertise, but expanding the USPSTF to include all disciplines concerned with prevention would have produced an unwieldy size. Instead, multidisciplinary input was sought through the outside review process, in which over 600 content experts from different fields participated. Notwithstanding these efforts, opportunities remain for expanding nonphysician involvement in USPSTF reviews.

The USPSTF model of a standing panel of generalists offers important advantages. Generalists with analytic expertise are often more capable of objectively assessing the evidence according to a systematic methodology and are less influenced by personal opinions and clinical background. Working on multiple topics over a period of years gives a standing panel added experience in guideline development and efficiencies of scale that are unlikely to reach maturity in panels that address only one topic. Generalists, however, may lack expertise and thereby misinterpret evidence, and their conclusions may be less credible to practitioners than those issued by opinion leaders. On the other hand, panels dominated by specialists are often subject to conflicts of interests, may be less experienced with the critical appraisal of evidence, and may be more likely to have preconceived biases about appropriate recommendations.

Liaisons from four primary care specialty societies were appointed to the second USPSTF panel to involve provider groups early in the development process. USPSTF staff in the Office of Disease Prevention and Health Promotion assumed a more central role in the construction of the analytic framework, review of evidence, and preparation of USPSTF documents (activities performed previously by panel members), thereby improving the efficiency and consistency of reviews. As with many expert panels, the staff operated under occasionally conflicting lines of authority, being employed by the sponsoring body (i.e. US Public Health Service) but also answering to the panel chair and panel members. This arrangement sometimes led to confusion over goals but provided an important counterbalance between the autonomous panel and the needs of the agency.

Topic Selection

Systematic topic selection is important to guideline developers to ensure that the most important health problems are prioritized, and not those that happen to be of interest to selected individuals or special interests. When it was established in 1984, the USPSTF used a formal group process (Delphi method) to select over 100 conditions for its initial evaluation. The list was later modified less systematically, with topics deleted because of time constraints or added to accommodate the interests of certain panelists. It was perhaps this ad hoc approach that led to the emphasis on adult medicine in the 1989 *Guide,* since there were few advocates on the panel to suggest otherwise. The second panel set six criteria for prioritizing topics: 1. severity of the target condition, 2. uncertainty about appropriate practice, 3. timeliness, 4. costs, 5. availability of data, and 6. feasibility of review. Topics were ranked according to the panel's assigned scores for each of these variables. Although the process helped identify new topics, the prioritzation scheme was ultimately abandoned, in part because the scores lacked validity. The panel had no basis for determining the correct score for subjective measures such as "uncertainty " or "timeliness," and thus priority rankings were unpredictable. Important pediatric topics received low priority scores, whereas screening for driving impairment and exercises to prevent low back pain received unexpectedly high scores. More effective strategies for topic prioritization have been outlined in a recent Institute of Medicine report (45).

The USPSTF intentionally selects topics by condition (e.g. breast cancer) rather than by intervention (e.g. mammography). Selecting conditions allows topics to be prioritized on the basis of public health priorities and to examine a broad range of potential interventions, enabling the USPSTF to move beyond traditional chronic-disease targets of prevention [e.g. coronary artery disease (CAD), cancer, stroke] to address other important conditions affecting the population (e.g. violence, injuries, depression). There are some disadvantages to this approach. It provides an awkward starting point for addressing risk factors that affect multiple conditions (e.g. smoking, unhealthy diet). Also, focusing on conditions led the USPSTF to examine only a handful of physical examination procedures. Breast examination was examined in relation to breast cancer, but cardiac auscultation, palpation of the spleen, and other physical examination procedures were not evaluated because they are not performed to prevent the conditions examined by the USPSTF. Critics mistakenly concluded that the physical examination recommended by the USPSTF included no more than a measurement of height, weight, and blood pressure and, in women, an examination of the breasts.

REVIEW OF EVIDENCE

Outcome Measures to Determine Effectiveness

An early task of the USPSTF was to define outcome measures for judging effectiveness. Due to the difficulty of conducting long-term trials with health outcomes such as morbidity or mortality, studies often use changes in surrogate or intermediate outcomes (e.g. cholesterol levels, bone-density) to infer effectiveness. Using intermediate, rather than health, outcomes involves important tradeoffs. Accepting surrogate endpoints opens the door to a larger body of research (e.g. pathophysiologic studies, short-term trials). This reduces the risk of a type II error (failing to detect a benefit when one exists), but *increases* the risk of a type I error (mistakenly concluding that an intervention is effective). Also, drawing inferences from short-term physiologic changes can lead to premature conclusions before long-term outcomes have been evaluated. There are well-known examples of treatments that appeared beneficial based on intermediate endpoints, only to be proven ineffective or harmful when definitive trials were conducted [e.g suppression of asymptomatic arrhythmias (13)]. The pitfalls of relying on intermediate endpoints in cancer screening have been well described: Due to lead-time and length biases, screening may produce spurious improvements in intermediate outcomes (e.g. increased early-stage cancers, prolonged survival) without providing any real mortality or morbidity benefit.

On the other hand, relying on clinical endpoints also has its limitations. It may be impossible to prove the benefits of interventions with relatively small or delayed effects (e.g. breast self-examination) but that may nonetheless be useful because they are inexpensive and target an important disease. (Conversely, recommending every measure that *might* be useful could quickly overwhelm both clinician and patient with many interventions of unproven effectiveness.) For many preventive services, the most important clinical outcome is reduced cause-specific mortality (e.g. reduction in breast cancer deaths); naturally, mortality is not a meaningful endpoint for nonfatal diseases (e.g. hearing loss). Even for leading causes of death (e.g. CAD, cancer), however, the emphasis on mortality over morbidity has been criticized on the grounds that some interventions may be beneficial even if they do not prolong life. Preventive interventions may reduce the need for unpleasant treatments and improve the quality of life, if not its length. The USPSTF readily accepted such outcomes as measures of effectiveness but found that validated scoring instruments were often lacking.

Ultimately, the USPSTF decided to consider a preventive service effective only if an improvement in meaningful health outcomes could be demonstrated, a requirement that led to early controversy. In its first publication in 1987, it reported that there was insufficient evidence to determine whether breast self-examination was effective in reducing morbidity or mortality from breast cancer, despite evidence that it could detect early-stage lesions (58). This stance brought the USPSTF into direct conflict with other organizations that placed greater weight on its beneficial effect on intermediate outcomes. In later years, the USPSTF would continue to encounter similar disagreements when it found that intermediate outcomes of importance to advocates of screening (e.g. increasing maternal hemoglobin levels during pregnancy, reducing mildly elevated blood lead levels during childhood, lowering serum cholesterol in young people) had no proven effect on health outcomes.

Causal Pathways

The USPSTF recognized that intermediate outcomes can be reasonable surrogates for health outcomes if the linkage between them is sufficiently strong. Definitive prospective studies with health outcomes may be an unattainable standard for some preventive interventions, where lengthy delays in benefits may make a trial unfeasible. There are no randomized studies showing that smoking cessation counseling lowers morbidity or mortality from cancer or heart disease. A multitude of studies, however, demonstrate that counseling can increase the number of persons who quit smoking, that smoking quantity and duration are associated with adverse health outcomes, and that these risks are lowered in those who quit smoking (86). Thus, although direct evidence of health benefits is lacking, combining the evidence from each of the linkages provides the necessary scientific support for the recommendation to counsel patients to stop smoking.

These observations led the USPSTF to develop explicit analytic diagrams to map out the linkages on which to base conclusions about effectiveness. These "causal pathways" were first described by Battista & Fletcher (7), members of the CTFPHE and USPSTF, and alternate evidence models have since been proposed by others (4, 40, 95). USPSTF staff expanded causal

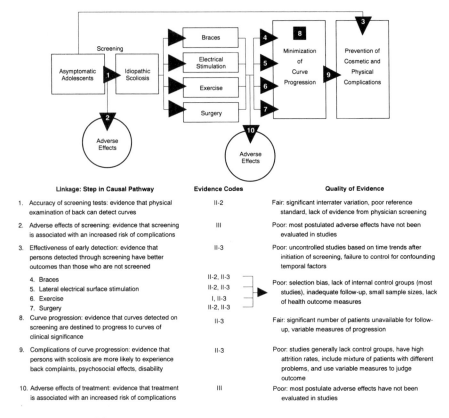

Figure 1 Examining the evidence on screening for idiopathic scoliosis along a causal pathway. Reproduced from JAMA 269:2664–66. 1993

pathways to incorporate complex models that frame the relationship between multiple intermediate and health outcomes. The causal pathway in Figure 1, for example, specifies the chain of assumptions that must be proven to infer that screening adolescents for scoliosis will improve health outcomes (83). The linkages represent the questions that must be answered by the literature review before the panel can reach conclusions about effectiveness.

Collecting the Evidence: Literature Searches

Searching the literature for relevant evidence can be labor-intensive and costly (57). In its first three years, the USPSTF examined evidence somewhat superficially, citing only selected review articles and the recommendations of other groups. When, in 1987, it became clear that evidence-based recommendations could not be made without examining all relevant evidence systematically, the pendulum swung in the other direction and it instituted comprehensive MED-LINE searches and screened tens of thousands of studies. Although gathering this information has generally been worthwhile, the staff's elaborate measures to ensure complete reviews (e.g. running searches under a variety of keywords, cross-checking against review articles) were probably unnecessary. The few studies overlooked in computerized searches would probably have been identified by outside reviewers familiar with the literature. A more important problem in reviewing evidence for hundreds of preventive services has been keeping pace with the rapidly expanding literature. For example, the efforts of the USPSTF to update its recommendations in time for a second edition of the *Guide* were threatened by the inability of staff to review all relevant studies. To solve this problem, it assigned the more straightforward topic updates to junior clinical scholars (residents, fellows) at institutions where panel members were based. Under USPSTF supervision, they examined the evidence and drafted revised chapters, which were reviewed and eventually adopted by the full task force. Even with this assistance, the second edition was published over a year behind schedule. As the medical information explosion continues in future years, the task of gathering evidence will become even more challenging and will require considerably more innovative solutions.

Evaluating Study Quality: The Evidence Codes

The USPSTF has always given special attention to the quality of studies, rather than accepting results on face value. Standard methodologic features (e.g. statistical power, sample selection, definition of interventions and outcomes) are used to judge quality. Although these criteria are well established, the USPSTF and other groups have encountered problems in finding a concise way to summarize a study's quality. In the 1970s, the CTFPHE introduced a hierarchical grading system, which ranked studies by design category. A modified version was adopted by both groups when the USPSTF was established in 1984 (Table 1). These evidence codes accompany most USPSTF recommendations.

Although evidence codes provide a useful shorthand for describing the evidence, they provide an incomplete description of quality, for several reasons. First, study design category is only one factor influencing quality. Implying that a randomized controlled trial (RCT) is "better" than a case-control study ignores the importance of research methods and study populations. A well-designed case-control study can be more persuasive than a poorly designed RCT. The strength of the evidence also depends on other factors, such as the magnitude and direction of the results and the consistency of the findings across studies (homogeneity). A uniform and validated coding system that

Table 1 U.S. Preventive Services Task Force Evidence Codes

I	Evidence obtained from at least one properly designed randomized controlled trial.
II-1	Evidence obtained from well-designed controlled trials without randomization.
II-2	Evidence obtained from well-designed cohort or case-control analytic studies, preferably from more than one center or research group.
II-3	Evidence obtained from multiple time series with or without the intervention. Dramatic results in uncontrolled experiments (such as the results of the introduction of penicillin treatment in the 1940s) could also be regarded as this type of evidence.
III	Opinions of respected authorities, based on clinical experience, descriptive studies, or reports of expert committees.

captures all of these variables has yet to be devised. Evidence codes, scores, and statistical techniques have been developed by others to address some of these issues (14, 16, 24), but none offers a validated measure of study quality. Second, the RCT may not always be the "gold standard." Although it is considered the most persuasive study design for evaluating interventions, it is inappropriate for assessing other important issues in prevention (e.g. the sensitivity and specificity of a screening test, the relative risk of health behaviors). Third, the USPSTF grading system makes no provision for meta-level study designs (e.g. meta-analysis, decision analysis). Fourth, the positioning of the RCT at the top of the hierarchy has fueled misconceptions that the USPSTF will only recommend preventive services that have been proven effective in such trials. In fact, many USPSTF recommendations (e.g. screening for cervical cancer or phenylketonuria) are supported by weaker evidence, such as controlled observational studies.

Finally, the quality of the evidence for a recommendation can rarely be described by a single evidence code, as was done frequently in early USPSTF and CTFPHE reports. The tables in the 1989 *Guide*, for example, provided only one code (category I) to describe the evidence for screening for diabetes mellitus (82). As the concept of causal pathways has evolved, it has become clear that the supporting evidence for a recommendation often includes separate bodies of data for each linkage in the causal pathway. Multiple evidence codes are often needed to fully describe the evidence for an intervention (see Figure 1).

Describing Results

Another challenge encountered in the review of multiple studies is summarizing the results. The simplest approach, a narrative description, has been the principal method used by the USPSTF. Other groups have made greater use of evidence tables and balance sheets (22). A powerful means of pooling data from multiple studies, meta-analysis, has been cited in USPSTF reviews when available in the published literature, but staff and resource constraints precluded performance of its own meta-analyses. Only two meta-analyses have been conducted by USPSTF members. More extensive use of meta-analysis might have helped the panel resolve uncertainties about the weight of the evidence, thereby prompting different recommendations, and thus future USPSTF support is expected to facilitate the performance of meta-analyses when needed.

MAKING RECOMMENDATIONS

The purest application of the evidence-based approach is to link recommendations directly to the evidence: Interventions are recommended when supporting evidence is available and are not recommended when evidence is lacking. The USPSTF was established with this intent in mind. A grading system (Table 2), adapted from CTFPHE codes (11), classified recommendations entirely on the basis of the supporting evidence. Using this approach, the USPSTF found that a number of clinical preventive services were supported by strong evidence of effectiveness. The decision to recommend these services was not difficult. The USPSTF encountered more problems, however, in determining whether to recommend interventions when the magnitude of benefit was uncertain and, in particular, when the relationship between benefits and harms was unclear.

Extrapolation

The effect of an intervention is often uncertain when data come from study populations and research settings that may not be generalizable to average patients in typical practice settings. Volunteers in clinical trials often differ from patients in the general population, investigators in research settings may

Table 2 U.S. Preventive Services Task Force Recommendation Codes

A	There is good evidence to support the recommendation that the condition be specifically considered in a periodic health examination.
B	There is fair evidence to support the recommendation that the condition be specifically considered in a periodic health examination.
C	There is insufficient evidence to make a recommendation for or against consideration in the periodic health examination.
D	There is fair evidence to support the recommendation that the condition be excluded from consideration in a periodic health examination.
E	There is good evidence to support the recommendation that the condition be excluded from consideration in a periodic health examination.

be more skilled than the average practitioner, and trials often include safeguards to minimize the adverse effects of treatments. How widely to generalize such results to community practice remains a contentious issue.

Traditionally, the USPSTF has taken a conservative stance on extrapolations, limiting recommendations to the specific population and conditions in the study. But it is unclear whether this dogmatism is justified. The USPSTF has argued, for example, that although there is compelling RCT evidence that lowering serum cholesterol is beneficial in middle-aged men with high cholesterol levels (27), the balance of benefits and risks may differ in other population groups (e.g. children, adolescents, the elderly). Evidence that risk factor modification can reverse atherosclerosis and improve mortality in men with preexisting CAD (59), the USPSTF has argued, may not be generalizable to asymptomatic persons to determine the balance of risks and benefits. However, although the reluctance to generalize beyond study conditions may be defensible on strict scientific grounds, it seems intuitive that other population groups would share similar atherogenetic mechanisms. It is also unrealistic to anticipate better data—clinical trials will not be repeated for every possible population subgroup—and thus some extrapolations are unavoidable. On the other hand, extrapolations cannot be made injudiciously, because conditions can differ significantly between populations and types of interventions. The effectiveness of counseling by dietitians or family therapists, for example, cannot necessarily be extrapolated to physicians.

Magnitude

Even when data are available for the population in question, it is often unclear whether the magnitude of the observed effect is "good enough" for a recommendation. Evidence, for example, that an intervention can achieve an absolute mortality reduction of 30% or 50% is certainly compelling, but is a statistically significant 0.5% reduction in mortality sufficient grounds for recommending a preventive service? Is the proven ability of lowered serum cholesterol to reduce the incidence of CAD (fatal and nonfatal events combined) (27) sufficient grounds for a recommendation if it has not been proven to reduce *all-cause* mortality in asymptomatic persons? Although this discrepancy is probably related to inadequate statistical power—larger samples and longer follow-up may reveal an effect on all-cause mortality—it has prompted the USPSTF and other groups to speculate on whether cholesterol-lowering drugs increase non-CAD mortality. That is, the harms of the intervention may outweigh its benefits, and thus both must be considered in the overall calculus.

Balancing Risks and Benefits

An interest in the potential harms of preventive services is one of the hallmarks of the USPSTF and CTFPHE. Both groups believe in a special ethical imperative to ensure that preventive services offered to asymptomatic persons do more good than harm. The USPSTF and CTFPHE explicitly consider a range of potential adverse effects of screening, such as psychological impact (e.g. anxiety, "labeling"), morbidity from follow-up testing, and unnecessary treatments precipitated by screening (28). Concerns about these "cascade" effects have prompted the USPSTF to take controversial conservative positions, refraining from recommending practices that others consider innocuous (and potentially beneficial), such as breast self-examination and digital rectal examination. While there are theoretical and anecdotal reasons for concerns about adverse effects, direct evidence of their importance is much harder to come by. Critics have raised the concern that the USPSTF gives greater weight to speculative harms than to benefits.

The USPSTF has also found it difficult to determine scientifically whether harms outweigh benefits. Trials often include beneficial effects on morbidity as primary endpoints (e.g. reduced nonfatal CAD or stroke), but relegate important adverse effects of treatment (e.g. nonfatal side-effects of medications or surgery) to secondary endpoints. Weighing the relative morbidity of different outcomes is often impossible. Decision analysis is used increasingly by researchers to calculate the overall balance of risks and benefits, using a common denominator such as quality-adjusted life years (30, 50). Because these analyses require a comparison of widely disparate outcomes (e.g. premature death vs impotence), however, they may be of limited value in estimating the potential benefit to an individual, who may value one outcome more than the average person. Furthermore, because the models are inherently complex and include numerous assumptions and sources of uncertainty, they are easy targets for criticism from opponents who disagree with inferences from sensitivity analyses and with the overall conclusions.

Thus, although the USPSTF reviewed findings from decision models, the evidence included in these models was usually too variable to influence its final recommendations. In many instances, the USPSTF would have preferred to conduct its own decision analysis to evaluate the data, but the demands of comprehensiveness (i.e. cataloguing the evidence for hundreds of preventive services) precluded such focused reviews. Even published decision analyses could not be cited as the primary basis for recommendations; USPSTF evidence codes (Table 1) made no provision for this class of evidence. The panel could not use a decision analysis prepared by two of its own members (and one CTFPHE member) (33) to recommend screening for abdominal aortic aneurysms, instead concluding that there was "insufficient evidence" to make a recommendation.

The USPSTF often struggled with the real possibility that an intervention that was beneficial under ideal conditions (i.e. efficacious) could lack effectiveness, resulting in no benefit or net harm, under typical practice conditions. For example, although a RCT demonstrated that carotid endarterectomy performed by skilled surgeons reduced the risk of stroke in patients with asymptomatic carotid artery stenosis, the net benefit was limited to settings with a low risk of operative complications (26). Since the complication rate was likely to be higher in the community, the net benefit of widespread population screening and increased surgery was unclear. The USPSTF often recommended such interventions only under specific conditions (e.g. settings with low operative mortality rates) rather than for all patients.

Costs

When it was established in 1984, the USPSTF was encouraged to exclude costs from its deliberations; recommendations were to be based largely on clinical benefits and harms. This policy stemmed from several concerns. First, including cost considerations could dilute the message to clinicians and policy makers that ineffective preventive services should be withheld on clinical grounds alone. Second, access to valid and reliable cost data was limited. Third, the science of evaluating the cost-effectiveness of preventive services was not sufficiently mature to justify valid comparisons of cost-effectiveness across different preventive services or between preventive and curative services (18, 66). Estimates of the cost-effectiveness of breast cancer screening, for example, have varied between $3400 to over $83,000 per life-year saved (10).

These early concerns about addressing costs have gradually been overtaken by the health care crisis and growing societal concerns about the costs of care. In the early 1990s, guideline developers began routinely including cost considerations in their evaluations of the evidence (22). With growing cost-consciousness, members of the USPSTF became reluctant to continue basing recommendations entirely on health outcomes. Without considering costs, its methodology provided no grounds for discouraging preventive services with any degree of effectiveness, however costly. The Office of Disease Prevention and Health Promotion began in-depth analyses of the issue in the early 1990s and, in 1992, formed the Panel on Cost Effectiveness in Health and Medicine to propose economic analytic methodologies for evaluating clinical preventive services (36). It also convened an interagency discussion group to facilitate coordination and information flow across US Public Health Service agencies. The examination of costs has been taken up by groups outside of government as well, such as projects to estimate the cost of providing the preventive services recommended by the USPSTF (15, 18).

Dealing with Insufficient Evidence

For many preventive services, the USPSTF concluded that current evidence was insufficient to recommend for or against routine inclusion in the periodic health exam ("C" recommendation). A variety of different circumstances underlie the numerous "C" recommendations included in the *Guide*: Available studies were inadequate to determine effectiveness (e.g. insufficient statistical power, unrepresentative populations, lack of clinically important endpoints); available studies produced conflicting results; evidence of significant benefits was offset by evidence of important harms; or studies of effectiveness had never been conducted. As a result, lack of evidence of effectiveness in these situations does not constitute *evidence of ineffectiveness*.

A vexing problem for the USPSTF was how to advise clinicians regarding preventive services that received "C" recommendations. The strictest interpretation of its evidence-based methodology was to take a purely neutral position, making no recommendation, either for or against the maneuver. Doing so presented a number of problems, the most obvious being that many clinicians found it unhelpful, giving no guidance in either direction. The scientific dogmatism seemed out of pace with the rest of medicine; much of what is done in clinical practice has not been proven to improve health outcomes. "C" recommendations were prone to misinterpretation, typically understood as a recommendation against the maneuver (rather than the absence of a recommendation). Panel members had additional problems with a neutral stance. For many procedures, especially those that impose important burdens of time or expense on patients and clinicians (e.g. routine colonoscopy), the USPSTF felt that the services should not be routinely offered in the absence of evidence of effectiveness. On the other hand, for interventions posing little cost or risk, a neutral position seemed overly nihilistic.

The solution in the first edition of the *Guide* was to use less explicit language to encourage "reasonable" interventions: e.g. "It is prudent to examine the uterine adnexa when performing gynecologic examinations for other reasons" (82, p. 81). "Clinically prudent" language was also used to remind clinicians to "remain alert" for conditions (e.g. depression) and to suggest screening in high-risk individuals (e.g. women with a family history of breast cancer), in whom a small reduction in risk might yield important benefits but be too small to be detected in prospective trials. This approach was criticized on several grounds. Stating that a procedure was clinically prudent was viewed as an implicit recommendation, seemingly in violation of the USPSTF rules of evidence. Furthermore, an intervention of uncertain effectiveness in low-risk persons is likely to be of uncertain effectiveness in high-risk persons as well.

The Distinction between Science and Practice Policy

These problems helped focus the USPSTF on the distinction between its dual missions: 1. giving clinicians information about current scientific knowledge and 2. advising them how to practice. Practice policy is dependent on more than scientific evidence. Other factors must be considered, including opinions about effectiveness, potential harms, personal preferences, costs, the serious-ness of the target condition, professional pressures, administrative or reim-bursement restrictions, and medicolegal concerns. Although scientific evidence is perhaps the most important variable, other factors warrant attention, espe-cially when there is insufficient evidence to determine the best choice on scientific grounds. A potentially beneficial maneuver may be appropriate if it is essentially harmless (e.g. taking a history), but, in the absence of proven benefits, can be inappropriate if it is potentially harmful or costly (e.g. routine amniocentesis). Reflecting these considerations, the second edition of the *Guide* (1995) retained the use of "C" recommendations but, where appropriate, added that recommendations for or against the maneuver could be made "on other grounds" (other than science). The "other grounds" could include argu-ments *for* performing the maneuver (e.g. low likelihood of harm, high burden of suffering from target condition) or *against* performing it (e.g. high likelihood of harms or costs).

OUTSIDE REVIEW

Professional organizations and over 600 experts from the United States, Can-ada, Europe, and Australia reviewed USPSTF draft recommendations. These reviews helped verify the accuracy and completeness of evidence summaries and provided useful input on recommendations. Groups with established po-sitions or special interests sometimes opposed the frequently conservative USPSTF recommendations and its strict interpretation of the evidence. The resulting dialogue over the scientific merits of opposing arguments has gen-erally had a positive effect, helping to build consensus (thereby reducing confusion about conflicting recommendations) and encouraging an examina-tion of data, rather than opinions, in defense of longstanding positions. The panel's call for better evidence, once a focus of criticism in a 1987 *Los Angeles Times* article (51), has since motivated some groups to collect better data (9).

COLLABORATION WITH OTHER GROUPS

Since its inception in 1984, the USPSTF has coordinated its work with the CTFPHE, using their common methodology to collaborate in shared meetings, background and methods papers, and books (37, 96). During 1992–1994, they worked concurrently on the publication of a *Guide* [*Guide to Clinical Preven-tive Services* (86) and *Canadian Guide to Clinical Preventive Health Care* (12)], with some chapters in each book based on the work of the other task force. (Similar cooperative relationships have been forged with other groups, as in USPSTF collaborations with the American College of Physicians and American Academy of Family Physicians.) The binational ties between the

USPSTF and CTFPHE have benefited both groups, improving efficiency through their combined experience. The collaboration has also underscored the limits of setting medical policy across borders, where health care systems and political conditions differ. Attempts by the two groups to issue joint recommendations were largely unsuccessful, despite similar interpretations of the data, because they faced different audiences in making recommendations.

EVALUATING THE IMPACT

The USPSTF has committed its energies to producing recommendations rather than evaluating their results. It has not formally monitored implementation of its recommendations. This preoccupation with production rather than use is a characteristic of many guideline development projects (5). Evidence that guidelines influence patient care is needed because their effectiveness in changing practice behaviors and improving health outcomes is widely questioned (94). In the case of the USPSTF, there is limited evidence that the guidelines have affected knowledge, attitudes about appropriate practice, or outcomes.

Knowledge

Efforts to disseminate USPSTF recommendations to clinicians have been extensive. The 1989 release of the *Guide* was covered heavily by the medical press and large-circulation medical journals (49, 74, 99). The *Guide* itself, a document in the public domain, was reprinted by private publishers (Williams & Wilkins), enabling broader dissemination and marketing. Over 64,000 copies have been sold, and the *Guide* has been translated for overseas distribution in Japan, Spain, Italy, Argentina, and Russia. The full text of the *Guide* is accessible online through a service of the National Library of Medicine. In 1989–1990, *American Family Physician*, a journal with a circulation of 150,000, reprinted chapters from the *Guide* in 18 monthly issues. *JAMA*, with an international circulation of 750,000, published most of the USPSTF background papers (38, 39, 41, 43, 46–48, 58, 61, 62, 68, 83–85, 98). USPSTF recommendation have also been presented at annual meetings of medical organizations and at medical and public health schools.

The extent to which these efforts have made clinicians aware of the USPSTF recommendations is unclear. Surveys of family physicians suggest that about 32–45% have read at least some of its recommendations, but 24% have not heard of the group (31, 76). A survey of 2600 internists found that only 17% were familiar with the *Guide*, whereas about 50–60% were familiar with American Cancer Society and National Cholesterol Education Program guidelines (78). Because clinicians were the primary target audience for the *Guide*, early efforts to disseminate the USPSTF recommendations to the public were limited. The 1989 release of the *Guide* was accompanied by a press conference and coverage by national television networks (Cable News Network, ABC News), a cover story in *U.S. News and World Report* (81), and articles in lay magazines (32, 69, 90) and newspapers (8, 55, 79). However, most Americans remain unaware of the USPSTF and are more familiar with, for example, the recommendations of the American Cancer Society. Consumer versions of the *Guide* have been developed, but only limited evaluations have been performed (77). Greater progress in public education about prevention guidelines may occur as part of the "Put Prevention into Practice" campaign (see below).

Attitudes

The extent to which clinicians agree with USPSTF recommendations is more difficult to assess. Its recommendations to counsel patients about health behaviors are readily accepted—75% of family physicians, for example, agree with recommendations to discuss dietary fat and cholesterol (72)—but physicians are often uncomfortable with its conservative stance on screening. A survey of 1784 family physicians in Ohio reported agreement with 88% of the recommendations overall (76), but only 23% agreed with a cluster of 67 more contentious recommendations (101). In particular, more than half disagreed with the group's neutral or negative positions on screening for oral, prostate, colorectal, and testicular cancer; testicular and skin self-examination; the age for discontinuing Papanicolaou smears; and routine vision testing.

A survey of 2600 internists suggested that, at the time of the survey (late 1991), the USPSTF recommendations had less credibility than other practice guidelines. Measured on a scale of 1–10, confidence in the USPSTF guidelines was rated 3.0. Higher scores were given to guidelines of the American College of Physicians, American Cancer Society, and other groups, but no organization received a score higher than 4.2 (78). Among internists and family physicians, the USPSTF appears to be more persuasive among those who are already familiar with the *Guide* and among those who are younger, recently graduated from medical school, or residency trained (76, 78, 101). No studies have examined the extent to which pediatricians, subspecialists, or nonphysician providers agree with USPSTF recommendations.

Outcomes

Direct evidence that USPSTF recommendations have changed practice behavior is limited. One study reported that patients at a residency program received 31% of the preventive services recommended by the USPSTF after physicians received instruction about the *Guide* (35), but the baseline rate before the intervention was not reported. Indirect evidence from physicians' self-reports of preventive practices provides equivocal information. A survey of 480 family physicians found that six of the seven preventive services that they ranked as most important for a hypothetical 53-year-old woman were recommended by the USPSTF (75). On the other hand, a survey of 698 New England physicians found that only 9–28% would omit from the periodic health examination a selection of eight tests not recommended by the USPSTF (52).

Although the impact of the USPSTF on practice behavior remains unclear, its effect on national health policy is readily apparent. In 1990, the USPSTF recommendations were cited explicitly in *Healthy People 2000*, the health objectives for the nation, as a benchmark for effective preventive care (80). USPSTF recommendations formed the basis for the clinical preventive services section of President Clinton's health care reform proposal and at least five separate Congressional plans. One survey found that 50% of Senate staff members had used the recommendations to structure prevention benefits, and 80% were familiar with them (67). Within organized medicine, USPSTF guidelines have been supported by several medical specialty societies (e.g. American Academy of Family Physicians, American College of Physicians, American College of Preventive Medicine).

In what may constitute its greatest impact on practice, the USPSTF recommendations have been used by purchasers of health care (insurers, managed care organizations, employers) to define preventive services benefits (42). For example, Champion International, a 27,000-employee corporation, gives $100 in health benefits to workers who receive the screening tests recommended by the USPSTF (88). The Pacific Business Group on Health, a coalition of health plans and major employers (including the State of California), recommends preventive services coverage based largely on USPSTF recommendations. The Washington Business Group on Health, an association of 200 large employers, is funded by the Robert Wood Johnson Foundation, Metropolitan Life Foundation, IBM, and others to develop an "Employers' Guide to Clinical Preventive Services" based on the *Guide* (S Muchnick-Baku, personal communication). Preventive services cited in the Health Plan Employer Data and Information Set (HEDIS), the measures developed by the National Committee for Quality Assurance (NCQA) to track health plan performance (17), were based in part on the USPSTF recommendations. The involvement of managed care affects preventive services for a large part of the population. For example, the minimum preventive services available to the 3.3 million members of CIGNA HealthCare, one of the nation's five largest managed care organizations, are based on the USPSTF report. Some of CIGNA's 55 managed care plans have used the recommendations more extensively. For example, free copies of the *Guide* were sent to all primary care providers participating with CIGNA Health Plan Mid-Atlantic and CIGNA HealthCare of California-Southern California. The latter, which serves 300,000 members, used the *Guide* to design health risk assessment and test-ordering forms for use by 160 primary care providers and to evaluate the delivery of preventive care at its 28 sites (KE Joslyn, personal communication).

The USPSTF has also influenced medical education. Medical and nursing schools and residency programs have used USPSTF materials in clinical clerkships and courses on preventive medicine and public health (87). The *Guide* is the most popular resource for teaching health promotion and disease prevention at family medicine residencies (63). Surveyed internal medicine residents affirm its relevance to clinical practice (89). Familiarity with USPSTF recommendations is tested in board-certification examinations, such as those of the American Board of Family Practice and American Board of Preventive Medicine. The USPSTF is also integrated into continuing medical education. Materials distributed nationally by "Put Prevention into Practice," the preventive services implementation campaign launched in 1994 by the US Public Health Service and private groups, include preventive services guidelines based largely on the work of the USPSTF (19).

Finally, the USPSTF methodology has influenced the practice guideline movement itself. When it was established in 1984, few groups were using an evidence-based approach to develop guidelines, but interest in such methods has grown dramatically in recent years (22, 44, 92). The USPSTF is routinely cited or consulted by the Agency for Health Care Policy and Research (93), Institute of Medicine (44), American Medical Association (3), and other groups for work on evidence-based methods. A report to the U.S. Congress stated that, "The prevention guidelines issued by the USPSTF in 1989 set a benchmark in the use of evidence to support guideline recommendations .... The USPSTF was the first major officially sanctioned group to produce practice guidelines linked directly to evidence, and its efforts were fundamental in establishing their practicality and acceptance" (57). The USPSTF rules of evidence are also used by other groups developing guidelines on prevention (25, 100) and other aspects of medicine (2, 56), as well as by reviewers conducting critical appraisals of evidence (6, 29, 34, 53, 54, 64).

UPDATING

When the USPSTF was disbanded in 1989 after completing the first edition of the *Guide*, the need to begin updating its recommendations had already become apparent. The mission of the second panel was dominated by the need to reevaluate preventive services for which there were new data and to produce a new edition of the *Guide* (97). However, the six years until the release of the second edition left a lengthy interim period during which its published positions became outdated. For example, shortly after the release of the first edition, many groups recommended that a second measles vaccination be given to all children. Although the USPSTF reviewed the evidence in 1992 and concurred with this recommendation, its position was not publicized until the second edition of the *Guide* was released in 1995. In the interim, its 1989 recommendations were quoted as evidence that it "disagreed" with a second vaccination (65).

SETTING A RESEARCH AGENDA

A key byproduct of evidence-based guideline development is focused attention on important priorities for future research. Stimulated in part by the USPSTF, debates among advocates and opponents of preventive services about the strength and limitations of supporting scientific evidence are helping to define a research agenda for both preventive medicine and guideline development. The specifics of the research agenda are outlined elsewhere (20) and warrant closer scrutiny by funding agencies (59).

LESSONS LEARNED

The experience outlined in this article highlights specific problems that require the attention of the USPSTF in its future work. These include the need for expanded input from nonphysician providers; more systematic topic selection; development of rules for extrapolation from relevant evidence; more systematic use of meta-analysis, decision analysis, and cost-effectiveness studies; improved consistency in judging the evidence for benefits and harms; and an ongoing mechanism for updating recommendations and the future research agenda. The dissemination and implementation of USPSTF guidelines deserve greater attention. Recent developments in government and managed care suggest that policy makers and health care delivery systems may be as important an audience as clinicians in putting preventive care recommendations into practice.

More broadly, the USPSTF experience suggests important lessons for all groups engaged in guideline development. Chief among these is an affirmation of the value of an explicit, evidence-based approach to making recommendations. Although the critical appraisal of evidence is resource-intensive, its contribution to the quality and credibility of the final product clearly justifies the investment. An explicit, evidence-based guideline can provide important information to clinicians and patients by clarifying what is known and not known about the benefits and harms of available options and by specifying when recommendations are based on evidence versus other factors (e.g. expert opinion, costs). Clarifying the goals and target audience is critical to the success of any guideline program. The most appropriate methodology and panel composition flow directly from these considerations. For the USPSTF, the goal was to develop guidelines on an array of services, predominately for primary care clinicians who were skeptical about the evidence. Thus, a panel composed largely of primary care clinicians, using a methodology that provided an internally consistent approach to choosing among multiple options based on data, was appropriate. Groups developing guidelines on a single procedure or condition, or targeted to a more narrow audience (e.g. subspecialists), may require more specific expertise and different decision rules. The goals and target audience also influence the design of the final product and dissemination and implementation strategies.

The USPSTF experience affirms the value of using causal pathways, or other evidence models, for structuring the analytic problem and organizing the literature review process. Although computerized literature searches are important, elaborate strategies to ensure comprehensiveness may be unnecessary if the reference list will undergo review by content experts. Systematic methods for judging the quality of studies are also important, but further research is needed to develop validated evidence codes or scoring systems that capture all aspects of quality.

A fundamental lesson learned by the USPSTF is the need for a policy on making recommendations when there is insufficient scientific evidence. Guideline developers must decide whether to maintain complete neutrality (making no recommendation) in such situations, or whether to give weight to other factors (e.g. expert opinion). When panels rely on considerations other than direct scientific evidence, they should develop explicit policies governing how these factors will be incorporated into recommendations, and they should clearly communicate these considerations to guideline users. When examining the evidence, measuring effectiveness on the basis of health outcomes, rather than on intermediate outcomes, and limiting extrapolations to other populations reduce the risk of type I errors (see earlier), but increase the risk of type II errors. Finally, potential adverse effects and costs must be examined along with benefits to determine whether the intervention will result in more good than harm.

Administrative lessons learned by the USPSTF include the importance of clarifying the roles of panel members, staff, and project directors. Productivity and efficiency can be enhanced through collaboration with other groups that share similar analytic methods, as in the close working relationship between the USPSTF and CTFPHE. The USPSTF also found that an organized network of contributing faculty and fellows at academic medical centers benefits both guideline developers and contributors, who gain academic advancement through their participation. The project has also underscored the value of sharing draft recommendations with content experts and organizations concerned with the content or implementation of guidelines.

Finally, and perhaps most importantly, the lack of data on the effect of the USPSTF on practice behavior emphasizes the need for guideline developers to commit greater resources to determining whether their recommendations are effective. Well-designed studies are needed to determine whether guidelines, or other quality improvement tools, are capable of improving outcomes and how to improve the effectiveness of guidelines. Only by this means will we know whether the efforts of the USPSTF and other guideline developers are successful in advancing the quality of patient care and promoting the overall health and well-being of the population.

Literature Cited

1. *AAP News.* 1990. Dr. Harvey examines pros, cons of task force recommendations. Feb., p. 2
2. Agency Health Care Policy Res. 1992. *Pressure Ulcers in Adults: Prediction and Prevention.* AHCPR Publ. No. 92–0047. Rockville, MD: Agency Health Care Policy Res.
3. Am. Med. Assoc. 1990. *Attributes to Guide the Development of Practice Parameters.* Chicago: Am. Med. Assoc.
4. Am. Soc. Anesthesiol. Task Force Pulm. Artery Catheter. 1993. Practice guidelines for pulmonary artery catheterization. *Anesthesiology* 78:380–94
5. Audet AM, Greenfield S, Field M. 1990. Medical practice guidelines: current activities and future directions. *Ann. Intern. Med.* 113:709–14
6. Bass JL, Christoffel KK, Widome M, Boyle W, Scheidt P, et al. 1993. Childhood injury prevention counseling in primary care settings: a critical review of the literature.*Pediatrics* 92:544–50
7. Battista RN, Fletcher SW. 1988. Making recommendations on preventive practices: methodological issues. *Am. J. Prev. Med.* 4:53–67 (Suppl.)
8. *Boston Globe.* 1989. Writing a new prescription for MDs. July 10, p. 27
9. Brown JC. 1994. Presidential address, Scoliosis Research Society: Dublin, Ireland, Sept. 1993. *Spine* 14:1546–48
10. Brown ML, Fintor L. 1993. Cost-effectiveness of breast cancer screening: preliminary results of a systematic review of the literature. *Breast Cancer Res. Treat.* 25:113–18
11. Can. Task Force Periodic Health Exam. 1979. The periodic health examination. *Can. Med. Assoc. J.* 121:1193–254
12. Can. Task Force Periodic Health Exam. 1994. *The Canadian Guide to Clinical Preventive Care.* Ottawa: Can. Commun.Group 1–1009
13. Cardiac Arrhythmia Suppression Trial (CAST) Investigators. 1989. Prelimi-

nary report. Effect of encainide and flecainide on mortality in a randomized trial of arrhythmia suppression after myocardial infarction. *N. Engl. J. Med.* 321: 406–12
14. Chalmers TC, Smith H Jr, Blackburn B, Silverman B, Schroeder B, et al. 1981. A method for assessing the quality of a randomized control trial. *Contr. Clin. Trials* 2:31–49
15. Chu RC, Trapnell GR. 1990. Costs of insuring preventive care. *Inquiry* 27: 273–80
16. Cook DJ, Guyatt GH, Laupacis A, Sackett DL. 1992. Rules of evidence and clinical recommendations on the use of antithrombotic agents. *Chest* 102(Suppl. 4):305–11S
17. Corrigan JM, Nielsen DM. 1993. Toward the development of uniform reporting standards for managed care organizations: the Health Plan Employer Data and Information Set (Version 2.0). *Jt. Comm. J. Qual. Improv.* 19:566–75
18. Davis K, Bialek R, Parkinson M, Smith J, Vellozzi C. 1990. Paying for preventive care: moving the debate forward. *Am. J. Prev. Med.* 6(Suppl. 2): 1–30
19. Dickey LL, Kamerow DB. 1994. The Put Prevention Into Practice campaign: office tools and beyond. *J. Fam.Pract.* 39:321–23
20. DiGuiseppi C, Atkins D. 1995. A research agenda for preventive medicine. *Am. J. Prev. Med.* In press
21. Eddy DM. 1982. Clinical policies and the quality of clinical practice. *N. Engl. J. Med.* 307:343–47
22. Eddy DM. 1992. *A Manual for Assessing Health Practices and Designing Practice Policies.* Philadelphia: Am. Coll. Phys.
23. Eddy DM, Billings J. 1988. The quality of medical evidence: implications for quality of care. *Health Aff.* 7:19–32

24. Eddy DM, Hasselblad V, Shachter R. 1990. A Bayesian method for synthesizing evidence: the Confidence Profile Method. *Int.J. Technol. Assess. Health Care* 6:31–55

25. Elster AB, Kuznets NJ, eds. 1994. *American Medical Association Guidelines for Adolescent Preventive Services(GAPS).* Baltimore: Williams & Wilkins

26. Exec. Comm. Asymptomatic Carotid Atherosclerosis Study. 1995. Endarterectomy for asymptomatic cartoid artery stenosis. *JAMA* 273:1421–28

27. Expert Panel Detect. Eval. Treat. High Blood Cholesterol Adults. 1993. Summary of the second report of the National Cholesterol Education Program (NCEP) Expert Panel on Detection, Evaluation, and Treatment of High Blood Cholesterol in Adults (Adult Treatment Panel II). *JAMA* 269:3015–23

28. Feldman W. 1990. How serious are the adverse effects of screening? *J. Gen. Intern. Med.* 5:S50–S53 (Suppl.)

29. Fiscella K. 1995. Does prenatal care improve birth outcomes? A critical review. *Obstet. Gynecol.*85:468–79

30. Fleming C, Wasson JH, Albertsen PC, Barry MJ, Wennberg JE, et al. 1993. A decision analysis of alternative treatment strategies for clinically localized prostate cancer. *JAMA* 269:2650–58

31. Flocke SA, Stange KC, Fedirko TL. 1994. Dissemination of information about the U.S. Preventive Services Task Force Guidelines. *Arch. Fam. Med.* 3:1006–8

32. *Forbes.* 1994. Expensive and ineffective. Sept.26, pp. 182–84

33. Frame PS, Fryback DG, Patterson C. 1993. Screening for abdominal aortic aneurysm in men ages 60 to 80 years: a cost-effectiveness analysis. *Ann. Intern. Med.*119:411–16

34. Gant NF. 1992. Infertility and endometriosis: comparison of pregnancy outcomes with laparotomy versus laparoscopic techniques. *Am. J. Obstet. Gynecol.* 166:1072–81

35. Geiger WJ, Neuberger MJ, Bell GC. 1993. Implementing the U.S. Preventive Services Guidelines in a family practice residency. *Fam. Med.* 25:447–51

36. Gold MR, Siegel JE, Russell LB, Weinstein MC, eds. 1996. Cost-Effectiveness in Health and Medicine. London: Oxford Univ. Press.

37. Goldbloom RB, Lawrence RS, eds. 1990. *PreventingDisease: Beyond the Rhetoric,* pp. 1–487. New York: Springer-Verlag

38. Greene JC, Louis R, Wycoff SJ. 1989. Preventive dentistry. I: dental caries. *JAMA* 262:3459–63

39. Greene JC, Louis R, Wycoff SJ. 1990. Preventive dentistry. II: periodontal diseases, malocclusion, trauma, and oral cancer. *JAMA* 263:421–25

40. Hadorn DC, McCormick K, Diokno A. 1992. An annotated algorithm approach to clinical guideline development. *JAMA* 267:3311–14

41. Harris SS, Caspersen CJ, DeFriese GH, Estes EH. 1989. Physical activity counseling for healthy adults as a primary preventive intervention in the clinical setting. *JAMA* 261:3588–98

42. Health Insur. Assoc. Am. 1992. *Good Health HIAA Prevention Initiative: Provider Affairs Report.* Washington, DC:Health Insur. Assoc. Am.

43. Horsburgh CR, Douglas JM, LaForce FM. 1987. Preventive strategies in sexually transmitted diseases for the primary care physician. *JAMA* 258:814–21

44. Inst. Med. 1992. *Guidelines for Clinical Practice: From Development to Use.* Washington, DC: Natl. Acad. Press

45. Inst. Med. 1995. *Setting Priorities for ClinicalPractice Guidelines.* Washington, DC: Natl. Acad. Press

46. Knight KK, Fielding JE, Battista RN. 1989. Occult blood screening for colorectal cancer. *JAMA* 261:586–93

47. Kottke TE, Battista RN, DeFriese GH, Brekke ML. 1988. Attributes of successful smoking cessation interventions in medical practice: a meta-analysis of 39 controlled trials. *JAMA* 259:2882–89

48. LaForce FM. 1987. Immunizations, immunoprophylaxis, and chemoprophylaxis to prevent selected infections. *JAMA* 257:2464–70

49. Lawrence RS, Mickalide AD, Kamerow DB, Woolf SH. 1990. Report of the U.S. Preventive Services Task Force. *JAMA* 263:436–37

50. Lenderking WR, Gelber RD, Cotton DJ, Cole BF, Goldhirsch A, et al. 1994. Evaluation of the quality of life associated with zidovudine treatment in asymptomatic human immunodeficiency virus infection. *N. Engl. J. Med.* 330:738–43

51. *Los Angeles Times.* 1987. New Task Force Questions Value of Breast Self-Exams. April 24, Sect. V, p. 1

52. Luckmann R, Melville SK. 1995. Periodic health evaluation of adults: a survey of family physicians. *J. Fam.Pract.* 40:547–54

53. Lurie P, Avins AL, Phillips KA, Kahn JG, Lowe RA, Ciccarone D. 1994. The cost-effectiveness of voluntary counsel-

ing and testing of hospital inpatients for HIV infection. *JAMA* 272:1832–38

54. Moyer VA, Grimes RM. 1990. Total and differential leukocyte counts in clinically well children. Information or misinformation? *Am. J. Dis. Child.* 144: 1200–3

55. *New York Times Magazine.* 1986. Challenging the annual physical. Sept. 28, pp. 36–40

56. NIH Consensus Dev. Panel Effect Corticosteroids Fetal Maturation Perinatal Outcomes. 1995. Effect of corticosteroids for fetal maturation on perinatal outcomes. *JAMA*273:413–18

57. Off. Technol. Assess., US Congr. 1994. *IdentifyingHealth Technologies That Work: Searching for Evidence.* Publ. No. OTA–H–608. Washington, DC: US GPO

58. O'Malley MS, Fletcher SW. 1987. Screening for breast cancer with breast self-examination: a critical review. *JAMA* 257:2196–203

59. Omenn GS. 1994. Prevention policy: perspectives on the critical interaction between research and policy. *Prev.Med.* 23:612–17

60. Ornish D, Brown SE, Scherwitz LW, Billings JH, Armstrong WT, et al. 1990. Can lifestyle changes reverse coronary heart disease? The Lifestyle Heart Trial. *Lancet* 336:129–33

61. Pels RJ, Bor DH, Woolhandler S, Himmelstein DU, Lawrence RS. 1989. Dipstick urinalysis screening of asymptomatic adults for urinary tract disorders. II: bacteriuria. *JAMA* 262:1220–24

62. Polen MR, Friedman GD. 1988. Automobile injury: selected risk factors and prevention in the health care setting. *JAMA* 259:76–80

63. Radecki SE, Brunton SA. 1992. Health promotion/disease prevention in family practice training: results of a national survey. *Fam. Med.* 24:534–37

64. Ratko TA, Burnett DA, Foulke GE, Matuszewski KA, Sacher RA. 1995. Recommendations for off-label use of intravenously administered immunoglobulin preparations. *JAMA* 273:1865–70

65. Robbins AS. 1993. Controversies in measles immunization recommendations. *West. J. Med.* 158:36–39

66. Russell LB. 1986. *Is Prevention Better thanCure?* pp. 1–34. Washington, DC: Brookings Inst.

67. Schauffler HH. 1994. Analysis of prevention benefits in comprehensive health care reform legislation in the 102nd Congress. *Am. J. Prev. Med.* 10: 45–51

68. Selby JV, Friedman GD. 1989. Sigmoidoscopy in the periodic health examination of asymptomatic adults. *JAMA* 261:594–601

69. *Self.* 1989. Getting physical. Aug., pp. 148–49

70. Sickles EA, Kopans DB. 1995. Mammographic screening for women aged 40 to 49 years: the primary care practitioner's dilemma. *Ann. Intern. Med.* 122:534–38

71. Smart CR. 1990. Critique of the early cancer detection guidelines of the U.S. Preventive Services Task Force and of the National Cancer Institute. *Mayo Clin. Proc.* 65:892–98

72. Soltesz KS, Price JH, Johnson LW, Tellijohann SK. 1995. Family physicians' views of the Preventive Services Task Force recommendations regarding nutritional counseling. *Arch. Fam.Med.* 4:589–93

73. Sox HC. 1995. Screening mammography in women younger than 50 years of age. *Ann. Intern. Med.* 122:550–52

74. Spitzer WO, Mann KV. 1989. The public's health is too important to be left to public health workers: a commentary on the *Guide to Clinical Preventive Services. Ann.Intern. Med.* 111:939–42

75. Stange KC, Fedirko T, Zyzanski SJ, Jaen CR. 1994. How do family physicians prioritize delivery of multiple preventive services? *J. Fam. Pract.* 38: 231–37

76. Stange KC, Kelly R, Chao J, Zyzanski SJ, Shank JC, et al. 1992. Physician agreement with U.S. Preventive Services Task Force recommendations. *J. Fam. Pract.* 34:409–16

77. Terry PE. 1994. The effect of a materials–based intervention on knowledge of risk-based clinical prevention screening guidelines. *J. Occup. Med.* 36:365–71

78. Tunis SR, Hayward RSA, Wilson MC, Rubin HR, Bass EB, et al. 1994. Internists' attitudes about clinical practice guidelines. *Ann. Intern. Med.* 120:956–63

79. *USA Today.* 1989. Disputed study urges cuts in medical tests. May 4, p. D4

80. US Dep. Health Hum. Serv. 1991. *Healthy People 2000: National Health Promotion and Disease Prevention Objectives,* p. 534. Washington, DC: GPO

81. *US News and World Report.* 1989. More talking, less testing. May 15, pp. 62–65

82. US Prev. Serv. Task Force. 1989. *Guide to Clinical Preventive Services: An Assessment of the Effectiveness of 169 Interventions,* pp. 1–419. Baltimore: Williams & Wilkins. 1st ed.

83. US Prev. Serv. Task Force. 1993. Screening for adolescent idiopathic scoliosis: policy statement. *JAMA* 269: 2664–66

84. US Prev. Serv. Task Force. 1993. Home uterine activity monitoring for preterm labor: policy statement. *JAMA* 270:369–70

85. US Prev. Serv. Task Force. 1993. Routine iron supplementation during pregnancy: policy statement.*JAMA* 270: 2846–48

86. US Prev. Serv. Task Force. 1995. *Guide to Clinical Preventive Services.* Baltimore: Williams & Wilkins. 2nded.

87. Vogel VG. 1991. A clinical cancer prevention curriculum in a comprehensive cancer center. *J. Cancer Educ.*6:133–39

88. *Wall Street Journal.* 1992. Workers get incentives to take medical tests. Nov. 11, p. B1

89. Walsh JM, Papadakis MA. 1994. Prevention training and medical residency. *Am. J. Prev. Med.* 10:168–71

90. *Woman's Day.* 1992. Do you have a hidden disease? June 2, pp. 42–45

91. Woo B, Woo B, Cook EF, Weisberg M, Goldman L. 1985. Screening procedures in the asymptomatic adult: comparison of physicians' recommendations, patients' desires, published guidelines, and actual practice. *JAMA* 254: 1480–84

92. Woolf SH. 1990. Practice guidelines: a new reality in medicine. I: Recent developments. *Arch. Intern. Med.* 150: 1811–18

93. Woolf SH. 1991. *Manual for Clinical Practice Guideline Development: A Protocol for Expert Panels Convened by the Office of the Forum for Quality and Effectiveness in Health Care.* AHCPR Publ. No. 91–0018. Rockville, MD: Agency Health Care Policy Res.

94. Woolf SH. 1993. Practice guidelines: a new reality in medicine. III. Impact on patient care. *Arch. Intern. Med.* 153: 2646–55

95. Woolf SH. 1994. An organized analytic framework for practice guideline development: using the analytic logic as a guide for reviewing evidence, developing recommendations, and explaining the rationale. In *Methodology Perspectives,* ed. KA McCormick, SR Moore, RA Siegel, pp. 105–13. AHCPR Publ. No. 95–0009. Rockville, MD: Agency Health Care Policy Res.

96. Woolf SH, Battista RN, Anderson GM, Logan AG, Wang E, et al. 1990. Assessing the clinical effectiveness of preventive maneuvers: analytic principles and systematic methods in reviewing evidence and developing clinical practice recommendations. A report by the Canadian Task Force on the Periodic Health Examination. *J. Clin. Epidemiol.* 43:891–905

97. Woolf SH, Sox HC Jr. 1991. The expert panel on preventive services: continuing the work of the U.S. Preventive Services Task Force. *Am. J. Prev. Med.* 7:326–30

98. Woolhandler S, Pels RJ, Bor DH, Himmelstein DU, Lawrence RS. 1989. Dipstick urinalysis screening of asymptomatic adults for urinary tract disorders. I: hematuria and proteinuria. *JAMA* 262: 1214–19

99. Young HF. 1989. *Guide to Clinical Preventive Services*: an overview. *Am. Fam. Phys.* 39:81, 84

100. Zazove P, Mehr DR, Ruffin MT 4th, Klinkman MS, Peggs JF, Davies TC. 1992. A criterion-based review of preventive health care in the elderly: Part 2. A geriatric health maintenance program. *J. Fam. Pract.* 34:320–47

101. Zyzanski SJ, Stange KC, Kelly R, Flocke S, Shank JC, et al. 1994. Family physicians' disagreements with the U.S. Preventive Services Task Force recommendations. *J. Fam. Pract.* 39: 140–47

102. *New York Times.* 1995. Health experts urge reduced use of some medical tests. Dec. 13, p. A12

103. *USA Today.* 1995. Let's talk: doctors should spend more time counseling. Dec. 13, p. D1

104. *Wall St. J.* 1995. Health panel recommends less testing. Dec. 13, pp. B1, B6

NOTE ADDED IN PROOF.

The authors thank Drs. J. Michael McGinnis (U.S. Deputy Assistant Secretary for Health, Disease Prevention and Health Promotion) and Harold C. Sox, Jr (chair, USPSTF, 1990–1995) for their review of this manuscript and for their excellent suggestions.

SUBJECT INDEX

539

CUMULATIVE INDEXES

CONTRIBUTING AUTHORS, VOLUMES 8–17

CHAPTER TITLES, VOLUMES 8–17

ENVIRONMENTAL AND OCCUPATIONAL HEALTH